JOSEPH D. DICKERMAN, M.D.
Professor of Pediatrics
University of Vermont
College of Medicine
Burlington, Vermont

JEROLD F. LUCEY, M.D.
Professor of Pediatrics
University of Vermont
College of Medicine
Burlington, Vermont

Smith's
The CRITICALLY ILL CHILD: Diagnosis and Medical Management

THIRD EDITION

W. B. SAUNDERS COMPANY
PHILADELPHIA LONDON TORONTO
MEXICO CITY RIO DE JANEIRO SYDNEY TOKYO

W. B. Saunders Company: West Washington Square
Philadelphia, PA 19105

1 St. Anne's Road
Eastbourne, East Sussex BN21 3UN, England

1 Goldthorne Avenue
Toronto, Ontario M8Z 5T9, Canada

Apartado 26370—Cedro 512
Mexico 4, D.F., Mexico

Rua Coronel Cabrita, 8
Sao Cristovao Caixa Postal 21176
Rio de Janeiro, Brazil

9 Waltham Street
Artarmon, N.S.W. 2064, Australia

Ichibancho, Central Bldg., 22-1 Ichibancho
Chiyoda-Ku, Tokyo 102, Japan

Library of Congress Cataloging in Publication Data

Main entry under title:

Smith's The Critically Ill Child.

1. Pediatric emergencies. I. Dickerman, Joseph D. II. Lucey, Jerold F., 1926– III. Title: Critically ill child. [DNLM: 1. Critical care—In infancy and childhood. 2. Emergency—In infancy and childhood. WS 366 C9335]

RJ370.S55 1985 618.92'0025 84–5396

ISBN 0–7216–8386–X

Listed here is the latest translated edition of this book together with the language of the translation and the publisher.

Portuguese (*2nd Edition*)—Editora Interamericana Ltda., Rio de Janeiro, Brazil

Smith's: The Critically Ill Child: Diagnosis and Medical Management ISBN 0–7216–8386–X

Last digit is the print number: 9 8 7 6 5 4 3 2

Contributors

DOROTHY J. BECKER, M.B.B.Ch., F.C.P. (Paed)
Associate Professor of Pediatrics, University of Pittsburgh School of Medicine; Children's Hospital of Pittsburgh, Pittsburgh, Pennsylvania.
Diabetic Ketoacidosis

C. WARREN BIERMAN, M.D.
Clinical Professor, Pediatrics, Chief, Division Allergy, University of Washington School of Medicine; Chief, Allergy, Children's Orthopedic Hospital and Medical Center, Seattle, Washington.
Status Asthmaticus

DENNIS R. BOARDMAN, M.D.
Clinical Instructor, Department of Pediatrics, Baylor College of Medicine; Texas Children's Hospital; Methodist Hospital; St. Luke's Episcopal Hospital; Woman's Hospital of Texas, Houston.
Acute Bacterial Meningitis

GEORGE R. BUCHANAN, M.D.
Associate Professor of Pediatrics, Director of Pediatric Hematology-Oncology, University of Texas Health Science Center at Dallas, Southwestern Medical School; Director, Pediatric Hematology-Oncology, Children's Medical Center of Dallas and Parkland Memorial Hospital, Dallas, Texas.
The Bleeding Child

JANICE K. BUSH, M.D.
Fellow in Adolescent Medicine, University of Maryland School of Medicine, Baltimore.
Acute Bacterial Meningitis

G. ROBERT DeLONG, M.D.
Assistant Professor of Neurology, Harvard Medical School; Associate Neurologist, Associate Pediatrician, Massachusetts General Hospital, Boston, Massachusetts.
Reye's Syndrome

DARRYL C. DeVIVO, M.D.
Sidney Carter Professor of Neurology, Professor of Pediatrics, Columbia University College of Physicians and Surgeons; Attending Neurologist, Attending Pediatrician, Director of Pediatric Neurology, Presbyterian Hospital in the City of New York, New York.
Head Injury

PHILIP R. DODGE, M.D.
Professor, Pediatrics and Neurology, Head, The Edward Mallinckrodt Department of Pediatrics, Washington University School of Medicine; Pediatrician-in-Chief, St. Louis Children's Hospital, St. Louis, Missouri.
Head Injury

ALLAN L. DRASH, M.D.
Professor of Pediatrics, University of Pittsburgh School of Medicine; Director of Division of Endocrinology, Children's Hospital of Pittsburgh, Pittsburgh, Pennsylvania.
Diabetic Ketoacidosis

RALPH D. FEIGIN, M.D.
Professor and Chairman, Department of Pediatrics, Baylor College of Medicine; Physician-in-Chief, Texas Children's Hospital; Physician-in-Chief, Pediatric Service, Harris County Hospital District; Chief, Pediatric Service, Methodist Hospital, Houston.
Acute Bacterial Meningitis

LAURENCE FINBERG, M.D.
Professor and Chairman, Department of Pediatrics, State University of New York Downstate Medical Center, College of Medicine; Chairman of Pediatrics, Kings County Hospital Center and State University Hospital, Brooklyn, New York.
Severe Dehydration Secondary to Diarrhea

CLIFTON T. FURUKAWA, M.D.
Clinical Associate Professor, Pediatrics, University of Washington School of Medicine; Allergy Education Coordinator, Division of Allergy, Children's Orthopedic Hospital and Medical Center, Seattle, Washington.
Status Asthmaticus

PIERRE GAUDREAULT, M.D.
Associate Professor of Clinical Pediatrics, University of Montreal Faculty of Medicine; Scientific Director, Poison Control Center, Hôpital Sainte-Justine, Montreal, Canada.
Acute Poisoning

WELTON M. GERSONY, M.D.
Professor of Pediatrics, Columbia University College of Physicians and Surgeons; Director, Division of Pediatric Cardiology, Presbyterian Hospital, New York, New York.
Cardiac Arrhythmias
Congestive Heart Failure

ALLAN J. HORDOF, M.D.
Associate Professor, Clinical Pediatrics, Columbia University College of Physicians and Surgeons; Associate Pediatrician, Presbyterian Hospital, New York, New York.
Cardiac Arrhythmias

SHELDON L. KAPLAN, M.D.
Associate Professor, Division of Infectious Disease, Department of Pediatrics, Baylor College of Medicine; Chief, Infectious Diseases Service, Texas Children's Hospital, Active Staff, Harris County Hospital District, Houston.
Endotoxin Shock

JOHN E. LEWY, M.D.
Professor and Chairman, Department of Pediatrics, Tulane University School of Medicine; Tulane Medical Center Hospital and Clinics, Charity Hospital of Louisiana, Children's Hospital, New Orleans.
Acute Renal Failure

FREDERICK H. LOVEJOY, JR., M.D.
Associate Professor of Pediatrics, Harvard Medical School; Associate Physician-in-Chief, Children's Hospital; Director, Massachusetts Poison Control System, Boston, Massachusetts.
Acute Poisoning

STEPHEN G. OSOFSKY, M.D.
Associate Professor, Department of Pediatrics, Tulane University School of Medicine; Medical Director, Children's Hospital; Tulane Medical Center Hospital and Clinics, Charity Hospital of Louisiana, New Orleans.
Acute Renal Failure

JOHN PEARN, M.D., Ph.D.
Head, Department of Child Health (University of Queensland) Royal Children's Hospital; Consultant Pediatrician, Royal Children's Hospital, Mater Misericordiae Children's Hospital, Hospital for Crippled Children, Brisbane Australia; Head, Department of Child Health, Faculty of Medicine, University of Queensland, Australia.
Drowning

HOWARD A. PEARSON, M.D.
Professor and Chairman, Department of Pediatrics, Yale University School of Medicine; Chief of Pediatrics, Yale–New Haven Hospital, New Haven, Connecticut.
Sickle Cell Disease and Its Crises

WILLIAM E. PIERSON, M.D.
Clinical Professor, Pediatrics and Environmental Health, University of Washington School of Medicine; Co-Director, Division of Allergy, Children's Orthopedic Hospital and Medical Center, Seattle, Washington.
Status Asthmaticus

RICHARD H. RAPKIN, M.D.
Professor of Pediatrics, University of Medicine and Dentistry, New Jersey Medical School; Medical Director, Children's Hospital of New Jersey, Newark.
Epiglottitis and Severe Croup

GAIL G. SHAPIRO, M.D.
Clinical Professor, Pediatrics, University of Washington School of Medicine; Clinical Professor, Division of Allergy, Children's Orthopedic Hospital and Medical Center, Seattle, Washington.
Status Asthmaticus

BENNETT A. SHAYWITZ, M.D.
Director, Pediatric Neurology, Associate Professor of Pediatrics, Neurology and The Yale Child Study Center, Yale University School of Medicine; Director, Pediatric Neurology, Attending Physician, Yale–New Haven Hospital, New Haven, Connecticut.
Diagnosis and Management of the Comatose Child

CARL N. STEEG, M.D.
Associate Professor of Clinical Pediatrics, Columbia University College of Physicians and Surgeons; Director, Pediatric Cardiovascular Laboratory, Columbia-Presbyterian Medical Center; Associate Attending Pediatrician, Babies Hospital, Columbia-Presbyterian Medical Center; New York.
Congestive Heart Failure

THOMAS A. VARGO, M.D.
Assistant Professor, Section of Cardiology, Department of Pediatrics, Baylor College of Medicine; Associate in Pediatric Cardiology, Texas Children's Hospital, Houston.
Endotoxin Shock

Preface
to the First Edition

Life is Short and the Art Long
The Occasion Instant
Experiment Perilous
Decision Difficult

Carved in stone on the wall of at least one medical school, the familiar words have given generations of medical students an unforgettable explanation of purpose. Many may have found such instant occasions less common than they expected in subsequent professional life. Some may wish their educations had given them wisdom and fortitude for the chronic situation rather than resourcefulness for the instant occasion. Nevertheless, all of us, if worth our salt, carry through life the hope of responding quickly and correctly to the critical problems that come our way.

Hence, when Dr. Morris Green, whose own writings have illuminated the area of less acute but often more trying disease, suggested to PEDIATRICS these articles on The Critically Ill Child, response was enthusiastic. Few of those asked to contribute did not rise to the challenge. Subscribers welcomed the monthly appearance of at least one article they could call "practical," because useful in the kind of pediatrics they hoped to practice. Now, through the interest of the W. B. Saunders Company, and with the particular assistance of Mr. Robert B. Rowan, these papers are here made available in one volume. May it help to reduce the peril of experiment and the difficulty of decision.

CLEMENT A. SMITH, M.D.

Preface
to the Third Edition

The third edition of this book differs significantly in form and in content from its two popular and critically acclaimed predecessors. The most common pediatric medical emergencies are exhaustively discussed and referenced with respect to Pathophysiology, Diagnosis and Management. In addition, flow diagrams or algorithms are presented to facilitate diagnosis and therapy. Only medical conditions that occur in critically ill children are discussed. Chapters dealing with surgical, psychiatric or neonatal problems, which appeared in the last two editions, have been omitted. It is hoped that the discussion of each topic in this book is sufficiently broad and detailed so that it will appeal to all physicians and medical students who care for critically ill children. The editors would like to express their deep appreciation to the many contributors who made this edition possible and to Dr. Jeffrey Horbar who provided valuable editorial assistance. We also wish to acknowledge our gratitude for the secretarial assistance of Donna Hergenrother, and the invaluable editorial guidance provided by Linda Belfus and her staff at W. B. Saunders Company.

JDD
JFL

Contents

CHAPTER

1

Epiglottitis and Severe Croup

Richard H. Rapkin, M.D.

A three-year-old white male child previously in good health became ill over several hours. He developed a fever, complained of a sore throat, began to drool and subsequently refused to lie down, talk, eat or drink. He was brought to the emergency room of a local community hospital, where he was noted to be acutely ill and apprehensive. He resisted examination, especially of the pharynx, and when forcibly examined had sudden cardiorespiratory arrest. A "code" was called, and closed chest massage and mouth-to-mouth resuscitation were performed. The patient was intubated with great difficulty because his trachea was obstructed by a large, red supraglottic swelling. Following intubation, he required mechanical ventilation. He was also given appropriate antibiotics. Obvious and permanent sequelae of hypoxic brain damage were subsequently noted.

An 18-month-old black female child on awakening from her nap had a fever and a "seal-like" cough. When the child inspired, a loud crowing sound was heard. A physician was consulted and recommended that she be exposed to high humidity. The patient's response to the high humidity was rapid and dramatic, accompanied by a substantial diminution of both the offending sound and associated distress. A vaporizer was used, fluids were offered and taken, and, although there was intermittent fever and distress for several days, she recovered with no further intervention.

It is obvious that these two illnesses as described are distinct and different in many respects. Yet it has been traditional in medical literature to discuss epiglottitis and viral croup together because of their anatomic proximity.[1–10] The pediatrician who correctly diagnoses and treats epiglottitis will save the life of a child,[11, 12] and viral croup is most often a benign, self-limiting disease that is unaffected by medical intervention.[13, 14]

I will review the croup syndrome, i.e., all acute, obstructive, infectious and noninfectious upper airway disease, emphasizing severe forms. It will be useful to discuss the two most important entities, epiglottitis and viral croup, in parallel, but the physician should seek to understand their remarkable disparities.

ETIOLOGY AND PATHOPHYSIOLOGY

Supraglottic Syndromes

The upper airway passage can be compromised under a variety of circumstances.[15–17] These can be divided into supraglottic and infraglottic and each can be subdivided into infectious and noninfectious. Above the glottis, the airway can be obstructed by infection of the soft tissues of the pharynx (i.e., retropharyngeal abscess, peritonsillar abscess and pharyngeal cellulitis). These obstructions are the sequelae of viral or bacterial pharyngitis with extension of infection into the soft tissue.[18] The group A streptococci can cause pharyngitis, which if untreated, can lead to parapharyngeal disease.[19] *Staphylococcus aureus* and anaerobes found in the mouth (e.g., *Peptococcus, Bacteroides*) can invade the same soft tissue after damage has occurred to the mucous membrane, presumably by a preceding viral infection.[20] Although uncommon, this swelling can lead to airway obstruction.[16] Another cause of supraglottic and subglottic obstruction is an infection by *Corynebacterium diphtheriae*.[1, 21, 22] This previously important and common type of croup, diphtheritic croup, has disappeared largely due to effective immunization practices. The Epstein-Barr virus can cause acute upper airway obstruction as part of the syndrome of infectious mononucleosis accompanied by lymphatic tissue swelling.[23]

Infection specifically of the epiglottis and its supportive structures can occur. This disease is called acute epiglottitis, sometimes supraglottitis, and is almost always caused by *Haemophilus influenzae* Type b.[24–29] Its pathogenesis will be discussed later.

Noninfectious supraglottic obstructive processes include hypopharyngeal and laryngeal foreign bodies, trauma, caustic poisoning, and less commonly, neoplasms and other entities (e.g., sarcoid).[16, 30–34] Another important disease process is angioneurotic edema of the glottis[35] due to the acute anaphylactic reaction to any of a variety of antigens.

Infraglottic Syndromes

Acute infectious airway obstruction syndromes below the glottis include the entity called viral croup. This disease has also been labeled acute laryngitis, acute laryngotracheitis and acute laryngotracheobronchitis.[8] It is caused by a variety of viral agents that are trophic to the ciliated epithelium of the airway.[36–38] Organisms identified and believed to be causative agents of viral croup include parainfluenza virus,[1, 3] influenza A and B viruses, measles virus, rhinovirus, adenovirus, respiratory syncytial virus, and *Mycoplasma pneumoniae*.[39–44] Secondary bacterial invaders may rarely play a role, giving rise to the recently redescribed and still controversial entity called bacterial tracheitis.[45, 46] The agents etiologically related to this syndrome have included *S. aureus, H. influenzae, Pneumococcus* and various streptococci including group A.[47–51]

Noninfectious subglottic airway compromisers include the following: esophageal and tracheal foreign bodies,[52, 53] acquired or congenital structural abnormalities such as tracheal stenosis and laryngomalacia, extrinsic mass lesions pressing upon the airway[15–17, 54, 55] and a not precisely understood, relatively common disease called spasmodic croup.[8] Spasmodic croup often seems to follow a viral upper respiratory illness, but there is little evidence of direct viral invasion of the trachea or bronchi. Rather there is swelling and edema, similar to the findings seen in the distal airway in asthma. It is postulated that this usually recurrent form of croup has an allergic pathogenesis, is triggered by a variety of noxious agents including pollutants and viral illness, and occurs because the target organ of the allergic process is the trachea.[56–59]

Epiglottitis

Epiglottitis is a rapidly developing cellulitis of the epiglottis[60] and its supporting structures, the aryepiglottic folds.[61–66] Sometimes there is subglottic inflammation as well. The causative organism is almost always *H. influenzae* Type b (HITB). Although other organisms have been incriminated occasionally, none has satisfied Koch's postulates.[67–71] HITB is able to invade by virtue of its antiphagocytic capsule, which is not present in the *H. influenzae* resident of normal pharyngeal flora.[72] Nontypable *H. influenzae* is present in the nasopharynx of 43 to 90 per cent of children.[73] HITB is acquired from human contact, usually with asymptomatic children, which rarely leads to symptoms.[74,75] Normal adults usually have antibodies to the capsular polysaccharide of HITB despite the absence of a recognizable childhood HITB infection such as meningitis or epiglottitis,[76] perhaps because asymptomatic acquisition of HITB is common or because of cross antigenicity to other bacteria (*Escherichia coli* serotype K1 and so forth).[77] Nevertheless, in some children acquisition of HITB leads to bacteremia and meningitis, and in others to epiglottitis, septic arthritis or cellulitis of the soft tissues.[64, 78] Children who develop epiglottitis rarely have other manifestations of HITB disease,[79] and most have not had an identifiable preceding viral respiratory infection.[3] Antibodies to HITB are usually found in the sera of patients who have recovered from epiglottitis.[80]

The *H. influenzae* organism reaches the epiglottis and attached structures either by direct extension from the nasopharynx[81] or as a result of bacteremia.[8] It is unclear which is the more common method. At the time of diagnosis, almost all patients with epiglottitis have HITB bacteremia,[8] but it has not been determined whether bacteremia is the cause or the result of the cellulitis.[8] The epiglottis becomes swollen and reddened, and its usually firm structure is softened initially and becomes floppy.[24, 82, 83] As an anterior structure, it tends to fall backward. The aryepiglottic folds surrounding the larynx also become swollen and inflamed.[3, 84] The airway is thereby compromised from above and circumferentially. This process is exceedingly rapid—it can occur in a few hours and almost always within 24 hours in a child[9, 62]; it takes somewhat longer in adults[85, 86]—and in the untreated patient leads to inspiratory obstruction followed inexorably by complete obstruction.[11, 12] Affected children cannot handle secretions, drool and refuse to talk and swallow. They maintain an upright position, usually lean forward with the neck extended and the arms behind them (tripoding), presumably to use gravity to keep the epiglottis from obstructing the glottis.

At the time of diagnosis of epiglottitis, hypoxemia is almost always present.[10, 87] Recent studies have demonstrated that this hypoxemia is probably the result of ventilation-perfusion and diffusion abnormalities,[87] rather than being secondary to hypoventilation because of upper airway obstruction, as was previously believed. Support for this contention comes from the finding of normal arterial CO_2 tension or hypocarbia (arterial $P_{CO_2} \leq 40$ torr) at the time of hypoxemia. If the airway obstruction was causing hypoventilation, hypercarbia would be seen instead. The reason for the ventilation-perfusion mismatch (perfusion of areas not well ventilated) is probably due to the atelectasis, pneumonia and pulmonary edema that may accompany epiglottitis. These conditions are likely the result of several factors: (1) occasional direct bacterial invasion of the lung causing pneumonia; (2) usual generation of high-negative intrathoracic pressure because of the partial upper airway obstruction, leading to interstitial edema and, in some instances, alveolar flooding and atelectasis; (3) increased cardiac output, leading to increased pulmonary hydrostatic pressure; and (4) bacteremia or endotoxemia, leading to increased capillary permeability.[87] Which of these factors is preeminent is not now known.

Sudden respiratory and occasionally cardiorespiratory arrest can occur unpredictably.[64, 88–90] Cardiac arrest is likely to be asystole, i.e., vagal or hypoxic. Putting the child into a supine position to examine the pharynx or to take a radiograph may precipitate arrest. The child who has appropriate therapeutic intervention, which most importantly includes bypassing the obstruction with an artificial airway (see "management"), is spared these complications.

Viral Croup

Viral croup follows the acquisition of a viral agent trophic to the ciliated epithelium of the larynx, trachea and bronchi. Such invasion causes damage to the mucosa and substantial disruption of the usually well-coordinated mechanisms of mucociliary clearance.[36–38] Because these structures have firm external support, any inflammation or edema extends inward, leading to a narrowing of the airway.[10, 91] In the small child, this can easily compromise the air flow. In the older child and adult, only extreme degrees of swelling and edema (not usually seen in viral croup) can significantly compromise the airway. It has been estimated that a circumferential narrowing by 1 mm of the airway of a small infant will cause a 75 per cent reduction in cross-sectional area, whereas a similar thickening of the mucous membrane of an adult will reduce the area by only 20 per cent.[10] The airway obstruction leads to the generation of a high negative intratracheal pressure during inspiration.[10] Since much of the trachea is extrathoracic and since the cartilagenous supports are flexible in the younger child, this unopposed intratracheal negative pressure causes collapse of the structure and inspiratory stridor. Hypoxemia is usually observed quite early[92] and it is initially associated with hypocarbia, indicating that the hypoxemia is not secondary to hypoventilation. Whether this hypoxemia results from ventilation-perfusion mismatch secondary to atelectasis or from subclinical pulmonary edema secondary to high negative intrathoracic pressure or both is not known.[10, 92–94] Whatever the specific pathophysiologic events, most patients who have viral croup severe enough to be hospitalized are initially hypoxemic and hypocarbic.[93] When observed in the hospital, the patient whose condition worsens will have ineffective ventilation. The initial hypocarbia becomes "normal" (in the presence of hypoxemia, normocarbia should be viewed as abnormal[94]) and then may progress to hypercarbia with signs of respiratory failure. In contradistinction to epiglottitis, the progression of viral croup is usually not sudden and total, but rather gradual and predictable.[2, 9] The decision to intervene with respiratory supportive measures can be determined by careful observation and measurement of respiratory parameters.[10]

Bacterial Tracheitis

Superinfection by resident bacterial flora is rare in viral croup. This occurrence, called bacterial tracheitis,[46] is probably the result of a variety of circumstances operating individually or in concert. In the pathogenesis of pneumonia, damage to the mucociliary clearance mechanism by viral illness has been shown to be responsible for the failure to clear normally aspirated pneumococci.[95] It is possible that when the larynx, trachea or bronchi are involved, secondary bacterial invasion can occur in a similar fashion.[45] Use of corticosteroids in viral croup may affect local defense mechanisms. Mechanical trauma from endotracheal tubes may also provide a site for superinfection. Forced inhalations, e.g., epinephrine by intermittent positive pressure breathing (IPPB), may lead to an increased likelihood of aspiration. Whether bacterial tracheitis can also be primary, i.e., direct bacterial invasion of the undiseased subglottic area of a previously normal host, is not known.[45–51]

DIAGNOSIS

Epiglottitis and viral croup should be easy to distinguish on clinical grounds.[62, 96] It has been estimated that 3 to 5 per cent of all children will have at least one episode of viral croup.[44, 97] Less than 10 per cent of them will need hospitalization and 2 per cent or less of those admitted to the hospital will require ventilatory support.[10] Epiglottitis is much less common than viral croup and because of its relative rarity may not be recognized. Epiglottitis represents approximately 0.1 per cent of hospital admissions to pediatric services.[10, 81] The relative frequency of admission to a pediatric intensive care service may be nearly the same for epiglottitis and severe viral croup (Table 1–1).

Epiglottitis

Epiglottitis has no true seasonal preponderance.[98] Males are more frequently affected than females. The age range is from early infancy to adulthood; the mean age is approximately 3½ years; the mode is two years.[8] The onset of epiglottitis is sudden and the disease progresses rapidly. The duration of illness prior to hospitalization can be very short (1–2 hours) and is almost always less than 24 hours. Preceding symptoms of upper respiratory infection occur infrequently.[3] Initial symptoms are sore throat and fever followed by dysphagia, drooling, respiratory distress, aphonia and, much less commonly, stridor or barking cough. The majority of patients have the peculiar syndrome of febrile dysphagia[24, 84] and appear acutely ill and frightened. They object to being disturbed, breathe with a soft muffled hissing sound, and maintain an upright posture by putting their arms behind them to steady themselves. Children may drool and have excessive mucus as a result of their refusal to swallow. They may have tachypnea and retractions. Often the initial attention of the physician is not directed to the airway. *Any child who has febrile dysphagia must be considered to have epiglottitis until proven otherwise.*

Physical examination is often unrevealing except for the throat. In some patients, the markedly swollen and cherry red epiglottis can be identified by direct visualizaiton.[96] This procedure is dangerous, however, since the child may try to resist, give up the posterior arm support (tripoding) to push the examiner away, fall back, and totally obstruct the airway. (I have seen this occur several times.) If the cooperative child can be induced to "show" the throat while sitting upright *(the examiner should never use a tongue blade),* a normal (or red but not swollen) epiglottis will be seen in 30 per cent of patients who have croup syndrome, thereby ruling out epiglottitis.[96] In the majority of patients, the epiglottis cannot be seen. In most patients with epiglottitis, this maneuver will not be helpful and may be dangerous. *In any patient with suspected epiglottitis, the throat should not be forcibly examined until an artificial airway can be provided.*[6, 9]

Radiographs of the airway can be useful in ruling out epiglottitis.[5, 63, 96, 99–101] The lateral neck film can be diagnostic but it has some controversial aspects.[100, 102] Sending an acutely ill patient to the radiology department may be dangerous and delay appropriate therapy; the patient may inappropriately be placed supine by the technician and the airway may become obstructed. The diagnosis of epiglottitis can be easily made on clinical grounds, and radiographs should only be confirmatory. In addition, most physicians do not have immediately available x-ray equipment and therefore cannot easily depend upon radiographs to assist in making this diagnosis with urgency. My view is that radiographs of the airway can be safely taken *provided the child is accompanied by a physician who is skilled in resuscitation and has the necessary equipment.* The child must remain upright.[103] The physician must have the radiograph taken as an urgent priority and read it himself or herself if there is no radiologist present. The film should be taken to rule out epiglottitis in a child who probably does *not* have the disease. *If the physician thinks that the child does indeed have epiglottitis, the child should go directly to the operating room for examination under anesthesia and provision of an airway if the diagnosis is confirmed* (see "management").

Usually when physicians are confronted by a patient who has upper airway obstructive symptoms, they can accurately rule out epiglottitis using clinical data. Less than 10 per cent of cases remain diagnostically puzzling,[96] and that group can be assessed by radiographs. The results of lateral neck radiographs are

Table 1–1. RELATIVE FREQUENCY OF VIRAL CROUP AND EPIGLOTTITIS

	Epiglottitis	Viral Croup
Incidence in children	1 in 10,000	50 in 1000
Admission to hospital	1 in 10,000	5 in 1000
Artificial airway needed	1 in 10,000	1 in 10,000

reliable and accurate in diagnosing epiglottitis and may spare the child an unnecessary trip to the operating room. Two findings on lateral radiographs are seen in virtually all cases of epiglottitis. The epiglottis is enlarged, usually to several times normal size, and the hypopharynx is distended with air.[63] In addition, subglottic edema may be seen on anteroposterior views.[104] On an adequate upright lateral radiograph taken with the child's neck extended (the preferred position in epiglottitis), a normal epiglottis and normal hypopharyngeal airway rule out the diagnosis of epiglottitis.[27, 96]

Cultures of the blood[65] and the surface of the epiglottis[28, 105, 106] are often helpful in confirming the etiology of epiglottitis. In addition, the sensitivity pattern of the organism, i.e., β-lactamase positive or negative, allows specific antibiotic therapy to replace the broader initial coverage. Growth of HITB in the blood can, by itself, establish the etiology. Nasopharyngeal or epiglottal surfaces have normal resident flora, and growth of such bacteria from these sites cannot determine etiology.[106] In more than 90 per cent of patients who have epiglottitis HITB will be identified from the blood or epiglottic culture.[8] No other organism has had a consistent relationship with the disease.

Viral Croup

The diagnosis of viral croup can also be made accurately by clinical assessment.[8, 96] The illness has its greatest frequency in late fall and early winter, but it also follows the epidemic peaks of its viral etiologies, i.e., parainfluenzae 1, 2 and 3 and influenza A and B.[44, 97, 107] The degree of air pollution has been related to epidemic peaks of viral croup.[108, 109] There is a substantially uneven sex ratio, with males predominating. The majority of patients are between six months and three years of age, with the mode being the second year of life.[2] The illness usually begins with symptoms and signs of an upper respiratory infection followed in one to two days by the gradual development of the typical seal-like cough and an associated change or loss of voice ("laryngitis"). Fever is common and may reach 105°F (40.5°C)[99], but the child is usually not considered "toxic." In some patients, there follows, or occurs simultaneously, the characteristic inspiratory crowing sound that may be associated with inspiratory dyspnea and retractions. The speed of progression and the degree of airway compromise are variable. In some patients, the illness ends with hoarseness and cough for a few days; in others a progression to severe respiratory distress occurs. The illness may last as long as ten days to two weeks. In most cases there is an intermediate course with variability of symptoms that may worsen and improve from one hour to the next without any progression.[107]

Physical examination reveals evidence of upper respiratory involvement (coryza) and commonly an inflamed pharynx. The epiglottis may be seen during examination in one-third of patients, and although sometimes reddened, it is always normal in size and never edematous or softened.[96] There are often signs of lower respiratory tract involvement, including rhonchi and rales. Tachypnea, retractions, tachycardia, restlessness and anxiety may be followed by cyanosis in the child with severe obstruction. Sometimes exhaustion accompanied by a reduction of obvious distress is misinterpreted as improvement. Determining whether stridor is present during quiet breathing or only with crying is often helpful in assessing the severity of the upper airway obstruction. Patients who have relatively minimal airway compromise may have stridor while crying (owing to the large negative intrathoracic pressure that is generated); this should not cause concern. However, the presence of stridor at rest in a patient is an ominous sign and indicates significant airway obstruction; such a patient should always be hospitalized and observed closely.

White blood cell counts often show leukocytosis with polymorphonuclear predominance.[2] Posterior-anterior or lateral radiographs of the neck will sometimes reveal a narrowed subglottic trachea.[5, 107] This finding is seen in less than 50 per cent of patients who have viral croup. Dynamic changes are also seen, i.e, on inspiration there is overdistention of the hypopharynx and narrowing of the upper trachea; on expiration the trachea becomes distended.[110] Blood gas analysis (mentioned

Table 1–2. CLINICAL FINDINGS IN EPIGLOTTITIS AND CROUP

	Epiglottitis	Viral Croup
Age	Infancy to adult	Six months to 3 years
Sex	M > F	M >> F
Season	Any	Fall to winter
Etiology	*H. influenzae* Type b	Variety of viral agents
Duration prior to hospitalization	Average of 8 hours	1–2 days
Preceding URI	Uncommon	Common
Dysphagia	Common	Uncommon
Drooling	Common	Rare
Excessive mucus	Common	Uncommon
Sore throat	Common	Common
Cough (seal-like)	Uncommon	Common
Stridor	Uncommon	Common
Initial respiratory distress	Variable	Common
Temperature	Usually elevated	100–105°F (37.8°–40.5°C)
Appearance	"Toxic"	"Nontoxic"
Position	Sitting up, "tripoding"	Any
Cyanosis	Uncommon early	Uncommon
Retractions	Uncommon early	Common
Inflamed pharynx	Common	Common
Red epiglottis	Always	Sometimes
Swollen epiglottis	Always	Never
Radiograph	Lateral view always shows supraglottic swelling	Anteroposterior and lateral views sometimes show subglottic narrowing
WBC count	Mean 24,000	Mean 12,000
Average per cent polymorphonuclear leukocyte	85%	63%
Course	Unpredictable; fatal if untreated	Gradual worsening or improvement

earlier) reveals hypoxemia and hypocarbia.[10] The latter may change to normocarbia or hypercarbia with the progression to respiratory failure.

The clinician will see many more patients who have viral croup than have epiglottitis. The symptoms of viral croup call attention to the airway. Those of epiglottitis do not. Viral croup is usually a benign and self-limiting condition whereas epiglottitis is always potentially lethal. It is therefore incumbent upon the clinician to be sure epiglottitis is not overlooked. Familiarity with the symptoms and signs will usually permit the physician to distinguish these entities without resorting to more diagnostic testing (Table 1–2).

Angioneurotic Edema

Angioedema produces a most serious airway compromise resulting from IgE-mediated sensitivity to foreign substances, or, in the hereditary type, from reduced levels of C1 esterase inhibitor (an inhibitor of the esterase activity of the C1 complement component). Reduction in C1 inhibitor levels leads to elevation of C1 esterase and increased capillary permeability.[35, 111] The causes in children are most commonly hymenopteran stings, "allergy shots" and penicillin allergies. After exposure to the offending antigen, the patient develops dysphagia, hoarseness, inspiratory stridor, wheezing, and sneezing as well as vascular instability, i.e., hypotension, tachycardia. Treatment is the same as that for anaphylaxis; airway maintenance via intubation or tracheostomy may be necessary.[112]

Foreign Body

A hypopharyngeal foreign body (laryngeal, tracheal or upper esophageal) must always be considered in the differential diagnosis of the croup syndrome. A history of sudden onset of choking, especially while eating nuts or carrots, coughing (especially paroxysmal coughing), and the absence of the usual signs of infection, e.g., fever, upper respiratory infection and so forth should suggest this possibility. Since delay in treatment can be most serious, the possibility of the presence of a foreign body should always be kept in mind.[10, 16, 52, 53] A hypopharyngeal foreign body may mimic epiglottitis, but since patients who are considered to have epiglottitis will have direct observation of the hypopharynx in the operating room, it is likely that appropriate care will be given even if the diagnosis of foreign body has not been made. In some patients, however, a paratracheal foreign body may cause recurrent or severe episodes of croup syndrome or both and may be missed.[17]

Bacterial Tracheitis

Bacterial tracheitis (see "Pathophysiology") is a confusing clinical entity, and there are several disparate descriptions.[45–51] In the largest recent series, 8 patients had the following clinical features: the age range was 4 months to 6 years; most cases occurred during the winter; and the illness began as typical viral croup except for the subsequent development of toxicity.[46] The signs of upper airway obstruction did not respond well to the usual therapy of viral croup. At endoscopy, the accumulation of thick purulent secretions was noted, and gram-positive cocci were seen on smear. *S. aureus* was grown in most cultures. Antibiotic therapy was followed by improvement. In another study of "membranous croup," the clinical findings were similar, but in addition lateral neck radiographs suggested irregular edema and membranous material in the trachea, which were confirmed at endoscopy.[47]

The remaining differential diagnostic possibilities[16] of croup syndrome are summarized in Table 1–3.

MANAGEMENT

Appropriate treatment of a hospitalized patient who has severe croup syndrome requires a stepwise diagnostic treatment plan that will allow diagnostic separation of clinical data into component parts simultaneous with treatment decisions. Before a discussion of the details of this approach, it is necessary to review specific issues about treatment for each illness.

Epiglottitis

The management of epiglottitis has its controversial aspects. The issues to be discussed here include the use of antibiotics, artificial airways, and the management of the child prior to availability of a physician who has airway

Table 1–3. DIFFERENTIAL DIAGNOSIS OF CROUP SYNDROME

Illness	Mimics Epiglottitis	Mimics Viral Croup	Diagnostic Aids
Severe pharyngitis	+	–	"Febrile dysphagia"
Infectious mononucleosis	+	–	"Febrile dysphagia"
Peritonsillar abscess	+	–	"Febrile dysphagia"
Retropharyngeal abscess	+	–	"Febrile dysphagia"
Caustic (e.g., lye) ingestion	+	–	History suggestive; patient usually afebrile
Pharyngeal neoplasm	+	–	Chronic; gradual onset
Hypopharyngeal foreign body	+	+	History suggestive; patient usually afebrile
Angioneurotic edema	+	+	History suggestive; patient usually afebrile
Trauma to neck	+	+	History suggestive; patient usually afebrile
Tetany	+	+	Seizures; hypocalcemia
Diphtheria	+	+	Membranous pharyngitis
Tracheo- (laryngo-) malacia	–	+	Chronic; nonprogressive
Laryngeal or tracheal foreign body	–	+	History suggestive; patient usually afebrile
Spasmodic croup	–	+	Patient afebrile
Measles	–	+	Rash; clinical course
Bacterial tracheitis	–	+	Prolonged and severe croup
Vascular ring	–	+	Chronic; nonprogressive
Mediastinal tumor	–	+	Chronic; gradual onset
Laryngeal tuberculosis	–	+	Gradual onset; PPD +
Chemical (e.g., smoke) inhalation	–	+	History suggestive
Congenital or acquired (post-intubation) tracheal stenosis	–	+	Recurrent or prolonged croup

expertise, i.e., in the emergency room or in the primary care physician's office. Other therapies such as those used in viral croup, i.e., nebulized epinephrine, corticosteroids, oxygen, humidification and hydration will be briefly mentioned.

Since the organism responsible for epiglottitis is HITB, therapy directed against this organism alone is appropriate. Unfortunately, antibiotic therapy for *H. influenzae* has become somewhat complicated because of the ability of *H. influenzae* to inactivate ampicillin and its congeners by the production of a β-lactamase.[113, 114] Choramphenicol remains effective against nearly all *H. influenzae* organisms; there have been rare reports of resistance.[115] It has the disadvantage of serious bone marrow toxicity, although this is rare. Second-generation cephalosporins (e.g., cefamandole) are effective against *H. influenzae,* but have not been widely studied in epiglottitis. These second-generation drugs do not enter the cerebrospinal fluid well and will not eradicate associated meningitis.[116] Third-generation cephalosporins (c.g., moxalactam, cefotaxime) have remarkable effectiveness against *H. influenzae,* but have not yet been adequately studied in epiglottitis.[117] The safest strategy appears to be the use of intravenous chloramphenicol alone, 50–100 mg/kg/day, every 6 hours until the sensitivity of the organism has been determined.[10] If ampicillin sensitivity is established, i.e., β-lactamase negative, chloramphenicol can be discontinued and ampicillin, 100–200 mg/kg/day, every 4–6 hours intravenously, can be substituted. The duration of therapy has not been rigorously studied but empiric observation suggests a total of five to seven days of initially parenteral, subsequently oral administration. Household contacts of the index case who are under the age of six years are at an increased risk of systemic HITB infection and rifampin prophylaxis may be indicated.[65, 118, 119] Dose and duration are similar to those for HITB meningitis contacts. The patient should also receive similar rifampin prophylaxis during or after primary therapy.

Respiratory failure commonly develops in epiglottitis, and the need for an artificial airway is unquestioned in that circumstance. The nature of airway insertion (nasotracheal or orotracheal intubation or tracheostomy) and the procedure of intubation are discussed in the section on viral croup. *Nasotracheal intubation has been assessed in treatment of epiglottitis and found to be the technique of choice, if a person with this expertise is available.*[120–128]

The major issue related to the artificial airway is whether one should be placed in every child with epiglottitis upon diagnosis or whether expectant therapy, as with viral croup, is appropriate.[129] There have been many studies of this problem, but none has been a prospective randomized comparison study. Despite the absence of such data, the circumstantial evidence is compelling that prophylactic intubation reduces morbidity and mortality.[11, 12, 64] Such prophylactic intubation may be indicated because epiglottitis does not progress in a predictable and observable fashion, as does viral croup; it is unpredictable.[130] A patient who is comfortable may suddenly and seemingly inexplicably suffer arrest.[90] Crisis intubation is always difficult and nearly impossible when there is a large obstructing epiglottis.[131] Although some experts have recommended observation in the intensive care unit where crisis intubation is a daily procedure,[132] the consensus is that crisis intubation depends so much upon the capability of the staff on duty that it is too risky. When an artificial airway is placed because of the progressive respiratory inadequacy, the mortality rate is 6 per cent or more.[11, 12] Prophylactic intubation reduces the morbidity and mortality of epiglottitis nearly to zero.[64, 133, 134] In epiglottitis, the expertise of the endoscopist should determine what kind of airway is used, i.e., nasotracheal tube or tracheostomy, not whether an airway is necessary.[135] *Prophylactic placement of an artificial airway is mandatory.* My preference is nasotracheal intubation.[136]

The duration of intubation is usually under 72 hours and some authorities state that the tube can be removed in as little as eight to twelve hours.[137, 138] Again, the expertise of a skilled endoscopist is the deciding factor.

One of the most frightening experiences in all of medical practice is having sole responsibility for a child who has acute upper airway obstruction, and who suffers respiratory arrest. It is likely that the physician will have a good idea that the patient has an infection, i.e., is febrile; if such a patient has a sudden cessation of effective respiratory effort, epiglottitis is the most common diagnosis. The patient must be kept alive until the acute upper airway obstruction protocol (discussed in a later section) can be instituted. A variety of methods have been suggested, none of which has been suitably studied. Cricothyroid stab tracheostomy has no evidence to support its use at present. Anecdotes abound regarding the use of a catheter or needle (12–14 gauge) placed through the cricothyroid membrane.[93] This procedure appears to be effective only when pressurized oxygen is attached to the needle. Bag and mask ventilation seems to be the most effective alternative on the basis of several uncontrolled studies.[139, 140] Since it is universally available, it is the treatment of choice for the patient who has sudden respiratory arrest caused by epiglottitis. Although artificial ventilation may allow the patient to survive, it is not sufficient by itself, and an artificial airway should be provided as soon as it is feasible.

The use of nebulized epinephrine has not been studied in epiglottitis. It is unlikely to be of any value and may delay diagnosis and therapy. The use of oxygen, humidification and hydration in epiglottitis do not differ from that in viral croup (discussed later). Systemic corticosteroids have not been rigorously studied in epiglottitis. They may be of marginal benefit,[141] but can quite possibly be harmful by interfering with normal defense mechanisms. I believe that they are, at best, superfluous.

Any discussion of the management of epiglottitis requires a brief note regarding the primary prevention of systemic HITB disease. A purified HITB capsular polysaccharide vaccine has been developed,[142] but it is not immunogenic in children less than 18 months of age.[143] There have been recent efforts to find a more potent antigen for the immunization of infants,[144] but at present there is no vaccine effective for the age group at risk.

Viral Croup

Therapies that have been used for the hospitalized patient who has viral croup include: (1) increased humidity, (2) oxygen, (3) hydration, (4) nebulized epinephrine, (5) corticosteroids, (6) antibiotics, and (7) artificial airway. Increased humidification, or mist therapy, has long been the favored therapeutic modality for viral croup.[145, 146] It is usually benign unless the mist is contaminated by hydrophilic bacteria, e.g., *Pseudomonas,*[147] or if the patient cannot be carefully watched because of the density of the mist. Mist by ultrasonic nebulization has also been associated with overhydration and water intoxication in infants.[148] Theoretically, mist should prevent drying of inflamed mucosa and keep secretions liquid.[149] It has been shown in experimental animals that there are mechanosensitive nerve endings within the mucosa of the larynx. Aerosol inhalation can produce reflex slowing of the rate of breathing, thereby slowing air flow and reducing turbulence.[150] Unfortunately, there has been no scientific evaluation of whether mist therapy is indeed beneficial in viral croup.[151] However, the combined anecdotal experience of pediatricians strongly supports use of this modality. The temperature of the mist is probably of little importance provided that it is neither too hot nor too cold.

Oxygen is warranted for the treatment of hypoxia, and it should always be humidified. Since almost all patients admitted to the hospital for croup are hypoxemic,[92] this therapy is, appropriately, nearly universal. The response of hypoventilation or ventilation-perfusion mismatch hypoxemia to oxygen administration may be salutory. Diffusion hypoxemia can also be expected to improve. It cannot be sufficiently stressed that oxygen, if needed, must be provided in a non-threatening way to a child who has viral croup because the development of excitement and anxiety in the child may intensify the degree of airway compromise and the amount of oxygen consumed.[10] Nursing experience can help assess whether the most effective device for a particular child is a mist tent, oxygen hood, nasal cannula or mask. Restraint and sedation usually make matters worse and should rarely, if ever, be used.[91]

Hydration has traditionally made good sense because it may contribute to liquefaction of tenacious secretions. I am not aware of data that prove this hypothesis. In lower respiratory disease, i.e., asthma, vigorous hydration (overhydration?) has not been beneficial and has even been associated with deterioration,[152] perhaps by reducing lung compliance. In addition, pulmonary edema has been observed as a complication of both viral croup and epiglottitis.[153–156] It has been postulated to result from a combination of factors, including (1) high negative intrathoracic pressure, which increases the capillary-to-alveoli pressure gradient and shifts blood volume from the systemic to the pulmonary circulation, (2) hypoxia leading to increased alveolar capillary permeability, and (3) failure of pulmonary lymphatics to clear the fluid.[156] These considerations would strongly suggest against vigorous or excessive hydration in the child who has acute upper airway obstruction. Dehydrated children, however, should receive sufficient fluids to repair and maintain them.

Nebulized, usually racemic, epinephrine delivered by intermittent positive pressure breathing has been reported by several investigators to be beneficial.[157–159] The initial studies on this modality were uncontrolled, but there appeared to be substantial reduction in the frequency of tracheostomies or intubations in patients who were so treated when compared with historical controls.[157, 158] A small quantity of a 2.25 per cent solution of epinephrine is added to sterile water or saline and delivered through a nebulizer. The quantity of epinephrine varies from 0.25 to 1.5 ml according to the size of the infant. Water or saline is added to make a total of 5 ml. Several carefully controlled prospective studies done in the past decade have shown the following: nebulized epinephrine (not necessarily racemic nor necessarily administered by IPPB) usually, but not always, leads to significant improvement when compared to saline or distilled water controls; improvement is short lived, lasting two hours or less, and the conditions of treated and untreated children are no different 24 to 36 hours later; repeated hourly treatments can be effective, but after several such treatments the benefit lessens and rebound may occur. The use of nebulized epinephrine, or a suitable congener such as phenylephrine, should be reserved for the hospitalized patient who has severe croup, since in some of these patients it may prevent the need for an artificial airway, but in many this need will only be forestalled.[10]

Systemic corticosteroids have been extensively studied,[160–162] but the great majority of these studies have been uncontrolled or poorly designed.[13] Some studies have had small numbers of patients in each comparison group (treated and untreated). In addition, almost all studies have failed to segregate spasmodic from viral croup,[163] and since the former is theoretically more likely to respond to systemic steroid administration, demonstrated benefit may be due to that subgroup's response alone. There have been few double-blind controlled studies. The most recent shows some benefit in the corticosteroid group.[161] The disadvantages of systemic steroids in infectious disease, i.e., alteration of defense mechanisms and increased incidence of superinfection, must be weighed against the, at best, marginal benefits shown by these studies. I believe steroids have little or no place in the management of viral croup, or epiglottitis (discussed previously). Other workers disagree.[164]

Antibiotics are not useful in the treatment of viral disease. In the past, it was assumed that when antibiotics were given during viral illness, subsequent bacterial illness might be prevented. Although this issue has not been specifically studied in viral croup, evidence from other viral respiratory infections indicates that it is more likely that antibiotics will select subsequent superinfecting bacterial species rather than prevent such infections from occurring. A possible justification for using antibiotics in viral croup is when it is unclear if the patient has epiglottitis or secondary bacterial tracheitis. As many as 85 per cent of patients who have viral croup receive antibiotics because of this type of rationalization,[8] and it exposes a substantial number of children to possibly toxic, certainly expensive and almost always useless therapy.[165] Antibiotics have no place in the management of patients who have typical viral croup. In contradistinction, the patient who has demonstrable bacterial tracheitis should receive antistaphylococcal antibiotic therapy until results of cultures of the purulent tracheal secretions allow greater precision.

The effective use of an artificial airway and mechanical ventilation, if necessary, has enabled even the sickest viral croup patient to survive and return to normality. It is most desirable that the physician try to predict the need for airway support before the situation becomes desperate, in order to avoid the crisis situation, which is often less than elegantly handled. The placement of an artificial airway in a child, whether orotracheal or nasotracheal intubation or tracheostomy, requires the skills of individuals with substantial experience. The care of any child who has severe viral croup requires that such consultants and intensive care nurses be immediately available until the situation has stabilized and provision of an airway is no longer necessary.

Unlike treatment of epiglottitis (mentioned earlier), the care of the patient who has viral croup can be expectant. Although clinical scoring systems have been used with some success,[14] the usual combination of clinical signs and blood gas data is sufficient in most patients to determine the need for further intervention. Absolute indications for ventilatory support include persistent cyanosis, hypotonia, absence of awareness of surroundings, and progression toward respiratory failure, i.e., increase of P_{CO_2} to "normal" or higher values. Other indications include unresponsive hypoxemia, inability to mobilize secretions, and increasing pulse and respiratory rates.[107, 166]

A prospective comparison of tracheostomy with oral or nasotracheal intubation has not been made for viral croup. There are data both pro and con for each modality.[6, 167–169] Nasotracheal or orotracheal intubation may intensify the inflammation in the narrowed subglottic region, making extubation difficult; tracheostomy has surgical risks and leaves a scar. At present, the type of airway intervention in the patients requiring it is best left to the expert present (anesthesiologist, otolaryngologist or pulmonologist-intensivist), since there are no clear data as to which method is preferable. My own preference is nasotracheal intubation because the data indicate that it is safer.[170] The details of airway management are also best handled by the subspecialist.[91]

If possible, tracheal intubation should be done in the operating room, and a patient who has an artificial airway should be managed in an intensive care unit where the staff is experienced in caring for infants and children. Intubation while the patient is awake is usually difficult and may be undesirable. The patient is anesthetized, usually while sitting up, using a mixture of halothane and oxygen by spontaneous inhalation. Laryngoscopy follows anesthesia, and an endotracheal tube of appropriate size is inserted. If tracheostomy is desired, it is done while the endotracheal tube is in place. The details of artificial airway management and methods of extubation have recently been described in detail elsewhere.[9, 91]

MANAGEMENT PROTOCOL

The synthesis of the previously discussed details into a useful plan is a worthwhile, perhaps essential, project for each hospital staff caring for children who have severe croup and epiglottitis. Since there are usually a number of people involved, and since these patients present with emergent needs, there is no time to debate the merits and debits of the controversies already discussed. A plan, agreed to in advance by all concerned, should be established and available for use at all times. Such a protocol ought to integrate both diagnostic and treatment modalities into a coordinated whole.

Several protocols have been published.[9, 84, 89, 171] The algorithm shows two branches: one is the management of a patient who has suspected epiglottitis and the other is the management of the patient with severe croup syndrome in which epiglottitis is clinically unlikely.

Management of Patient with Suspected Epiglottitis

When epiglottitis cannot be ruled out clinically by the evaluating physician or triage nurse, the following protocol should be followed.

1. A history and brief physical examination by the physician have indicated that this patient with acute upper airway obstruction syndrome may have epiglottitis.
2. Examination of the hypopharynx is now prohibited and the patient is permitted and encouraged to remain sitting up and leaning forward. *Until epiglottitis has been ruled out, the patient will not be forced into or placed in a supine position.*
3. The epiglottitis team is summoned and the operating room staff is notified. The team consists of a prearranged group who has participated in the development of the local protocol. It usually includes the pediatric surgeon or otolaryngologist, the pediatric intensivist and the anesthesiologist. This group must be available on 15 minutes' notice.
4. While awaiting the arrival of the team, the patient in moderate to severe respiratory distress is offered oxygen by mask held near or upon the face of the patient by the parent. If the oxygen increases the distress of the patient, it should not be forced.
5. If respiratory arrest occurs, the patient will be supported by bag and mask ventilation until arrival of the team.
6. If the patient is not in a facility that has an upper airway team, he or she will be transferred, by emergency ambulance, to such a facility. The patient is kept sitting up, is offered oxygen, and is accompanied by the parent(s) and personnel capable of bag and mask ventilation.
7. When the team arrives or the patient is transported to the receiving facility, and the clinical diagnosis is accepted by the experienced observers, the patient is brought directly to the operating room by the team. The parent accompanies the patient until the operating room is entered. If the team disagrees with the clinical diagnosis, i.e., they doubt the diagnosis of epiglottitis, the patient should be managed as in no. 3 of "Management of Patient in Whom Epiglottitis Is Unlikely."
8. In the operating room, direct laryngoscopy is performed using general anesthesia. If the diagnosis of epiglottitis is confirmed, an artificial airway is placed. Samples for cultures of the epiglottis are obtained as well as for blood cultures, blood counts, and necessary biochemical tests. An intravenous infusion is begun and chloramphenicol is administered. It should be noted that blood sampling and even an intravenous line have been deferred until the airway has been secured.

ALGORITHM FOR THE TREATMENT OF EPIGLOTTITIS AND SEVERE CROUP

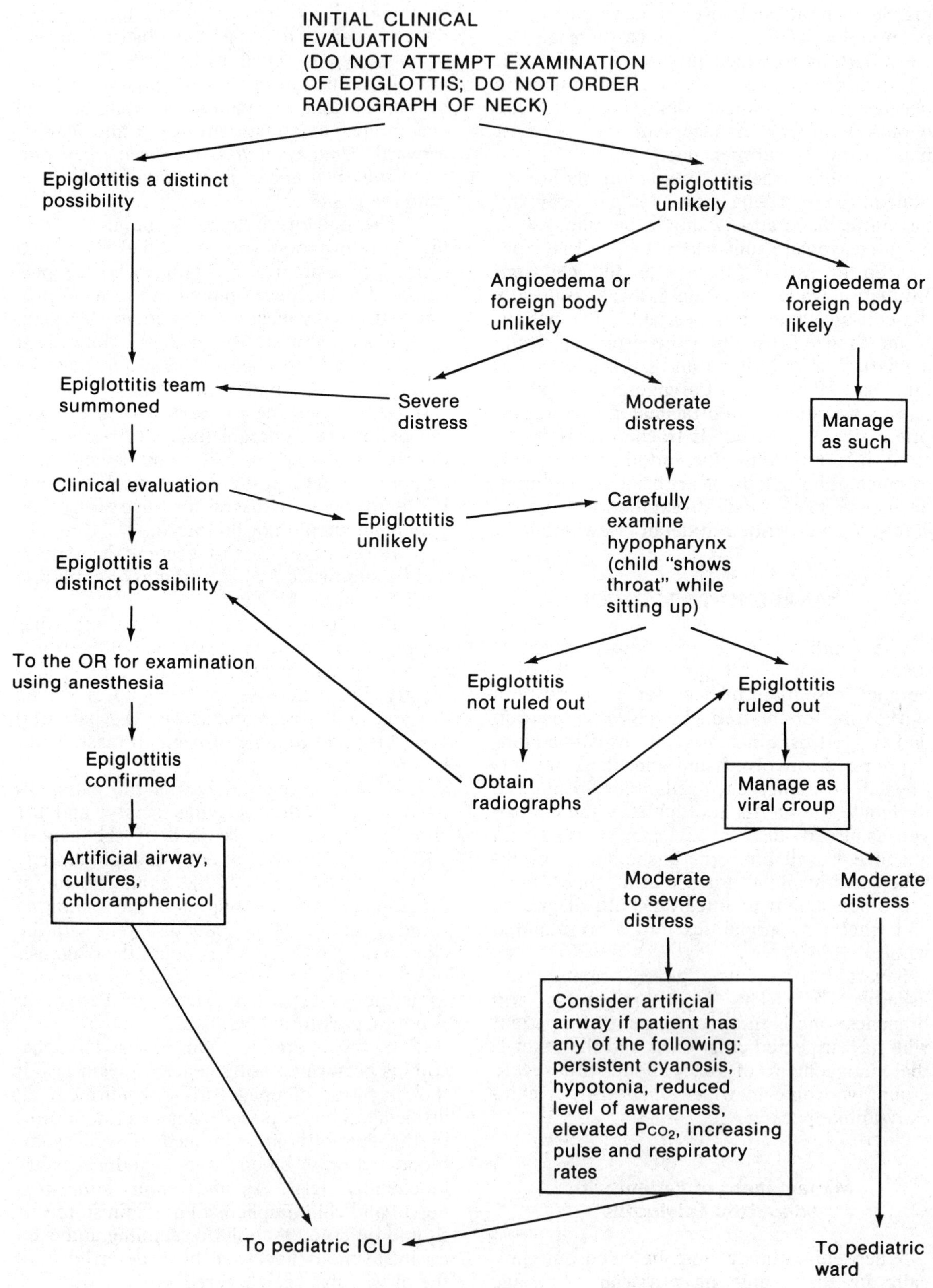

9. If the diagnosis of epiglottitis is not confirmed and viral croup or another condition is diagnosed, an assessment of the patient's respiratory status is made and arterial blood gas analysis is obtained. The team determines whether an artificial airway should be immediately placed or whether the child can be taken to the pediatric ICU for additional observation and management in hopes of avoiding an artificial airway.

Management of Patient in Whom Epiglottitis Is Unlikely

When the patient has severe croup, and epiglottitis is thought to be clinically unlikely by the examining physician the following protocol should be followed.

1. The history and brief physical examination have indicated that this patient with acute upper airway obstruction syndrome is unlikely to have epiglottitis. There is no history of choking on food suggestive of a foreign body, nor of bee sting or environmental exposure suggestive of angioneurotic edema.

2. If the patient is in severe distress, the epiglottitis team is summoned as in "Management of Patient with Suspected Epiglottitis."

3. If the patient is in moderate distress, the hypopharynx is not forcibly examined, but gentle encouragement of the patient to "show" the throat while sitting up may allow the epiglottis to be visualized and confirmed as not swollen, although it may be inflamed. If it is determined that the epiglottis is not swollen, the pharynx is now examined carefully, with the patient supine, to rule out parapharyngeal infection, and therapy for acute viral croup is begun. The patient is then admitted either to the hospital ward or to the pediatric ICU or transferred to a facility with such a unit as the patient's condition requires.

4. If the distress is moderate and the epiglottis is not seen on physical examination, or the epiglottitis team does not consider epiglottitis likely, oxygen is offerred as for epiglottitis, discussed previously, and appropriate radiographs are obtained. When the radiologist is not available the films are read by the most experienced physician in attendance. If epiglottitis is ruled out, the child is admitted to the hospital ward or pediatric ICU as the child's condition warrants. If epiglottitis is suspected, proceed as in Management of Patient with Suspected Epiglottitis.

COMPLICATIONS AND PROGNOSIS

The complications and prognosis of viral croup and epiglottitis include problems that are common to both conditions and those that are unique to either epiglottitis or croup. Common to both are complications associated with respiratory failure, such as respiratory arrest and the sequelae of anoxic damage and their management. Mechanical ventilation may lead, in a small percentage of patients, to problems such as atelectasis, pneumothorax, and pneumomediastinum, in addition to postintubation sequelae such as tracheal stenosis.[9, 91, 172, 173] Secondary bacterial infection of the trachea (bacterial tracheitis, discussed previously) or of the lungs, i.e., pneumonia, may occur. As previously noted, acute pulmonary edema has also occurred in both conditions before and after artificial airway placement.[153, 154] Pulmonary edema has also been reported in acute non-inflammatory airway obstruction, e.g., strangulation.[156] Its development should be anticipated although its actual occurrence is uncommon.

Specific to epiglottitis is the possibility of other manifestations of infection with HITB.[78, 79, 174] These conditions include pneumonia, cervical adenitis and meningitis. The "pneumonia" associated with epiglottitis may be infection of the lung parenchyma with HITB or, more likely, may represent atelectasis, pulmonary edema, or both.[87] Cervical adenitis has been described by some investigators as an unusual diffuse soft tissue cellulitis rather than true adenitis.[175] It is also not uncommon. Meningitis is distinctly rare in association with epiglottitis and probably relates more to the nature of the host than to the organism's tropism, but the explanation for this lack of association still is unclear.[72, 78]

Specific to viral croup is the peculiar tendency to persistence or recurrence in some patients. Two such groups of patients are identifiable. In the first group the problem is airway hyper-reactivity, i.e., spasmodic croup that has been diagnosed initially as viral croup.[57] In the second group, persistence or recurrence is related to congenital or acquired structural abnormalities of the trachea or surrounding tissues such as congenital stenosis or retained foreign body.[16, 32, 53, 55] All patients who have recurrent or persistent croup should be evaluated by appropriate surgical and radiologic consultants. Endoscopy may be needed to identify the cause.

SUMMARY

Croup syndrome is a common problem, which has two major causes. Epiglottitis, when untreated, is a uniformly fatal disease. Diagnosis and treatment, if appropriate and timely, can lead to recovery without sequelae. Viral croup is usually self-limiting and only occasionally requires medical intervention in order to forestall or treat the rare occurrence of respiratory failure. It is the physician's responsibility to be able to recognize and treat both—not failing to aggressively intervene in a sophisticated manner and avoiding unnecessary potentially harmful manipulation.[176]

REFERENCES

1. Rabe EF. Infectious croup: I. Etiology. Pediatrics 1948; *2*:255–265.
2. Rabe EF. Infectious croup: II. "Virus" croup. Pediatrics 1948; *2*:415–427.
3. Rabe EF. Infectious croup: III. *Hemophilus influenzae* type b croup. Pediatrics 1948; *2*:559–566.
4. Davison FW. Acute laryngeal obstruction in children. JAMA 1959; *171*:1301–1305.
5. Dunbar JS. Epiglottitis and croup. J Can Assoc Radiol 1961; *12*:86–95.
6. Fried MP. Controversies in the management of supraglottitis and croup. Pediatr Clin North Am 1979; *26*:931–942.
7. Rowe LD. Advances and controversies in the management of supraglottitis and laryngotracheobronchitis. Am J Otolaryngol 1980; *1*:235–243.
8. Cherry JD. Acute Epiglottitis, Laryngitis, and Croup. *In:* Remington JS and Swartz MN, eds. Current Clinical Topics in Infectious Diseases, vol. 2. New York: McGraw-Hill, 1981:1–30.
9. Davis HW, Gartner JC, Galvis AG, et al. Acute upper airway obstruction: croup and epiglottitis. Pediatr Clin North Am 1981; *28*:859–880.
10. Levison H, Tabachnik E, Newth CJL. Wheezing in infancy, croup and epiglottitis. Curr Prob Pediatr 1982; *12*:1–65.
11. Rapkin RH. Tracheostomy in epiglottitis. Pediatrics 1973; *52*:426–429.
12. Margolis CZ, Ingram DL, Meyer JH. Routine tracheotomy in *Hemophilus influenzae* type b epiglottitis. J Pediatr 1972; *81*:1150–1153.
13. Cherry JD. The treatment of croup: continued controversy due to failure of recognition of historic, ecologic and clinical perspectives. J Pediatr 1979; *94*:352–354.
14. Taussig LM, Castro O, Beaudry PH, et al. Treatment of laryngotracheobronchitis (croup): use of intermittent positive pressure breathing and racemic epinephrine. Am J Dis Child 1975; *129*:790–793.
15. Quinn-Bogard AL, Potsic WP. Stridor in the first year of life. Clin Pediatr 1977; *16*:913–919.
16. Maze A, Block E. Stridor in pediatric patients. Anesthesiology 1979; *50*:132–145.
17. Holinger LD. Etiology of stridor in the neonate, infant and child. Ann Otolaryngol 1980; *89*:397–400.
18. Stern RC. Retropharyngeal Abscess. Peritonsillar and Retrotonsillar Abscess. *In:* Vaughn VC, McKay RJ, Behrman RE, eds. Nelson Textbook of Pediatrics. 11th ed. Philadelphia: WB Saunders, 1979:1173–1174.
19. Markowitz M. Streptococcal Infections: Group A Beta Hemolytic Streptococci. *In:* Rudolph AM, Hoffman JIE, eds. Pediatrics. 17th ed. Norwalk, Conn.: Appleton-Century-Crofts, 1982:556–560.
20. Yamauchi T, Ferrieri P, Anthony BF. The aetiology of acute cervical adenitis in children. J Med Microbiol 1980; *13*:37–43.
21. Neftson AH. Acute Laryngotracheobronchitis. New York: Grune & Stratton, 1949:1–193.
22. Fischer GW. Diphtheria. *In:* Wedgewood RJ, Davis SD, Ray CG, Kelley VC, eds. Infections in Children. Philadelphia: Harper and Row, 1982:652–662.
23. Plotkin SA, Henle W. Infectious Mononucleosis. *In:* Vaughn VC, McKay RJ, Behrman RE, eds. Nelson Textbook of Pediatrics. 11th ed. Philadelphia: WB Saunders, 1979:886–890.
24. Jones HM. Acute epiglottitis. Practitioner 1975; *215*:732–739.
25. Benjamin B, O'Reilly B. Acute epiglottitis in infants and children. Ann Otol Rhinol Laryngol 1976; *85*:1–8.
26. Editorial. Acute epiglottitis. Lancet 1978; *1*:1294–1295.
27. Bottenfield GW, Arcinue EL, Sarnaik A, Jewell MR. Diagnosis and management of acute epiglottitis—report of 90 consecutive cases. Laryngoscope 1980; *90*:822–825.
28. Diaz JH, Lockhart CH. Early diagnosis and airway management of acute epiglottitis in children. South Med J 1982; *75*:399–403.
29. Margolis CZ, Colletti RB, Grundy G. *Hemophilus influenzae* type b: the etiologic agent in epiglottitis. J Pediatr 1975; *87*:322–323.
30. Vauthy PA, Reddy R. Acute upper airway obstruction in infants and children. Ann Otol Rhinol Laryngol 1980; *89*:417–418.
31. Morris P, Shaw EA. Acute upper respiratory tract obstruction complicating childhood leukemia. Br Med J 1974; *2*:703–704.
32. Tauscher JW. Esophageal foreign body: an uncommon cause of stridor. Pediatrics 1978; *61*:657–658.
33. Toomey JM, Synder GG, Maenza RM, Rothfield NF. Acute epiglottitis due to systemic lupus erythematosus. Laryngoscope 1974: *84*:522–527.
34. Kirschner BS, Holinger PH. Laryngeal obstruction in childhood sarcoidosis. J. Pediatr 1976; *88*:263–264.
35. Donaldson VH, Rosen FS. Hereditary angioneurotic edema: a clinical survey. Pediatrics 1966; *37*:1017–1027.
36. Richards L. A further study of the pathology of acute laryngotracheobronchitis in children. Ann Otol Rhinol Laryngol 1938; *47*:326–341.
37. Reed SE, Boyde A. Organ cultures of respiratory epithelium infected with rhinovirus of parainfluenzae virus studied in a scanning electron microscope. Infect Immun 1972; *6*:68–76.
38. Klein JD, Collier AM. Pathogenesis of human parainfluenzae type 3 virus infection in hamster tracheal organ culture. Infect Immun 1974; *10*:883–888.
39. Denny FW. The replete pediatrician and the etiology of lower respiratory tract infections. Pediatr Res 1969; *3*:464–470.

40. Blahova O, Mertenova J, Pecenkova I. Acute obstructive laryngotracheobronchitis due to myxovirus infection. Acta Paediatr Acad Sci Hung 1973; *14*:139–143.
41. Monto AS. The Tecumseh study of respiratory illness. V. Patterns of infection with the parainfluenzae viruses. Am J Epidemiol 1973; *97*:338–348.
42. Glezen WP, Denny FW. Epidemiology of acute lower respiratory disease in children. N Engl J Med. 1973; *288*:498–505.
43. Hall CB, Geiman JM, Breese BB, Douglas RG. Parainfluenzae viral infections in children: correlation of shedding with clinical manifestations. J Pediatr 1977; *91*:194–198.
44. Chapman RS, Henderson FW, Clyde WA, et al. The epidemiology of tracheobronchitis in pediatric practice. Am J Epidemiol 1981; *114*:786–797.
45. Orton HB, Smith EL, Bell HO, Ford RA. Acute laryngotracheobronchitis: analysis of 62 cases with report of autopsies in 8 cases. Arch Otolaryngol 1941; *33*:926–960.
46. Jones R, Santos JI, Overall JB. Bacterial tracheitis. JAMA 1979; *242*:721–726.
47. Han BK, Dunbar JS, Striker TW. Membranous laryngotracheobronchitis (membranous croup). AJR 1979; *133*:53–58.
48. Liston SL, Gehrz RC, Jarvis CW. Bacterial tracheitis. Arch Otolaryngol 1981; *107*:561–564.
49. Denneny JC, Handler SD. Membranous laryngotracheobronchitis. Pediatrics 1982; *70*:705–707.
50. Davidson S, Barzilay Z, Yahav J, Rubinstein E. Bacterial tracheitis—a true entity? J Laryngol Otol 1982; *96*:173–175.
51. Hefelfinger DC. Croup vs. epiglottitis vs. tracheitis. JAMA 1981; *246*:1087.
52. Rothmann BF, Boeckman CR. Foreign bodies in the larynx and tracheobronchial tree in children. Ann Otol Rhin Laryngol 1980; *89*:434–436.
53. Smith PC, Swischuk LE, Fagan CJ. An elusive and often unsuspected cause of stridor or pneumonia (the esophageal foreign body). Am J Roentgenol Radium Ther Nucl Med 1974; *122*:80–89.
54. Kahn A, Baran D, Spehl M. et al. Congenital stridor in infancy: clinical lessons derived from a survey of 31 instances. Clin Pediatr 1977; *16*:19–26.
55. Fearon B, Crysdale WS, Bird R. Subglottic stenosis of the larynx in the infant and child. Ann Otol Rhinol Laryngol 1978; *87*:1–4.
56. Loughlin GM, Taussig LM. Pulmonary function in children with a history of laryngotracheobronchitis. J Pediatr 1979; *94*:365–369.
57. Zach M, Erben A, Olinsky A. Croup, Recurrent croup, allergy and airways hyperreactivity. Arch Dis Child 1981; *56*:336–341.
58. Zach M, Schnall RP, Landau LI. Upper and lower airway hyperreactivity in recurrent croup. Am Rev Respir Dis 1980; *121*:979–983.
59. Gurwitz D, Corey M, Levison H. Pulmonary function and bronchial reactivity in children after croup. Am Rev Respir Dis 1980; *122*:95–99.
60. Thiesen CF. Angina epiglottidea anterior. Albany Med Ann 1900; *21*:395–401.
61. Jones HM, Camps FE. Acute epiglottitis. Practitioner 1957; *178*:223–229.
62. Berenberg W, Kevy S. Acute epiglottitis in childhood: a serious emergency readily recognized at the bedside. N Engl J Med 1958; *258*:870–874.
63. Poole CA, Altman DH. Acute epiglottitis in children. Radiology 1963; *80*:798–805.
64. Baxter JD. Acute epiglottitis in children. Laryngoscope 1967; *77*:1358–1367.
65. Dajani AS, Asmar BI, Thirumoorthi MC. Systemic *Hemophilus influenzae* disease: an overview. J Pediatr 1979; *94*:355–364.
66. Cherry JD. Invasive Hemophilus infections: epiglottitis and cellulitis. Ann Otol Rhinol Laryngol 1981; *90*:19–22.
67. Kessler HA, Schade R, Trenholme GM, et al. Acute pneumococcal epiglottitis in immunocompromised adults. Scand J Infect Dis 1980; *12*:207–210.
68. Schwartz RH, Knerr RJ, Hermansen K, Wientzen RL. Acute epiglottitis caused by beta hemolytic group C streptococci. Am J Dis Child 1982; *136*:558–559.
69. Schwenzfeier CW, Fechner RE. Herpes simplex of the epiglottis. Arch Otolaryngol 1976; *102*:374–376.
70. Johnson RH, Rumans LW. Unusual infections caused by *Pasteurella multocida.* JAMA 1977; *237*:146–147.
71. Berthiaume JT, Pien FD. Acute Klebsiella epiglottitis: considerations for initial antibiotic coverage. Laryngoscope 1982; *92*:799–800.
72. Whisnant JK, Rogentine GN, Gralnick MA, et al. Host factors and antibody response in *Hemophilus influenzae* type b meningitis and epiglottitis. J Infect Dis 1976; *133*:448–455.
73. Roseburg T. Bacteria Indigenous to Man. *In:* Dubos RJ, Hirsch JG, eds. Bacterial and Mycotic Infections of Man, 4th ed. Philadelphia: JB Lippincott, 1965:334.
74. Michaels RH, Norden CW. Pharyngeal colonization with *Hemophilus influenzae* type b: a longitudinal study of families with a child with meningitis or epiglottitis due to *H. influenzae* type b. J Infect Dis 1977; *136*:222–228.
75. Sell SHW. The clinical importance of *Hemophilus influenzae* infections in children. Pediatr Clin North Am 1970; *17*:415–426.
76. Robbins JB, Schneerson R, Argaman M, Handzel ZT. *Hemophilus influenzae* type b: disease and immunity in humans. Ann Intern Med 1973; *78*:259–269.
77. Bradshaw WM, Parke JC, Schneerson R. Bacterial antigens cross reactive with capsular polysaccharide of *Hemophilus influenzae* type b. Lancet 1971; *1*:1095.
78. Walker SH. Influenza b epiglottitis and meningitis. Pediatrics 1981; *67*:581–582.
79. Molteni RA. Epiglottitis: incidence of extraepiglottic infection: report of 72 cases and review of the literature. Pediatrics 1976; *58*:526–531.
80. Norden CW, Michaels R. Immunologic response in patients with epiglottitis caused by *Hemophilus influenzae* type b. J Infect Dis 1973; *128*:777–780.
81. Daum RS, Bates JR, Smith AL. Epiglottitis (supraglottitis). *In*: Feigin RD, Cherry RD, eds. Textbook of Pediatric Infectious Diseases. Philadelphia: WB Saunders, 1981:138–146.
82. DuBois PG, Aldrich CA. *H influenzae* type b laryngitis with bacteremia. J. Pediatr 1943; *23*:184–188.
83. Davis HV. Obstructive laryngitis in children caused by *Hemophilus influenzae* bacillus type b. J Kans Med Soc 1947; *48*:105–108.
84. Blanc VF, Weber MC, Leduc C, Laberge R, et al. Acute epiglottitis in children: management of 27 consecutive cases with nasotracheal intubation,

with special emphasis on anesthetic considerations. Can Anaesth Soc J 1977; *24*:1–10.

85. Ossoff RH, Wolff AP. Acute epiglottitis in adults. JAMA 1980; *244*:2639–2640.
86. Hawkins DB, Miller AH, Sachs BG, Benz RT. Acute epiglottitis in adults. Laryngoscope 1973; *83*:1211–1220.
87. Costigan DC, Newth CJL. Respiratory status of children with and without an artificial airway. Am J Dis Child 1983; *137*:139–141.
88. Olinson GK, Sullivan JL, Bishop LA. Acute epiglottitis: review of 55 cases and suggested protocol. Arch Otolaryngol 1974; *100*:333–337.
89. Faden HS. Treatment of *Hemophilus influenzae* type b epiglottitis. Pediatrics 1979; *63*:402–407.
90. Rapkin RH. Acute epiglottitis: pitfalls in diagnosis and management. Clin Pediatr 1971; *10*:312–314.
91. Duncan PG. Management of Upper Airway Disease in Children. *In*: Gregory GA, ed. Respiratory Failure in the Child. New York: Churchill-Livingstone, 1981:53–66.
92. Newth CJL, Levison H, Bryan HC. The respiratory status of children with croup. J Pediatr 1972; *81*:1068–1073.
93. Wesley AG. The acid base balance of infective croup. So Afr Med J 1972; *46*:729–731.
94. Wesley AG. Interpretation of arterial carbon dioxide tension in laryngotracheobronchitis. So Afr Med J 1974; *48*:1152–1154.
95. Hoeprich PD. Bacterial Pneumonias. *In*: Hoeprich PD, ed. Infectious Diseases. 7th ed. Hagerstown, Md.: Harper and Row, 1977:295–308.
96. Rapkin RH. The diagnosis of epiglottitis: simplicity and reliability of radiographs of the neck in the differential diagnosis of the croup syndrome. J Pediatr 1972; *80*:96–98.
97. Cherry JD. Croup. *In*: Feigin RD, Cherry JD, eds. Textbook of Pediatric Infectious Diseases. Philadelphia: WB Saunders, 1981:146–155.
98. Lewis JK, Galvis AG, Michaels RH. Occurrence of Hemophilus epiglottitis. Am J Dis Child 1978; *132*:424–426.
99. Podgore JK. The "thumb sign" and "little finger sign" in acute epiglottitis. J Pediatr 1976; *88*:154–155.
100. Margolis CZ. Are lateral neck x-rays a waste of time? Pediatrics 1981; *68*:469.
101. Swischuk LE. Acute respiratory distress in the infant. Radiol Clin North Am 1978; *16*:77–90.
102. Edelson PJ. Radiographic examination in epiglottitis. J Pediatr 1972; *81*:1036.
103. Rapkin RH. Radiographic examination in epiglottitis. Reply. J Pediatr 1972; *81*:1036–1037.
104. Shackelford G, Siegel MJ, McAlister WH. Subglottic edema in acute epiglottitis in children. Am. J Roentgenol 1978; *131*:603–605.
105. Miller AH. *Hemophilus influenzae* type b epiglottitis or acute supraglottic laryngitis in children. Laryngoscope 1948; *58*:514–526.
106. Andrew JD, Tandon OP, Turk DC. Acute epiglottitis: challenge of a rarely recognized emergency. Br Med J 1968; *3*:524–526.
107. Hall CB, Hall WJ. Viral croup (acute laryngotracheobronchitis). *In*: Hoekelman RA, ed. Principles of Pediatrics. New York: McGraw-Hill, 1978:1747–1751.
108. Jaklin RH, Bender SW, Becker F. Environmental factors in croup syndrome. Z Kinderheilkd 1971; *111*:85–94.
109. Emmerich H, Bender SW, Jaklin RH, Emmerich W. The effect of atmospheric sulfur dioxide on croup syndrome. Z Kinderheilkd 1972; *113*:111–121.
110. Currarino G, Williams B. Lateral inspiration and expiration radiographs of the neck in children with laryngotracheitis (croup). Radiology 1982; *145*:365–366.
111. Auerbach VH. C1 Esterase Inhibitor. *In*: Vaughn VC, McKay RJ, Behrman RE, eds. Nelson Textbook of Pediatrics. Philadelphia: WB Saunders, 1979:553.
112. Ellis EF. Anaphylaxis. *In*: Vaughn VC, McKay RJ, Behrman RE, eds. Nelson Textbook of Pediatrics. Philadelphia: WB Saunders, 1979:640–641.
113. Nelson JD. The increasing frequency of β-lactamase producing *Hemophilus influenzae* B. JAMA 1980; *244*:239.
114. Riley HD. The dilemma of invasive disease due to *Hemophilus influenzae.* South Med J 1977; *70*:133–135.
115. Long SS, Phillips SE. Chloramphenicol resistant *Hemophilus influenzae.* J Pediatr 1977; *90*:1030.
116. Azimi PH, Chase PA. The role of cefamandole in the treatment of *Hemophilus influenzae* infections in infants and children. J Pediatr 1981; *98*:995–1000.
117. Thirumoorthi MC, Kobos DM, Dajani AS. Susceptibility of *Hemophilus influenzae* to chloramphenicol and eight beta-lactam antibiotics. Antimicrob Agents Chemother 1981; *20*:208–213.
118. Handler SD, Plotkin SA, Potsic WP, Downes JJ. *Hemophilus influenzae* epiglottitis occurring concurrently in two siblings. Clin Pediatr 1982; *21*:634–635.
119. CDC. Prevention of secondary cases of *Hemophilus influenzae* type b disease. Morbidity Mortality Weekly Rep. 1982; *31*:672–680.
120. Smith RM. Diagnosis and treatment: nasotracheal intubation as a substitute for tracheostomy. Pediatrics 1966; *38*:652–654.
121. Heldtander P, Lee P. Treatment of acute epiglottitis in children by long-term intubation. Acta Otolaryngol 1973; *75*:379–381.
122. Sweeney DB, Allen TH, Steven IM. Acute epiglottitis—management by intubation. Anesth Intensive Care 1973; *1*:526–528.
123. Tos M. Nasotracheal intubation in acute epiglottiditis. Arch Otolaryngol 1973; *97*:373–375.
124. Milko DA, Marshak G, Striker TW. Nasotracheal intubation in the treatment of acute epiglottitis. Pediatrics 1974; *53*:674–677.
125. Coker SB, Scherz RG. Safe alternative to tracheostomy in acute epiglottitis. Am J Dis Child 1975; *129*:136.
126. Battaglia JD, Lockhart CH. Management of acute epiglottitis by nasotracheal intubation. Am J Dis Child 1975; *129*:334–336.
127. Rapkin RH. Nasotracheal intubation in epiglottitis. Pediatrics 1975; *56*:110–112.
128. Weber ML, Desjardins R, Perreault G, et al. Acute epiglottitis in children—treatment with nasotracheal intubation: report of 14 consecutive cases. Pediatrics 1976; *57*:152–155.
129. Smith DS. Editorial. J Pediatr 1972; *81*:1153.
130. Bass JW, Steele RW, Wiebe RA. Acute epiglottitis. A surgical emergency. JAMA 1974; *229*:671–675.
131. Scheidemandel HHE, Page RS. Special considerations in epiglottitis in children. Laryngoscope 1975; *85*:1738–1745.

132. Wetmore RF, Handler S. Epiglottitis: evolution in management during the last decade. Ann Otol Rhinol Laryngol 1979; *88*:822–826.
133. Cohen SR, Chai J. Epiglottitis. 20-year study with tracheotomy. Ann Otol Rhinol Laryngol 1978; *87*:1–7.
134. Myers MG. More on treatment of epiglottitis. J Pediatr 1973; *83*:168–169.
135. Cantrell RW, Bell RA, Morioka WT. Acute epiglottitis: intubation vs. tracheostomy. Laryngoscope 1978; *88*:994–1005.
136. Lazoritz S, Saunders BS, Bason WM. Management of acute epiglottitis. Crit Care Med 1979; *7*:285–290.
137. Phelan PD, Mullins GC, Landua LI, et al. The period of nasotracheal intubation in acute epiglottitis. Anesth Intensive Care 1980; *8*:402–403.
138. Schultz RL, Morrison WV. Short-term intubation in children with acute epiglottitis. South Med J 1982; *75*:158–160.
139. Glicklich M, Cohen RD, Jona JZ. Steroids and bag and mask ventilation in the treatment of acute epiglottitis. J Pediatr Surg 1979; *14*:247–251.
140. Szold PD, Glicklich M. Children with epiglottitis can be bagged. Clin Pediatr 1976; *15*:792–793.
141. Strome M, Jaffe B. Epiglottitis—individualized management with steroids. Laryngoscope 1974; *84*:921–928.
142. Anderson P, Peter G, Johnson RB, et al. Immunization of humans with polyribosephosphate, the capsular antigen of *Hemophilus influenzae* type b. J Clin Invest 1972; *51*:39–44.
143. Peltola H, Kayhty H, Sivonen A, Makaela PH. *Hemophilus influenzae* type b capsular polysaccharide vaccine in children; a double blind field study of 100,000 vaccinees 3 months to 5 years of age in Finland. Pediatrics 1977; *60*:730–737.
144. Pichichero ME, Anderson P, Loeb M, Smith DH. Do pili play a role in pathogenicity of *Hemophilus influenzae* type b? Lancet 1982; *2*:960–962.
145. Davison FW. Some observations on control of temperature and humidity in oxygen tents. Ann Otol Rhinol Otolaryngol 1940; *49*:1083–1090.
146. Avery ME, Galina M, Nachman R. Mist therapy. Pediatrics 1967; *39*:160–165.
147. Moffet HL, Allan D. Colonization of infants exposed to bacterially contaminated mists. Am J Dis Child 1967; *114*:21.
148. Rossiter MA, Boryzskowski M, Bower BD. Water intoxication and mist tent therapy. Lancet 1974; *1*:935.
149. Parks CR. Mist therapy: rationale and practice. J Pediatr 1970; *76*:305–313.
150. Sasaki CT, Suzuki M. The respiratory mechanism of aerosol inhalation in the treatment of partial airway obstruction. Pediatrics 1977; *59*:689–694.
151. Gardner HG, Powell KR, Roden VJ, Cherry JD. The evaluation of racemic epinephrine in the treatment of infectious croup. Pediatrics 1973; *52*:52–55.
152. Stalcup SA, Mellins RB. Mechanical forces producing pulmonary edema in acute asthma. N Engl J Med 1977; *297*:592–595.
153. Travis KW, Todres ID, Shannon DC. Pulmonary edema associated with croup and epiglottitis. Pediatrics 1977; *59*:695–698.
154. Galvis AG, Stool SE, Bluestone CD. Pulmonary edema following relief of acute upper airway obstruction. Ann Otol Rhinol Laryngol 1980; *89*:124–128.
155. Hurley RM, Kearns JR. Pulmonary edema and croup. Pediatrics 1980; *65*:860.
156. Oswalt CE, Gates GA, Holmstrom FMG. Pulmonary edema as a complication of acute airway obstruction. JAMA 1977; *238*:1833–1835.
157. Adair JC, Ring WH, Jordan WS, Elwyn RA. Ten year experience with IPPB in the treatment of acute laryngotracheobronchitis. Anesth Analg 1971; *50*:649–655.
158. Singer OP, Wilson WJ. Laryngotracheobronchitis: 2 years' experience with racemic epinephrine. Can Med Assoc J 1976; *115*:132–134.
159. Westley CR, Cotton EK, Brooks JG. Nebulized racemic epinephrine by IPPB for the treatment of croup. Am J Dis Child 1978; *132*:484–487.
160. Eden AN, Kaufman A, Yu R. Corticosteroids and croup. JAMA 1967; *200*:133–134.
161. James JA. Dexamethasone in croup. Am J Dis Child 1969; *117*:511–516.
162. Leipzig B, Oski FA, Cummings CW, et al. A prospective randomized study to determine the efficacy of steroids in treatment of croup. J Pediatr 1979; *94*:194–196.
163. Tunnessen WW, Feinstein AR. The steroid croup controversy: an analytic review of methodologic problems. J Pediatr 1980; *6*:751–756.
164. Hawkins DB. Corticosteroids in the management of laryngotracheobronchitis. Otolaryngol Head Neck Surg 1980; *88*:207–210.
165. Tercero-Talavera FI, Rapkin RH. Antibiotic usage in the management of acute laryngotracheobronchitis (croup). Clin Pediatr 1974; *13*:1074–1076.
166. Wesley AG. Indications for intubation in laryngotracheobronchitis in black children. So Afr Med J 1975; *49*:1126–1128.
167. Wesley AG, Desai S, Holloway R, Thambiran AK. Nasotracheal intubation in the management of infective croup. So Afr Med J 1972; *46*:839–842.
168. Schuller DE, Birck HG. The safety of intubation in croup and epiglottitis: an eight year follow-up. Laryngoscope 1975; *85*:32–46.
169. Thomson PD, Olinsky A. Nasotracheal intubation in acute laryngotracheobronchitis. So Afr Med J 1975; *49*:785–788.
170. Orlowski JP, Ellis NG, Amin NP, Crumrine RS. Complications of airway intrusion in 100 consecutive cases in a pediatric ICU. Crit Care Med 1980; *8*:324–331.
171. Oh TH, Motoyama EK. Comparison of nasotracheal intubation and tracheostomy in management of acute epiglottitis. Anesthesiology 1977; *46*:214–216.
172. Jordan WS, Graves CL, Elwyn RA. New therapy for postintubation laryngeal edema and tracheitis in children. JAMA 1970; *212*:585–588.
173. Waterman PM, Smith RB. Acute laryngeal obstruction in children following intubation. Ear Nose Throat Monthly 1973; *52*:173–177.
174. Baugh R, Baker SR. Epiglottitis in children. Otolaryngol Head Neck Surg 1982; *90*:157–162.
175. Simpson GT, McGill TIJ, Healy GB. *Hemophilus influenzae* type b soft tissue infections of the head and neck. Laryngoscope 1981; *91*:17–29.
176. Davison FW. Acute laryngeal obstruction in children. A fifty year review. Ann Otol Rhinol Laryngol 1978; *87*:1–8.

CHAPTER

2

Acute Bacterial Meningitis

Ralph D. Feigin, M.D.
Dennis R. Boardman, M.D.
Janice K. Bush, M.D.

Bacterial meningitis remains a very common and significant medical problem despite the fact that antibiotics capable of eradicating the organisms that cause the disease are available. Although the reported fatalities from infectious diseases such as scarlet fever, measles, and tuberculosis decreased 10- to 200-fold between 1935 and 1968, the number of deaths from bacterial meningitis were only halved during this period. Rather than diminishing in incidence, bacterial meningitis has increased in absolute frequency during the past several decades, largely as a result of a striking rise in the frequency of meningitis caused by *Haemophilus influenzae* Type b (HITB)[1–5] and group B β-hemolytic streptococcal infections.[1, 2, 4]

Although any bacterial organism may produce meningitis in a susceptible host, HITB, *Streptococcus pneumoniae,* and *Neisseria meningitidis* are the responsible microorganisms in approximately 95 per cent of children over 2 months of age. HITB accounts for more than 60 per cent of all cases.[6] In 1972, the Centers for Disease Control (CDC) estimated that there were 29,000 cases of meningitis caused by HITB, 4800 cases of pneumococcal meningitis, and 4600 cases of meningococcal meningitis.[7] More recently, 235 patients were enrolled in a prospective study (initiated at Washington University School of Medicine and continued at Baylor College of Medicine) of bacterial meningitis in children who were between 1 month and 15 years of age. Of these, 151 (64%) had *H. influenzae* Type b meningitis, 35 (15%) had pneumococcal meningitis, and 26 (11%) had meningococcal meningitis. Twenty-three (10%) had meningitis caused by other organisms (unpublished data).

Other less common bacterial agents causing meningitis are β-hemolytic streptococcus, other streptococci, *Staphylococcus aureus,* and gram-negative bacilli. The more unusual gram-negative organisms have been found, particularly in cases of meningitis secondary to trauma or in association with underlying diseases such as brain tumors and congenital defects. Gram-negative enteric organisms remain a major cause of meningitis in the neonatal period. Group B streptococcal meningitis is primarily a disease of the neonatal period, although it has been reported to occur in children as old as 6 months.

EPIDEMIOLOGY

Haemophilus Influenzae

H. influenzae are small pleomorphic, gram-negative coccobacilli. There are six antigenically distinct capsular types (Types a–f) and other, non-typable (non-encapsulated) strains; the majority of colonizing strains are non-typable. Invasive disease, such as meningitis, generally is caused by encapsulated strains, primarily strain b. The source of the organism often is the upper respiratory tract. Carriage of HITB occurs in children of the same age group, in whom the disease occurs with the greatest frequency.[1] The mode of transmission is person-to-person direct contact through infected droplets of respiratory tract secretions; the precise period of communicability is unclear but may be considered to be equivalent to the period during which the organism is present in the upper respiratory tract. The period of incubation generally is less than ten days. Invasive disease is most common in children 3 months to 3 years of age. It may occur in older children and, on occasion, in adolescents and adults.

Meningitis is twice as common in males as in females, is more common in black children than in white children, and generally is more common in the poor, in large families, and in urban dwellers. Children less than 4 years of age who are in contact with children with invasive disease caused by HITB are at significant risk for serious infection from this organism; contact may be in the household or in other closed communities such as day care centers and chronic care facilities. The incidence of invasive disease including bacteremia, pneumonia, and meningitis in household contacts of patients with *H. influenzae* Type b meningitis is approximately five per cent in children under 2 years of age. Thus, the risks of spread of infection and serious disease caused by *H. influenzae* and *N. meningitidis* are similar except that secondary cases caused by *H. influenzae* are unlikely to occur in older children or adults.[6, 8] The incidence of cases of invasive *H. influenzae* Type b disease in contacts of patients with *H. influenzae* Type b infection is four per cent in children under 12 months of age, 2.1 per cent in children under 4 years of age, and 0.5 per cent in children under 6 years of age.[8]

The risk of a child's developing meningitis due to HITB by 5 years of age has been estimated to be from 1 in 400 to 1 in 2000. This risk is greatest in the age group from 6–12 months; this age distribution has remained unchanged for the past 40 years.[7] An absolute increase in frequency of this organism has occurred over the past 35 to 40 years; several large hospital centers (St. Louis Children's, Columbus Children's, and Pittsburgh Children's Hospitals) reported a 400 to 1000 per cent increase in the incidence of *H. influenzae* Type b infection during a period of time (1940–1970) in which there was only a 100 to 200 per cent increase in hospital admissions (unpublished data).

Statistics compiled by Mortimer[9] in 1968 revealed that the age-corrected death rate for children under 5 years of age for *H. influenzae* Type b meningitis was 3.8 in 100,000; this rate equalled or exceeded the crude death rate for each of the disorders for which immunizing agents are now available (e.g., diphtheria, pertussis, tetanus, polio, or measles).[9]

The occurrence of *H. influenzae* infection in older patients should prompt efforts to exclude the possibility of predisposing factors such as otitis media, other parameningeal foci of infection, a leak of cerebrospinal fluid (CSF), an immunodeficiency disorder, sickle cell disease, and splenectomy. Current morbidity rates vary from 2 to 14 per cent[2, 3, 4, 5, 7]; most deaths occur during the first few days of illness.

Streptococcus Pneumoniae

Streptococcus pneumoniae are lancet-shaped, gram-positive diplococci. There are 84 serotypes of this microorganism; serotypes 1, 3, 6, 7, 14, 17, 19, and 23 are the most common causes of sepsis and meningitis. Immunity is type specific and long lasting. The pneumococcus is ubiquitous; many persons carry this organism in their upper respiratory tracts without symptoms. Transmission is person-to-person, usually by direct contact. The infection is communicable presumably as long as the organism appears in respiratory discharges. Effective antibiotic therapy generally renders secretions free of this organism within 24 hours.[10]

The incubation period may be as short as one to three days. Infection is most common in the very young and the old. Pneumococcal infections are more prevalent during the seasons of the year when viral respiratory diseases occur in a particular community. Infection due to *S. pneumoniae* has a higher incidence in the black population and is independent of income or population density. Statistical analysis reveals a 5- to 36-fold increase in pneumococcal infection in blacks when compared with whites and a 314-fold increase in blacks with sickle cell disease when compared with whites.[7] The greatest mortality occurs in very young and very old patients and has been estimated to be 20 to 60 per cent.[2, 3, 4, 5, 7] This high mortality rate, in part, can be accounted for by the presence of concomitant potentially fatal illness, advanced age, bacteremia, and delay in instituting medical therapy.

Meningitis due to *S. pneumoniae* is extremely rare after the age of 10 years, and one should suspect a parameningeal focus (mastoiditis, sinusitis, brain abscess, rupture, or CSF leak), sickle cell disease, immunodeficiency disease, asplenia (from surgical removal, congenital defect, or disease), otitis media, pneumonia, or a skull fracture.[11] Pneumococcal infections also can occur in association with a predisposing viral upper respiratory tract infection or when a strain of *S. pneumoniae* of apparently enhanced virulence is prevalent in a community.

Meningococcal Infections

Neisseria are biscuit-shaped gram-negative diplococci. *Neisseria meningitidis* can be grouped serologically on the basis of capsular polysaccharides; the common serogroups are A, B, C, D, X, Y, Z, 29E, and W–135. Groups B, C, Y, and W–135 are currently the most prevalent serogroups causing disease in the United States. The source of meningococcal infection is the upper respiratory tract of humans. Transmission is person-to-person by direct contact through infected droplets of respiratory tract secretions often from asymptomatic carriers. The majority of persons exposed to pathogenic meningococci become carriers. They may respond to carriage of the organism by forming a bactericidal antibody and are thereby rendered immune to a specific serogroup. The period of communicability is probably the duration of the presence of the organism in the upper respiratory tract. The incubation period most commonly is less than four days.[12]

Disease occurs most frequently in children less than 5 years of age, with a peak attack rate in the 6- to 12-month-old age group. A second, much lower peak occurs among adolescents; less than ten per cent of the cases occur in patients over 45 years of age. In most series, the peak incidence of invasive disease occurs in the late winter and early spring. Invasive meningococcal infection usually results in meningococcemia or meningitis or both. In meningitis the manifestations of fever, altered mental status, seizures in some patients, and meningeal irritation are indistinguishable from those of acute meningitis caused by other bacteria unless the petechial or purpuric rash of meningococcemia occurs. Similar lesions, however, may be seen in patients with aseptic meningitis due to ECHO virus type 9 and acute staphylococcal endocarditis. They are very rare in patients with pneumococcal, *H. influenzae,* or streptococcal meningitis.[2]

Fatalities usually occur in patients who have the fulminant form of the disease. The duration of overt illness in these individuals may be measured in terms of hours. Approximately 50 per cent of those hospitalized within the first 24 hours of their illness die, some within a few hours of the onset of symptoms. Presenting features of meningococcal infection associated with a poor prognosis include the following: petechiae for less than 12 hours, systolic hypotension with systolic blood pressure (BP) less than 70 mm Hg, peripheral white blood cell (WBC) less than 10,000/mm^3, erythrocyte sedimentation rate (ESR) less than 10 mm/hr, and absence of meningitis (< 20 WBC/mm^3 in CSF).

Meningococcal infections tend to be more prevalent in urban dwellers, and in closed communities including day care centers, nursery schools, and camps for military recruits. Patients with a deficiency of terminal complement components C5 through C8, and those with a complement-depleting underlying illness, may be at particular risk for invasive disease.[13, 14]

PATHOPHYSIOLOGY

Meningitis denotes inflammation of the meninges, whereas *leptomeningitis,* perhaps a more specific term, denotes inflammation of the arachnoid and pia mater, the usual distribution of meningitis. Meningitis may be caused by noninfectious disorders as well as by virtually all microorganisms.

In most cases of meningitis caused by bacteria, the organisms are thought to reach the subarachnoid space by way of the blood stream. The pathogenesis of bacterial meningitis has been studied using a number of animal models. In the rat model it has been shown that following intranasal inoculation of *H. influenzae,* bacteremia could be documented hours before meningitis could be defined histologically by detection of fluorescent-tagged antibody to *H. influenzae* capsular wall antigens. These findings support the concept that meningitis follows hematogenous dissemination from a nasopharyngeal site of infection or colonization.[15] The choroid plexuses of the cerebral ventricles presumably are the initial site of entry of blood-borne bacteria into the CSF. Bacteria also may be inoculated directly into the subarachnoid space through dural defects of congenital or traumatic origin or from parameningeal suppurative foci such as chronic sinusitis and mastoiditis.

The development of meningitis is influenced by the interaction of a number of factors, including the host, the organism, and the environment.

Host Factors[1, 2, 11, 16]

There is good evidence that males suffer central nervous system (CNS) infections more frequently than females of all ages with the possible exception of neonatal group B streptococcal infections.[1, 2, 11, 16] Meningitis occurs with greatest frequency and severity in the very young and very elderly. The presence of congenital (physiologic or pathologic) or acquired deficiencies in the immunologic (B, T cell) response of the host to infection is an important factor that may predispose to the occurrence of severe bacterial disease including infection of the CNS. Disorders of granulocyte motility and function or of the complement system also predispose the host to serious infections. Congenital asplenia and sickle cell disease have been associated with a higher incidence of meningitis due to *S. pneumoniae.*[17] It has been suggested that this increased incidence of septicemia and meningitis following splenectomy may be related more closely to the type and severity of the disease process that necessitated removal of the spleen than to the absence of the spleen per se.[17] There is a small but distinct risk of septicemia following removal of the spleen when it is necessitated by trauma.[18]

Other hereditary and acquired diseases that predispose the host to an increased incidence and severity of serious infection include malignancies of the reticuloendothelial system, such as leukemia, lymphoma, multiple myeloma, and Hodgkin's disease.[11] The use of irradiation or immunosuppressive agents and anti-metabolites also predisposes the host to infections of the CNS.[11] Anatomic defects (dermal sinus tracts, dermoids, congenital heart disease, etc.), old age, chronic illness, alcoholism, diabetes mellitus, renal failure, cystic fibrosis, adrenal insufficiency, hypoparathyroidism, exudative enteropathy, cardiac and neurological surgery, and burns all may play an important role in the increased susceptibility to infection of the CNS in the debilitated host.[11] It also has been shown that nutrition may profoundly affect the progress of infection within the host regardless of baseline nutritional status.[19]

The Organism[1, 2, 11, 16, 20, 21]

The importance of bacterial virulence factors in meningitis is reflected in the marked proclivity of *H. influenzae,* pneumococci, and meningococci for causing meningeal infection. Many other bacteria that inhabit the oropharynx (streptococci) and that frequently cause bacteremia almost never cause meningitis. Virulence appears to be related to the specific serotype (for pneumococci and *H. influenzae*) or serogroup (for meningococci), that, in turn, is determined by the chemical composition of the polysaccharide in the bacterial capsule.

Meningitis due to HITB has occurred with greater frequency in recent decades, but the most susceptible individuals are between 3 months and 3 years of age.[1] Earlier studies suggested that infants or older children and adults were protected from developing *H. influenzae* meningitis by the passive transfer or later acquisition of bactericidal antibody to HITB.[22] This finding has been disputed by more recent experiences in our own institution (unpublished to date), which have shown that 30 to 75 per cent of normal newborn infants and 30 to 80 per cent of normal adults lack bactericidal antibody to this organism. The development of detectable concentrations of HITB bactericidal antibody in adults appears to be dependent upon contact with patients who have *H. influenzae* infections.[1] In children, the prolonged presence in the nasopharynx of *H. influenzae* in the absence of disease also has been associated with high titers of bactericidal antibody to HITB.[1] Feigin and associates [23] have shown that the presence of high titers of bactericidal antibody does not prevent the development of *H. influenzae* bacteremia or meningitis in animals or in children.[23]

The pathogenicity of HITB may relate, in part, to its capsular antigen. In one study, children who experienced sequelae of *H. influenzae* meningitis had concentrations of polyribose phosphate (PRP) capsular antigen within the CSF and serum that were significantly higher than those found in children whose course was uneventful.[23] Morbidity correlated positively with the magnitude and duration of exposure to capsular PRP. Anti-PRP antibody, which can be detected by radioimmunoassay, appears to protect against *H. influenzae* Type b infections in animals and humans.[1] In general, anti-PRP antibody has not been found at the time of hospital admission in children with *H. influenzae* meningitis. Few children less than 17 months of age appear to develop anti-PRP antibody even following exposure to PRP antigen during the course of infection or following immunization with currently available experimental vaccines.[23]

The relationship of virulence and capsular polysaccharide antigen also has been studied extensively in patients with *Escherichia coli* infection. It was shown that 84 per cent of *E.*

coli isolated from CSF of newborn infants with meningitis contained a K1 capsular polysaccharide antigen (identified by agglutination immunoelectrophoresis).[24] In contrast, *E. coli* with K1 antigen accounted for only 31 per cent of *E. coli* in blood cultures of infants without meningitis, 14 per cent of *E. coli* in blood cultures of adults, 11 per cent of *E. coli* in adult urine, and 12 per cent of *E. coli* in normal stool cultures.[24] The large number of K1 antigen–containing *E. coli* recovered from patients with meningitis, coupled with its antigenic similarities to meningococcal serogroups B, C, D, pneumococcal types 1, 2, 4, 7, 10, 33, HITB, and group B streptococci, suggests that its invasive properties are related to capsular polysaccharide configuration.[2]

Certain other organisms produce meningitis infrequently except under conditions in which the host has been compromised. Neurosurgical treatment of hydrocephalus in which a ventriculoperitoneal or ventriculoatrial shunt has been placed may be followed by meningitis due to *Staphylococcus epidermidis*.[25] The host whose lymphoid or reticuoendothelial system is functioning imperfectly may be infected by bacteria such as diphtheroids, *Pseudomonas, Proteus, Serratia,* and *Listeria.*[11]

The Environment

Environmental influences are important in a consideration of the pathogenesis of CNS infection involving a wide variety of microorganisms. The most notable association between the environment and the development of meningitis has been described for *N. meningitidis.* Although meningococcal meningitis can occur at any age in the normal host, its incidence is markedly greater in situations where individuals are in close contact with one another.[1, 2, 21, 26]

PATHOLOGY[1, 2, 6, 7, 16, 27, 28, 29]

An awareness of the alteration in the structure of the nervous system is crucial to an understanding of the many clinical phenomena encountered in meningitis; the fundamental process is an inflammation of the leptomeninges.

In the first stage of this process, hyperemia of the meningeal vessels occurs and is followed by migration of neutrophils into the subarachnoid space, creating an exudate that rapidly increases and extends into the sheaths of cortical blood vessels and along cranial and spinal nerves. The meningeal exudate is probably the result of bacteria and their toxins, which induce vascular congestion, increase vascular permeability, and engender a leukocyte response. The exudate produced varies from essentially none to an amount several millimeters in thickness. The purulent material has been found in a wide distribution but tends to accumulate over the convexity of the brain (as with pneumococcal disease), in the depths of the sulci, in the sylvian fissures, and along the major veins and venous sinuses. Along the undersurfaces of the brain (as in *H. influenzae* meningitis), the exudate is concentrated within the basal cisterns and about the cerebellum. The spinal cord has been found encased in pus in a number of cases, although its general distribution is over the dorsum of the cord. Purulent material has been found within the ventricles, and subdural empyema also has been described.

During the first few days of illness, polymorphonuclear leukocytes, often containing phagocytized bacteria, predominate. As time progresses, these cells degenerate and are removed by macrophages that are derived from meningeal histocytes or monocytes, both of which subsequently become the principal cell types. During this time, exudation of fibrinogen and other blood proteins occurs.

In the second week of infection, the subarachnoid exudate consists of two layers of cells—an outer layer of neutrophils and fibrin and an inner layer, next to the pia, of lymphocytes, macrophages, and plasma cells. Fibroblasts also are present and aid in the organization of the exudate. With resolution, cells disappear in the order of their initial appearance. Complete resolution depends upon the stage at which infection is arrested. If it is controlled early, little residua may be present, but following an infection lasting several weeks, there is permanent fibrous overgrowth of the meninges resulting in adhesive arachnoiditis and permanent and progressive hydrocephalus.

Once established, meningeal infection spreads along the leptomeningeal investments of penetrating cortical vessels, causing arterial endothelial cell swelling and proliferation. The adventitial layers of the vessels become infiltrated by neutrophils and other round cells, creating necrotic foci within the arterial walls, which lead to arterial thromboses. A similar process occurs in the veins, and focal necrosis and mural thrombi develop, resulting in occlusion of the lumen. In meningitis, venous thrombosis is much more common than arterial thrombosis. Perineural sheaths of spinal and cranial nerves often become infiltrated by inflammatory cells; occasionally the endoneurium is infiltrated, and degenerating myelinated fibers become evident with fat-laden macrophages and proliferating Schwann cells and fibroblasts.

When the fibrinopurulent exudate accumulates in large quantity around the midbrain, pons, and spinal cord, the spinal subarachnoid space becomes obstructed, causing hydrocephalus. Hydrocephalus may be a complication of meningitis. When it occurs, hydrocephalus generally is of the communicating type, and is the result of adhesive arachnoidal thickening about the cisterns at the base of the brain and the arachnoid villi. Occasionally the aqueduct of Sylvius or the foramina of Magendie and of Lushka become obstructed by reactive gliosis and fibrosis, causing hydrocephalus of the noncommunicating type.

As a result of the inflammatory reaction (which may reduce absorption of CSF) in the vicinity of the perivascular spaces, edema of the superficial cortex occurs. In addition, toxins in the purulent exudate alter the integrity of brain cell membranes, causing increased levels of intracellular sodium, decreased levels of cellular potassium, and elevated cellular water. This type of brain edema is cytotoxic and may compromise cerebral circulation to such an extent that uncal herniation and death may ensue.

There is ample evidence to suggest that in meningitis excessive secretion of antidiuretic hormone occurs, which causes water retention and sodium loss via the kidney. This combination of factors places the patient at greater risk for developing increased intracranial pressure or seizures.[30] Cellular electrolyte disturbances may depolarize the neuronal membranes, resulting in a predisposition to seizure activity.[31] Increased glucose oxidation and lactate production associated with depletion of high energy compounds, such as phosphocreatine and ATP, also are observed. The choroid plexuses, ependyma, and pia mater respond to the inflammation of the subarachnoid space by becoming more permeable to serum protein, thus producing an increase in CSF protein.

Hypoglycorrhachia results primarily from the decreased transport of glucose across the inflamed choroid plexus as well as from increased utilization of glucose by host tissue. Utilization of glucose by bacteria and polymorphonuclear leukocytes is relatively less important in producing low levels of CSF glucose.[31]

Another effect of meningitis is a reduction in the cerebral blood flow and in the utilization of available oxygen. A loss of cerebral vascular autoregulation, which in some cases is restored by hypocapnia, is believed to be caused by tissue acidosis.

In summary, a variety of factors such as necrosis of cerebral tissue, occlusion of vascular vessels, circulatory disturbances, metabolic waste products, bacteria, bacterial toxins, edema, and hypoxia may combine to produce nerve damage manifested by cranial nerve signs, focal cerebral signs, seizures, or generalized encephalopathy. Impaired consciousness (lethargy, stupor, coma), impaired intelligence, permanent cranial nerve deficits, hemiparesis or quadriparesis, or death may ensue.

PATHOLOGIC-CLINICAL RELATIONS[2, 4, 7, 16, 27, 28, 29, 31]

Signs and symptoms associated with fully developed meningitis, regardless of the etiology, include fever, headache, nausea, vomiting, nuchal and spinal rigidity, alterations of sensorium, convulsions, cranial nerve palsies, disturbances in vision and hearing, and, rarely, papilledema and ataxia.[31] This variety of neurologic findings may be evident during the acute phase of bacterial meningitis, may occur after a few days as complications of the meningitic process, or may be late sequelae of the infection.

In acute meningitis, pure pia-arachnoiditis (involving the vessels and nerve roots—especially pain-carrying fibers of the fifth cervical nerve) may result in headache, stiff neck, and Brudzinski and Kernig signs. There signs depend on the activation of protective reflexes, which shorten and mobilize the spine (extension of the head and neck and flexion of the hips and knees reduce stretch in inflamed spinal structures). These findings also can occur secondary to increased intracranial pressure with resultant nerve root distortion and irritation and hence pain-carrying fiber irritation. These signs are accompanied by hyperesthesia and photophobia. Currently there is no satisfactory pathophysiologic explanation for photophobia. Papilledema is rare in meningitis, probably because of the brief duration of increased intracranial pressure. When papilledema is noted, associated conditions including brain abscess, subdural empyema, and venous sinus occlusion should be considered.

Sub-pial encephalopathy probably is toxic or metabolic in origin because bacteria generally do not penetrate the pia. It may be manifested by alterations in sensorium including confusion, stupor, coma, and seizures. Seizures may be both generalized and focal. Generally, when focal signs are noted, cortical necrosis or occlusive vasculitis or thrombosis of the cortical veins has occurred. Inflammatory involvement or vascular compromise of the cranial nerve roots may result in cranial nerve palsies (cranial verves III, IV, VI are most commonly involved), facial weakness, and deafness. Thrombosis of meningeal vessels or cortical necrosis may result in focal convulsions or focal cerebral defects such as hemiparesis. These signs may appear during the first three or four days or less commonly, may occur after the first or second week of infection.

Complications of meningitis may occur and include ventriculitis, hydrocephalus, subdural effusion, and paralysis. Infections of the ventricular system may be primary or may be secondary to the spread of organisms from the subarachnoid spaces or the migration of motile bacteria. When ventriculitis is accompanied by an obstruction of the aqueduct of Sylvius the infection may behave as an abscess. Obstructive or communicating hydrocephalus may be due to purulent exudate around the base of the brain, to meningeal fibrosis, or rarely to aqueductal stenosis. Variable degrees of impairment may be seen when hydrocephalus develops. In the mildest form psychomotor retardation, unsteadiness of gait, and incontinence may be seen. In more severe forms of hydrocelphalus, decorticate posturing, grasping and sucking reflexes, and sphincter incontinence may occur.

Subdural effusion occurs with sufficient frequency that we consider it a normal event of the disease rather than a complication. Effusions generally occur over the frontoparietal region, although localized collections do occur over the occipital region. The etiology may be related to thrombophlebitis of the veins bridging the subdural space, small tears in the vessels secondary to shifting of the brain, or spread of an infection from arachnoiditis. Subdural fluid has a disproportionately high albumin to globulin ratio. The effusion usually is bilateral and generally asymptomatic. Its incidence is proportional to the vigor with which it is sought by the clinician. Subdural effusions are seen with all organisms but most commonly with *H. influenzae, S. pneumoniae,* and *N. meningitidis* infections, in decreasing order of frequency. Subdural effusions may cause focal neurologic signs, persistence of fever, seizures, or vomiting. Extensive venous or arterial infarction may result in hemiplegia, decorticate or decerebrate rigidity, cortical blindness, seizures, and coma.

Blindness and optic atrophy may be related to optic arachnoiditis. Spastic paraparesis with sensory loss in the lower extremities may be secondary to meningomyelitis.

A general deficit in intellectual function may be manifested as persistent mental retardation or behavioral disturbances. The pathogenesis of this intellectual function deficit may be complicated and may include not only damage from the meningitis itself but also damage resulting from shock and hypoxia that may aggravate the acute illness.

All sequelae of bacteria meningitis occur more commonly in children than in adults. Pessimism about sequelae observed when the patient is discharged from the hospital at the conclusion of therapy is unwarranted, however. Even major neurologic sequelae have a tendency to clear with time.[23, 53]

PARAMENINGEAL SUPPURATIVE FOCI

In many cases, parameningeal and meningeal infections occur concurrently.[32] The neurologic expression of the various parameningeal infections depends on the site of the lesion(s), which in turn is determined by how the intracranial or intraspinal infection was established.[2, 27] Some of the important suppurative foci to be discussed are the brain, subdural and epidural (empyema) abscesses, spinal epidural abscess, and intracranial thrombosis.

Brain Abscess[33–37]

Brain abscesses are approximately twice as common in males as in females. Brain abscesses occur in infants, children, and adults; the incidence in some series is higher in infancy and early childhood because of the high incidence of congenital cyanotic disease.[33] In other series, brain abscesses rarely are reported in children less than 2 years of age.[35] Although brain abscesses are not common, awareness of their occurrence is extremely important because they are potentially curable lesions if identified early in their development.

The pyogenic organisms gain access to the brain by several routes: (1) through the blood stream from a distant focus of infection or from septicemia, (2) extension from contiguous infections of the middle ear, mastoids, and paranasal sinuses, osteomyelitis of adjacent bone or from inflammation of the small bridging veins (thrombophlebitis) or both, (3) as a complication of a penetrating wound, and (4) in association with a cardiopulmonary malformation such as an intracardiac right-to-left shunt or a pulmonary arteriovenous fistula.[35]

The most common causative organisms of brain abcesses are *Staphylococcus aureus,* anaerobic streptococci, β- and α-hemolytic streptococci. Pneumococci and *H. influenzae* are less prevalent. A variety of gram-negative microorganisms also have been isolated.[33–37]

Anaerobic isolates have composed two-thirds of the microorganisms found in brain abscesses when strict techniques for their collection, transportation, and cultivation have been employed.[34] The location of abscesses may be random when they result from hematogenous spread, or they may be localized to areas of the brain that are in close proximity to a parameningeal focus of infection such as sinusitis or mastoiditis.

Predisposing factors include acute or chronic otitis, mastoiditis, dental abscess, sinusitis, pulmonary infection, cyanotic congenital heart disease, pulmonary arteriovenous fistula, and bacterial endocarditis.[33–37]

The earliest stage of the development of a brain abscess is cerebritis, i.e., septic encephalitis, which represents an edematous area, usually within the white matter and accompanied by hyperemia, petechial hemorrhages, and inflammatory cell infiltrates. The center becomes liquefied with subsequent formation of purulent material comprising the abscess. Initially, the wall is ill-defined, but gradually a firmer, thicker wall encapsulates the lesion, and profound edema of the white matter surrounding the capsule appears. This process of encapsulation requires a minimum of four to six weeks.[36]

Brain abscesses are identified less often during infancy. Frequently, the only sign may be a rapidly enlarging head without focal neurologic signs. In older children, the initial manifestations may be nonspecific, reflecting the presence of cerebritis, and may include headache, vomiting, fever, listlessness, disorientation, neck pain, stiffness, and seizures. If the abscess enlarges, specific neurologic signs may become apparent and may include: hemiparesis, lateralizing signs, ocular palsies, papilledema, increased deep tendon reflexes, extensor plantar responses, pupillary changes, homonymous hemianopia, aphasia, stupor, coma, and death.[33–37] These signs will vary depending on where the abscesses are located. For example, headaches, vomiting, drowsiness, and homonymous hemianopia may result from an abscess involving radiations of the optic tract; coordination disturbances, i.e., dysmetria, nystagmus, and ataxia, may occur with cerebellar abscesses; posterior-frontal or anterior-parietal lobe abscesses often may cause focal motor or sensory seizures on the contralateral side, and temporal and/or cerebellar abscesses and frontal lobe abscesses may be, respectively, otogenic or rhinogenic in origin. A brain abscess can be surprisingly silent from a clinical standpoint, especially when it is located in the frontal lobe. Brain abscesses rarely can complicate primary bacterial meningitis when the diagnosis of meningitis is delayed and the infection is not treated properly. Untreated, the infection usually is fatal. Death may result from increased intracranial pressure or from the sudden rupture of the abscess into the ventricular system.[33–35]

Computerized axial tomography (CAT) is the diagnostic method of choice.[34, 37] Generally, it reveals a mass lesion with a contrast-enhanceable margin and a zone of decreased density around the margin. Electroencephalograms (EEGs) may reveal high-voltage slow wave activity. Brain scans (useful especially during the stage of acute cerebritis when CAT scan may reveal only an isodense mass) and cerebral angiographic studies also may be of some value in delineating the brain abscess focus.[33–37]

A lumbar puncture (LP) should not be considered as an initial diagnostic procedure in a patient with a suspected brain abscess because of the danger of herniation. When the LP is performed, CSF pressure and cell count may be elevated. The results of Gram stain and culture may be positive if the abscess ruptures into the ventricular system.[34, 37] Treatment often entails open surgical drainage or removal of necrotic brain tissue coupled with appropriate antibiotic therapy,[33, 34, 35, 37] as well as anticonvulsant therapy when needed.[36] When the diagnosis of brain abscess is established early, antibiotic therapy alone may suffice. Residual defects may include seizure activity, localized neurologic abnormalities, hydrocephalus, and mental retardation.[35] The mortality rate in one recent large study was 22 per cent.[37]

Subdural Empyema Abscess[38–43]

Subdural empyema occurs with greater frequency in males than in females.[33, 42] Subdural empyema may develop at any age but is most common during the second and third decades of life. The pathogenesis of subdural empyema mimics, to some extent, that of brain abscess. Subdural empyema may result from sepsis or from an extension (via thrombophlebitis or osteomyelitis) of an infection like otitis media, mastoiditis, frontal and ethmoidal sinusitis, or orbital cellulitis, or from bacterial contamination of a subdural effusion in meningitis.[38, 41] Frontal and ethmoidal sinusitis, otitis media, and pneumococcal meningitis are common sources of organisms in subdural abscesses in older children, whereas in children less than one year of age the most common predisposing factor is primary leptomeningitis.[40] In the younger child, the etiologic agent usually is *Streptococcus pneumoniae, H. influenzae,* or gram-negative bacilli. The microorganisms implicated most commonly in the older child usually are anaerobic or aerobic streptococci or *Staphylococcus aureus.*[40]

The infection generally occurs over the convexity of the brain. Lesions arising secondary to frontal sinusitis often are located over the corresponding frontal pole and extend back variable distances over the frontal convexity. Lesions of otogenic origin frequently are located primarily in the temporal region but may occur in the cerebellar region. Most subdural empyemas are unilateral in location, although some are found interhemispherically.[41] Focal osteomyelitis or epidural abscess or both may be found concomitantly.

Clinical manifestations generally include fever, headache, vomiting, papilledema, increased intracranial pressure, focal neurologic signs, and focal seizures, with the more focal findings occurring anytime from a day to several weeks after the presentation of nonspecific findings.[38–42]

The diagnosis of subdural empyema ideally is made by a CAT scan, which reveals a band of decreased radiolucency adjacent to the skull, sometimes with an ill-defined zone of increased density medial to the lesion. One recent study found CAT scan unreliable for detecting primary subdural empyema.[43] Angiography or brain scanning was recommended when clinical findings suggested subdural empyema but the CAT scan was negative.

CSF changes are nonspecific. Lumbar punctures should be perfomed with great care because of the danger of the tonsillar herniation.[38–42] Angiographic studies show displacement of vessels away from the inner table of the skull or the falx.

Early diagnosis, prompt chemotherapy along with surgical aspiration, drainage, or excision are imperative. Long-term neurologic sequelae may include residual hemiparesis, seizures, deficits in the child's school performance, and behavioral problems. The overall morbidity rate varies from 25 to 45 per cent.[38–42]

Epidural Abscess[44]

Infection of the epidural space is rare in childhood. The etiology, pathogenesis, and bacteriology of intracranial epidural abscess are identical to those described for intracranial subdural empyema. Common predisposing factors include otitis media, mastoiditis, and sinusitis. *S. aureus* is the principal etiologic agent.

Epidural abscesses usually are less aggressive than subdural empyemas. An epidural abscess can remain clinically silent, or increased intracranial pressure, headache, and vomiting may be noted. These findings may be followed by other focal neurologic signs or by seizures. Generally, if focal signs or signs suggesting significant elevation of intracranial pressure are present, a brain abscess or venous thrombosis exists concomitantly.

Subdural empyema also is present in a large percentage of cases of epidural abscess. CAT scanning will reveal an abscess that generally is more constricted than that found with a subdural abscess, and the lesion generally is bounded medially by a thick, dense ring. Arteriography will outline an avascular mass with inward displacement of cortical vessels and venous sinuses. CSF usually is sterile, and CSF changes are nonspecific. The danger of tonsillar herniation is present; thus, lumbar puncture should be deferred. The treatment is identical to that suggested for subdural empyema.

Spinal Epidural Abscess

Spinal epidural abscess is an uncommon lesion in children, especially those less than 10 years of age.[45] Epidural abscess most often is the result of the hematogenous spread of bacteria. Direct extension from cerebral osteomyelitis is a less common cause. Cutaneous furunculosis is the most common identifiable infection antedating a spinal epidural abscess.[45] The vast majority of cases are due to penicillin-resistant *S. aureus*[45]; however aerobic and anaerobic streptococci and gram-negative bacilli have been recovered from selected patients.

Spinal epidural abscess most commonly is located in the midthoracic or lower lumbar regions. In children, the cervical and lumbar regions are involved most frequently.[45] Suppuration usually is located on the dorsal surface of the spinal dura.[45,46] Some children with spinal epidural abscess have no history of significant antecedent events, whereas others have had a preceding bacterial infection or an injury with blunt trauma to the back. Deep-aching pain, at or near the site of the involved level of the spine, is the usual initial symptom of the disease. This discomfort may worsen to such an extent that spinal rigidity and localized vertebral tenderness to percussion become evident. Fever, headache, vomiting, and nuchal rigidity may occur. Subsequently, radicular pain from nerve root irritation results. The pain may be followed by weakness of the lower extremities, sensory deficits, or hyperesthesias of the legs or feet, and abnormalities of bowel or bladder function. At this stage, back pain may be so severe that the child refuses to walk or may be unable to walk because of paralysis.[45,46]

Useful diagnostic parameters may include a leukocytosis with a left shift and an elevated ESR. Blood cultures may be of help in identifying the organism, but roentgenographic evidence of osteomyelitis rarely may be present.[45]

The diagnosis can be established by successful needle drainage of the epidural abscess after CAT scan of the area has been performed. A lumbar puncture generally will reveal marked CSF pleocytosis and elevated CSF protein concentration. A myelogram using metrizamide (water-soluble contrast dye), which can be performed concomitantly, will confirm the presence and level of a block caused by an extradural mass.

A laminectomy with decompression and drainage should be carried out as soon as the diagnosis is made, in order to avoid permanent paralysis or death, and the patient should be started on antibiotic therapy. Therapy should be continued for at least two weeks postoperatively[45] and up to four to six weeks if vertebral osteomyelitis is demonstrated roentgenographically or by nuclear scan techniques. Morbidity occurs in approximately 10 to 20 per cent of cases.

Intracranial Vasculitis (Thrombophlebitis, Arteritis)[47–49]

Septic intracranial thrombophlebitis most frequently follows an infection of the paranasal sinuses, middle ear, mastoid, or orpharynx; it also may occur in association with an epidural abscess, subdural empyema, or meningitis, or may be the result of an infection that spreads hematogenously from a focus elsewhere within the body. Septic intracranial thrombophlebitis may begin within veins or venous sinuses and may involve additional vessels. Cerebral angiography has revealed vascular lesions in children with bacterial meningitis. Abnormalities that have been identified include arteritis, thrombosis, thrombophlebitis, and vascular narrowing.[49] The offending organisms usually are *Staphyloccus aureus,* with a minority of cases due to streptococci (including *Streptococcus pneumoniae*) and gram-negative bacilli.[47,48]

Septic intracranial thrombophlebitis may involve the cortical vessels, cavernous sinus, lateral sinus, superior sagittal sinus, and superior and inferior petrosal sinus. Inflammation of these vessels eventually may result in occlusion with secondary edema, hemorrhagic infarction, and necrosis that may be responsible for brain, epidural, and subdural abscess formation or communicating hydrocephalus.

Septic intracranial thrombophlebitis appears as sepsis without neurologic signs or with stupor and focal neurologic signs in the presence of intracranial infection. The symptoms of venous sinus occlusion depend upon the venous sinus involved. Cavernous sinus thrombosis most commonly follows a facial infection or paranasal sinusitis.[47] Clinically, the child appears quite ill with a combination of systemic symptoms and local signs that include high spiking fevers, chills, headache, vomiting, lethargy, severe stabbing ocular pain, chemosis, exophthalmos, ophthalmoplegia, pupillary dilatation, retinal venous engorgement, and papilledema. Signs and symptoms of cerebral involvement may include hemiparesis or seizures from cortical vein involvement.

The diagnosis generally is made on clinical grounds. Leukocytosis and elevated ESR may be noted. Skull films may reveal sinusitis. Lumbar puncture may reveal increased CSF pressure, a slight lymphocytosis, and increased CSF protein concentration. Radionuclide scan, CAT scan, and angiography all may be required in individual patients to establish a diagnosis. Carotid angiography may reveal focal arteritis or obstruction, and the venous phase may show delayed filling or non-visualization of the cavernous sinus.

Treatment of septic cavernous sinus thrombosis requires administration of high doses of antibiotics in addition to other supportive measures for a critically ill child. Control of infection may require urgent surgical drainage of intra- or extracranial abscesses.

Lateral sinus thrombosis most commonly follows otitis media, mastoiditis, or, rarely, pharyngitis.[48] Clinically, earache and mastoid tenderness followed by a generalized headache may be noted. Generally, there is a paucity of neurologic signs, but lateral rectus weakness, facial dysesthesias, increased intracranial pressure with papilledema, and temporal lobe seizures may occur.

Diagnosis and treatment are established in a similar manner to that described previously. Skull radiographs may reveal evidence of mastoiditis.

Brain infarction, in association with bacterial meningitis, is more common in children less than one year of age, in males, in children infected with *S. pneumoniae,* and in patients with severe hypoglycorrhachia whose clinical course is complicated by seizures.[49]

CLINICAL MANIFESTATIONS[50, 51]

The clinical manifestations that usually are associated with acute bacterial meningitis include nausea, vomiting, anorexia, irritability, lethargy, photophobia, headache, and alterations of sensorium. Nuchal rigidity and positive Kernig and Brudzinski signs occur relatively late in the young child. Kernig sign is present when the leg is flexed 90 degrees at the hip and cannot be extended more than 135 degrees. Brudzinski's sign is present if the thighs and legs are flexed involuntarily when the neck is flexed. Nuchal rigidity may not be elicited in comatose patients or when signs of focal or diffuse neurologic impairment are present. In the infant, only minimal signs of meningeal inflammation may be noted; lethargy, irritability, or poor feeding may be reported.

Generally, fever is present, although its absence, in our experience, does not exclude the possibility of bacterial meningitis; the elevation of the fever is variable. The patient may complain of headache, which may be related to inflammation of the meningeal vessels or to an increase in intracranial pressure or both. Increased intracranial pressure may be manifest by a bulging anterior fontanelle and diastasis of sutures in the infant. Papilledema usually is not a clinical feature of bacterial meningitis. If it is noted, venous sinus occlusion, subdural empyema, or brain abscess should be considered.

Another common finding, especially in meningococcal meningitis, is a petechial or purpuric rash. These rashes may accompany any infectious or noninfectious disease process in which vasculitis is present.

Myalgias, arthralgias, and evidence of cardiac involvement all have been noted and reflect the systemic nature of the disease. Arthritis has been associated most often with meningococcal disease but may accompany disease due to any organism. Pericardial effusions may be present, but studies have indicated that they usually are not of clinical significance and resolve without antimicrobial drug therapy.[50]

Obtundation, stupor, coma, seizures, cranial nerve involvement, and focal neurologic signs may be associated with bacterial meningitis. Cranial nerve involvement is caused by both local inflammation and impaired vascular supply to the nerves. Cranial nerves most commonly affected are III, IV, and VI; the paralysis may be transient or permanent. Deafness or disturbances in vestibular function also are noted frequently, but optic nerve involvement with blindness is rare. Involvement of the eighth cranial nerve may reflect disease at the cochlear and vestibular end organs or may be related to concomitant infection of the inner ear.[51]

In one study, 14 per cent of children with meningitis had focal neurologic signs at the time of admission. The presence of focal neurologic signs was predictive of a poor outcome; they were correlated significantly ($P < 0.01$) with abnormal neurologic findings even one year following discharge.[23]

In the same study, seizures occurred prior to admission in approximately 20 per cent of children with bacterial meningitis.[23] Overall, 30 per cent of children had seizures at some time during their illness. Seizures that occurred during the first few days of illness had no prognostic significance. Seizures that were difficult to control or persisted beyond the fourth hospital day, as well as seizures that were noted for the first time late in the hospital course, appeared to be more significant and were associated with the permanent sequelae of meningitis.[51]

During the acute illness, subdural effusions or collections of fluid in the subdural space have been noted frequently; they can be demonstrated in up to 50 per cent of children and almost always are sterile.[31] In a prospective study, subdural effusions were noted in 35 per cent of children with *H. influenzae* meningitis, 19 per cent of children with pneumococcal meningitis, 8 per cent of children with meningococcal meningitis, and 23 per cent of children with meningitis due to other organisms or from whom no organism was recovered.[1] However, when appropriate statistical corrections were made to normalize differences in age, the incidence of subdural effusions was shown to be independent of the bacterial organisms causing the meningitis. Subdural effusions either are more frequent in the very young child, more readily detectable in infants, or both.[51]

Frequently, meningitis is associated with an increased secretion of antidiuretic hormone (ADH).[16, 23, 30, 51] When excess fluid is provided, there may be a greater increase in intracranial pressure and brain edema, and the symptoms are those of water intoxication.

Shock has been found in 5.8 per cent of children and meningococcal meningitis and 5.5 per cent of children with *H. influenzae* meningitis in one prospective study.[51] Signs of disseminated intravascular coagulation may accompany the hypotension in these patients.

Differential Diagnosis

When the signs and symptoms described previously are observed, the physician must entertain the possibility of acute meningeal inflammation, but none is pathognomonic for a bacterial process or even for meningitis. Many pathologic processes, including aseptic meningitis, tuberculous meningitis, fungal meningitis, brain abscess, bacterial endocarditis with embolism, and brain tumors may mimic the clinical manifestations of bacterial meningitis. The specific diagnosis of each of these processes may be accomplished using a variety of studies; the most important of these is the examination of CSF. Specific immunologic, roentgenographic, and isotopic studies are available to assist in the differentiation of these disorders. A systematized approach to the diagnosis and treatment of bacterial meningitis and its complications is presented in the algorithm.

DIAGNOSIS

The definitive diagnosis of acute bacterial meningitis rests upon the results of the lumbar puncture (LP). The opening pressure and the total number of white blood cells should be noted, and a differential cell count performed. The CSF protein should be measured, and the CSF glucose should be compared with a blood glucose obtained concomitantly. In a young child, particularly one who has an open anterior fontanelle, or whose sutures can be split by increased intracranial pressure, there is no contraindication to the performance of an LP in the presence of suspected bacterial meningitis. In older children, when signs and symptoms suggest a significant increase in intracranial pressure but the possibility of bacterial meningitis exists, an LP may be performed by an experienced clinician utilizing a #26 needle. Under these circumstances, an intravenous line should be established prior to the procedure. If the pressure appears to be extremely elevated when the needle enters the subarachnoid space, mannitol, 1 gm/kg, should be infused through the intravenous line immediately; the stylet should be replaced in the needle, and the needle should not be removed until the CSF pressure has been reduced.

Smears should be Gram stained for bacteria and Kenyoun stained for mycobacteria. The CSF should be cultured on blood agar, chocolate agar, in Fildes or Leventhal media, and in broth. Chocolate agar facilitates the growth of *N. meningitidis*. Fildes or Leventhal media provide for optimal growth of *H. influenzae*.

Generally, patients with bacterial meningitis have an increased number of WBCs within the CSF and a predominance of polymorphonuclear leukocytes (PMNs). An increase in protein usually is seen as well as a depression of CSF glucose and of the CSF to blood glucose ratio. The Gram stain may reveal microorganisms.

At times, however, it is impossible to make a definitive diagnosis from either the clinical presentation or CSF chemical and morphologic findings. In these cases, additional laboratory data can be helpful. Blood cultures should be obtained. In one prospective study, 80 to 90 per cent of children with bacterial meningitis had blood cultures that grew the same organism as was identified within the CSF.[23, 51] Cultures of the throat and nasopharynx are of no value. Smears of petechial lesions, when present, may reveal microorganisms on Gram stain.[51]

Text continued on page 34.

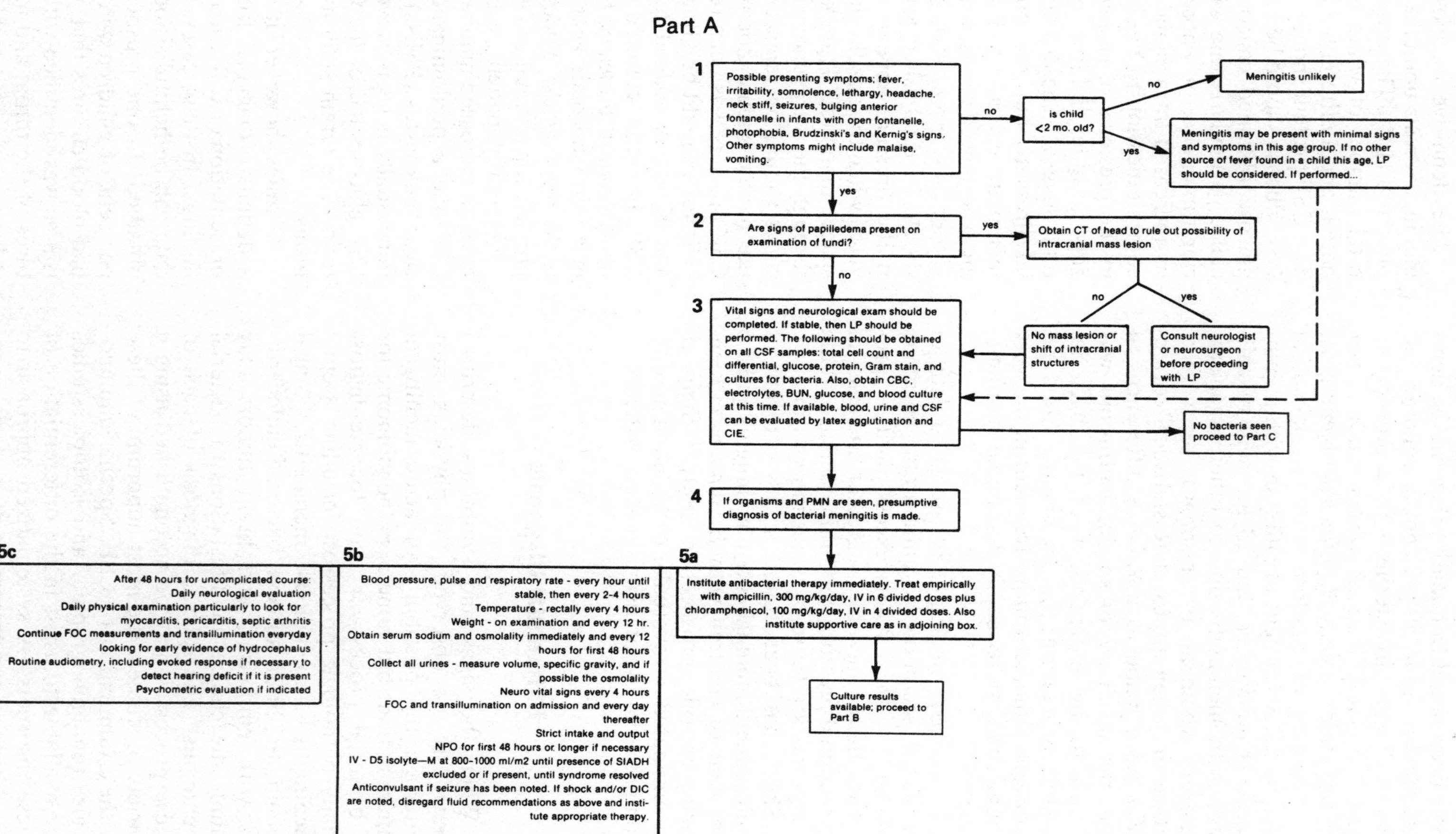
ALGORITHM
DIAGNOSIS AND THERAPY OF ACUTE BACTERIAL MENINGITIS
Part A
1
Possible presenting symptoms; fever, irritability, somnolence, lethargy, headache, neck stiff, seizures, bulging anterior fontanelle in infants with open fontanelle, photophobia, Brudzinski's and Kernig's signs. Other symptoms might include malaise, vomiting.
no
is child <2 mo. old?
no
Meningitis unlikely
yes
Meningitis may be present with minimal signs and symptoms in this age group. If no other source of fever found in a child this age, LP should be considered. If performed...
yes
2
Are signs of papilledema present on examination of fundi?
yes
Obtain CT of head to rule out possibility of intracranial mass lesion
no
No mass lesion or shift of intracranial structures
yes
Consult neurologist or neurosurgeon before proceeding with LP
no
3
Vital signs and neurological exam should be completed. If stable, then LP should be performed. The following should be obtained on all CSF samples: total cell count and differential, glucose, protein, Gram stain, and cultures for bacteria. Also, obtain CBC, electrolytes, BUN, glucose, and blood culture at this time. If available, blood, urine and CSF can be evaluated by latex agglutination and CIE.
No bacteria seen proceed to Part C
4
If organisms and PMN are seen, presumptive diagnosis of bacterial meningitis is made.
5a
Institute antibacterial therapy immediately. Treat empirically with ampicillin, 300 mg/kg/day, IV in 6 divided doses plus chloramphenicol, 100 mg/kg/day, IV in 4 divided doses. Also institute supportive care as in adjoining box.
Culture results available; proceed to Part B
5b
Blood pressure, pulse and respiratory rate - every hour until stable, then every 2-4 hours
Temperature - rectally every 4 hours
Weight - on examination and every 12 hr.
Obtain serum sodium and osmolality immediately and every 12 hours for first 48 hours
Collect all urines - measure volume, specific gravity, and if possible the osmolality
Neuro vital signs every 4 hours
FOC and transillumination on admission and every day thereafter
Strict intake and output
NPO for first 48 hours or longer if necessary
IV - D5 isolyte—M at 800–1000 ml/m2 until presence of SIADH excluded or if present, until syndrome resolved
Anticonvulsant if seizure has been noted. If shock and/or DIC are noted, disregard fluid recommendations as above and institute appropriate therapy.
5c
After 48 hours for uncomplicated course:
Daily neurological evaluation
Daily physical examination particularly to look for myocarditis, pericarditis, septic arthritis
Continue FOC measurements and transillumination everyday looking for early evidence of hydrocephalus
Routine audiometry, including evoked response if necessary to detect hearing deficit if it is present
Psychometric evaluation if indicated

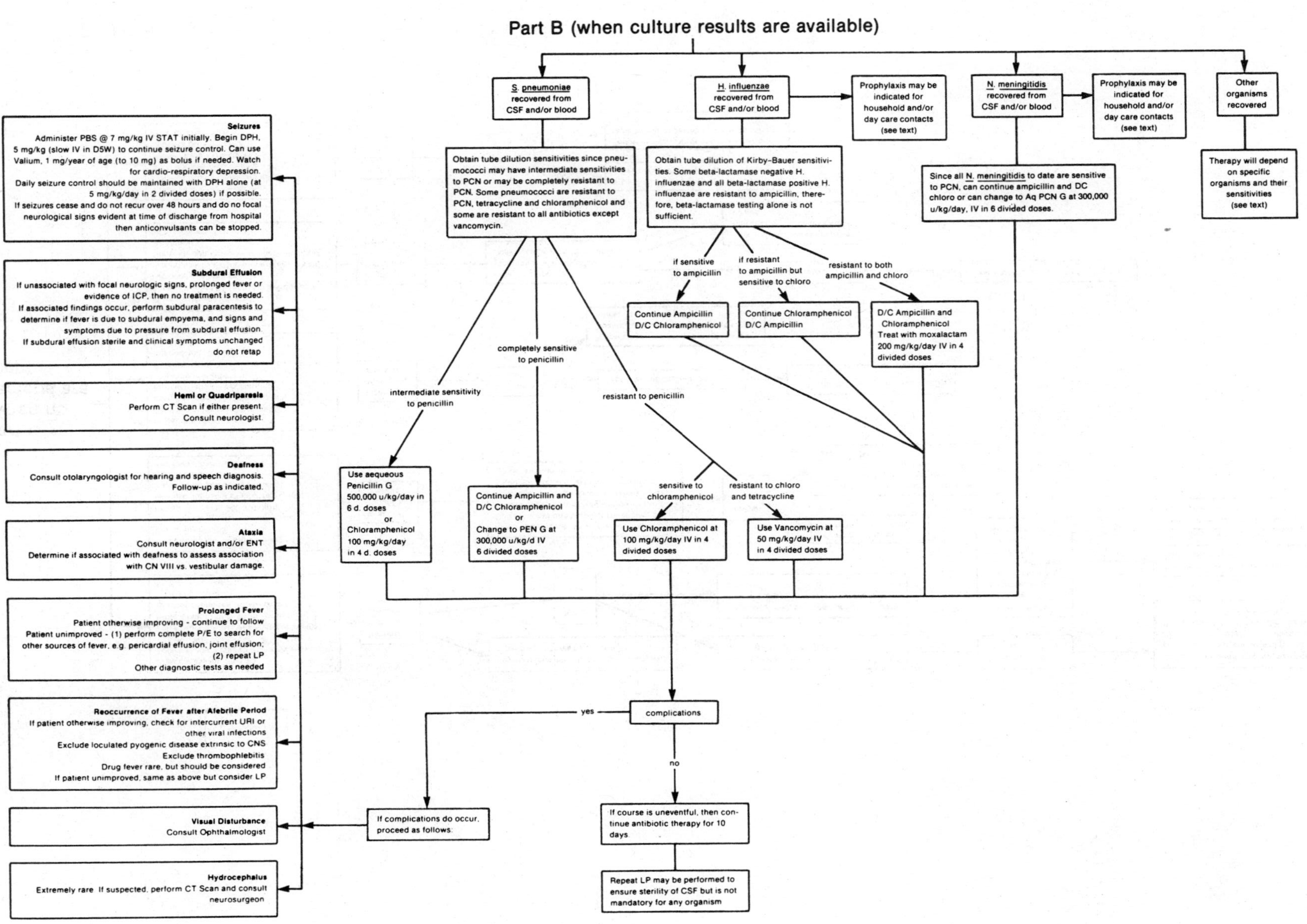
Part B (when culture results are available)
S. pneumoniae recovered from CSF and/or blood
H. influenzae recovered from CSF and/or blood
Prophylaxis may be indicated for household and/or day care contacts (see text)
N. meningitidis recovered from CSF and/or blood
Prophylaxis may be indicated for household and/or day care contacts (see text)
Other organisms recovered
Therapy will depend on specific organisms and their sensitivities (see text)
Obtain tube dilution sensitivities since pneumococci may have intermediate sensitivities to PCN or may be completely resistant to PCN. Some pneumococci are resistant to PCN, tetracycline and chloramphenicol and some are resistant to all antibiotics except vancomycin.
Obtain tube dilution of Kirby-Bauer sensitivities. Some beta-lactamase negative H. influenzae and all beta-lactamase positive H. influenzae are resistant to ampicillin, therefore, beta-lactamase testing alone is not sufficient.
Since all N. meningitidis to date are sensitive to PCN, can continue ampicillin and DC chloro or can change to Aq PCN G at 300,000 u/kg/day, IV in 6 divided doses.
if sensitive to ampicillin
if resistant to ampicillin but sensitive to chloro
resistant to both ampicillin and chloro
Continue Ampicillin D/C Chloramphenicol
Continue Chloramphenicol D/C Ampicillin
D/C Ampicillin and Chloramphenicol Treat with moxalactam 200 mg/kg/day IV in 4 divided doses
completely sensitive to penicillin
intermediate sensitivity to penicillin
resistant to penicillin
Use aequeous Penicillin G 500,000 u/kg/day in 6 d. doses or Chloramphenicol 100 mg/kg/day in 4 d. doses
Continue Ampicillin and D/C Chloramphenicol or Change to PEN G at 300,000 u/kg/d IV 6 divided doses
sensitive to chloramphenicol
resistant to chloro and tetracycline
Use Chloramphenicol at 100 mg/kg/day IV in 4 divided doses
Use Vancomycin at 50 mg/kg/day IV in 4 divided doses
complications
yes
no
If complications do occur, proceed as follows:
If course is uneventful, then continue antibiotic therapy for 10 days.
Repeat LP may be performed to ensure sterility of CSF but is not mandatory for any organism
Seizures
Administer PBS @ 7 mg/kg IV STAT initially. Begin DPH, 5 mg/kg (slow IV in D5W) to continue seizure control. Can use Valium, 1 mg/year of age (to 10 mg) as bolus if needed. Watch for cardio-respiratory depression.
Daily seizure control should be maintained with DPH alone (at 5 mg/kg/day in 2 divided doses) if possible.
If seizures cease and do not recur over 48 hours and do no focal neurological signs evident at time of discharge from hospital then anticonvulsants can be stopped.
Subdural Effusion
If unassociated with focal neurologic signs, prolonged fever or evidence of ICP, then no treatment is needed.
If associated findings occur, perform subdural paracentesis to determine if fever is due to subdural empyema, and signs and symptoms due to pressure from subdural effusion.
If subdural effusion sterile and clinical symptoms unchanged do not retap
Hemi or Quadriparesis
Perform CT Scan if either present. Consult neurologist.
Deafness
Consult otolaryngologist for hearing and speech diagnosis. Follow-up as indicated.
Ataxia
Consult neurologist and/or ENT
Determine if associated with deafness to assess association with CN VIII vs. vestibular damage.
Prolonged Fever
Patient otherwise improving - continue to follow
Patient unimproved - (1) perform complete P/E to search for other sources of fever, e.g. pericardial effusion, joint effusion; (2) repeat LP
Other diagnostic tests as needed
Reoccurrence of Fever after Afebrile Period
If patient otherwise improving, check for intercurrent URI or other viral infections
Exclude loculated pyogenic disease extrinsic to CNS
Exclude thrombophlebitis
Drug fever rare, but should be considered
If patient unimproved, same as above but consider LP
Visual Disturbance
Consult Ophthalmologist
Hydrocephalus
Extremely rare. If suspected, perform CT Scan and consult neurosurgeon

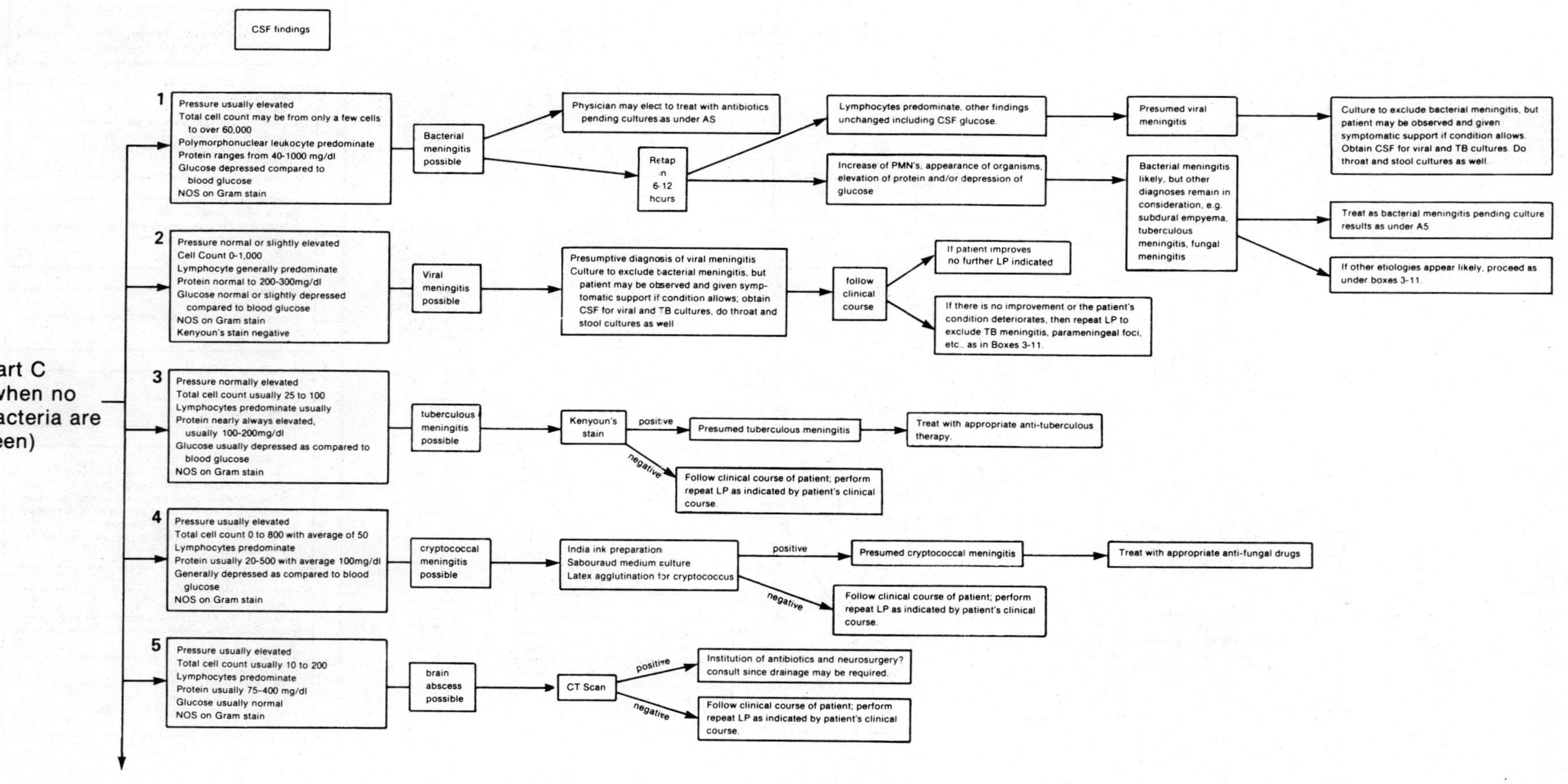
Part C (when no bacteria are seen)
CSF findings
1
Pressure usually elevated
Total cell count may be from only a few cells to over 60,000
Polymorphonuclear leukocyte predominate
Protein ranges from 40-1000 mg/dl
Glucose depressed compared to blood glucose
NOS on Gram stain
Bacterial meningitis possible
Physician may elect to treat with antibiotics pending cultures as under AS
Retap in 6-12 hours
Lymphocytes predominate, other findings unchanged including CSF glucose.
Presumed viral meningitis
Culture to exclude bacterial meningitis, but patient may be observed and given symptomatic support if condition allows. Obtain CSF for viral and TB cultures. Do throat and stool cultures as well.
Increase of PMN's, appearance of organisms, elevation of protein and/or depression of glucose
Bacterial meningitis likely, but other diagnoses remain in consideration, e.g. subdural empyema, tuberculous meningitis, fungal meningitis
Treat as bacterial meningitis pending culture results as under A5
If other etiologies appear likely, proceed as under boxes 3-11.
2
Pressure normal or slightly elevated
Cell Count 0-1,000
Lymphocyte generally predominate
Protein normal to 200-300mg/dl
Glucose normal or slightly depressed compared to blood glucose
NOS on Gram stain
Kenyoun's stain negative
Viral meningitis possible
Presumptive diagnosis of viral meningitis
Culture to exclude bacterial meningitis, but patient may be observed and given symptomatic support if condition allows; obtain CSF for viral and TB cultures, do throat and stool cultures as well
follow clinical course
If patient improves no further LP indicated
If there is no improvement or the patient's condition deteriorates, then repeat LP to exclude TB meningitis, parameningeal foci, etc., as in Boxes 3-11.
3
Pressure normally elevated
Total cell count usually 25 to 100
Lymphocytes predominate usually
Protein nearly always elevated, usually 100-200mg/dl
Glucose usually depressed as compared to blood glucose
NOS on Gram stain
tuberculous meningitis possible
Kenyoun's stain
positive
Presumed tuberculous meningitis
Treat with appropriate anti-tuberculous therapy.
negative
Follow clinical course of patient; perform repeat LP as indicated by patient's clinical course.
4
Pressure usually elevated
Total cell count 0 to 800 with average of 50
Lymphocytes predominate
Protein usually 20-500 with average 100mg/dl
Generally depressed as compared to blood glucose
NOS on Gram stain
cryptococcal meningitis possible
India ink preparation
Sabouraud medium culture
Latex agglutination for cryptococcus
positive
Presumed cryptococcal meningitis
Treat with appropriate anti-fungal drugs
negative
Follow clinical course of patient; perform repeat LP as indicated by patient's clinical course.
5
Pressure usually elevated
Total cell count usually 10 to 200
Lymphocytes predominate
Protein usually 75-400 mg/dl
Glucose usually normal
NOS on Gram stain
brain abscess possible
CT Scan
positive
Institution of antibiotics and neurosurgery? consult since drainage may be required.
negative
Follow clinical course of patient; perform repeat LP as indicated by patient's clinical course.
(see 6)

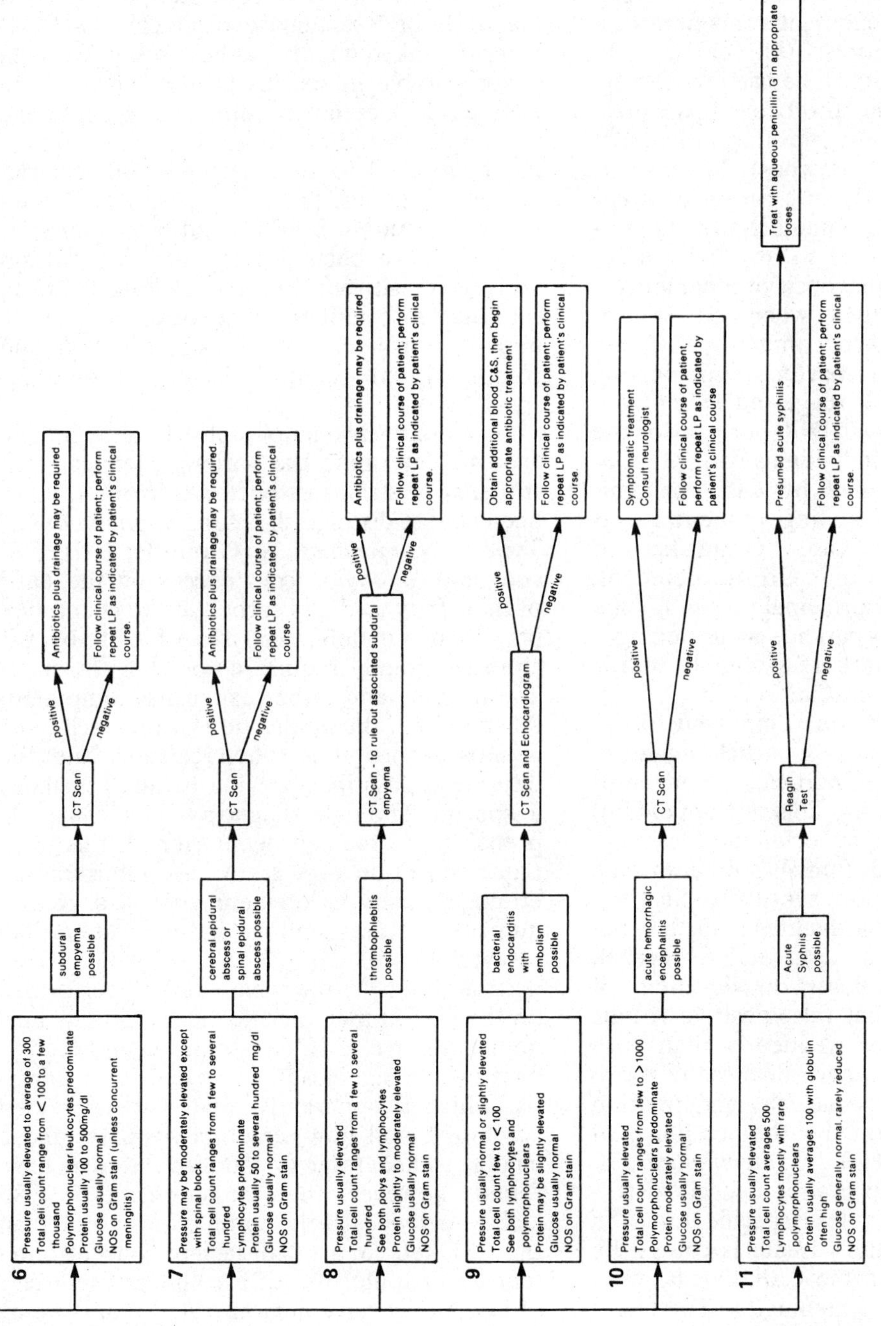
6
Pressure usually elevated to average of 300
Total cell count range from < 100 to a few thousand
Polymorphonuclear leukocytes predominate
Protein usually 100 to 500mg/dl
Glucose usually normal
NOS on Gram stain (unless concurrent meningitis)
subdural empyema possible
CT Scan
positive
Antibiotics plus drainage may be required
negative
Follow clinical course of patient; perform repeat LP as indicated by patient's clinical course.
7
Pressure may be moderately elevated except with spinal block
Total cell count ranges from a few to several hundred
Lymphocytes predominate
Protein usually 50 to several hundred mg/dl
Glucose usually normal
NOS on Gram stain
cerebral epidural abscess or spinal epidural abscess possible
CT Scan
positive
Antibiotics plus drainage may be required.
negative
Follow clinical course of patient; perform repeat LP as indicated by patient's clinical course.
8
Pressure usually elevated
Total cell count ranges from a few to several hundred
See both polys and lymphocytes
Protein slightly to moderately elevated
Glucose usually normal
NOS on Gram stain
thrombophlebitis possible
CT Scan - to rule out associated subdural empyema
positive
Antibiotics plus drainage may be required
negative
Follow clinical course of patient; perform repeat LP as indicated by patient's clinical course.
9
Pressure usually normal or slightly elevated
Total cell count few to < 100
See both lymphocytes and polymorphonuclears
Protein may be slightly elevated
Glucose usually normal
NOS on Gram stain
bacterial endocarditis with embolism possible
CT Scan and Echocardiogram
positive
Obtain additional blood C&S, then begin appropriate antibiotic treatment
negative
Follow clinical course of patient; perform repeat LP as indicated by patient's clinical course.
10
Pressure usually elevated
Total cell count ranges from few to > 1000
Polymorphonuclears predominate
Protein moderately elevated
Glucose usually normal
NOS on Gram stain
acute hemorrhagic encephalitis possible
CT Scan
positive
Symptomatic treatment
Consult neurologist
negative
Follow clinical course of patient, perform repeat LP as indicated by patient's clinical course
11
Pressure usually elevated
Total cell count averages 500
Lymphocytes mostly with rare polymorphonuclears
Protein usually averages 100 with globulin often high
Glucose generally normal, rarely reduced
NOS on Gram stain
Acute Syphilis possible
Reagin Test
positive
Presumed acute syphilis
Treat with aqueous penicillin G in appropriate doses
negative
Follow clinical course of patient; perform repeat LP as indicated by patient's clinical course.

A variety of techniques have been employed that may aid in establishing a specific diagnosis of bacterial meningitis more rapidly than isolation by the usual culture techniques. In addition, prior antibiotic therapy does not interfere with the results of the newer rapid diagnostic tests.

One of the most useful techniques for rapid diagnosis of bacterial meningitis is countercurrent immunoelectrophoresis (CIE). The technique is very specific; it can be used to identify bacteria, viruses, and protozoan parasites. Antisera directed against capsular antigens of HITB, *S. pneumoniae* (84 types), *N. meningitidis* (Groups A, C, D), and Group B *Streptococcus* are available commercially. Generally, CIE can be applied to any body fluid, The specific etiologic diagnosis of meningitis is established most effectively when CSF, serum, and urine are screened concomitantly.[52] In one prospective study of bacterial meningitis, Gram stain of the CSF suggested *H. influenzae,* Type b meningitis in 84.6 per cent of the patients. In the same individuals, CSF, blood, and urine were screened by CIE concomitantly; the diagnosis of meningitis due to HITB was established in every case.[23] Gram stains of CSF are more sensitive than CIE for detection of *N. meningitidis;* the principal reason for the poor results of CIE in patients with meningococcal disease is the lack of a reliable source of group B meningococcal antisera.[52]

Another useful technique employed to detect microorganisms is latex particle agglutination. In this test, latex particles absorb antisera for specific antigens. This test appears to be a sensitive and specific technique for detection of bacterial and fungal polysaccharide antigens and is even more sensitive than CIE. However, there are disadvantages in that the test must be repeated sequentially for each antigen sought. In addition, the sensitivity of the test is so great that false-positive results are encountered more frequently than with CIE. We believe that wherever these tests are available, CIE or latex particle agglutination tests should be performed if the possibility of disease caused by HITB, *N. meningitidis, S. pneumoniae,* or Group B streptococci exists.

The limulus test (a less specific test), in which gelation of limulus lysate is caused by endotoxin produced in the CSF, can be used to detect gram-negative meningitis. The test is rapid, sensitive, and reliable for detection of endotoxin in both untreated and partially treated patients with gram-negative bacterial meningitis but is unable to distinguish among the gram-negative organisms. Generally, it is believed that the *Limulus* lysate assay offers little diagnostic help.[53]

An enzyme radioisotopic assay (ERIA) has been developed to measure the activity of β-lactamase, an enzyme produced by many pathogenic bacteria.[54] Though not generally available, this assay offers potential for rapid diagnosis of β-lactamase producing bacteria. Enzyme-linked immunosorbent assay (ELISA) is comparable in sensitivity and specificity to ERIA but does not require use of expensive equipment or radioisotopes. ELISA technique has been used for the detection of bacteria, viruses, fungi, and protozoan parasites. Assays for the detection of HITB and *S. pneumoniae* antigens have been developed. These assays are very sensitive but require as long as five to six hours to complete (compared with 5 to 30 minutes for latex particle agglutination and countercurrent immunoelectrophoresis, respectively).

Gas-liquid chromatography is a technique used to determine the various chemical constituents of strains of bacteria. Workers have been able to distinguish among *S. pneumoniae,* Type 3, *N. meningitidis,* Group B, HIBT, *E. coli,* and *Staphylococcus aureus* on the basis of their fatty acid and carbohydrate chemotyping. Unfortunately, analyses of CSF by gas chromatography require a very lengthy preparation time and rather expensive equipment. At this time, the application of this technique is most appropriate when cultures and the other tests described previously fail to establish a specific etiologic diagnosis. If the sample preparation time can be shortened, this technique would be very useful in establishing an etiologic diagnosis of meningitis in a greater number of cases and in settings other than research.[53]

In addition to the usual studies performed on the CSF, other specific measurements may be informative. CSF lactate has been noted to be elevated significantly in bacterial meningitis, which is apparently related to decreased cerebral blood flow, cerebral hypoxia, and a change to anaerobic metabolism. Studies have found, however, that measurement of CSF lactate provides little more information than the CSF cell count; CSF lactate concentration tends to parallel the CSF cellular response.[55] Other studies have demonstrated that in some individuals with aseptic meningitis, the CSF lactate concentration was within the range reported for patients with bacterial meningitis. Thus, determination of CSF lactate cannot be used to reliably differentiate viral from bacterial meningitis in the individual patient.[56] Depression of CSF pH also has been reported in patients with bacterial meningitis; it is more transient than the elevation of CSF lactate and, therefore, it less valuable in differential diagnoses.[15]

Lactic dehydrogenase (LDH), glutamic oxalacetic transaminase, and creatine phosphokinase may be elevated in patients with bacterial meningitis. Total LDH activity within CSF may be similar in patients with bacterial and aseptic meningitis. LDH isoenzyme analysis may permit differentiation of viral from bacterial meningitis, but this procedure is cumbersome, is time-consuming, and does not permit a specific etiologic diagnosis.[52, 57]

Despite the availability of all of these methods, situations arise in which differentiation of bacterial from aseptic meningitis remains problematic. In these cases, usually a predominance of polymorphonuclear leukocytes is found in the CSF, the CSF cell count is less than 1000 cells/mm^3, the CSF glucose level is normal or nearly so, and the Gram stain result is negative. In addition, the patient who exhibits some of the signs and symptoms of meningitis does not appear acutely ill. Some investigators have suggested withholding antibiotic therapy in these individuals, and repeating the LP after 6 to 12 hours of close clinical observation. This course of action is *not* recommended if the patient has been pre-treated with antibiotics. The repeated LP usually will either substantiate the impression of aseptic meningitis (a shift to a lymphocytic differential will be noted) or point more conclusively to a bacterial process.[58, 59]

Tuberculous meningitis patients may present with signs and symptoms similar to those seen in almost any meningeal process. LP generally will reveal less than 1000 cells/mm^3 with a predominance of lymphocytes. Early in the course of tuberculous meningitis, however, polymorphonuclear leukocytes may predominate. CSF protein may be elevated with CSF to blood glucose ratio reduced. Gram stain results are negative. Kenyoun stain may be positive in selected cases. A definitive diagnosis is established by culturing *Mycobacterium tuberculosis* from the CSF. A diagnosis of tuberculous meningitis may be considered more likely if no bacteria grow on routine culture after 72 hours. the clinical condition of the patient continues to deteriorate, and repeated LP shows a predominance of lymphocytes with a CSF protein concentration that is greater than that noted following the original LP. A CSF glucose concentration is lower than that in the first LP sample.

Partial Treatment of Meningitis

Many children who are suspected of having bacterial meningitis have received antimicrobial therapy before a definitive diagnosis has been established. Generally, one dose to several days of oral antibiotic therapy does not reduce markedly the percentage of culture-positive CSF specimens (93 to 97 per cent in one study),[60] nor alter significantly other CSF findings.[51, 61] Pre-treatment may render the CSF sterile in patients with pneumococcal or meningococcal meningitis but rarely affects CSF culture results in patients with *H. influenzae* meningitis. In addition, since the advent of rapid diagnostic techniques that detect antigen rather than viable bacteria, identification of the microorganism may be established even when the culture fails to grow.

Recurrent episodes of bacterial meningitis are encountered most often in patients who have anatomic defects involving the CNS or who have immunologic deficiency states. Any patient who has multiple episodes of meningitis may be treated initially as one with a new episode of meningitis, but CNS and immunologic abnormalities should be sought.

TREATMENT

The management of acute bacterial meningitis in patients one month to 18 years of age includes the provision of appropriate antibiotic therapy in sufficiently high dosage to maintain effective CSF concentrations, and specific measures designed to reverse systemic and neurologic complications.

Prompt administration of antibiotics to the patient with suspected meningitis is essential. The choice of antibiotic depends on the causative organism, but one should never wait for culture results before initiating therapy. Generally, treatment is started empirically with intravenous ampicillin at a dose of 300 mg/kg/day in six divided doses; an initial bolus of 100 mg/kg is given. Intravenous chloramphenicol also is given in a dose of 100 mg/kg/day in four divided doses. These antibiotics will provide effective treatment for most of the organisms most commonly causing bacterial meningitis.

(e.g., *Streptococcus pneumoniae, N. meningitidis,* and most strains of *H. influenzae*).

The use of both ampicillin and chloramphenicol initially is required, since strains of HITB that are resistant to ampicillin but sensitive to chloramphenicol (28% in some areas) have been encountered in every state. Selected strains of *H. influenzae* are resistant to chloramphenicol, but these strains usually remain sensitive to ampicillin. Recently, strains of *H. influenzae* resistant to both ampicillin and chloramphenicol have been detected. Fortunately, these organisms are sensitive to newer antimicrobials that have been developed (e.g., moxalactam, cefotaxime). Moxalactam can be provided in a dose of 200 mg/kg/day in four divided doses, intravenously. A loading dose of 75 mg/kg may be provided. Pneumococci resistant to penicillin are encountered infrequently.

After culture results are known, antibiotic therapy can be altered accordingly. If the organism is HITB and resistant to ampicillin (always resistant if it produces β-lactamase, but sometimes resistant even when it doesn't), the chlorampenicol is continued and ampicillin is discontinued. When *H. influenzae* is susceptible to ampicillin, chloramphenicol is discontinued. In the rare cases of resistance to both ampicillin and chloramphenicol, moxalactam provides effective therapy.

Moxalactam is a β-lactamase antibiotic that has been evaluated recently. *In vitro* strudies suggested that moxalactam would be effective in killing all isolates of *H. influenzae,* including those resistant to ampicillin and chloramphenicol. Studies in children have shown that moxalactam penetrates the CSF readily.[62] An ongoing prospective study to evaluate moxalactam further has shown that a daily dose of 200 mg/kg/day in four divided doses is effective therapy for *H. influenzae* meningitis.

Cefotaxime also has been shown to be effective against *H. influenzae* and other gram-negative organisms *in vitro* and *in vivo.* This drug has been approved for use and it may be helpful when organisms are resistant to conventional therapy. Ceftriaxone also possesses a broad spectrum of activity. Its use has been followed by rapid sterilization of the CSF in patients with both gram-negative and gram-positive meningitis. This drug has not been approved for use in treating meningitis at this time.

When meningitis is caused by pneumococci, tube dilution sensitivity tests must be performed; these organisms no longer are susceptible uniformly to penicillin. Some pneumococci are sensitive to penicillin only in concentrations of 0.1-1 units/ml. If this is the case, the dosage of penicillin should be increased to 500,000 units/kg/day, intravenously, and given in six divided doses. If the organism is resistant to penicillin but sensitive to chloramphenicol, chloramphenicol would be the treatment of choice. Most recently, multiply resistant pneumococci have been implicated as a cause of disease in various parts of the United States; they originally were identified as a cause of disease in South Africa. These organisms have retained their sensitivity to vancomycin, which should be given in a dose of 50 mg/kg/day, intravenously, in four divided doses.[63] To date, all strains of *N. meningitidis* have been sensitive to penicillin. In patients with meningitis due to this organism, ampicillin can be continued alone, or aqueous penicillin G at a dose of 300,000 units/kg/day in six divided doses, intravenously, may be substituted.

If the meningitis is due to *Streptococcus pyogenes,* ampicillin alone is effective. When meningitis is caused by *S. aureus* (generally resistant to penicillin), oxacillin, methicillin, or nafcillin at 200 mg/kg/day, intravenously, in six divided doses should be used. Meningitis due to other organisms is less frequent.

Recommendations for antibiotic therapy of meningitis caused by various microorganisms are provided in Table 2–1.

Generally, all antibiotics given to a child with meningitis should be given intravenously. Some investigators have advocated the use of oral chloramphenicol following several days of intravenous therapy because studies have shown that comparable plasma levels of chloramphenicol are obtained with the oral and the intravenous preparations.[64] The controversy concerning this approach is related not to lack of efficacy or oral therapy but rather to the possibility that the risk of idiosyncratic bone marrow arrest is more common following use of the oral palmitate preparation. This concept has been challenged recently; several cases of aplastic anemia associated with use of intravenous chloramphenicol have been reported.[65] There have been no prospective studies comparing the efficacy of oral and intravenous chloramphenicol therapy for bacterial meningitis, particularly with regard to long-term sequelae. Oral chloramphenicol (in the same doses as the intravenous form) can be used for an in-patient (to ensure compliance), and to treat a serious infection when administration

Table 2–1. CURRENT RECOMMENDATIONS FOR ANTIBIOTIC THERAPY

Organism	Antibiotic	Recommended Dosage
Bacteroides fragilis	Chloramphenicol Metronidazole	100 mg/kg/day in 4 dd Not established
Bacteroides, other than *B. fragilis*	Penicillin G	300,000 units/kg/day in 6 dd
Clostridium	Penicillin G	300,000 units/kg/day in 6 dd
Corynebacterium	Penicillin G Erythromycin	300,000 units/kg/day in 6 dd 50 mg/kg/day in 4 dd
Enterobacter	Gentamicin Carbenicillin Cefotaxime Moxalactam	7.5 mg/kg/day in 3 dd 600 mg/kg/day in 6 dd Not established (150 mg/kg in 4 dd has been used) 200 mg/kg/day in 4 dd
Escherichia coli	Ampicillin Gentamicin Kanamycin Moxalactam Cefotaxime	300 mg/kg/day in 6 dd 7.5 mg/kg/day in 3 dd 15–30 mg/kg/day in 3 dd 200 mg/kg/day in 4 dd Not established (150 mg/kg in 4 dd has been used)
Haemophilus influenzae	Ampicillin Chloramphenicol Moxalactam	300 mg/kg/day in 6 dd 100 mg/kg/day in 4 dd 200 mg/kg/day in 4 dd
Klebsiella	Gentamicin Kanamycin	7.5 mg/kg/day in 3 dd 15–30 mg/kg/day in 3 dd
Listeria monocytogenes	Ampicillin Gentamicin Kanamycin	300 mg/kg/day in 6 dd 7.5 mg/kg/day in 3 dd 15–30 mg/kg/day in 3 dd
Neisseria meningitidis	Penicillin G	300,000 units/kg/day in 6 dd
N. gonorrhoeae	Penicillin G	300,000 units/kg/day in 6 dd
Proteus mirabilis Indole-negative	Ampicillin	300 mg/kg/day in 6 dd
P. mirabilis Indole-positive	Gentamicin Kanamycin Carbenicillin	7.5 mg/kg/day in 3 dd 15–30 mg/kg/day in 3 dd 600 mg/kg/day in 6 dd
Pseudomonas	Gentamicin Carbenicillin Amikacin Cefotaxime	7.5 mg/kg/day in 3 dd 600 mg/kg/day in 6 dd 15 mg/kg/day in 3 dd Not established (150 mg/kg in 4 dd has been used)
Salmonella	Ampicillin Gentamicin Chloramphenicol	300 mg/kg/day in 6 dd 7.5 mg/kg/day in 3 dd 100 mg/kg/day in 4 dd
Staphylococci Penicillinase-negative	Penicillin G	300,000 units/kg/day in 6 dd
Staphylococci Penicillinase-positive	Methicillin, nafcillin, or oxacillin	200 mg/kg/day in 6 dd
Streptococcus pneumoniae	Penicillin G Chloramphenicol Vancomycin	300,000 units/kg/day in 6 dd 100 mg/kg/day in 4 dd 50 mg/kg/day in 4 dd
Unknown	Ampicillin and chloramphenicol (both drugs) Methicillin (or nafcillin) if question of staphylococcal infection Gentamicin if question of *Pseudomonas*	300 mg/kg/day in 6 dd 100 mg/kg/day in 4 dd 200 mg/kg/day in 6 dd 7.5 mg/kg/day in 3 dd

of the intravenous form is impossible. We generally do not advocate its broad use at this time.

When patients with suspected or proven meningitis have a significant allergy to penicillin (urticaria, exfoliative dermatitis, anaphylaxis), then chloramphenicol should be administered alone. If the organism proves to be *S. aureus,* vancomycin may be preferable.[51]

The appropriate antibiotic should be continued intravenously until the patient has been afebrile for at least five days; however, the total treatment period must be a minimum of ten days; in instances of meningitis due to *N. meningitidis,* therapy for seven days may be adequate.

If clinical improvement is noted and the child has an uneventful course, *repeated LP is not necessary*. If improvement is not noted, or if clinical deterioration occurs, repeated LP is indicated.

There is controversy regarding the performance of a spinal tap at the completion of antimicrobial therapy. Some clinicians advocated repeating LP at completion of therapy to document bacterologic sterility of the CSF.[51] Other investigators have reviewed the results of CSF examinations in individuals who later had recurrent or recrudescent meningitis and who had repeated examination of CSF at the conclusion of therapy. The investigators found that this routine procedure did not permit the prediction of relapse of meningitis.[66, 67] In the study of Schaad and coworkers,[66] however, repeated LP was performed to document sterilization of CSF during the course of therapy. We favor the use of repeated LP at the conclusion of treatment to document sterility, but it is not mandatory. Re-treatment is mandatory if cultures are not sterile and may be suggested if more than ten per cent of the cells found within CSF at the conclusion of therapy are polymorphonuclear leukocytes.[51]

HITB has been recovered from the throats of patients following completion of a course of treatment for meningitis caused by this organism. For this reason, when children 4 years of age or less are members of the household to which the patient will return, the patient should be given rifampin, 20 mg/kg once daily for four days, to prevent potential secondary cases.

Supportive Care

Although administration of appropriate antibiotics is a mainstay of therapy, supportive care given to the patient with bacterial meningitis, especially during the first 48 hours of the illness, must be meticulous. Blood pressure, pulse, and respiratory rate should be measured as often as necessary initially, sometimes every 15 minutes, until the patient is stable. Subsequently, vital signs may be followed less frequently (every 4 hours). Temperature should be measured rectally every four hours.

Neurologic examination is performed upon initial assessment and it should be repeated often. Complete neurologic examinations daily with frequent brief assessments several times each day during the first several days of therapy are indicated.

In addition to the routine and neurologic vital signs that must be assessed immediately, the following laboratory data are suggested for children if results of the LP suggest bacterial meningitis: total peripheral WBC count and differential, hemoglobin concentration, hematocrit value, and platelet count. Body weight should be measured carefully. Serum electrolyte levels, serum and urine osmolalities, urine volume and urine specific gravity should be obtained (to be discussed).

Anemia associated with *H. influenzae,* Type b septicemia due to immune hemolysis of red blood cells (RBCs) that are coated with soluble bacterial antigens has been reported recently.[68] Shurin and Anderson[68] found an abrupt decline in hemoglobin concentration in 17 of 19 children within three days of admission for *H. influenzae,* Type b septicemia. Following a detailed investigation, they concluded that the anemia related to *H. influenzae,* Type b septicemia was a result of injury to RBCs by interaction of adsorbed soluble bacterial antigens with host immune mechanisms whose function is to ensure bacterial clearance.

Generally, intravenous fluids only should be provided for the first 48 hours. Aspiration is best avoided if the child does not vomit, and fluid balance can be documented more accurately. A multiple electrolyte solution (e.g., Isolyte/M or ME–75) may be given at an appropriate rate intravenously.

The syndrome of inappropriate secretion of antidiuretic hormone (SIADH) is a frequent concomitant of bacterial meningitis. The effect of SIADH can be avoided most readily by proper management. If hyponatremia and concomitant serum hypo-osmolality are noted in a patient who is receiving appropriate quantities of fluid intravenously or orally, SIADH is suggested. If moderate or severe hypo-osmolality exists, and the urine is not maximally dilute or the osmolality is not less than that of a serum specimen obtained simultaneously, ADH secretion is inappropriately elevated.[69]

In a prospective study of bacterial meningitis, 88 per cent of the children enrolled had documented SIADH (unpublished data).[51] When SIADH is suspected or confirmed, fluids should be restricted to 800 to 1000 ml/m^2/day. This restriction should be continued until it can be proven that either SIADH is not a factor or, if it is present, that the effect of inappropriate ADH secretion has dissipated. The most reliable indications of fluid retention in excess of solute are body weight and serum sodium level; therefore, these measurements, as well as serum electrolyte levels, serum and urine osmolalities, urine volume, and urine specific gravity should be obtained initially and every 12 hours for the first 48 hours. As the serum sodium level approaches normal (140 mEq/L), fluid administration may be liberalized to normal maintenance rates of 1500 to 1700 ml/m^2/day.[51]

A special problem arises when a child with bacterial meningitis also is hypotensive. Sufficient fluid to maintain adequate circulation and blood pressure is mandated, but brain swelling must be prevented. The patient should receive only those fluids sufficient to maintain the systolic blood pressure at 80 to 90 mmHg, a urine output of at least 500 ml/m^2/day, and adequate cerebral perfusion, as evidenced by an improved mental status. Dopamine and isoproterenol, or other similar agents, may be useful in increasing peripheral perfusion and blood pressure without administration of large quantities of fluid. The most osmotically active fluid should be provided (plasma, whole blood, etc.), and the smallest possible volume utilized.

A more complete discussion of septic shock and associated disseminated intravascular coagulation is found in chapter 3.

Seizures occur so frequently during the course of meningitis that prompt recognition of seizure activity is necessary. When seizures are noted, an adequate airway must be ensured. Oxygen and endotracheal intubation may be necessary. The stomach should be emptied with a nasogastric tube. Anticonvulsants should be given intravenously immediately. Phenobarbital sodium (7–10 mg/kg IV stat) may be given and repeated if the seizures are not controlled. It produces a prolonged anticonvulsant effect, but effective brain concentrations are achieved slowly (in 20–60 min); immediate cessation of seizures should not be expected.

Phenytoin (Dilantin) is effective in about 80 per cent of patients with status epilepticus. This drug penetrates the brain rapidly and stops the seizures in 5 to 30 minutes. There are two advantages to the use of phenytoin in the meningitis patient: it causes little or no sedation and it may inhibit the secretion of ADH. Phenytoin may be administered in a dose of 7–10 mg/kg, intravenously. When used, it should be infused slowly (not more rapidly than 25 to 50 mg/minute) to avoid induction of cardiac arrhythmias; electrocardiographic monitoring always should be used. Phenytoin never should be given intramuscularly; absorption is erratic and unpredictable.[70]

If seizures remain uncontrolled, a bolus of intravenous diazepam (1 mg/kg/year of age to a maximum of 10 mg) can be used. The anticonvulsant effect of diazepam is short-lived; thus, it must be used with a second anticonvulsant to achieve a sustained effect. Diazepam can produce significant sedation and if used with phenobarbital can precipitate marked respiratory and cardiovascular depression.[71] After the acute seizure episode is controlled, it is preferable to maintain seizure control with daily phenytoin (5 mg/kg/day IV in 2 divided doses). If seizure activity is no longer noted after the second hospital day, and there are no focal neurologic signs at the time of discharge from the hospital, anticonvulsants may be discontinued. It is important to note that both phenytoin and phenobarbital can induce hepatic microsomal enzymes; their use may increase the rate of chloramphenicol metabolism, possibly significantly lowering the serum concentration of chloramphenicol.[72] Therefore, monitoring the serum concentration of chloramphenicol is suggested when these anticonvulsants are administered.

It is not necessary to perform an electroencephalogram (EEG) in all patients who have seizures with meningitis. However, there are many situations in which an EEG is indicated. They include the presence of focal seizures, seizures that persist longer than 72 hours after hospitalization, and seizures that first occur within 72 hours in the hospital. If there is a subdural effusion or prolonged alteration of sensorium, an EEG also may be important. An EEG also may be of value in distinguishing abnormal intermittent posturing from the movements associated with seizure activity.

Subdural effusions should be sought routinely and may be suspected when the infant has vomiting, persistent fever, distended head veins, full fontanelles, and enlarging head size. The head circumference should be measured at the time of admission, and similar measurements should be repeated daily. Transillumination of the head should be performed on the same schedule. If a subdural effusion is noted or suspected, generally, no treatment is required. When a patient has persistent fever, or signs of increased intracranial pressure, or is suspected of having effusions that may be responsible for seizure activity or focal neurologic signs, a subdural paracentesis should be performed. If the effusion is sterile, and the clinical symptoms remain unchanged, no further taps are needed.[51] In our own large prospective study of bacterial meningitis performed to date, subdural effusion has been noted in 138 of 256 children studied; subdural empyema was only found in one patient (unpublished data). CAT scannings may be helpful in detecting large subdural effusions or hydrocephalus. In children with hemi- or quadriparesis, a CAT scan may document cerebrovascular abnormalities. A CAT scan should be obtained in children with papilledema or on an emergency basis before proceeding with the initial LP.

In some children, persistent fever (lasting longer than the eighth day of illness) may be noted.[73] Fever of this type frequently is related to an intercurrent nosocomial, usually viral, infection. Suppurative complications, however, including septic arthritis, subdural or pleural empyema, and pericarditis should be sought carefully. Fever also may be due to thrombophlebitis or may be related to the severity of the disease process. "Drug fever" is often cited but rarely is the cause of prolonged fever and is a diagnosis of exclusion. Repeated LP to exclude a poor therapeutic response must be considered on a case by case basis.

SEQUELAE AND PROGNOSIS

The outcome of meningitis depends primarily on six factors: (1) the nature of the infectious agent and severity of the initial process, (2) the age of the patient, (3) the duration of symptoms before diagnosis and institution of intensive antibiotic therapy, (4) the number of organisms or quantity of capsular polysaccharide material present within the meninges and CSF at the time of diagnosis, (5) the presence of disorders that may compromise host response to infection, and (6) the type and amount of antibiotic used.[15, 51] The younger the patient and the greater the antigenic load at the time of admission, the worse the prognosis.

Although antibiotic therapy has reduced the mortality rate for all forms of bacterial meningitis, sequelae are still encountered in as many as 50 per cent of survivors. Specific sequelae of bacterial meningitis include the following: deafness, blindness, hemiparesis, quadriparesis, muscular hypertonia, ataxia, permanent seizure disorders, mental retardation, learning disabilities, and the development of obstructive hydrocephalus.[51]

The most common, significant persistent sequela of bacterial meningntis is impairment of hearing. In one prospective study, impairment of hearing determined by an audiologic evaluation with abnormal results was noted in 25 per cent of children who had had bacterial meningitis.[74] More severe hearing impairment that interfered with development of normal speech was found less frequently. The incidence of hearing loss and major hearing handicaps varied with the organism causing meningitis; nine per cent of children who had *H. influenzae* meningitis had hearing handicaps, whereas 33 per cent of children with meningitis due to *Streptococcus pneumoniae* had impairment of auditory activity. There was no correlation between loss of hearing and either the age of the patient at the onset of meningitis or duration of illness prior to admission. There was a significant correlation of hearing loss with the presence of seizures prior to admission, the duration of fever in the hospital after therapy had been initiated, a positive identification of an organism in the CSF as determined by CIE, and a depressed ratio of CSF to blood glucose at the time of admission. Hearing loss frequently is already present at the time when children with bacterial meningitis are admitted to the hospital.[74] Early diagnosis and treatment will not invariably prevent this disability.

In another prospective study, a small group of children with postmeningitis ataxia were studied with detailed neurologic, audiologic, and neurovestibular evaluations; severe to profound sensorineural hearing losses were present in the majority of these children.[29] Generally, the ataxia persisted, but steady improvement was observed in all the children.[29] Since hearing deficits are so common in patients with bacterial meningitis, hearing evaluation, utilizing evoked response audiometry when necessary, is recommended strongly at the time of or shortly after discharge from the hospital. Repeated audiometric evaluation is recommended after discharge if the initial examination results were abnormal. It is important to distinguish hearing deficits due to conductive disturbance from those related to damage to the eighth cranial nerve. Some children who have had repeated episodes of otitis media may experience conductive loss unrelated to the meningitis.

In one prospective study, neurologic sequelae were reported in 38.7 per cent of children with bacterial meningitis at the time of discharge.[51] Specific deficits were noted in only 9.1 per cent of this same group of children two years after hospital discharge. Hemiparesis or quadriparesis was noted in eight per cent of children initially, but one year later these significant deficits were detected in only two per cent of the group.[51]

Intelligence quotients (IQs) of postmeningitic children were studied and compared with control children of the same age and with the closest in age of patients with meningitis. No significant differences in mean IQ were observed. A significantly greater proportion of children who recovered from meningitis, however, had IQs less than 80 than did children from control groups.[51]

Retrospective reviews by workers who have evaluated sequelae of bacterial meningitis reveal the same type of sequelae. The frequency with which each deficit has been reported varies somewhat from study to study.[75–78]

Prospective studies have facilitated assessment of factors present at the time of admission that are predictive of sequelae of meningitis. Evidence of SIADH correlated significantly ($P < 0.0001$) with abnormal neurologic examinations three months after discharge and with poor psychometric performance ($P < 0.01$). Focal neurologic findings detected at the time of admission were shown to be a most reliable predictor of permanent sequelae of bacterial meningitis, including poor psychometric performance ($P < 0.001$).[51]

PROPHYLAXIS

Haemophilus influenzae

The Report of the Committee on Infectious Diseases of the American Academy of Pediatrics states that prophylaxis is indicated for adults and children less than 4 years old who are household and day care center contacts of children with *H. influenzae* disease.[79] A recent re-evaluation of the available data has resulted in a modification of the recommendation with regard to day care centers. The newest recommendation suggests that prophylaxis is not required for day care center contacts unless two or more cases of *H. influenzae* have occurred within the day care center. Antimicrobials effective in treating invasive disease often are ineffective in eliminating the carrier state. Ampicillin, erythromycin-sulfisoxazole, cefaclor, and trimethoprim-sulfamethoxazole all have been shown to be ineffective in eliminating *H. influenzae* from the pharynx.[80] Although rifampin-resistant strains of *H. influenzae* have been reported, they are rare; thus, rifampin is the agent of choice. Rifampin should be given in a dose of 20 mg/kg/day, orally, once daily for four days.

The recommendations are somewhat controversial. Only one prospective study with placebo controls has been performed in an attempt to determine whether rifampin can prevent the spread of *H. influenzae,* Type b disease.[81] This study was coordinated by Band[81] at the CDC in Atlanta, Georgia. A multi-center, prospective, placebo-controlled trial among household and day care center contacts of persons with invasive *H. influenzae,* Type b disease was conducted. A total of 1356 household members and 584 day care classmates of 325 index patients were enrolled. Pretreatment *H. influenzae,* Type b carriage rates were similar in the treatment groups. Four of 839 placebo-treated contacts developed secondary disease, whereas none of the 1101 rifampin-treated contacts developed disease, a difference significant at $P = 0.03$. The investigators concluded that prophylaxis of close contacts with rifampin in households or day care centers with at least one individual at risk (< 6 years of age) can significantly reduce the risk of secondary *H. influenzae,* Type b disease.

Several concerns have been expressed since these data first were presented in November of 1981. To date, the details of this report have not been published nor subjected to critical peer review. During the course of the trial, several groups who had agreed to participate during its initial phases withdrew from the study. In addition, the dose of rifampin recommended for prophylaxis was changed during the time that the study was carried out from 10 mg/kg given twice a day to 20 mg/kg given once a day. Rifampin provided in a dose of 20 mg/kg/day has proved more effective in eradicating *H. influenzae* carriage than a 10 mg/kg regimen. These methodologic problems notwithstanding, it also should be noted that if one placebo-treated patient who developed disease was moved to the rifampin-treated group, the study would lose its statistical significance. All of these factors have contributed to the controversy among infectious disease experts concerning the merits of rifampin prophylaxis for household and day care center contacts of children with *H. influenzae* invasive disease.

Nevertheless, most authorities agree that rifampin prophylaxis will diminish the number of secondary cases to some extent. It should be emphasized that it would be advantageous for physicians to follow the present recommendation put forth by the Committee on Infectious Diseases of the American Academy of Pediatrics.[79] It must be emphasized, however, that the parents of children who have been in intimate contact with a patient who has invasive *H. influenzae* infection should be requested to bring their child to the attention of a physician if any symptoms whatsoever become apparent, irrespective of whether or not rifampin prophylaxis has been prescribed.

Neisseria meningitidis

Most authorities advocate the use of chemoprophylaxis for all household contacts of a patient with meningococcal meningitis and for all day care center contacts. It usually is not necessary to give prophylactic medication to schoolroom classmates or hospital contacts. Rifampin is the drug of choice for prophylaxis unless the strain causing the disease in the index patient is known to be susceptible to the sulfonamides. Rifampin should be given in a dosage of 600 mg twice daily for four doses in adults, and of 10 mg/kg twice daily for four doses in children between 1 and 12 years of age. For infants 3 to 12 months old, the dosage is 5 mg/kg twice daily for four doses.[82] The index case also should receive rifampin because therapy of invasive disease does not invariably eradicate nasopharyngeal carriage of *N. meningitidis*.

PREVENTION

Haemophilus influenzae

Administration of *H. influenzae,* Type b capsular polysaccharide has been followed by a long-lasting serum antibody response in patients over 18 months of age. In individuals at greatest risk of disease (< 18 months of age), however, the response has been relatively poor. These data suggest the need for preparation of better vaccines designed to improve immunogenic responses in children less than 18 months of age. The efficacy of this approach remains in doubt; only a small number of children who acquire *H. influenzae* meningitis during the first 15 months of life develop anticapsular antibody following recovery from naturally acquired invasive diseases.[51]

Neisseria meningitidis

Four meningococcal polysaccharide vaccines are licensed in the United States for use on a selective basis: monovalent Group A, monovalent Group C, bivalent Groups A and C, and quadrivalent Groups A, C, Y and W–135. Group A vaccine is effective in children 3 months of age and older. Group C vaccine is effective in children 2 years of age and older. Vaccine may be used as an adjunct to chemoprophylaxis in members of households and day care centers where outbreaks of disease have occurred caused by these serotypes. Military recruits currently receive bivalent A/C or quadrivalent A, C, Y and W–135 vaccine routinely.[82]

REFERENCES

1. Feigin RD, Dodge PR. Bacterial meningitis: newer concepts of pathophysiology and neurologic sequelae. Pediatr Clin North Am 1976; *23*:541–556.
2. Feigin RD, Dodge PR. Bacterial and fungal infections of the Central Nervous System. *In:* Tower DB, ed. The Nervous System, vol. 2: The Clinical Neurosciences. New York: Raven Press, 1975:89–104.
3. Finland M, Barnes MW. Acute bacterial meningitis at Boston City Hospital during 12 selected years—1935–1972. J Infect Dis 1977; *136*:400–415.
4. Fraser DW, Henke CE, Feldman, RA. Changing patterns of bacterial meningitis in Olmstead County, Minnesota 1935–1970. J Infect Dis 1973; *128*:300–307.
5. Geiseler PJ, Nelson KE, et al. Community-acquired purulent meningitis: a review of 1316 cases during the antibiotic era 1954–1976. J Infect Dis 1980; *2*:725–744.
6. Filice GA, Andrews JS Jr, Hudgins MP, et al. Spread of *Hemophilus influenzae*—secondary illness in household contacts of patients with *H. influenzae* meningitis. Am J Dis Child 1978; *132*:757–759.
7. Smith DH, Ingram DL, et al. Bacterial meningitis—a symposium. Pediatrics 1973; *52*:586–600.
8. Ward JI, Fraser DW, Baraff LN, et al. *Hemophilus influenzae* meningitis—a national study of secondary spread in household contacts. N Engl J Med 1979; *301*:122–126.
9. Mortimer EA Jr. Immunization against *Hemophilus influenzae*. Pediatrics 1973; *52*:633–635.
10. Stiehm ER, Damrosch DS. Factors in the prognosis of meningococcal infection. J Pediatr 1966; *68*: 457–467.
11. Feigin RD, Shearer WT. Opportunistic infections in

children, I–III. J Pediatr 1975; *87*:507–514, 677–694, 852–866.

12. Glode MP, Smith AL. Meningococcal Disease. *In:* Feigin RD, Cherry RD, eds. Textbook of Pediatric Infectious Diseases. Philadelphia: WB Saunders, 1981:916–928.
13. Peter G, Weigert MB, Bissel AR, et al. Meningococcal meningitis in familial deficiency of the fifth component of complement. Pediatrics 1981; *67*: 882–886.
14. Ellison RT III, Kohler PF, Curd JG, et al. Prevalence of congenital or acquired complement deficiency in patients with sporadic meningococcal disease. N Engl J Med 1983; *308*:913–916.
15. Weil ML. Infections of the Nervous System. *In:* Menkes JH, ed. Textbook of Child Neurology. Philadelphia: Lea and Febiger, 1980:276–304.
16. Feigin RD, Dodge PR. Central Nervous System Infections. *In:* Eliasson S, Prensky AL, eds. Pathophysiology of Nervous System Diseases. New York: Oxford University Press, 1974:310–333.
17. Eraklis AJ, Kevy SV, Diamond LK, et al. Hazard of overwhelming infection after splenectomy in childhood. N Engl J Med 1967; *276*:1225–1229.
18. Singer DB. Postsplenectomy Sepsis. *In:* Rosenberg HS, Bolande RP, eds. Perspectives in Pediatric Pathology. Chicago: Yearbook Medical Publishers Inc., 1973:285–311.
19. Feigin RD. Interaction of nutrition and infection: plans for future research. Am J Clin Nutr 1977; *30*:1553–1563.
20. Feigin RD, Richmond D, Hosler DW, et al. Reassessment of the role of bactericidal antibody in *Hemophilus influenzae* infection. Am J Med Sci 1971; *262*:338–346.
21. Feldman WE, Ginsburg CM, McCracken GH Jr, et al. Relation of concentrations of *Hemophilus influenzae* type b in cerebrospinal fluid to late sequelae of patients with meningitis. J Pediatr 1982; *100*: 209–212.
22. Fothergill LD, Wright J. Influenzal meningitis: the relation of age incidence to the bactericidal power of blood against the causal organism. J Immunol 1933; *24*:273–284.
23. Feigin RD, Stechenberg BW, et al. Prospective evaluation of treatment of *Hemophilus influenzae* meningitis. J Pediatr 1976; *88*:542–548.
24. McCracken GH Jr, Sarff LD. Current status and therapy of neonatal *E. coli* meningitis. Hosp Pract 1974; *9*:57–64.
25. Schoenbaum SC, Gardner P, Shillito J. Infections of cerebrospinal fluid shunts: epidemiology, clinical manifestations and therapy. J Infect Dis 1975; *131*:543–552.
26. Feigin RD, Baker CJ, et al. Epidemic meningococcal disease in an elementary school classroom. N Engl J Med 1982; *307*:1255–1257.
27. McGee ZA, Kaiser AB. Acute Meningitis. *In:* Mandell GL, Douglas RG Jr, Bennett JE, eds. Principles & Practice of Infectious Disease. New York: John Wiley & Sons, 1979:738–760.
28. Adams RD, Victor M, eds. Infections of the Nervous System (Nonviral). *In:* Principles of Neurology. New York: McGraw-Hill, 1977:618–654.
29. Kaplan SL, Goddard J, Van Kleeck M, et al. Ataxia and deafness in children due to bacterial meningitis. Pediatrics, 1981; *68*:8–13.
30. Garcia H, Kaplan SL, Feigin RD. Cerebrospinal fluid concentration of arginine vasopressin in children with bacterial meningitis. J Pediatr 1981; *98*:67–70.
31. Dodge, PR, Swartz MN. Bacterial meningitis—a review of selected aspects. II. Special neurologic problems, postmeningitic complications and clinicopathological correlations. N Engl J Med 1965; *272*:954–960, 1003–1009.
32. Bell WE, Menezes, AH. Focal suppurative diseases of the central nervous system. *In:* Kelley V, ed. Practice of Pediatrics. Philadelphia: J. B. Lippincott, Company, 1983:1–28.
33. Beller AJ, Sahar A, Praiss I, et al. Brain abscess: review of 89 cases over a period of 30 years. J Neurol Neurosurg Psychiatry 1973; *36*:757–768.
34. Brook I. Bacteriology of intracranial abscess in children. J Neurosurg 1981; *54*:484–488.
35. Samson DS, Clark K. A current review of brain abscess. Am J Med 1973; *54*:201–210.
36. Schurr P. Brain abscess in childhood. Dev Med Child Neurol 1965; *7*:433–435.
37. Yang S-Y. Brain abscess: a review of 400 cases. J. Neurosurg 1981; *55*:794–799.
38. Bhandari YS, Sarkari NBS. Subdural empyema: a review of 37 cases. J Neurosurg 1970; *32*:35–37.
39. Coonrod JD, Dans PE. Subdural empyema. Am J Med 1972; *53*:85–91.
40. Farmer TW, Wise GR. Subdural empyema in infants, children and adults. Neurology 1973; *49*:254–261.
41. Hitchcock E, Andreadis A. Subdural empyema: a review of 29 cases. J Neurol Neurosurg Psychiatry 1964; *27*:422–434.
42. Kaufman DM, Miller MH, Steigbigel NH. Subdural empyema: an analysis of 17 recent cases and review of the literature. Medicine 1975; *54*:485–498.
43. Luken MG III, Whelan AM. Recent diagnostic experience with subdural empyema. J Neurosurg 1980; *52*:764–771.
44. Handel SF, Klein WC, Kim YW, et al. Intracranial epidural abscess. Radiology 1974; *111*:117–120.
45. Baker CJ. Primary spinal epidural abscess. Am J Dis Child 1971; *121*:337–339.
46. Hulme A, et al. Spinal epidural abscess. Br Med J 1954; *1*:64–68.
47. Brown P. Septic cavernous sinus thrombosis. Johns Hopkins Med J 1961; *109*:68.
48. Greer M, Berk MS. Lateral sinus obstruction and mastoiditis. Pediatrics 1963; *31*:840–844.
49. Snyder RD, Stovring J, Cushing AH, et al. Cerebral infarction in childhood bacterial meningitis. J Neurol Neurosurg Psychiatry 1981; *44*:581–585.
50. Laird WP, Nelson RD, Huffines FD. The frequency of pericardial effusions in bacterial meningitis. Pediatrics 1979; *63*:764–770.
51. Feigin RD. Central Nervous System Infections. I. Bacterial Meningitis beyond the Neonatal Period. *In:* Feigin RD, Cherry JD, eds. Textbook of Pediatric Infectious Diseases. Philadelphia: WB Saunders, 1981:293–308.
52. Kaplan SL, Feigin RD. Rapid identification of the invading microorganism. Pediatr Clin North Am 1980; *27*:783–804.
53. Feigin RD, Kaplan SL. Bacterial Meningitis. *In:* Appel SH, ed. Current Neurology. Philadelphia: WB Saunders, 1982: 255–279.
54. Yolken RH, Hughes WT, Stopa PJ. Rapid diagnosis of infections caused by B-lactamase-producing bacteria by means of an enzyme radioisotopic assay. J Pediatr 1980; *97*:715–720.
55. Rutledge J, Benjamin D, Hood L, Smith A. Is the CSF lactate measurement useful in management of children with suspected bacterial meningitis? J Pediatrics 1981; *98*:20–24.

56. Komorowski RA, Farmer SG, et al. Cerebrospinal fluid lactic acid in diagnosis of meningitis. J Clin Microbiol 1978; *8*:89–92.
57. Neches W, Platt M. Cerebrospinal fluid LDH in 287 children, including 53 cases of meningitis of bacterial and non-bacterial etiology. Pediatrics 1968; *41*:1097–1103.
58. Feigin RD, Shackelford PG. Sequential lumbar puncture as a diagnostic aid in aseptic meningitis. N Engl J Med 1973; *289*:571–574.
59. Adair CV, Gauld RL, Smadel JE. Aseptic meningitis, a disease of diverse etiology: clinical and etiologic studies on 854 cases. Ann Intern Med 1953; *39*:675–704.
60. Mandal BD. The dilemma of partially treated bacterial meningitis. Scand J Infect Dis 1976; *8*:185–188.
61. Feldman WE. Effect of prior antibiotic therapy on concentrations of bacteria in CSF. Am J Dis Child 1978; *132*:672–674.
62. Kaplan SL, Mason EO Jr, Garcia H et al. Pharmacokinetics and cerebrospinal fluid penetration of moxalactam in children with bacterial meningitis. J Pediatr 1981; *8*:152–157.
63. Ward J. Antibiotic-resistant *Streptococcus pneumoniae:* clinical and epidemiologic aspects. Rev Infect Dis 1981; *3*:254–266.
64. Yogev R, Kolling WM, Williams T. Pharmacokinetic comparison of intravenous and oral chloramphenicol in patients with *Haemophilus influenzae* meningitis. Pediatrics 1981; *67*:656–660.
65. Lietman PS. Oral chloramphenicol therapy. J Pediatr 1981; *99*:905–906.
66. Schaad UB, Nelson JC, McCracken GH. Recrudescence and relapse in bacterial meningitis of childhood. Pediatrics 1981; *67*:188–195.
67. Jacob J, Kaplan RA. Bacterial meningitis, limitations of repeated lumbar puncture. Am J Dis Child 1977; *131*:46–48.
68. Shurin SB, Anderson P. Anemia associated with *H. influenzae* b (Hib) septicemia is due to immune hemolysis of RBC coated with soluble bacterial antigens. Pediatr Res 1983; *17*:932.
69. Kaplan SL, Feigin RD. The syndrome of inappropriate secretion of antidiuretic hormone in children with bacterial meningitis. J Pediatr 1978; *92*:758–761.
70. Gold AP, Carter S. Neurology. *In:* Shirkey HC, ed. Pediatric Therapy, 6th ed. St. Louis: The CV Mosby Company, 1980: 897–918.
71. Oppenheimer EY, Rosman NP. Seizures in childhood: an approach to emergency management. Pediatr Clin North Am 1979; *26*:837–855.
72. Powell DA, Nahata MC, Durrell DC, et al. Interactions among chloramphenicol, phenytoin, and phenobarbital in a pediatric patient. J Pediatr 1981; *98*:1001–1003.
73. Balagtas RC, Levin S, Nelson KE, Gotoff SP. Secondary and prolonged fevers in bacterial meningitis. J Pediatr 1970; *77*:957–964.
74. Feigin RD, Kaplan SL, Catlin FI, et al. Prospective studies of bacterial meningitis in children: hearing evaluation (submitted for publication).
75. Sell SHW, Merrill RE, Doyne EO, Zimsky, EP. Long-term sequelae of *Hemophilus influenzae* meningitis. Pediatrics 1972; *49*:206–211.
76. Lombardi N. Central nervous system infections: long-term complications and management. Pediatr Ann 1977; *6*:12:785–796.
77. Sproles ET III, Azewad J, Williamson C, et al. Meningitis due to *Hemophilus influenzae:* long-term sequelae. Pediatrics 1969; *75*:782.
78. Sell S, Warren W, Pate J, et al. Psychological sequelae to bacterial meningitis: two controlled studies. Pediatrics 1972; *49*:212.
79. Klein JO, ed. *Hemophilus influenzae* Infections. *In:* Report of the Committee on Infectious Diseases, 19th ed. Evanston, Illinois: American Academy of Pediatrics, 1982:105–107.
80. Shapiro ED. Prophylaxis for contacts of patients with meningococcal or *Haemophilus influenzae* type b disease. Pediatr Infect Dis 1982; *1*:132–138.
81. Band JD, and the *Haemophilus influenzae* Disease Study Group. Prevention of *Haemophilus influenzae,* type b (Hib) disease by rifampin. 21st Interscience Conference on Antimicrobial Agents and Chemotherapy, November 4–6, 1981.
82. Klein JO, ed. Meningococcal Infections. *In:* Report of the Committee on Infectious Diseases, 19th ed. Evanston, Illinois: American Academy of Pediatrics, 1982:139–141.

CHAPTER

3

Endotoxin Shock in Children

Sheldon L. Kaplan, M.D.
Thomas A. Vargo, M.D.

Endotoxin or septic shock is a state of inadequate tissue perfusion accompanied by a wide variety of adverse metabolic, physiologic, and hematologic consequences in association with localized or generalized infection.[1–3] Most frequently, the organisms associated with septic shock are gram-negative and have endotoxin or lipopolysaccharide (LPS) within their cell walls. The most common gram-negative organisms responsible for endotoxin or septic shock include *Escherichia coli, Klebsiella* and *Enterobacter, Pseudomonas* species, *Neisseria meningitidis*, and *Haemophilus influenzae*, Type b. However, other microorganisms such as *Staphylococcus aureus, Streptococcus pneumoniae*, Group B *Streptococcus*, viruses, rickettsiae, and fungi are also associated with septic shock.

The incidence of septic shock in adults is thought to be increasing, and it is estimated to be 20-fold that of two decades ago. A number of factors may be responsible for this increased incidence.[4] Patients with previously rapidly fatal diseases are surviving longer owing to immunosuppressive agents, corticosteroids, and antibiotics; and these patients are at increased risk for bacteremia. The more aggressive and sophisticated medical and surgical therapy practiced in intensive care units (ICUs) with the use of indwelling vascular lines, urinary catheters, and ventilators increases the likelihood of bacteremia and ensuing shock. The incidence of gram-negative bacteremia or septic shock has not been carefully studied in children. Dupont and Spink[5] reviewed bacteremia caused by gram-negative organisms over an eight year period in 172 children 1 month to 16 years of age. The genitourinary and gastrointestinal tracts, skin and wounds, and respiratory tract were the most common sources of bacteremia. The portal of entry could not be established in 30 per cent of the children. Hospital-acquired infections were almost five times more frequent than non–hospital-acquired infections. Almost 75 per cent of the children had an ultimately fatal underlying disease. Shock occurred in 25 per cent of the bacteremic children, and the mortality rate for children with shock was 98 per cent. Corrigan and coworkers observed shock in 31 per cent of children (8 of 11 <1 year of age) with septicemia caused by a wide variety of organisms.[6] In meningococcal disease, 11 to 16 per cent of children develop shock.[7, 8] Early onset Group B streptococcal disease in the neonate and overwhelming *S. pneumoniae* infection in the asplenic host are associated with shock in a high percentage of cases. *Staphylococcus aureus* may be associated with hypotension with or without other manifestations of toxic-shock syndrome.[9, 10] We have observed a 5.5 per cent incidence of shock associated with meningitis caused by *H. influenzae*, Type b (unpublished data).

PATHOPHYSIOLOGY

The pathophysiology of endotoxin shock is very complex and still not completely understood. Most of the data from which the proposed sequence of events leading to septic shock has been developed are derived from animal models using purified endotoxin or live bacteria. Although human disease is not accurately simulated by these animal models, much of what has been determined in the animal can be corroborated in humans. Endotoxin is one important component for the development of septic shock, and all gram-negative organisms have endotoxin or lipopolysaccharide (LPS) as part of the outer membranes of their cell walls. Endotoxin has three basic components: (1) terminal side chains of repeating oligosaccharides, which are responsible for the antigenic specificity of O antigens and thus, differ greatly from strain to strain of bacteria, (2) a core LPS that is very similar in hexose composition and antigenic determinants among gram-negative microorganisms, and (3) lipid-A that also is very similar among different strains and is responsible for most of the biologic properties of endotoxin.[11]

Animal Models of Endotoxin Shock

After the administration of purified endotoxin or live gram-negative organisms, a large number and variety of events occur in subhuman primates. Endotoxin stimulates the release of endogenous pyrogen from leukocytes, which results in fever. Initial cardiovascular effects are decreased peripheral resistance with pooling of blood and diminished venous return to the heart, decreased cardiac output, and decreased systemic pressure.[12, 13] The peripheral pooling of blood is, in part, related to the generation of bradykinin, serotonin, and histamine, which are potent vasodilators. Endotoxin activates Hageman factor, which in turn initiates the enzymatic steps leading to kinin production.[14] Prostaglandins, endorphins, and vasoactive anaphylatoxins released by complement activation also contribute to the peripheral pooling of blood and decreased venous return to the heart.[15, 16] Endorphins and ACTH have the same parent molecule, the release of which is stimulated by stress. Endorphins are increased five-fold in dogs after endotoxin treatment and are potent vasodilators.[17] As the shock state persists, alterations in blood flow are observed. Coronary artery flow is diminished, resulting in a significant depression of myocardial function.[18] In the dog, immediately following endotoxin administration, cerebral blood flow and cerebral perfusion pressure fall and cerebral ischemia develops.[19] Cerebral vascular resistance initially decreases but then progressively increases over the baseline value, indicating intact cerebral autoregulation.

The pathophysiology associated with septic shock due to gram-positive organisms, which do not possess LPS in their outer membranes, is not well understood nor as carefully studied as the pathophysiology of septic shock due to gram-negative organisms. In one report, complement levels were depressed in hypotensive newborns with sepsis caused by Group B *Streptococcus*.[20] Certain isolates of *Staphylococcus aureus* elaborate an exotoxin that may be associated with the development of shock.[21]

Numerous metabolic changes have been associated with endotoxin shock in animals. Hyperglycemia and hypoinsulinemia are consistently demonstrated in primates injected with *E. coli*.[22] The hypoinsulinemia appears to be mediated through α-adrenergic receptors and correlates with survival, i.e., those animals with hypoinsulinemia survived a significantly shorter time than euinsulinemic animals. Along with the progression of shock, hypoglycemia results from the inhibition of hepatic gluconeogenesis and increased glucose utilization by peripheral tissues, especially skeletal muscles.[23, 24] Alanine and glycine concentrations are elevated, indicating that glucogenic amino acids are not being converted to glucose via gluconeogenesis.[25] Furthermore, endotoxin may have an insulin-like action on tissues, which increases glucose oxidation.[26] Inducible hepatic enzymes such as tryptophan oxygenase and phosphoenolpyruvate carboxykinase are altered.[27] Growth hormone, vasopressin, and serum copper concentrations rise while levels of iron, transferrin, and zinc fall in association with the presence of endotoxin.[11, 28] Hypertriglyceridemia and impaired lipid disposal mechanisms as well as elevated free fatty acids are noted in primates given endotoxin.[29] The fatty acid elevations are important factors, since fatty acids are precursors to prostaglandins, and rats rendered deficient in essential fatty acids are much less susceptible to the lethal effects of endotoxin than normal rats.[30]

Endotoxin probably does not have a direct effect on the central nervous system (CNS) in the presence of an intact blood-brain barrier.[31] However, direct injection of endotoxin into the ventricular fluid of dogs results in hyperventilation and lowering of cardiac output and blood pressure.[32] When given intravenously, endotoxin lessens total and regional cerebral blood flow, alters glucose utilization, and increases cerebral oxygen consumption.[33] Cerebrospinal fluid (CSF) concentrations of lactate are elevated, and pyruvate levels are diminished, indicating that the brain has shifted from aerobic to anaerobic metabolism.[34]

The effect of endotoxin or gram-negative bacteremia on the lungs of experimental animals is a subject of intense interest. Pathologic examination of the lungs of *E. coli*–treated monkeys shows congestive atelectasis and polymorphonuclear leukocytes (PMNS) in the alveoli. Capillary beds are engorged with PMNs and platelets, and capillary permeability is increased.[35, 36] Complement activation through C5a and circulating PMNs are essential factors in the genesis of the capillary permeability changes.[36] In addition, fibrin split products, which may be elevated during shock, can cause platelet aggregation and sequestration by many organs including the lung, where the platelets may help in recruiting PMNs.[37] Other pathologic findings of endotoxin shock in experimental animals include: (1) PMNs within hepatic sinusoids, hepatocyte vacuolization, and centrilobular congestion, (2) edematous hepatocytes with loss of glycogen stores and mitochondrial edema, and (3) dilatation of the proximal convoluted tubules of the kidney.[35]

Endotoxin Shock in Humans

In humans, gram-negative bacteremia may be followed by an early decrease in systemic vascular resistance and mean arterial blood pressure but an increase in cardiac output, all of which suggest peripheral pooling of blood and a hyperdynamic state.[38, 39] Gram-positive bacteremia is usually associated with a greater cardiac output than gram-negative bacteremia.[38, 40] Maintenance of a high or adequate cardiac output (>3.1 L/min/m^2) is related to increased survival in adults, but the progression of bacterial shock is characterized by a decline in cardiac output. This decline is accompanied by greater concentrations of blood lactate, decreased arterial blood pH, and lower survival rates in adults.[41] Similar data are not available for older children, who might be expected to maintain a greater than normal cardiac index for a longer time than adults with underlying myocardial dysfunction.

Coagulation and metabolic alterations in the human host are similar to those in the experimental animal with endotoxin shock. Mason and coworkers found markedly depleted levels of Hageman factor, kallikreinogen, and kallikrein inhibitor in adult patients with gram-negative bacteremia and hypotension.[42] Coagulation abnormalities such as disseminated intravascular coagulation (DIC) stem in part from activation of Hageman factor.

Concentrations of C3 in bacteremic hypotensive patients are diminished compared with those in normal adults or those patients with normotensive bacteremia.[43] Furthermore, C5, C6, C9, properdin, and factor B levels are lowered significantly in endotoxin shock. These measurements are consistent with activation of the complement cascade, which occurs primarily through the alternative pathway; this activation occurs in and contributes to the shock of the human host with gram-negative bacteremia.[44] Fenton and Strunk performed serial measurements of CH_{50}, C3, C4, and factor B in three newborns with Group B streptococcal sepsis.[20] All three had hypotension, prolonged coagulation times, neutropenia, and respiratory failure. Factor B, C3, C4, and CH_{50} were depressed 30 to 100 per cent in these newborns compared with their own cord blood levels (obtained from the placentas but on the babies' side) recorded at birth or with levels determined in their unaffected twins or in control infants. In acute meningococcal disease in children, Tubbs found a mean C3 level (as a percentage of normal) of 132 ± 21 per cent for survivors *versus* 91 ± 21 per cent for children who died.[45] There was no correlation between endotoxin and C3 levels. Some data support the occurrence of complement activation in children with septic shock.

Hyperglycemia followed by hypoglycemia is a common metabolic response to overwhelming sepsis complicated by shock.[46] Patients with underlying liver disease and decreased glycogen stores are most susceptible to the development of hypoglycemia. As tissue perfusion remains diminished, lactic acidosis ensues, and concentrations of lactic acid are significantly higher in nonsurvivors or those patients with "low-flow states" (lower cardiac output) compared with survivors or patients with "high-flow states." Clowes and colleagues described a group of adult patients with low-flow septic shock (mean cardiac index [CI] = 2.4 L/min/m^2) in whom serum insulin concentrations were 12 μU/ml, compared with 42 μU/ml in patients with high-flow septic shock (mean CI = 4.6 L/min/m^2), and suggested that low blood insulin concentrations may adversely affect the myocardium.[47] Glucose, insulin, and potassium infusions to the low-flow group resulted in higher cardiac output and blood pressure with a concomitant lowering of central venous and pulmonary wedge pressures.

Hypertriglyceridemia and elevated free fatty acids develop during gram-negative bacteremia in adults.[48] Patients with high-flow states have normal free fatty acid concentrations whereas those with low-flow states have greatly elevated free fatty acid concentrations.[47]

Presumably, the low insulin concentration in the low-flow patients favors lipolysis. Other metabolic alterations that have been documented in humans with septic shock include:

1. Elevated cortisol and growth hormone levels.[49]

2. A decrease in ionized calcium that correlates directly with cardiac output.[50]
3. Depression of circulating T3 and T4 levels associated with poor nutrition.[51]
4. Elevation in total plasma amino acid concentrations caused mainly by high levels of aromatic amino acids (phenylalanine and tyrosine) and the sulfur-containing amino acids. Patients who survive sepsis had higher levels of alanine and branched-chained amino acids compared with nonsurvivors.[52]

Adult respiratory distress syndrome (ARDS), or "shock lung" is a major cause of morbidity and mortality in patients with septic shock. Several investigative groups have reported that "shock lung" occurs in children as well as adults and that septic shock is a common precursor of this complication.[53, 54] Characteristic pathologic changes in the lungs of children with ARDS include increased lung weight with congestion and atelectasis, alveoli lined with hyaline membranes and debris, microthrombi, hemorrhage, and interstitial edema.[53] Using ^{131}I-labeled human serum albumin (^{131}I-HSA), Anderson and coworkers found significantly greater clearance of the radionuclide from plasma into bronchial secretions in patients with pulmonary edema associated with sepsis than in controls.[55] A rise in pulmonary microvascular permeability was proposed as the explanation for the greater clearance. Dantzsker and colleagues, employing ventilation-perfusion techniques, demonstrated that the hypoxemia of ARDS in humans could be explained entirely by large intrapulmonary shunts and not by diminished diffusion.[56] Positive end expiratory pressure (PEEP) lessened perfusion to the unventilated portions of lung, which is one reason why PEEP is useful in ARDS treatment. The pathogenesis of the increased capillary permeability appears to be related to C5a, an activated component of complement, which causes PMN aggregation *in vitro*. Hammerschmidt and coworkers determined C5a levels in 61 patients (16 with sepsis) at risk for ARDS.[57] Thirty-one of the 33 patients who ultimately developed ARDS had positive C5a assays *versus* only 5 of 28 patients who did not develop ARDS ($P<.000001$). Presumably, high circulating levels of C5a lead to pulmonary leukostasis and subsequent damage to the pulmonary microvascular endothelium through the superoxide anion and hydrogen peroxide released by PMNs.

Bacterial shock is one of the most common causes of DIC in children. Endotoxin directly, or endothelial damage produced by bacteria, may activate Hageman factor, which initiates the coagulation cascade. DIC is characterized by hypofibrinogenemia, thrombocytopenia, and reduction in the concentration of coagulation factors II, V, and VIII. Restoration of blood pressure and tissue perfusion improves these coagulation parameters.[58, 59] In most patients, DIC does not lead to significant bleeding or microvascular thrombosis. Nevertheless, serious hemorrhages into the lungs or central nervous system can be associated with DIC. Thrombocytopenia is a common occurrence during septicemia of any etiology and may be related to platelet-associated IgM in some patients. Corrigan found that 57 per cent of children with gram-negative and 77 per cent of children with gram-positive septicemia had thrombocytopenia ($<150{,}000/mm^3$).[60]

The effects of septic shock alone on the CNS have not been examined critically in humans; therefore, findings in experimental animals must be applied to the human host. More investigations using modern techniques such as nuclear magnetic resonance and the use of stable isotopes to measure regional and total cerebral blood flow and regional cerebral glucose utilization may provide important information in regard to the pathophysiology of altered cerebral function during endotoxin shock. In a histologic study, Graham and coworkers described acute hemorrhagic leukoencephalitis in six adults with gram-negative bacteremia, septic shock, and neurologic abnormalities, predominantly coma.[61] Microscopic findings of the brain at necropsy showed the following: (1) necrosis of vessel walls with fibrin exuding into and through the walls into the perivascular space, (2) perivascular edema particularly of white matter, (3) PMN infiltrates into abnormal areas of the brain, (4) perivascular tissue destruction, and (5) ball or ring hemorrhages. The investigators postulated that the acute hemorrhagic leukoencephalitis seen in these patients could be due to an endotoxin-mediated Shwartzman reaction and activated complement that lead to endothelial cell damage, which explains the damage to the small vessels. The generalized Shwartzman reaction in rabbits is characterized by fibrin deposition, particularly in the kidney, thrombosis of small vessels, and a consumptive coagulopathy. Endotoxemia also has been linked by several groups of workers to the pathogenesis of acute renal failure associated with gram-negative bacteremia.[61, 62]

Bohm summarized the pathologic findings

in ten children who died of fulminating meningococcemia.[63] In all of these patients, the adrenal glands showed hemorrhagic changes, microthrombi, and hemorrhage; microthrombi were also seen in the skin. All of the hearts had evidence of pronounced diffuse vasculitis and myocarditis. Endothelial cells were edematous and detached from the basement membrane. In the kidney, microthrombi were seen in some glomeruli. Pathologic findings that are indicative of small blood vessel and endothelial cell damage are common in fatal septic shock due to a wide variety of gram-negative organisms.

CLINICAL PRESENTATION AND DIAGNOSIS

During the treatment of a hypotensive child, knowledge of an underlying disease or preceding injury or surgical procedure that is associated with gram-negative bacteremia should alert the physician to the possibility of septic shock. The presence of shock in a female with a recent menstrual period and a history of tampon use suggests the possibility of toxic-shock syndrome. Fever, chills, nausea, vomiting, and an altered mental state may be among the first signs and symptoms manifested by a child with septic shock.[1] A variety of rashes may be noted. Petechiae are nonspecific and are associated with vasculitis of any etiology including bacteremia and viremia. Purpura is a much more ominous finding and frequently indicates meningococcemia. Pyogenic skin infections may be the foci for septicemia due to *Staphylococcus aureus* or *S. pyogenes*. Erythema gangrenosum generally indicates *Pseudomonas aeruginosa* is the etiologic agent. The skin overlying plastic catheters may be erythematous, and purulent material may ooze from around the catheter if the line or tract is infected. Oral thrush in a compromised host could mean that gastrointestinal colonization with *Candida* is a source of fungemia. Signs of meningeal irritation or increased intracranial pressure (ICP) are very important to observe because fluid management of shock must be modified if either meningitis or increased ICP is found.

In the early stages of shock, the skin feels warm and the patient may look flushed. An older child may be apprehensive. Hyperventilation precedes the onset of hypotension and can be an early clue to circulatory insufficiency.[64] Careful auscultation of the heart may reveal a pericardial friction rub associated with infectious pericarditis. Abdominal distension and guarding are evidence of peritonitis. Palpation of an abdominal mass could suggest genitourinary obstruction or an intra-abdominal abscess as the source of bacteremia.

Cold clammy skin, a weak pulse, tachycardia, tachypnea, diaphoresis, hypotension, and diminished urine output are indications that shock is progressing. Cyanosis of the extremities, ear lobes, and the tip of the nose may be noted. Rales on auscultation of the lungs may signify pneumonia or pulmonary edema.

The physical findings in septic shock are nonspecific, although the sudden appearance of petechiae or purpura in a child in shock certainly points towards meningococcemia as the etiologic cause. Shock in a child can be divided into three fundamental types: (1) hypovolemic, (2) cardiogenic, and (3) distributive.[1] Hypovolemic shock, a lowering of circulating blood volume, may be due to acute internal or external blood loss, fluid and electrolyte losses usually through the gastrointestinal tract, burns with massive extravasation of fluid, adrenal insufficiency, and many other causes. Intracardiac surgery, severe congestive heart failure, dysrhythmias, drug intoxication, tension pneumothorax, and pericardial effusion with tamponade are some of the events that lead to cardiogenic shock, which is due to decreased myocardial contractility. Distributive shock is a result of abnormal blood flow distribution leading to inadequate tissue perfusion. Septic shock falls within this category. Other important causes of distributive shock include anaphylaxis and drug intoxication.

Laboratory Evaluation

The laboratory evaluation of a child with endotoxin shock provides important information for diagnosis and optimal management. The hemoglobin and hematocrit values may aid in distinguishing between hemorrhagic and septic shock. Either leukocytosis or leukopenia usually is present in septic shock. Severe neutropenia generally signifies an overwhelming infection and is a poor prognostic sign in meningococcemia as well as any other overwhelming infection. A peripheral blood smear may show fragmented red blood cells, which are evidence of DIC, or it may show Howell-Jolly bodies, indicating asplenia or splenic dysfunction. Gram stain of a buffy coat smear may suggest the etiologic agent; this technique is particularly useful in the asplenic child with suspected pneumococcemia.[66] Meningococcus may be seen in a Gram stain of a petechial lesion. Thrombocytopenia alone is common during sepsis but may signify DIC. Prolongation of thrombin time and partial thromboplastin time and the presence of fibrin split products and hypofibrinogenemia are classic laboratory findings in DIC.

Hyponatremia is common and may provide some prognostic information. Nishijima and colleagues noted in adult patients with shock induced by gram-negative bacteremia that the survival rate was decreased when the serum sodium concentration was below 130 mEq/L.[41] Depression of the serum bicarbonate concentration in such patients usually indicates metabolic acidosis, a result of inadequate tissue perfusion and higher lactic acid level. Monitoring of lactic acid concentration and arterial pH is useful for assessing the adequacy of therapy in restoring tissue perfusion. If the lactic acid concentration continues to rise and the arterial pH does not improve during therapy, tissue perfusion is not being restored. Hyperglycemia or hypoglycemia may be noted, depending upon the duration and severity of the illness as well as the age, size, and underlying disease of the patient. Small infants with liver dysfunction are likely to become hypoglycemic owing to septic shock. Serum calcium concentrations, and preferably ionized calcium levels, should be checked because hypocalcemia can contribute to poor myocardial contractility.

Initially, arterial blood gas measurements during endotoxin shock disclose evidence of respiratory alkalosis. hypocapnea, and elevated pH, which may be the first clue of impending shock and usually occurs prior to the development of hypotension.[64, 67] At this point, the patient has a mixed metabolic acidosis and respiratory alkalosis. Adult patients who survive endotoxin shock have significantly greater initial arterial pH values (mean pH 7.48) than patients who die (mean pH 7.3).[41] As the shock state progresses, additional lactic acid is produced, metabolic acidosis worsens, and the patient becomes acidotic because ventilatory mechanisms cannot fully compensate for acid production. If the patient tires from continued hyperventilation, respiratory failure is imminent. Hypoxemia is the primary consequence of ARDS. The chest roentgenogram commonly shows bilateral, diffuse, hazy infiltrates located in the perihilar and basilar regions; opacifications of all lung fields is usually seen in the later stages of ARDS.

The presence of many white blood cells (WBCs) or WBC casts in the urine may suggest that the genitourinary tract is the source of bacteremia. Gram-negative bacteria seen on Gram stain of unspun urine correlates with a quantitative colony count of 10^5 CFU/ml or more. Decreased perfusion of the kidney results in a reduction in the glomerular filtration rate, which is indicated by increases in blood urea nitrogen and serum creatinine levels. A urine to plasma osmolality ratio less than 1.5 was associated with progressive renal failure in adults with shock in one study.[68] In contrast, urine to plasma osmolality ratio greater than 1.5 was associated with the remote likelihood of progressive renal failure. Dilute urine (osmolality <150 mOsm/L) also reflects the probable preservation of renal function.

Every attempt must be made to establish the agent responsible for septic shock so that the most appropriate antibiotics can be administered. Obviously, blood, CSF, and urine cultures should be obtained, preferably before any antibiotic therapy. Gram stain and culture of sputum and tracheal aspirates should be performed when an intubated child deteriorates suddenly without explanation. Blood for cultures that is drawn through infected lines is more commonly positive than the usual blood drawn peripherally in line-related sepsis.[69] Rapid diagnostic techniques such as countercurrent immunoelectrophoresis or latex agglutination may identify the responsible etiologic bacteria within an hour.[70] Bacterial polysaccharides from *H. influenzae*, Type B, Group B *Streptococcus, S. pneumoniae*, and *N. meningitidis* serogroups A, C, D, Y and W-135 can be detected reliably in sera, CSF, urine, or virtually any body fluid by these techniques. Unfortunately, *N. meningitidis*, Group B is responsible for over 50 per cent of meningococcal disease in the United States but cannot be detected by these immunologic methods using commercially available antisera. Although the K1-associated antigen of *E. coli* can be detected with research antisera, there are no routine rapid diagnostic tests for other gram-negative enteric bacteria. Blood cultures processed anaerobically are indicated when a child has a suspected intra-abdominal focus of infection. Joint, pleural, and peritoneal fluids should be obtained for analysis and culture when appropriate. Detection of endotoxin using the limulus lysate assay is nonspecific in terms of etiology, and the large number of false-positive results also contributes to the limited clinical usefulness of this test.

Children with C5, C6, C7, or C8 deficiency

are at greater risk for infection due to *N. meningitidis* and repeated episodes of meningococcal disease.[71, 72] Although it is not directly applicable to the management of the child in septic shock, a total hemolytic complement determination after the acute illness has resolved is useful with infection due to *N. meningitidis* occurs. If a complement deficiency is documented, the patient or the family should be counseled that immediate medical attention is required whenever fever or petechiae develop.

MANAGEMENT

The major objectives in the management of a child with endotoxin shock are four-fold: (1) to eradicate the infection, (2) to restore adequate tissue perfusion, (3) to maintain adequate ventilation, and (4) provide other supportive measures.

Eradicate the Infection

As soon as endotoxin shock is suspected, antibiotics should be administered after suitable cultures are obtained. Appropriate antibiotic therapy will significantly reduce fatality rates even when administered after shock complicates gram-negative bacteremia.[73] The selection of antibiotics is dependent upon the clinical situation (Table 3–1). Children who are more than one month of age with septic shock complicating presumed bacterial meningitis should have standard initial antibiotic therapy for meningitis, ampicillin, 300–400 mg/kg/day in six divided doses, plus chloramphenicol, 100 mg/kg/day in four divided doses. Chloramphenicol can be cardiotoxic, thus, serum concentrations of chloramphenicol must be monitored carefully, particularly in the child with septic shock. Antistaphylococcal agents such as nafcillin, 200 mg/kg/day in six divided doses, or vancomycin, 40–60 mg/kg/day in four divided doses intravenously for the penicillin-allergic patient, is included if preceding pyogenic skin lesions are present or if other evidence points to *Staphylococcus aureus* sepsis.

Aminoglycosides plus an extended spectrum of penicillins (carbenicillin, ticarcillin, and piperacillin) is appropriate therapy for the immunosuppressed child who is at risk for gram-negative sepsis.[74] The combination of aminoglycosides plus broad spectrum semisynthetic penicillins is frequently synergistic *in vitro* against gram-negative enterics, *Pseudomonas aeruginosa* in particular; and a synergistic combination of antibiotics may be desirable for treating gram-negative infections in leukopenic patients. Lau and coworkers reported that in leukopenic patients, therapy with a combination of antibiotics was associated with increased survival when *in vitro* studies demonstrated synergy of the antibiotics against the microorganisms isolated from the patient.[75] Which combination of antibiotics to use is somewhat arbitrary because no specific combination has been proved superior to another. In general, carbenicillin, 400–600 mg/kg/day, plus gentamicin, 4.5–7.5 mg/kg/day, depending on the patient's age, will adequately cover most gram-negative infections. However, one must be familiar with the antibiotic susceptibility patterns within the community as well as in one's own hospital in order to select the most appropriate antibiotic therapy. Proper management of nosocomial infections clearly requires knowledge of current hospital antibiograms. For example, the child without underlying illness who has not received antibiotics is more likely to have a gentamicin-susceptible gram-negative organism that is responsible for septicemia than the child with leukemia who has recently undergone gentamicin therapy in the hospital for a previous febrile episode.[76] In hospitals where gentamicin resistant gram–negative organisms are common, tobramycin, 6–7.5 mg/kg/day, or amikacin 15–20 mg/kg/day should be administered from the outset. Intra-abdominal sepsis suggests an anaerobic etiology, and antibiotics to which anaerobes are susceptible should be included in the initial therapy. A combination of ampicillin, gentamicin, and clindamycin 30–40 mg/kg/day will cover virtually all bacteria associated with perforated bowel, ruptured appendix, or intra-abdominal abscesses. Surgical drainage of intra-abdominal or other abscesses is mandatory for the optimal management of such infections and should be performed as soon as the child's condition allows.

Moxalactam, cefotaxime, and other third-generation cephalosporins are newer antibiotics that are effective against a wide variety of aerobic and anaerobic gram-negative organisms. They penetrate well into the CSF and may be very useful in selected patients. An important advantage of the newer agents is their lack of renal toxicity compared with aminoglycosides, which require careful monitoring especially when administered to children with

Table 3–1. ANTIBIOTIC TREATMENT OF SEPTIC SHOCK IN CHILDREN

Selected Organisms	Antibiotics	Dosage	Interval (hours)	Comments
Gram-negative Enterics				
Escherchia coli	Gentamicin	7.5 mg/kg/day (<5 yrs. of age)	6–8	Serum levels must be monitored; oto- and nephrotoxic; and requires altered dose in renal failure.
Klebsiella		6.0 mg/kg/day (>5, <10 yrs. of age)	6–8	
Enterobacter		4.5 mg/kg/day (>10 yrs. of age)	6–8	
Proteus				
Serratia				
Pseudomonas	Tobramycin	7.5 mg/kg/day	6–8	
	Amikacin	15–20 mg/kg/day	6–8	
	Carbenicillin	400–600 mg/kg/day	4	Synergy with aminoglycosides against gram-negatives, especially *Pseudomonas;* Na load: Carb >Tic >Pip; and covers anaerobes.
	Ticarcillin	200–300 mg/kg/day	4	
	Piperacillin	200–300 mg/kg/day	4	
Other Organisms				
Bacteroides	Clindamycin	30–40 mg/kg/day	6–8	Pseudomembraneous enteritis is rare in children (for clindamycin)
	Chloramphenicol	50–100 mg/kg/day	6–8	
	Cefoxitin	120–160 mg/kg/day	6–8	
Staphylococcus aureus	Nafcillin	200 mg/kg/day	4	Nafcillin preferred for use in renal failure and methicillin in hepatic failure. For *S. aureus* methicillin-resistant, use vancomycin.
	Methicillin			
	Vancomycin	40–60 mg/kg/day	6	
Streptococcus pneumoniae	Penicillin	100,000–300,000 units/kg/day	4	
Haemophilus influenzae Type b	Ampicillin	300 mg/kg/day	4	For ampicillin-resistant HITB, use chloramphenicol, moxalactam or cefotaxime
	Chloramphenicol	100 mg/kg/day	6	
	Moxalactam	150–200 mg/kg/day	6	
	Cefotaxime	150–200 mg/kg/day	6	

renal impairment. These agents are not reliably effective against *P. aeruginosa.*

The serum half-life (T½β) of a drug is the duration of time required for one-half of the total body amount of the drug to be eliminated. The T½β of gentamicin in children with renal dysfunction and stable serum creatinine concentration can be estimated by the formula T½β = 4 × serum creatinine concentration.[77] A standard dose of gentamicin can be given every two to three serum half-lives as the initial dosage interval. Modification of the dose is then based on the serum peak and trough levels. Guidelines for estimating the dose of antibiotics to be given to adult patients with various degrees of renal impairment can be used initially in children until serum levels have been obtained.[78] Since vancomycin is not appreciably cleared by dialysis, it is a convenient drug to use if *Staphylococcus aureus* is the possible cause of septic shock in a child with prior or recent onset of renal failure. The dose of vancomycin for the anuric child is 10–15 mg/kg every seven to ten days and serum levels determine how frequently one must administer the vancomycin.

Amphotericin B is the antifungal agent of choice when *Candida* species are thought to be responsible for septic shock. Amphotericin B is mixed with 5 per cent glucose to a maximum concentration of 10 mg/100 ml. An initial dose of 0.25–0.30 mg/kg should be given without delay rather than a test dose when the patient is thought to be critically ill owing to the fungemia. The drug is administered over three to six hours intravenously every 24 hours, and blood pressure, pulse, respiratory rate, and temperature are carefully monitored during the infusion.[79] Depending upon how well the patient tolerates the drug, the dose is gradually increased by 0.1–0.25 mg/kg increments until a total daily dose of 0.5–1.0 mg/kg (not to exceed 50 mg) is reached. For *Candida* septicemia, 10 to 14 days of amphotericin B are curative in many patients. Adverse reactions to amphotericin B are numerous and include fever, chills, phlebitis, hypotension or hypertension, and cardiac arrhythmias (ventricular tachycardia and fibrillation).[79] Because nephrotoxicity and hypokalemia are commonly noted with amphotericin B administration, serum electrolyte, blood urea nitrogen, and serum creatinine values should be checked at least three times per week.[79] Potassium supplementation may be required if hypokalemia is detected. The dose of amphotericin B is altered when renal function is diminished. Removal of infected intravenous or bladder catheters is imperative for eradication of the candidemia.

Restore Tissue Perfusion

Intravenous infusion of fluid is the cornerstone of reestablishment of good tissue perfusion in endotoxin shock. The type of fluid initally administered is probably not as critical as the volume of fluid provided to the patient. Ten to 20 ml/kg of isotonic crystalloid solutions such as normal saline and lactated Ringer's solution are satisfactory for the initial restoration of the intravascular volume. Although isotonic colloid solutions such as albuminized saline and fresh-frozen plasma provide greater expansion of the intravascular space than crystalloid solutions, the colloid may leak out of damaged capillaries from the intravascular compartment, shifting water to the interstitial space. If hypoproteinemia is documented, fresh-frozen plasma should be administered. A total serum solids value of less than 4.5 gm/100 ml as measured by refractometer is indicative of hypoproteinemia; unless the initial fluid challenge returns perfusion to normal, all patients should have a central venous pressure (CVP) line to guide the physician in deciding how much volume to infuse. In infants and young children CVP lines are usually most easily inserted in the inguinal area via percutaneous puncture of the femoral vein. In larger children (>20 kg) most CVP lines are inserted via venous cutdown in the antecubital fossa. Many surgeons, anesthesiologists, and intensivists will insert a CVP line using an internal jugular, axillary, or subclavian vein, but this procedure requires special training.

In children without primary heart disease, the CVP provides a reasonable estimate of the left ventricular filling pressure and the relative ability of the right ventricle to eject venous return. A low CVP reading in a child with low cardiac output usually reflects an inadequate circulating blood volume. Therefore, in a hypotensive child, if the CVP reading is less than 5 to 6 mmHg, a second 10–20 ml/kg volume of isotonic fluid should be infused over ten minutes. If the CVP is between 6 and 10 mmHg, a second 5–10 ml/kg aliquot of isotonic fluid should be infused until perfusion improves or the CVP exceeds 10 mmHg. Excessive fluid administration may be hazardous owing to the risk of vascular overload and development of pulmonary edema. It is especially likely to occur if the CVP is greater than 10 mmHg, or the patient develops an increase in pulmonary capillary permeability. If the hematocrit is less than 30 per cent, blood should be infused to maintain the hematocrit between 35 and 40 per cent.

If poor perfusion persists with a CVP greater than 10 mmHg, or pulmonary edema develops, a pulmonary artery catheter should be inserted. Pulmonary artery catheterization can be performed safely in children by experienced personnel with or without fluoroscopy.[80] Complications of pulmonary artery catheterization include pneumothorax, hemorrhage from the vascular access site, hypotension, arrhythmias, cardiac perforation, and tamponade. The pulmonary capillary wedge pressure [(PCWP), balloon inflated in the pulmonary artery] correlates well with the left ventricular end-diastolic pressure (left ventricular pre-load) and provides a more accurate measure of left ventricular pre-load than the CVP, particularly when the intrathoracic pressure is high when positive pressure ventilation is being delivered.

The normal CVP is 1 to 4 mmHg and the normal PCWP is 6 to 7 mmHg.[81, 82] However, these values are much less than what we recommend in the treatment of shock. Many children in septic shock require excessive fluid to maintain an effective circulating blood volume, and the increased vascular volume causes the elevated CVP and PCWP values. As mentioned previously, the main complication of excessive fluid administration is the development of pulmonary edema. Usually, pulmonary edema does not occur if the CVP is 10 mmHg or less or if the PCWP is 12 mmHg or less. However, some children will develop pulmonary edema at lower levels and may require intensive respiratory support (described later).

If the PCWP is less than 8 mmHg, a 10–20 ml/kg fluid challenge can be administered. If the PCWP changes less than 3 mmHg with the fluid challenge and the patient remains in shock, an additional fluid challenge can be infused.[1, 83] Since children with endotoxin shock frequently develop pulmonary edema, even at relatively low PCWP levels, one should strive for the lowest PCWP or fluid volume that provides an adequate cardiac output.

There are patients who remain in shock with a PCWP of ≥12 mmHg. In these instances, we usually continue to infuse additional fluid as long as the fluid challenge continues to result in clinically improved perfusion and greater cardiac output, and any pulmonary edema that develops is adequately controlled. Sometimes this procedure requires PCWPs as high as 20 mmHg, and such patients need exceedingly intensive, sophisticated supportive care.

Cardiovascular Medications in Endotoxin Shock

If the cardiac output remains low despite adequate fluid therapy, or if pulmonary edema has developed, medication to enhance cardiovascular performance is required. Pulmonary edema is usually secondary to overzealous fluid administration, poor cardiac contractility or ARDS.[83] In any case, improving cardiac contractility will lower left atrial pressure and improve the pulmonary edema. The decision to use cardiovascular drugs should be based primarily upon clinical findings. However, a CVP of greater than 10 mmHg, a PCWP of more than 12 mmHg, or a cardiac output of less than 2.5 L/min/m^2 supports the decision to use such medication.

Cardiac output in shock is measured using a pulmonary artery thermodilution catheter.[1, 84, 85] Cold saline is injected through the catheter into the right atrium, and as the atrial blood together with cold saline flows through the pulmonary artery, the temperature is measured by a thermistor on the distal end of the catheter. The cardiac output is automatically calculated by a computer, which can be attached to the catheter.

The cardiac output in normal children, indexed to one square meter of body surface area, is 4.4 ± 0.95 L/min/m^2 (mean ± SD), with approximately 2.5 L/min/m^2 being the lowest normal value.[86]

Catecholamines (sympathomimetic amines) are the medications of choice for improving cardiac contractility in patients with shock.[83–85] We routinely use vasoactive drugs for the patient in shock if the cardiac output is less than 2.5 L/min/m^2 and frequently use them even if the cardiac output is normal but the patient clinically continues to remain in shock. Because catecholamines are rapid-acting, have a short half-life, and are effective immediately, the doses can be adjusted to the patient's response. All catecholamines are extremely potent and can cause serious complications, including fatal arrhythmias, if an excessive dose is given. Sympathomimetic amines must be administered via a constant infusion pump through a line that is neither flushed nor temporarily interrupted. Extravasation of catecholamines into the subcutaneous tissues can cause severe necrosis. Thus, catecholamine infusions require a separate central venous line for their use, with different venous lines for fluid replacement, infusion of other drugs, and so forth. However, in emergency situations catecholamines can be administered through a peripheral venous line.

Catecholamine therapy increases oxygen consumption of the myocardium.[87] While this is a possible therapeutic consideration, it is usually of minimal concern in children with septic shock. Nevertheless, the increase in oxygen consumption must be considered when one is treating shock, especially if cardiac contractility does not improve or if it worsens during catecholamine infusion. Also, the electrocardiogram (ECG) must be closely monitored for signs of myocardial damage such as ST segment and T-wave changes. Cardiac contractility can be assumed to be improving if the patient's clinical status improves, cardiac output increases, and PCWP decreases.

Whenever catecholamine therapy is used, careful monitoring of the clinical status, CVP, PCWP, and cardiac output is mandatory because of the many different effects catecholamines can have in individual patients. Catecholamines are less effective if the patient is acidemic; conversely, alkaline solutions inactivate the drug. Therefore, the patient's acidemia should be corrected to a pH greater than 7.2, and the intravenous solution containing the catecholamine should not be mixed with sodium bicarbonate or other alkaline solutions.[88] The three sympathomimetic amines primarily used in shock therapy are dopamine, isoproterenol, and dobutamine.[83, 84, 88, 89] Briefly, dopamine is used when the urine output is diminished, isoproterenol when the patient has bradycardia and persistent acidemia, and dobutamine as a substitute for isoproterenol when the patient has tachycardia. The main complication of all catecholamines is the development of arrhythmia. Many reports suggest that dopamine and dobutamine are less effective in infants during the first year of life.[88, 89] However, our clinical impression is that they are effective drugs for this age group.

Dopamine has different effects depending

upon the dose used.[84, 85, 90] Although these effects overlap, the dopaminergic response predominates at lower doses, the β-adrenergic response predominates in the median therapeutic dose range, and the α-adrenergic response predominates at the higher doses. In general, we have found these effects to occur at slightly lower doses than are reported in most texts.[84, 85] The dopaminergic response, which includes renal, coronary, intracerebral, and mesentery arterial vasodilatation, begins at 2 μg/kg/min and increases until the β-adrenergic effect supersedes it. Renal vasodilatation usually results in a significant increase in urinary output. At 5–10 μg/kg/min, the β-adrenergic activity begins and predominates until the α-adrenergic activity begins at approximately 15 μg/kg/min. β-adrenergic activity causes an increase in cardiac inotropy and usually causes a mild to moderate rise in systemic vasodilatation. In our patients with septic shock we have found doses of 10–15 μg/kg/min cause the greatest elevation in cardiac output. At doses greater than 15–20 μg/kg/min, the α-adrenergic effect causes peripheral vasoconstriction, which increases as the dose is augmented. The renal vasoconstriction causes a decline in urine output. A greater systemic vascular resistance increases cardiac afterload, resulting in diminished cardiac output. Therefore, we rarely use dosages greater than 15 μg/kg/min. We routinely use dopamine early in the treatment of all but the mildest cases of shock, beginning with a dose of 2–5 μg/kg/min and usually rapidly raising it to 10 μg/kg/min.

Isoproterenol is a β-adrenergic drug that causes a significant increase in cardiac contractility along with a usually marked systemic vasodilatation and a rapid increase in the heart rate. It is, therefore, the agent we use in patients who have bradycardia and those who have acidosis secondary to peripheral vasoconstriction with inadequate tissue perfusion. Marked vasodilatation occurs with isoproterenol, and as a result, intravascular deficits and hypovolemia must be corrected prior to its use. The usual dosage of isoproterenol is 0.05–1.5 μg/kg/min beginning with an initial dose of 0.1 μg/kg/min.[83, 85, 88] It must be remembered, especially when using larger doses, that isoproterenol causes the most tachycardia and is the most arrhythmogenic of the three catecholamines used for shock.

Dobutamine is a myocardial β_1-adrenergic agent, which compared with isoproterenol has a similar effect in increasing cardiac contractility but causes only minimal changes in heart rate and systemic vascular tone.[92] Dobutamine therapy has been studied extensively in adults, but there have been relatively few reports of its use in children.[90, 92, 93] In children, it is effective in increasing cardiac contractility and output in shock without causing a rise in heart rate. Dobutamine's effects on other cardiovascular parameters in children have not been agreed upon. Our clinical experience suggests that it does mildly lower systemic vascular resistance in children with shock. In most children with significant cardiac dysfunction, we use a combination of dopamine and dobutamine. After a dopamine dosage of 10 μg/kg/min is achieved, we begin dobutamine at 2 μg/kg/min and usually increase it to 10 μg/kg/min. We find in most cases that this combination results in good renal blood flow, mild vasodilatation, a significant increase in cardiac contractility, and a lowering of both the CVP and PCWP. Again, it is important to modify the dose according to the patient's response.

If cardiac contractility or cardiac output remains inadequate despite catecholamine therapy, use of vasodilator therapy should be considered. Vasodilators are usually used in shock therapy in combination with catecholamines to have maximum vasodilation from the vasodilator plus increased cardiac contractility from the catecholamines.[94] Nitroprusside is the primary vasodilator used in children because of its rapid onset and short duration.[95] It should only be used when the patient has poor peripheral perfusion, the blood pressure is at least near normal value or elevated, the patient has an adequate intravascular volume, and systemic vascular resistance is elevated.

Determination of systemic vascular resistance requires measuring the cardiac output, CVP, and systemic arterial pressure and is calculated by the following formula:

$$\mathrm{SVR} = \frac{\mathrm{SAP} - \mathrm{CVP}}{\mathrm{CO}} \times 80$$

where SVR = systemic vascular resistance in dynes/sec/cm^{-5}, SAP = mean systemic arterial pressure in mmHg, which usually has to be measured by an indwelling arterial line connected to an electronic transducer, CVP = central venous pressure in mmHg, CO = cardiac output in L/min, and 80 = conversion factor. Normal systemic vascular resistance in children is 1000–1600 dynes/sec/cm^{-5}.[82]

When using nitroprusside, we regulate the dose to maintain the SVR at normal levels, but in some children slightly below normal values are maintained if the cardiac output is

ALGORITHM FOR THE TREATMENT OF ENDOTOXIN SHOCK IN CHILDREN

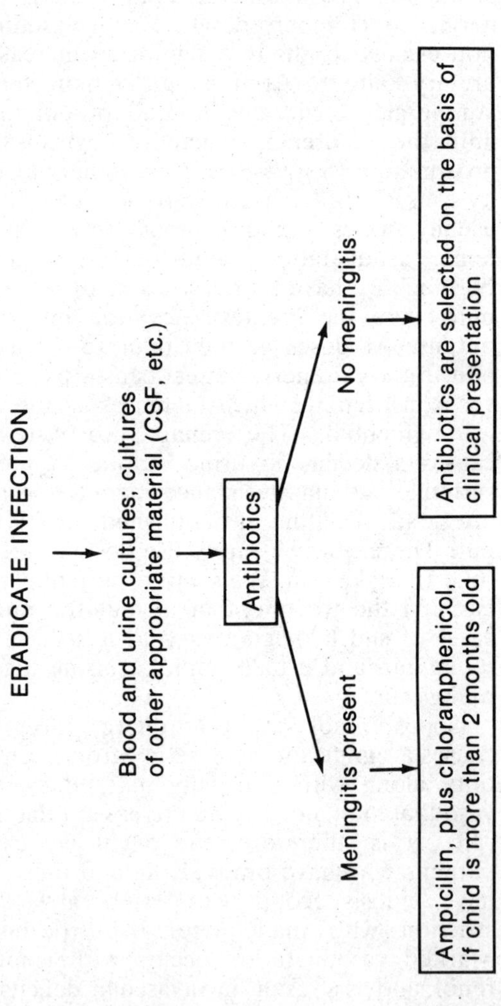

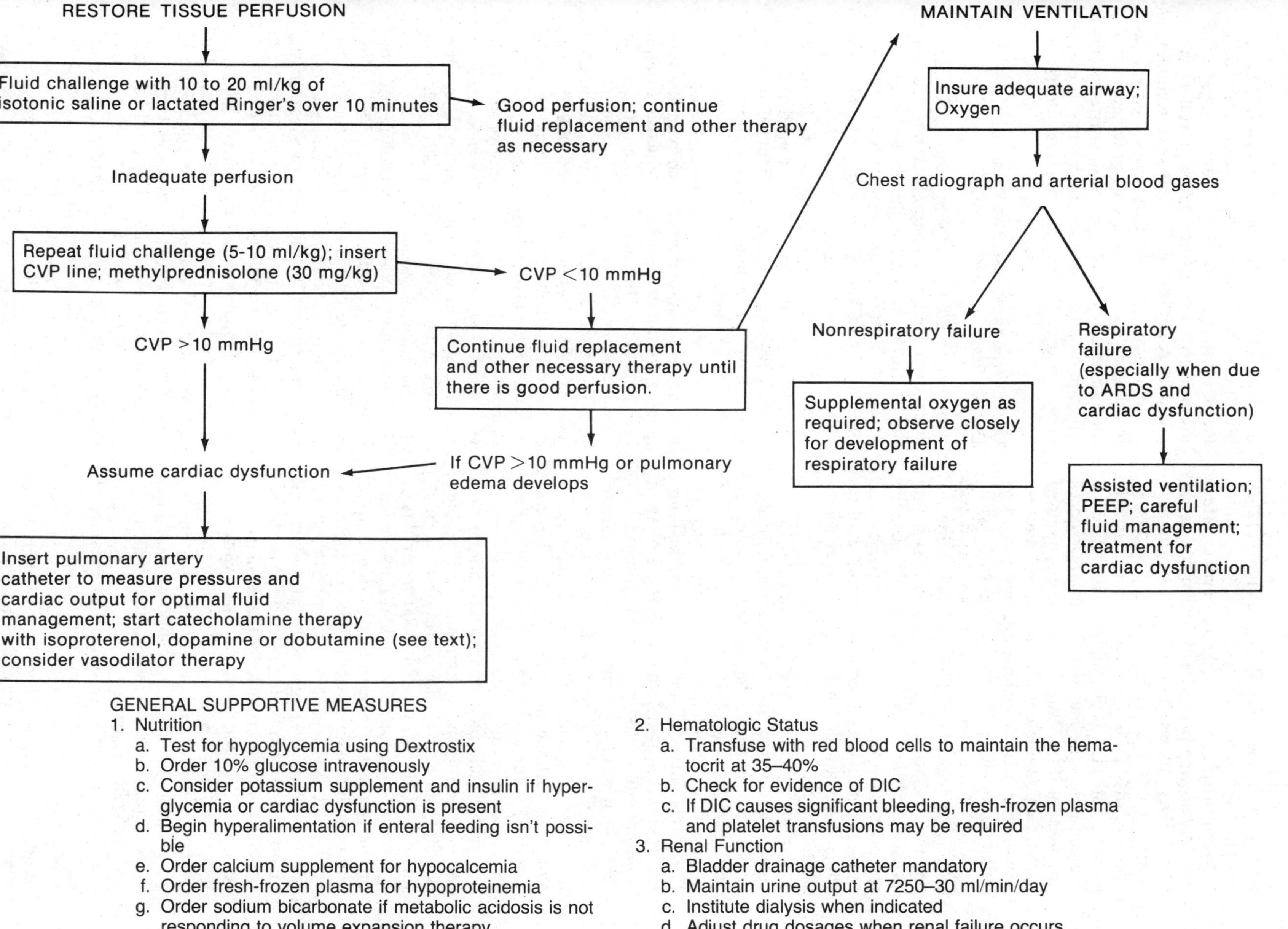

GENERAL SUPPORTIVE MEASURES

1. Nutrition
   a. Test for hypoglycemia using Dextrostix
   b. Order 10% glucose intravenously
   c. Consider potassium supplement and insulin if hyperglycemia or cardiac dysfunction is present
   d. Begin hyperalimentation if enteral feeding isn't possible
   e. Order calcium supplement for hypocalcemia
   f. Order fresh-frozen plasma for hypoproteinemia
   g. Order sodium bicarbonate if metabolic acidosis is not responding to volume expansion therapy
2. Hematologic Status
   a. Transfuse with red blood cells to maintain the hematocrit at 35–40%
   b. Check for evidence of DIC
   c. If DIC causes significant bleeding, fresh-frozen plasma and platelet transfusions may be required
3. Renal Function
   a. Bladder drainage catheter mandatory
   b. Maintain urine output at 7250–30 ml/min/day
   c. Institute dialysis when indicated
   d. Adjust drug dosages when renal failure occurs

normal and the PCWP is elevated (12–20 mmHg or greater).

Nitroprusside has no direct cardiac effect but, by reducing peripheral vascular resistance (after-load), allows the inadequately pumping heart to contract more effectively. The dosage of nitroprusside is 0.5–8 μg/kg/min, usually starting with 1.0 μg/kg/min. Thiocyanate or cyanide poisoning may develop if larger doses are used, or if the drug is used for a prolonged period. Thiocyanate poisoning causes nausea, vomiting, muscle twitching, and sweating. Cyanide poisoning results in persistent metabolic acidosis. If nitroprusside is of benefit, it will usually be evident clinically within 10 minutes, and the cardiac output and peripheral systemic vascular resistance should improve. We usually reserve the use of nitroprusside for those cases of significantly depressed cardiac contractility, which have not responded to any other therapeutic intervention.

Various formulas have been devised to calculate the dosage of catecholamines in children. We have found the method of Holbrook and coworkers helpful.[88] We mix 60 mg of dopamine or dobutamine in 100 ml of D5W. When this mixture is infused at 1 ml/kg/hour, the dose is 10 μg/kg/min. Similarly, 0.6 mg of isoproterenol in 100 ml of D5W infused at 1 ml/kg/hour results in a dose of 0.1 μg/kg/min.

Generally, the patient's mental status and urine output improve when circulation is restored. Metabolic acidosis may not be corrected by volume replacement alone, in which case sodium bicarbonate at 1–2 mEq/kg can be given. Additional bicarbonate administration is based upon the patient's ongoing base deficits. Once circulation is restored, a maintenance fluid rate of 1500–2000 ml/m^2/day is reasonable. Adjustments in fluid rates depend on the patient's temperature, urine output, and ongoing losses of body fluid. In the presence of cerebral edema or increased intracranial pressure, which might occur when bacterial meningitis is complicated by endotoxin shock, volume restoration must be the primary concern with the realization that the overzealous use of fluid rates may exacerbate cerebral edema.[96] In such situations, the early use of pharmacologic agents to support perfusion may decrease the volume of fluid that might ordinarily be required.

Urine output is a very important measure of adequate tissue perfusion. A urine output that exceeds oliguric volumes (250–300 ml/m^2/day) usually indicates satisfactory renal perfusion. Bladder catheterization and accurate recording of urine output are essential to the management of a child with endotoxin shock. Complications of bladder catheterization are bacterial or fungal infections, hemorrhage, and urethral irritation. Since gastric bleeding is a possible complication of any overwhelming acute illness, a nasogastric tube should be inserted to facilitate the early recognition of this potentially fatal event. Nasogastric administration of antacids or cimetidene may prevent major gastric bleeding due to stress ulcers.

Unproven Cardiovascular Therapies During Septic Shock

In many patients with septic shock, adequate circulation cannot be restored despite vigorous fluid restoration and administration of cardiovascular pharmacologic agents. In some cases, the CVP or PCWP is elevated, and additional volume cannot be given. Under these conditions, less conventional approaches to restoring tissue perfusion should be considered. As previously discussed, some patients with septic shock have inadequate cardiac output ("low-flow" state), elevated systemic vascular resistance, and depressed serum insulin concentration.[47] In one study, when such patients were given a 10 minute infusion of glucose, insulin, and potassium, there was a dramatic rise in blood pressure, cardiac output, and urine output. There was a concomitant drop in the CVP and PCWP. Presumably, such therapy improves myocardial function by unknown mechanisms.[97] *Obviously, glucose-insulin-potassium therapy requires close monitoring of the serum glucose level to prevent hypoglycemia!* Bedside determination of serum glucose levels by Dextrostix can be accomplished easily with minimal quantities of blood.

β-endorphins possibly contribute to the pathogenesis of endotoxin shock, and naloxone, a specific opiate antagonist, can reverse hypotension in experimental animals injected with endotoxin. On the basis of these animal studies, Peters and colleagues administered naloxone to 13 adult patients with shock (11 septic).[98] Dopamine and supportive measures were continued unchanged. Three patients had received steroids. Naloxone was injected intravenously at an initial dose of 0.4 mg and increased every five minutes until the systolic blood pressure reached 100 mmHg or a total dose of 8 mg was given. Eight of nine patients not receiving corticosteroids had an immediate and impressive elevation in blood pressure associated with the naloxone administration (mean increase 30.4 ± 5.1 mmHg). The three patients who had received high doses of steroids and one who had hypoadrenocorticotropism following pituitary irradiation did not respond with an elevated blood pressure. No apparent adverse effects of naloxone were observed. Presumably, naloxone was not effective in the steroid pre-treated group because of suppression of ACTH and endorphin release from the pituitary. Similar reports for children are not available. The dose of naloxone in children with septic shock has not been established, but an initial dose of 0.4 mg/1.73 m^2 seems reasonable. The recommended initial dose of naloxone in children for narcotic antagonism is 0.005–0.01 mg/kg. This drug might be worth trying if the septic shock is not responding to fluids, vasopressors, and other supportive measures. Although lidocaine and indomethacin improve the survival of baboons given lethal doses of endotoxin, there is insufficient evidence to support the use of these agents in humans at the present.[99]

An intriguing approach to the treatment of endotoxin shock is the administration of antiserum to the core LPS–lipid-A complex of endotoxin, which is very similar in all gram-negative organisms. Ziegler and coworkers evaluated the efficacy of human antisera to a mutant *E. coli* strain in the treatment of gram-negative bacteremia and shock.[100] Human antisera to core LPS-lipid–A were prepared by vaccinating adult volunteers with the J5 mutant *E. coli,* which lacks oligosaccharide side chains in its endotoxin molecule. In a randomized, prospective, controlled trial, patients with presumed gram-negative infection and recent deterioration received either preimmune or J5 antisera. *E. coli* and *P. aeruginosa* were the most common organisms isolated from the 212 patients evaluated. *N. meningitidis* and HITB were isolated from 12 and 7 patients, respectively. Twenty-one patients had meningitis. Age, underlying disease, other risk factors, sources of infection, and type of bacteria isolated were the same in both groups. The number of children enrolled in the study was not stated. Approximately 40 per cent of patients in both groups had profound septic shock and 50 per cent received high-dose steroids. The mortality rate for all patients who received the J5 antisera was 22 per cent, which was significantly less (P = .011) than the 39 per cent rate in the non-immune sera group. Data were analyzed from patients in profound septic shock and 26 of 34 (76%) of the preimmune sera patients died compared to 17 of 37 (46%) of the J5 antisera group (P = .009). Thus, from this study, it does appear that human J5 antisera could substantially reduce mortality from gram-negative bacteremia and endotoxin shock. Limited availability of such antisera is the major drawback to its routine use.

STEROIDS

Perhaps no other aspect of the management of endotoxin shock has stirred as much controversy as the role of corticosteroids. There is a vast medical literature showing that steroids given prior to or concomitantly with endotoxin or live bacteria in animal models prevent many of the metabolic, hemodynamic, complement-mediated, and lethal effects of septic shock. However, extrapolation of the results of such studies to humans is hazardous because the models do not really approximate clinical situations when bacteremia and shock occur before any treatment. Hinshaw and associates have evaluated steroids in a baboon model of endotoxin shock, which mimics the human situation closely, except that these animals are healthy prior to the experiments and in the human, gram-negative bacteremia and shock usually occur if the host's resistance is altered in some way.[101, 102] Nevertheless, these studies are the best approximation of human disease to date. In one study, 14 adult baboons were divided into three treatment groups after they were injected with approximately 2–3 × 10^{10} live *E. coli*/kg over two hours. Group A (5) animals were not treated. The five animals in group B received methylprednisolone, 15–30 mg/kg, after approximately 50 per cent of the organisms had been infused. Gentamicin, 4.5–9 mg/kg also was administered to these animals. The four animals in group C were treated with gentamicin only at the same dose as group B. Gentamicin was initially given to groups B and C after completion of the live *E. coli* infusion; subsequent doses were given every 12 hours. All five animals given no therapy died within an average of 19 hours (range 3–42 hours). The four baboons given gentamicin died within an average of 24 hours (range 15–23 hours). All five baboons who received steroid and gentamicin treatment (group B) were survivors (P = .025). Animals in all groups became hypotensive within two hours of the completion of *E. coli* infusion, but animals in groups A and C sustained hypotension, and the animals in group B regained relatively normal blood pressures within four hours. Furthermore, only group B animals maintained serum glucose and insulin concentrations within or above normal levels.

In a second experiment to study corticosteroid and antibiotic effectiveness, Hinshaw and workers allowed 16 baboons to become hypotensive for two hours after an LD_{100} dose of *E. coli* before treating the animals using doses of gentamicin and methylprednisolone similar to those used in the first study.[102] All eight untreated baboons died within 42 hours. Five of eight treated animals survived, and again, treated animals had significantly greater ($P<.05$) blood glucose and insulin concentrations than controls. Unfortunately, antibiotics alone were not compared with the combination of aminoglycosides and methylprednisolone in this study.

The evidence that steroids are beneficial in human septic shock is based almost entirely on one study. Schumer reported a randomized, prospective, double-blinded clinical investigation comprising 172 consecutive patients in septic shock enrolled over eight years.[103] Study treatment was either saline (100 ml), 3 mg/kg dexamethasone phosphate (DMP) in 100 ml, or 30 mg/kg methylprednisolone succinate (MPS) in 100 ml, in addition to standard supportive measures. Treatment was repeated only once, four hours after the first dose, if the patient remained in shock. Forty-three patients received DMP, 43 received MPS, and 86 received saline. The groups were comparable in age, severity of shock, and underlying diseases. The mortality rate of the saline-treated patients was 38.4 per cent (33 of 86) *versus* 10.4 per cent (9 of 86) in the steroid-treated group ($P=.001$). No significant difference in the complication rate was noted among the groups. No information was given concerning adjunctive measures, and the antibiotics administered changed in the middle of the study. Currently, there is insufficient evidence for the Federal Drug Administration to include septic shock as an indication for the use of high dose corticosteroids.[104] Nevertheless, we routinely recommend one to two doses of corticosteroids for endotoxin shock, considering that the adverse reactions are minimal and the drug is possibly beneficial. If steroids are to be administered, then dexamethasone, 3 mg/kg, or methylprednisolone, 30 mg/kg, which are the agents and doses with some proven efficacy, provided once or twice appears reasonable.

Maintenance of Adequate Ventilation

One of the most important aspects in the management of children with septic shock is maintaining a clear airway and avoiding any interference with adequate ventilation. Periodic suctioning of the patient's hypopharynx to remove pooled secretions may be necessary. Early institution of oxygen therapy is indicated even before any blood gas values have been obtained to document hypoxemia. The method by which the oxygen is administered depends upon the patient's condition. If the patient is able to maintain a low Pa_{CO_2} and has a Pa_{O_2} greater than 100 mmHg assisted ventilation usually is not necessary. One should intervene with intubation and assisted ventilation immediately if the child shows evidence of impending respiratory failure such as prolonged hyperventilation, retention of CO_2, or severe hypoxemia.

The development of "shock lung" or ARDS during the course of septic shock may greatly complicate the patient's management. Inability to maintain adequate blood oxygen tensions in the patient because of ARDS characteristically occurs 24 to 72 hours after the onset of septic shock but can occur earlier. Positive end expiratory pressure (PEEP) and mechanical ventilation should be instituted as soon as ARDS is recognized. PEEP appears to improve oxygenation by lowering ventilation perfusion inequalities and increasing functional residual capacity.[56] The general approach to using PEEP is to increase it until the concentration of inspired oxygen is 50 per cent or less, in an attempt to maintain the $Pa_{O_2} \geq 60$ mmHg. Since PEEP alters many cardiovascular parameters such as venous return, it is preferable to carefully monitor the cardiac output by a pulmonary artery catheter. Greater fluid administration is usually required as the PEEP is increased. Placement of a radial artery catheter facilitates frequent sampling for blood gas measurements. Fresh red blood cells should be transfused to maintain a hematocrit of 35 to 40 per cent to optimize oxygen delivery to tissues and increase venous return. Pneumothorax is the most common of the many complications of barotrauma due to high PEEP. Detailed guidelines for the use of PEEP in children with ARDS have been published.[53, 54]

Hydrostatic pulmonary edema associated with poor myocardial contractility or excessive fluid administration also may cause inadequate oxygenation and ventilation. Children with this problem have an elevated PCWP or CVP, and their ventilation is managed as that of a patient with ARDS.

In addition to PEEP, oxygen, and careful attention to cardiovascular parameters, steroids have been advocated as useful therapeutic agents in ARDS. Sladen reported that methylprednisolone, at a dose of 30 mg/kg every 6 hours for 48 hours, decreased the mortality rate of ten patients with ARDS to 10 per cent compared with previously reported rates of 60 to 90 per cent.[105] Sibbald and coworkers studied the effect of corticosteroid administration on alveolo-capillary permeability during septic shock in humans.[106] Nineteen patients with ARDS secondary to sepsis were studied using the appearance of ^{131}I-HSA administered intravenously into broncho-alveolar secretions as a measure of capillary permeability. Subjects were studied before and after a large dose of methylprednisolone (30 mg/kg) or dexamethasone (4 mg/kg) was given. In 14 of the 19 patients, steroids significantly decreased ($P<.001$) the clearance of ^{131}I-HSA compared with pretreatment values. The mechanism of action for the steroids in ARDS may involve the interaction of PMNs and C5a. Methylprednisolone and dexamethasone block the binding of chemotactic factors to receptors on PMNs, preventing PMN aggregation.[107] Methylprednisolone was more potent than dexamethasone in this activity. Theoretically, corticosteroids may inhibit PMN aggregation and leukostasis in the lungs and thereby prevent endothelial damage by the oxygen radicals released by the PMNs. Steroids would seem most beneficial in ARDS when administered very early during this process and may prevent rather than reverse lung damage.

General Supportive Care

The nutritional and metabolic requirements of children with endotoxin shock should not be neglected.[1, 83, 108] Caloric requirements are greatly increased in septic states compared with the resting metabolic state. Also, inadequate nutrition contributes to alterations in host defense mechanisms. Ten per cent glucose infusions may be necessary to prevent hypoglycemia, although hyperglycemia may develop at this concentration of glucose. As soon as the child is able to tolerate enteral feeding, provision of nutrients by this route should be attempted. A wide variety of commercial liquid formulas are available for tube feedings.[108] Unfortunately, the optimal amount and composition of nutrients needed by septic patients have not been established. For example, septic patients receiving standard concentrations of amino acids and glucose by hyperalimentation continue to release amino acids from peripheral tissues despite a positive nitrogen balance.[109] Administration of parenteral amino acid mixtures enriched with branched-chain amino acids resulted in the improvement of the plasma amino acid patterns and metabolic encephalopathy in five patients with overwhelming sepsis.[52] Hypocalcemia, specifically a reduction in ionized serum calcium level, is an indication for supplemental calcium. Calcium chloride contains 27 per cent elemental calcium or 14 mEq/gm $CaCl_2$, and a standard dose of calcium chloride is 5–10 mg/kg initially, followed by 300 mg/kg every 24 hours. If renal failure results from septic shock, dialysis is indicated when standard criteria are met such as symptomatic uremia, hyperkalemia, fluid overload, and pulmonary edema. If significant bleeding associated with DIC does occur in septic shock, marked thrombocytopenia or depleted coagulation factors may require replacement by platelet transfusion or infusion of fresh frozen plasma.

SUMMARY

The prognosis for children with septic shock treated in modern pediatric ICUs is unknown. The age, underlying disease, and specific microorganisms causing the endotoxin shock are major factors for predicting ultimate morbidity and mortality. The early institution of therapy as outlined in this chapter should certainly decrease the mortality rate of 98 per cent reported by Dupont and Spink.[5] Future developments, such as human antisera to endotoxin, may further reduce mortality due to septic shock in children. As with almost every infectious disease, prevention is the key to diminishing the fatalities related to septic shock. Vaccines for endotoxin or related components of gram-negative bacteria may be developed. For now, careful attention to maintaining indwelling lines and catheters and other important details of intensive care may prevent some cases of bacteremia. Although unproven, the use of prophylactic antibiotics and the pneumococcal polyvalent vaccine for children over 2 years of age may prevent overwhelming septicemia in children with asplenia or splenic dysfunction.

REFERENCES

1. Perkin RM, Levin DL. Shock in the pediatric patient. Part 1. J Pediatr 1982; *101*:163–169.
2. Schumer W. Septic shock. JAMA 1979; *242*:1906–1907.
3. Hardaway RM. Endotoxemic shock. Dis Colon Rectum 1980; *23*:597–604.

4. Kreger BE, Craven DE, Carling PC, McCabe WR. Gram-negative bacteremia. III. Reassessment of etiology, epidemiology and ecology in 612 patients. Am J Med 1980; *68*:332–343.
5. Dupont HL, Spink WW. Infections due to gram-negative organisms: an analysis of 860 patients with bacteremia at the University of Minnesota Medical Center, 1958–1966. Medicine 1969; *48*:307–332.
6. Corrigan JJ, Ray WL, May N. Changes in the blood coagulation system associated with septicemia. N Engl J Med 1968; *279*:851–856.
7. Stiehm ER, Damrosch DS. Factors in the prognosis of meningococcal infection. J Pediatr 1966; *68*:457–467.
8. Edwards MS, Baker CJ. Complications and sequelae of meningococcal infections in children. J Pediatr 1981; *99*:540–545.
9. Shulman ST, Ayoub EM. Severe staphylococcal sepsis in adolescents. Pediatrics 1976; *58*:59–66.
10. Todd J, Fishant M, Kapral F, Welch T. Toxic-shock syndrome associated with Phage-Group I Staphylococci. Lancet 1978; *2*:1116–1118.
11. McCabe WR. Endotoxin: Microbiological, Chemical, Pathophysiologic and Clinical Correlations. *In:* Weinstein L, Fields BN, eds. Seminars in Infectious Disease. Vol. 3. New York: Thieme-Stratton Inc, 1980:38–88.
12. Guenter CA, Fiorica V, Hinshaw LB. Cardiorespiratory and metabolic responses to live *E. coli* and endotoxin in the monkey. J Appl Physiol 1969; *26*:780–786.
13. Reichgott MJ, Melmon KL, Forsyth RP, Greineder D. Cardiovascular and metabolic effects of whole or fractionated gram-negative bacterial endotoxin in the unanesthetized rhesus monkey. Circ Res 1973; *33*:346–352.
14. Miller RL, Reichgott MJ, Melmon KL. Biochemical mechanisms of generation of bradykinin by endotoxin. J Infect Dis 1973; *128*:Suppl:144–156.
15. Kessler E, Hughes RC, Bennett EN, Nadela SM. Evidence for the presence of prostaglandin-like material in the plasma of dogs with endotoxin shock. J Lab Clin Med 1973; *81*:85–93.
16. Faden AL, Holaday JW. Experimental endotoxin shock: the pathophysiologic function of endorphins and treatment with opiate antagonists. J Infect Dis 1980; *142*:229–238.
17. Bone RC, Jacobs ER, Potter DM, et al. Endorphins in endotoxin shock. Microcirculation 1981; *1*:285–295.
18. Hinshaw LB. Myocardial function in endotoxin shock. Circ. Shock Suppl 1979; *1*:43–51.
19. Parker JL, Emerson TE. Cerebral hemodynamics, vascular reactivity, and metabolism during canine endotoxin shock. Circ Shock 1977; *4*:41–53.
20. Fenton LJ, Strunk RC. Complement activation and group B streptococcal infection in the newborn: similarities to endotoxin shock. Pediatrics 1977; *60*:901–907.
21. Schlievert PM, Kelly JA. Staphylococcal pyrogenic exotoxin C: further characterization. Ann Intern Med 1982; *96*(Part 2):982–986.
22. Cryer PE, Coran AG, Soda J, et al. Lethal *Escherichia coli* septicemia in the baboon: alpha-adrenergic inhibition of insulin secretion and its relationship to the duration of survival. J Lab Clin Med 1972; *79*:622–638.
23. Filkins JP, Cornell RP. Depression of hepatic gluconeogenesis and the hypoglycemia of endotoxin shock. Am J Physiol 1974; *227*:778–781.
24. Romanosky AJ, Bagby GJ, Bockman EL, Spitzer JJ. Increased muscle glucose uptake and lactate release after endotoxin administration. Am J Physiol 1980; *239*:E311–316.
25. Woolf LI, Groves AC, Duff JH. Amino acid metabolism in dogs with *E. coli* bacteremic shock. Surgery 1979; *85*:212–218.
26. Witek-Janusek L, Filkins JP. Insulin-like action of endotoxin: antagonism by steroidal anti-inflammatory agents. Circ Shock 1981; *8*:573–583.
27. Berry LJ, Rippe DF. Effect of endotoxin on induced liver enzymes. J Infect Dis 1973; *128*:Suppl 118–121.
28. Wilson MF, Brackett DJ, Hinshaw LB, et al. Vasopressin release during sepsis and septic shock in baboons and dogs. Surg Gynecol Obstet 1981; *153*:869–872.
29. Kaufmann RL, Matson CF, Beisel WR. Hypertriglyceridemia produced by endotoxin: role of impaired triglyceride disposal mechanisms. J Infect Dis 1976; *133*:548–555.
30. Cook JA, Wise WC, Callihan CS. Resistance of essential fatty acid-deficient rats to endotoxic shock. Circ Shock 1979; *6*:333–342.
31. Trippodo NC, Jorgensen JH, Priano LL, Traber DL. Cerebrospinal fluid levels of endotoxin during endotoxemia. Proc Soc Exp Bio Med 1973; *143*:932–937.
32. Simmons RL, Anderson RW, Ducker TB, et al. The role of the central nervous system in septic shock: II. Hemodynamic, respiratory and metabolic effects of intracisternal or intraventricular endotoxin. Ann Surg 1968; *167*:158–167.
33. Raymond RM, Emerson TE. Cerebral metabolism during endotoxin shock in the dog. Circ Shock 1978; *5*:407–414.
34. Raymond RM, Harkema JM, Emerson TE. Cerebrospinal fluid composition during endotoxin shock in the dog. Adv Shock Res 1979; *2*:249–256.
35. Coalson JJ, Archer LT, Hall NK, et al. Prolonged shock in the monkey following live *E. coli* organism infusion. Circ Shock 1979; *6*:343–355.
36. Hill SL, Eblings VB, Lewis FR. Changes in lung water and capillary permeability following sepsis and fluid overload. J Surg Res 1980; *28*:140–150.
37. Manwaring D, Curreri PW. Platelet and neutrophil sequestration after fragment D–induced respiratory distress. Circ Shock 1982; *9*:75–80.
38. Blain CM, Anderson TO, Pietras RJ, Gunnar RM. Immediate hemodynamic effects of gram-negative vs. gram-positive bacteremia in man. Arch Intern Med 1970; *126*:260–265.
39. Weil MH, Nishijima H. Cardiac output in bacterial shock. Am J Med 1978; *64*:920–922.
40. Winslow EJ, Loeb HS, Rahimtosla SH, et al. Hemodynamic studies and results of therapy in 50 patients with bacteremic shock. Am J Med 1973; *54*:421–432.
41. Nishijima H, Weil MH, Shubin H, Canavilles J. Hemodynamic and metabolic studies on shock associated with gram-negative bacteremia. Medicine 1973; *52*:287–294.
42. Mason JW, Kleeberg V, Dolan P, Colman RW. Plasma kallikrein and Hageman factor in gram-negative bacteremia. Ann Intern Med 1970; *73*:545–551.
43. McCabe WR. Serum complement levels in bacter-

emia due to gram-negative organisms. N Engl J Med 1973; *288*:21–23.
44. Fearon DT, Ruddy S, Schur PH, McCabe WR. Activation of the properdin pathway of complement in patients with gram-negative bacteremia. N Engl J Med 1975; *292*:937–940.
45. Tubbs HR. Endotoxin in meningococcal infections. Arch Dis Child 1980; *55*:808–819.
46. Miller SI, Wallace RJ, Musher DM, et al. Hypoglycemia as a manifestation of sepsis. Am J Med 1980; *68*:649–654.
47. Clowes GHA, O'Donnell TF, Ryan NT, Blackburn GL. Energy metabolism in sepsis: treatment based on different patterns in shock and high output stage. Ann Surg 1974; *179*:684–696.
48. Gallin JI, Kaye D, O'Leary WM. Serum lipids in infection. N Engl J Med 1969; *281*:1081–1086.
49. Beisel WR. Metabolic Response of Host to Infections. *In*: Feigin RD, Cherry J, eds. Textbook of Pediatric Infectious Diseases. Philadelphia: WB Saunders Company, 1981.
50. Woo P, Carpenter MA, Trunkey D. Ionized calcium: the effect of septic shock in the human. J Surg Res 1979; *26*:605–610.
51. Richmond DA, Molitch ME, O'Donnell TF. Altered thyroid hormone levels in bacterial sepsis: the role of nutritional adequacy. Metabolism 1980; *29*:936–942.
52. Freund HR, Ryan JA, Fischer JE. Amino acid derangements in patients with sepsis. Ann Surg 1978; *188*:423–430.
53. Holbrook PR, Taylor G, Pollack MM, Fields AI. Adult respiratory distress syndrome in children. Pediatr Clin North Am 1980; *27*:677–685.
54. Pfenninger J, Gerber A, Tschappeler H, Zimmermann A. Adult respiratory distress syndrome in children. J Pediatr 1982; *101*:352–357.
55. Anderson RR, Holliday RL, Driedger AA, et al. Documentation of pulmonary capillary permeability in the adult respiratory distress syndrome accompanying human sepsis. Am Rev Respir Dis 1979; *119*:869–877.
56. Dantzsker DR, Brook CJ, Hehart P, et al. Ventilation-perfusion distributions in the adult respiratory distress syndrome. Am Rev Respir Dis 1979; *120*:1039–1052.
57. Hammerschmidt DE, Weaver LJ, Hudson LD, et al. Association of complement activation and elevated plasma-C5a with adult respiratory distress syndrome. Pathophysiological relevance and possible prognostic value. Lancet 1980; *1*:947–949.
58. Corrigan JJ. Jordan CM. Heparin therapy in septicemia with disseminated intravascular coagulation. N Engl J Med 1970; *283*:778–782.
59. Corrigan JJ. Disseminated intravascular coagulopathy. Pediatrics 1979; *64*:37–45.
60. Corrigan JJ. Thrombocytopenia: a laboratory sign of septicemia in infants and children. J Pediatr 1974; *85*:219–221.
61. Graham DI, Behan PO, More IAR. Brain damage complicating septic shock. Acute hemorrhagic leukoencephalitis as a complication of the generalized Shwartzman reaction. J Neurol Neurosurg Physchiatry 1979; *42*:19–28.
62. Warde EN. Endotoxinaemia and the pathogenesis of acute renal failure. Q J Med 1975; *44*:389–398.
63. Bohm N. Adrenal, cutaneous and myocardial lesions in fulminating endotoxinemia (Waterhouse-Friderichsen syndrome). Pathol Res Pract 1982; *174*:92–105.
64. Blair E. Hypocapnea and gram-negative bacteremic shock. Am J Surg 1970; *119*:433–438.
65. Christy JH. Pathophysiology of gram-negative shock. Am Heart J 1971; *81*:694–701.
66. Bisno AL, Freeman JC. The syndrome of asplenia, pneumococcal sepsis, and disseminated intravascular coagulation. Ann Intern Med 1970; *72*:389–393.
67. Blair E. Acid-base balance in bacteremic shock. Arch Intern Med 1971; *127*:731–739.
68. Jones LW, Weil MH. Water, creatinine and sodium excretion following circulatory shock with renal failure. Am J Med 1971; *51*:314–318.
69. Shapiro ED, Wald ER, Nelson KA, Spiegelman KN. Broviac catheter–related bacteremia in oncology patients. Am J Dis Child 1982; *136*:679–681.
70. Kaplan SL, Feigin RD. Rapid identification of the invading microorganism. Pediatr Clin North Am 1980; *27*:783–803.
71. Peterson BH, Lee TJ, Snyderman R, Brooks GF. *Neisseria meningitidis* and *Neisseria gonorrhoeae* bacteremia associated with C6, C7 or C8 deficiency. Ann Intern Med 1979; *90*:917–920.
72. Ellison RT, Kohler PF, Curd JG, et al. Prevalence of congenital or acquired complement deficiency in patients with sporadic meningococcal disease. N Engl J Med 1983; *308*:913–916.
73. Kreger BE, Craven DE, McCabe WR. Gram-negative bacteremia. IV. Reevaluation of clinical features and treatment in 612 patients. Am J Med 1980; *68*:344–354.
74. Pizzo PA. Infectious complications in the child with cancer. I. Pathophysiology of the compromised host and the initial evaluation and management of the febrile cancer patient. J Pediatr 1981; *98*:341–354.
75. Lau WK, Young LS, Black RE, et al. Comparative efficacy and toxicity of amikacin/carbenicillin versus gentamicin/carbenicillin in leukopenic patients. A randomized prospective trial. Am J Med 1977; *62*:959–966.
76. Guerrant RL, Strausbaugh LJ, Wenzel RP, et al. Nosocomial bloodstream infections caused by gentamicin-resistant gram-negative bacilli. Am J Med 1977; *62*:894–901.
77. Sirinavin S, McCracken GH, Nelson JD. Determining gentamicin dosage in infants and children with renal failure. J Pediatr 1980; *96*:331–334.
78. Bennett WM, Muther RS, Parker RA, et al. Drug therapy in renal failure: dosing guidelines for adults. Part 1. Antimicrobial agents, analgesics. Ann Intern Med 1980; *93*:63–89.
79. Utz JP. Chemotherapy of the systemic mycoses. Med Clin North Am 1982; *66*:221–233.
80. Pollack MM, Reed TP, Holbrook PR, Fields AI. Bedside pulmonary artery catherization in pediatrics. J Pediatr 1980; *96*:274–276.
81. Rowe RD. Cardiac Catheterization. *In*: Keith JO, Rowe RD and Vlad PI, eds. Heart Disease in Infancy and Childhood. New York: MacMillan Publishing Co Inc, 1978:81–115.
82. Krovetz LJ, Goldbloom S. Normal standards for cardiovascular data. II. Pressure and vascular resistances. Johns Hopkins Med J 1972; *130*:187–195.
83. Perkin RM, Levin DL. Shock in the pediatric patient. Part II. Therapy. J Pediatr 1982; *101*:319–332.
84. Holbrook PR. Care of the Critically Ill Child. *In*: Shoemaker WC and Thompson WL, eds. Critical Care State of Art. Fullerton, California: The Society of Critical Care Medicine, 1980:1–49.

85. Levin DL, Patz J, Stein P. Shock. *In*: Levin DL, Morris FC, Moore GC, eds. A Practical Guide to Pediatric Intensive Care. St. Louis, Missouri: CV Mosby, 1979:58–63.
86. Graham TP, Jarmakani JM, Canent RU, Morrow MN. Left heart volume and estimation in infancy and childhood. Reevaluation of methodology and normal values. Circulation 1971; *43*:895–904.
87. Vasu Ma, O'Keefe GZK, Vezeredis MP. Myocardial oxygen consumption: effects of epinephrine, isoproterenol, dopamine, norepinephrine and dobutamine. Am J Physiol 1978; *235*:H237–241.
88. Holbrook PR, Mickell J, Pollack MM, Fields AI. Cardiovascular resuscitation drugs for children. Crit Care Med 1980; *8*:77–78.
89. Driscoll DJ, Pinsky WW, Entman ML. How to use inotropic drugs in children. Drug Ther 1979; *39*:124–135.
90. Perkin RM, Levin DL, Webb R, et al. Dobutamine: a hemodynamic evaluation in children with shock. J Pediatr 1982; *101*:977–983.
91. Driscoll DJ, Gillette PC, McNamara DG. The use of dopamine in children. J Pediatr 1978; *92*:309–314.
92. Tuttle RR, Mills J. Development of a new catecholamine to selectively increase cardiac contractility. Circ Res 1975; *36*:185–196.
93. Driscoll DJ, Gillette PC, Duff DF, et al. Hemodynamic effects of dobutamine in children. Am J Cardiol 1979; 43:581–584.
94. Stephenson LW, Edmunds HL, Raphaely R, et al. Effects of nitroprusside and dopamine on pulmonary arterial vasculature in children after cardiac surgery. Circulation 1979; *60*:104–110.
95. Luderer J, Hayes AH, Dubynsky O, Berlin CM. Long-term administration of sodium nitroprusside in childhood. J Pediatr 1977; *91*:490–491.
96. Kaplan SL, Feigin RD. The syndrome of inappropriate secretion of antidiuretic hormone in children with bacterial meningitis. J Pediatr 1978; *92*:758–761.
97. Weisul JP, O'Donnell TF, Stone MA, Clowes GHA. Myocardial performance in clinical septic shock: effects of isoproterenol and glucose potassium insulin. J Surg Res 1975; *18*:357–363.
98. Peters WP, Friedman PA, Johnson MW, Mitch WE. Pressor effect of naloxone in septic shock. Lancet 1981; *1*:529–532.
99. Fletcher JR, Ramwell PW. Lidocaine or indomethacin improves survival in baboon endotoxin shock. J Surg Res 1978; *24*:154–160.
100. Ziegler EJ, McCutchan JA, Fierer J, et al. Treatment of gram-negative bacteremia and shock with human antiserum to a mutant *Escherichia coli.* N Engl J Med 1982; *307*:1225–1230.
101. Hinshaw LB, Archer LT, Beller-Todd BK, et al. Survival of primates in LD_{100} septic shock following steroid/antibiotic therapy. J Surg Res 1980; *28*:151–170.
102. Hinshaw LB, Beller-Todd BK, Archer LT, et al. Effectiveness of steroid/antibiotic treatment in primates administered LD_{100} *Escherichia coli.* Ann Surg 1981; *194*:51–56.
103. Schumer W. Steroids in the treatment of clinical septic shock. Ann Surg 1976; *184*:333–341.
104. Sheagren JN. Septic shock and corticosteroids. N Engl J Med 1981; *305*:456–458.
105. Sladen A. Methylprednisolone. Pharmacologic doses in shock lung syndrome. J Thorac Cardiovasc Surg 1976; *71*:800–806.
106. Sibbald WJ, Anderson RR, Reid B, et al. Alveolo-capillary permeability in human ARDS. Chest 1981; *79*:133–142.
107. Skubitz KM, Craddock PR, Hammerschmidt DE, August JT. Corticosteroids block binding of chemotactic peptide to its receptor on granulocytes and cause disaggregation of granulocyte aggregates *in vitro*. J Clin Invest 1981; *68*:13–20.
108. Reimer SL, Michener WM, Steiger E. Nutritional support of the critically ill child. Pediatr Clin North Am 1980; *27*:647–660.
109. Clowes GHA, Heidman M, Lindberg B, et al. Effects of parenteral alimentation on amino acid metabolism in septic patients. Surgery 1980; *88*:531–543.

CHAPTER

4

Severe Dehydration Secondary to Diarrhea

Laurence Finberg, M.D.

Diarrhea, a symptom of a variety of disorders affecting infants, often leads to marked physiologic disturbances. Vomiting is a common accompanying symptom, which adds to and modifies the disturbances produced by diarrheal disease. Enteric infections produce these symptoms more often than all other causes combined. The cause occasionally is noninfectious. Consideration of the management of diarrhea will be limited to the physiologic disturbances that accompany excessive loss of water and salts from the gastrointestinal tract. Etiologic considerations, however important they may be, will not be presented. This emphasis is appropriate because survival following critical dehydration depends far more upon the correction of the physiologic disturbance than upon the removal of its cause.

The management of serious, life-threatening dehydration will be discussed. The management of less severe degrees of dehydration is omitted. Oral rehydration will not be presented other than to point out that the oral route can be used with great success in most infants who do not have circulatory impairment and will drink proffered oral solution.

A critical stage in diarrheal disease occurs when a volume of fluid equal in mass to about ten per cent of the body weight has been lost over a period of one or two days. Clinically this fluid loss usually occurs shortly after the illness has precluded oral intake because of anorexia or vomiting. At this stage of the illness, parenteral fluid therapy should be employed. Oral intake should be curtailed during the early hours of therapy. The use of milk or other food high in calories and solute often markedly increases stool water loss and complicates management. Even when severe undernutrition coexists with the diarrhea, the first few hours of therapy should be a period of brief starvation; parenteral glucose will provide emergency calories.

Although routes of administration such as intragastric drip and subcutaneous infusion have been employed successfully, their use should be restricted to institutions where a deficiency of supplies or trained personnel interdicts the preferred parenteral route—continuous intravenous infusion. With modern equipment, skilled house officers and pediatricians should be able to use venipuncture with only rare recourse to venisection (cutdown).

PATHOPHYSIOLOGY[1]

Dehydration, as the word is used in clinical medicine or in physiology, refers to a loss of extracellular fluid, i.e., water and solute, primarily sodium and chloride ions. When one wishes to refer to water loss alone, the disturbance is called "hypernatremic dehydration," a condition in which the water loss occurs primarily from cellular water. The terminology is an historical convention; the chemical anatomy and the mechanisms that determine the types of losses are fundamental to understanding water and electrolyte changes in any state, normal or diseased.

Body water volume is equal to 70 per cent of the lean body mass in children in good health after about one week of age (for those born at term). As adipose tissue is added the percentage of body weight as water diminishes so that the well-nourished young adult has about 60 per cent of weight as water, but still has a body water volume equal to 70 per cent of lean body mass.

The body water volume is distributed into extracellular fluid (ECF) and intracellular fluid (ICF), two aqueous phases with very different solutes. The separate compositions are maintained by an energy dependent, active transport system that extrudes sodium ions from cell water. The extracellular water is further subdivided into an intravascular phase, the plasma, and interstitial water. The respective volumes of these fluids in infancy are 45 per cent of lean body mass in ICF, 25 per cent of lean body mass in ECF, plasma 6 per cent, and interstitial fluid 19 per cent of lean body mass. The integrity of the plasma volume is sustained by the relative impermeability of the plasma protein, creating an oncotic pressure as described by Starling.

From the foregoing brief account of chemical anatomy and the mechanisms for maintaining the "spaces," it follows that the body content of the plasma proteins, and of sodium and chloride ions, determines the distribution of body water. In addition, the ICF principal cation, potassium, must also be present to sustain ICF volume. All of these substances then must be considered in a rational therapeutic plan.

Increased loss of stool leads to loss of base (bicarbonate) from the body because the stool water is mildly alkaline. In addition, when extracellular depletion is developing, plasma volume drops eventually, leading to a diminished peripheral perfusion and later to a reduced renal blood flow. The diminished peripheral perfusion leads to tissue hypoxia and thus to anaerobic oxidation with lactic acid accumulation. The reduced renal blood flow prevents the kidney from excreting nonvolatile acids. This last event is the most important one in bringing about acidosis and acidemia in diarrheal disease. When plasma volume is restored, the kidney will restore acid base homeostasis in most instances.

In most circumstances (60–70 per cent of the cases in the United States) loss and intake that are influenced by many homeostatic compensations result in an isotonic constriction of fluids with a normal osmolality and normal plasma (serum) concentrations of sodium. For reasons that will become apparent in the following discussion "classic dehydration" is also referred to at times as "isonatremic dehydration." The important concept is that the body salts are reduced proportionately with the loss of ECF and of plasma volume especially, causing most of the objective signs.

During the course of the illness, when oral replacement of water without salt occurs (while both water and electrolytes are being lost) a hyponatremic dehydrated state ensues. The patient has a relative rise in ICF and a relative lowering in ECF including plasma. Hence circulatory signs appear with lesser volume losses and are progressively more severe with greater degrees of loss.

When water is lost in excess of sodium from either dilute stool loss, from excessive insensible losses, or simply from marked water deprivation, hypernatremic dehydration follows. In this disturbance the ECF is relatively well preserved and the ICF bears the greater loss. The consequences of the loss in the ICF affect the central nervous system (CNS).

Owing to tight junctions between the vascular endothelial cells in the nervous system, the sodium and chloride ions—indeed all passively diffusing solutes—do not equilibrate as rapidly as do water molecules. Osmotic gradients between the nervous system and the plasma are initially resolved by the movement of water alone, which changes nervous tissue volume. This change in volume in turn causes the brain to shrink (when the solute concentration is higher in the plasma) and the capillaries to expand, which sometimes rupture, leading to hemorrhage and thrombosis, serious complications of hypernatremia.

Another more complex phenomenon that occurs is the breakdown of intracellular protein to non-diffusible amino acids such as taurine ("idiogenic osmols"), which limit water loss from cells but make the same cells vulnerable to suddenly available water by causing swelling.

All of the previous mechanisms should be considered when diagnosing and treating dehydration. Care must be taken to restore plasma volume rapidly and the other spaces gradually. In hypernatremic states, water intoxication in particular should be avoided by means of very gradual replacement.

DIAGNOSIS

The plan for therapy begins with clinical assessment of the patient. When available, laboratory analyses add valuable complementary assistance. Even if chemical analyses cannot be performed for many hours, an initial blood sample should be obtained to be analyzed for urea nitrogen, Na^+, Cl^-, and K^+ levels, and CO_2 content. If enough blood and a sufficiently versatile laboratory are available, tests for pH, P_{CO_2}, and Ca^{++} levels are also of value. The role of each of these determinations will be discussed later individually. Since the body weight of the patient (accurately determined and repeated at intervals) constitutes the most important and useful measurement, as much attention should be paid to the technique of weighing as to the laboratory procedures.

Clinical evaluation may be divided into five points of appraisal, in decreasing order of immediate importance: volume, osmolality, hydrogen ion status, intracellular ion deficits, and calcium ion homeostasis (Table 4–1). Each of these points may be discussed usefully in terms of the type of clinical evaluation, usefulness of laboratory measurements, and calculation for physiologic correction during each of the three phases of critical therapy: emergency, initial repletion, and early recovery. First, a 24-hour period of therapy will be considered followed by a breakdown for the first hour, the next six to eight hours, and the remaining hours of the first 24. For the more seriously ill infants, a plan for the second day will be outlined, which will complete the critical therapy of dehydration.

Volume

Water volume repletion and maintenance constitute the most important facets in the treatment of dehydration. Assessment of the therapeutic volume requires three considerations: (1) the deficit, (2) the ongoing usual requirements for normal maintenance, and (3) continuing abnormal losses.

The Deficit

Deficit refers to a loss of volume or mass of water from the hydrated state. When diarrhea causes loss of water and salt in physiologic proportions (about two-thirds of the time in North American experience), clinical signs first appear when about five per cent of the body mass (7% of the body fluid) has been lost over a one or two day period. Tachycardia and dryness of the mucous membranes appear as the earliest signs. Earlier symptoms, such as thirst and a dry feeling in the mouth, are not useful in infants; moreover, thirst may be obscured by nausea. Cessation of tearing and reduced urine output may be noticed early by parents or other observers. Next in order of appearance are evidences of advancing circulatory insufficiency and changes in the elasticity of the skin and subcutaneous tissue. Thus, by the time the deficit has progressed to the order of ten per cent of the weight, the extremities show cyanosis or mottling and diminished temperature. The pulse rate may be very rapid, even for the fever that may also be present. Oliguria becomes manifest. The fontanelle, if open, will be depressed, and the eyeballs appear sunken. The skin and subcutaneous tissue of the abdomen in the infant will show loss of elasticity by sustaining folds when pinched and

Table 4–1. CLINICAL APPRAISAL OF PROBLEMS OF HYDRATION*

Point of Appraisal	Clinical Symptoms and Signs*	Laboratory Determination of Greatest Value
Volume	Circulatory impairment, skin, eye, and fontanelle changes, oliguria.	Body weight; SUN
Osmolality	Hypernatremia: CNS signs are disturbance of consciousness, hypertonicity of muscles, increased reflexes, marked thirst, "inapparent dehydration" with good circulation for degree of loss. Hyponatremia: exaggeration of the signs listed under volume.	Serum Na^+
Hydrogen ion status	Hyperpnea in acidemia.	CO_2 content (serum HCO_3); P_{CO_2}; pH
Intracellular ion deficits	Abdominal distention; muscle weakness; diminished reflexes.	Serum K^+ (limited use); ECG
Calcium ion homeostasis	Tetany, convulsions.	Serum Ca^{++} (complex interpretation); ECG

*Only the symptoms and signs of dehydration have been given in this table. A companion group of signs for the corresponding disturbances of overhydration has been omitted for simplicity. The same points of appraisal and the same laboratory determinations may be used advantageously.

loss of turgor by the slow return of color after pressure. After the age of about 2 years, subcutaneous tissue composition will differ from that of infants, and these last signs usually cannot be elicited. When water loss exceeds ten per cent of body weight, circulatory failure becomes more pronounced, so that at an acute weight loss of about 15 per cent, a moribund, irreversible state may occur.

In the preceding discussion, the repeated reference to weight makes it evident that this measurement delineates the volume deficit. Because pre-illness weight is seldom known, a clinical estimate according to the criteria discussed may be employed usefully with reasonable accuracy. If the previous weight is known, it should be used. A clinical axiom, applicable without significant error, is that changes in body weight within any 24-hour period may be considered to be water. However, one must remember not to extend this period beyond one day, because clinically insignificant deviations within 24 hours may be cumulative and highly significant over longer intervals.

Normal Ongoing Losses (Maintenance)

Although weight constitutes the direct measure of water deficit, normal maintenance requirements of water are a simple function not of mass but rather of energy expenditure. Because the infant and the young child have a higher rate of metabolism per unit of mass than older, large individuals, their obligate water losses, and hence maintenance requirements, are also greater per unit of mass. One hundred calories expended result in 100 ml of water loss through skin, lungs, urine, and stool. This relationship, in which obligate water losses directly follow energy expenditure, roughly parallels the surface area relation to mass, a fact that has led some workers to use surface area in calculation. In fact, neither surface area nor caloric expenditure measurements are made on clinical services. Each system requires for practical application that a table of estimates, such as Table 4–2 or a nomogram, be used to derive from the weight a quantity of water per unit mass appropriate for age and size. The weight remains the practical measurement available.

The fact that two distinct bases, namely the metabolic expenditure and the loss in weight, are necessary for the volume calculation remains the most fundamental contribution by pediatric clinicians to the field of hydration therapy.[2] No single reference base may be used; weight, calories, or surface area alone will not be accurate over a range of ages and sizes. I prefer to use calories rather than surface area for maintenance calculations for two reasons: (1) for clarity of thinking in terms of physiology to stress the fundamental relationship, and (2) because the newborn state and a few other states (edematous and obesity) are exceptions to a simple surface area relationship. If these matters are understood, surface area nomogram enthusiasts may use their nomograms with results equal to those obtained by the scheme proposed here.

Using a value for caloric expenditure at basal conditions from a table requires an additional interpretation of the patient's actual state. If one allows for usual activity, temperature variation, and rate of breathing, as well as observed urine formation, energy expenditure ordinarily may be assumed to be one and one-half times the basal rate. Persistent high fever warrants the doubling of the basal figure; and the extreme combination of persistent high body temperature, hyperventilation, and convulsive muscular activity might triple the basal allotment.

Abnormal Losses

Continued abnormal losses, the third factor in assessing volume requirements, are measured by direct collection and include tube drainages as well as estimated stool losses.

In addition to weight, but much less useful, is a measurement of serum urea nitrogen (SUN) concentration, which helps in assessing volume depletion. The level of this determination depends upon the duration as well as the quantity of deficit, since it reflects the effect of glomerular filtration failure, roughly indicating the degree of severity of ECF loss. Because that compartment sustains most of the loss of volume when water and sodium salts are lost together in physiologic proportion, and in the absence of complicating primary renal disease, the SUN level may be used for retrospective and prognostic estimates.

To illustrate the application of the foregoing discussion, consider a 5½-month-old infant who weighs 5000 gm (5 kg) in the dehydrated state with clinical features suggesting a loss of ten per cent of body weight. This information leads to an estimate of a 500 ml (gm) deficit. For convenience the dehydrated weight justifiably may be used by ignoring the subtraction of a value for the water of oxidation, rather than adding a value for the hydrated weight.

At the age of the patient in the example, these quantities would be of equal arithmetic magnitudes in opposite directions. Estimating the usual requirement figure at this patient's age and size (5 kg × 65 ml/kg, basal × 1½ correction factor) adds about another 500 ml per day (see Table 4–2). Together these values total 1000 ml if the volume of the deficit is to be restored in one day. Continual abnormal losses are observed and added. Details concerning segments are best considered after the remainder of the appraisal is completed. In general, however, except as noted, a volume of water roughly equal to one-half the volume allotment for the first 24 hours (500 ml) will have been administered in six to eight hours; the remaining 500 ml plus the volume of any abnormal losses will have been administered by the end of 24 hours.

Osmolality

Osmolality of body fluids is the second most important general element in evaluation. In a somewhat simplified sense, the content of sodium salts in the body determines the physiologically significant osmolality because Na^+ and Cl^-, owing to their relative exclusion from ICF, by their content in the body determine the distribution of body water into its two main compartments, ECF and ICF. Therefore, sodium concentration constitutes a more clinically relevant determination than the actual osmolality because those solutes that are distributed evenly in body water do not affect the relative size of the compartments.

This knowledge, together with the patient's clinical appearance and course, has led to a classification of dehydration on the basis of sodium concentration in serum. In North America, isonatremic dehydration occurs in about 75 per cent of patients, hypernatremic dehydration in 15 per cent, and hyponatremic dehydration in about 10 per cent of those admitted to hospitals with dehydration. These incidence values vary from one region to another and also with the season and the prevailing feeding practices. In countries where dry whole milk was promoted and made available as an inexpensive food for infants, the incidence of hypernatremic dehydration was higher.[3]

A high sodium concentration, defined as greater than 150 mEq/L of serum, implies relative cellular desiccation and relative preservation of ECF volume; conversely, a low sodium concentration, less than 132 mEq/L, denotes relatively greater ECF depletion per unit volume lost. Hypernatremic dehydration then has, for a given degree of loss in volume, less than the expected evidence of circulatory failure and subcutaneous tissue changes, frequently justifying the description "deceptively inapparent" dehydration. The cellular desiccation produced by hypernatremia leads to a preponderance of CNS symptoms, signs, and pathologic damage. These manifestations usually occur at about the same volume loss as do the circulatory signs of classic or isonatremic dehydration.

Certain features from the history and physical findings enable one to recognize hypernatremia prior to confirmation by laboratory test results. Younger infants have a higher incidence of hypernatremia. Intake usually has stopped abruptly fairly early in the course of the disease. Less constant features that suggest the possibility of hypernatremia include a high solute intake (e.g., full-strength skim milk) just before cessation of intake, persistent high fever, a hot, dry environment (e.g., heated apartment in winter), and hyperventilation. On physical examination, disturbance of consciousness usually is manifested by a peculiar combination of marked lethargy or somnolence, with hyperirritability when the infant is stimulated by touch, noise, or light. Hypertonicity of muscles, often producing mild nuchal rigidity, may occur. More extreme manifestations of CNS involvement include muscle twitchings, tremors, and frank convulsions. The abdominal skin has a velvety feel and, inconstantly, a "doughy" consistency. Circu-

Table 4–2. APPROXIMATE BASAL WATER REQUIREMENTS IN RELATION TO AGE, WEIGHT, AND SURFACE AREA

			Minimal Basal Water Requirement		
Age	**Weight (kg)**	**Surface area (m^2)**	***ml/kg or cal/kg/24 hr***	***ml/m²/24 hr***	***ml/24 hr***
Newborn	2.5–4.0	0.20–0.23	50	750	125–200
1 week–6 months	3.0–8.0	0.20–0.35	65–70	1000–1100	200–250
7 months–12 months	8.0–12.0	0.35–0.45	50–60	1000–1050	500–600
12 months–24 months	10.0–15.0	0.45–0.60	45–50	1000–1050	500–750

lation usually is maintained, but when dehydration exceeds ten per cent of body weight, or when the hypernatremia is very severe (Na^+ > 180 mEq/L), shock may complicate even this variety of dehydration.[1]

Hyponatremic dehydration is most likely to appear when protracted stool losses have produced large electrolyte losses, and especially when this circumstance is accompanied by an ample water intake that is very low in solute (i.e., water without electrolyte). Its clinical manifestation consists of an increase of circulatory failure per unit of volume lost. Thus extreme shock may appear at an earlier stage of volume deficit. The low sodium concentration in patients with kwashiorkor represents a different and more complex phenomenon requiring a therapeutic approach not applicable in this discussion of a better nourished population.

The most common osmolal occurrence in dehydration, a normal concentration of sodium (isonatremia), produces the well-known condition of extracellular depletion with moderate circulatory deficit when about ten per cent of body weight has been lost over a day or two. In isonatremic dehydration, electrolyte balance studies have shown losses of Na^+ in the order of 8 to 15 mEq/kg.[4] Patients with hypernatremic dehydration have lost as little as two to five mEq/kg; hyponatremic patients may have deficits of up to 20 mEq/kg.

With regard to solute loss, hence osmolality, treatment should take into account not only the magnitude of sodium loss, but also the important fact that brain swelling results when dilute solutions of electrolyte are administered rapidly. When the solute requirement is low in hypernatremic dehydration, deficit replacement should be spread evenly over a period of at least 48 hours in order to avoid CNS insult or edema from excessive isotonic ECF expansion.

Except as noted in hypernatremic dehydration, the sodium salt replacement should be planned to take place during the first 24 hours of therapy. During this period, the deficit of sodium so exceeds the amount necessary for normal maintenance that no provision need be made for sodium "requirement." In the 5-kg infant not thought to have hypernatremia in our previous example, the sodium deficit of about 12 mEq/kg (range 8–15 mEq/kg) would be 5 kg × 12 mEq/kg, or 60 mEq (or a range of 40–75 mEq). Administration of this amount of sodium to the infant would produce the necessary expansion of ECF to carry out life functions, including urine formation. The average concentration of sodium in the first day's therapy would thus be 60 mEq/L (range, 40–75 mEq/L). If the hypothetical patient was diagnosed as hypernatremic, the recommended average concentration would be lower, e.g., 25–40 mEq/L. The sodium administered to patients with hypernatremia may even have to exceed the deficit slightly in order to avoid too rapid infusion of water without electrolyte, a circumstance that produces brain swelling.

If restoration of volume and sodium replacement are achieved in patients with reasonably intact, functioning renal and pulmonary systems, the remaining three points of assessment will require little or no attention other than the oral provision of intracellular ions.

Hydrogen Ion Status

Patients with diarrhea usually have a primary excess of H^+ for four reasons: (1) stool water may contain a relatively large amount of HCO_3^-; (2) starvation and dehydration lead to increased production of keto-acids (non-volatile acid production); (3) diminished perfusion of tissue causes increased lactic acid release; and (4) perhaps most importantly, progressive reduction of renal function leads to retention of non-volatile acids (H^+). In spite of compensatory "blowing off" of CO_2, which reduces the P_{CO_2}, pH may fall. The CO_2 content of the serum will be low. PCO_2Cl^- concentration is usually raised in this type of acidosis.

Unless these changes are very severe (CO_2 content < 3 mEq/L) or some persistent impairment of kidney or lung exists, no specific administration of alkali ordinarily will be required. The physiologic proportion of basic anions to the total in ECF is about 1:5 or 1:4. Thus, all deficit repair solutions for acidotic states and all maintenance solutions should have from one-fifth to one-quarter of the anions as base. Although this may with safety be elevated slightly in diarrheal disease, experience shows that this extra base usually is not necessary as long as volume and osmolality needs are met and, very importantly, urine formation occurs. For this reason, the emergency phase of therapy will be optimal if it promotes urine formation.

Intracellular Ion Deficits

The loss of potassium from cells, first demonstrated more than 30 years ago, has proved to be an important cause of the physiologic disturbance of severe diarrheal disease.[5] All infants with severe diarrheal disease will sustain potassium loss, and replacement is necessary during the phases of repletion and early recovery. Clinical signs often not seen until unmasked by initial hydration include hypotonia of muscles, abdominal distention, and weakness. The level of K^+ in serum may be high because of poor glomerular filtration, even in severe K^+ deficit. Because the myocardium is quite sensitive to small (absolute) changes in K^+ levels in serum, caution is required in its administration, particularly prior to the establishment of urine output. Even afterwards, parenteral K^+ must be given carefully, and experience has shown that the safer oral route may be employed in most instances. The magnitude of the deficit may be as much as 10 mEq/kg.[4] This deficit does not necessarily represent a corresponding volume of loss of ICF, because probably not all the K^+ is osmotically active.

Generally, 3 mEq/kg per day is a reasonably effective and safe rate of replacement. If parenteral K^+ must be given, concentrations greater than 40 mEq/L should be avoided, and rates greater than 4 mEq/hr should be avoided. Rates greater than 4 mEq/hr may be risky for small infants.

Correcting Mg^{++} and PO_4 deficits has not been shown to be clinically important.

Calcium Homeostasis

Calcium homeostasis occasionally goes awry during dehydration especially with hypernatremia, resulting in hypocalcemia. However, it rarely leads to tetany.[3] For this reason, during the management of hypernatremic dehydration, the addition of 10 ml of ten per cent calcium gluconate to every 500 ml of intravenous solution has seemed a wise precaution.

MANAGEMENT

Having presented the principles, let us return to the example. At this point a volume of 1000 ml has been tentatively established for administration during the first 24 hours of treatment. The sodium content will be approximately 60 mEq and the potassium content will be about 15mEq. The 75mEq of anions should be apportioned approximately 55 mEq as chloride and 20 mEq as base, e.g., bicarbonate, lactate, or acetate. The sodium solution should also include glucose to supply calories.

As previously stated, this therapy should be considered in three phases: emergency, repletion, and early recovery.

Phase 1—Emergency

Immediate infusion of a volume of fluid over 10 to 15 minutes to expand the intravascular compartment and thus restore circulation should be the beginning of therapy for every patient in circulatory distress. The following fluids have been used successfully: whole blood, single donor plasma, five per cent albumin, and a ten per cent glucose solution with a sodium concentration of 75 mEq/L, bicarbonate of 20 mEq/L, and chloride of 55 mEq/L. Blood and plasma have fallen into mild disfavor because of suspected problems with hepatitis and actual problems of availability. The albumin solutions are not available everywhere but have proved particularly useful for the coincidence of shock and hypernatremia, a potentially deadly combination. I prefer hypertonic glucose (10%) to plain electrolyte solutions (e.g., lactated Ringer's) because of the more immediate expansion of the intravascular space and the empiric impression of more rapid urine formation. Solutions containing albumin are preferred for malnourished infants and for infants with hypernatremia plus circulatory deficit.

The volume of these rapid infusions should be 20 ml/kg of body weight for blood, plasma, or five per cent albumin and 40 ml/kg for the solution of ten per cent glucose with 75 mEq/L of sodium. The larger volume (40 ml/kg) will require 30 to 40 minutes for administration.

Phase 2—Repletion

The remaining water volume with electrolytes may now be combined as a single solution for the rest of the 24 hours, with the rate adjusted appropriately. The glucose concentration now should be reduced to five per cent. In the example of the 5-kg infant with an estimated deficit of 500 ml, if the amount already administered in Phase 1 was 40 ml/kg, then 200 ml subtracted from 1000 ml leaves 800 ml to be infused. Fifteen milliequivalents of sodium have been given, leaving 45 to be given. Potassium will be added after urine formation has been assured by clinical observation; 15 mEq will be added in a concentration not to exceed 40 mEq/L. The anions for Na^+ and K^+ combined should be approximately one-quarter base (HCO_3^-, acetate, or lactate) and three-quarters chloride. The rate of administration should be adjusted to deliver the remaining one-half of the estimate for the first 24 hours, 300 ml (500 − 200 = 300 ml), by the time eight hours have elapsed from the onset of therapy. Even though body composition remains abnormal, the circulation and renal function will be adequately restored, enabling physiologic mechanisms to operate maximally in the final recovery phase. Because ongoing losses have occurred, the patient's water volume remains somewhat less than the estimated normal.

Note that all of the plan as outlined has been based on clinical observations and general principles. If laboratory values are available during this phase of therapy, suitable adjustments may be made if, for instance, the Na^+ concentration is in an unexpected range or the acidosis is more severe than supposed. Only occasionally will such adjustments be truly necessary, since the model permits treatment of a fairly wide latitude of disturbances narrowed by decisions derived from clinical data.

In the hospitals where only commercial polyionic solutions are available, they may be readily modified to the compositions indicated herein. Small differences, even up to 20 per cent in concentration values, need not be adjusted. I do not use these solutions because of the inflexibility their exclusive use imposes.

If the example given had been a patient suspected of having hypernatremia, the rate of fluid administration would have been slower during repletion, which then would have been planned for a 48-hour period. In that event, the Na^+ concentration of the intravenous infusion would be at the lower level (25–40 mEq/L), and K^+ salts would be added at the earliest safe moment. The selected rate should then deliver the deficit volume plus two days' maintenance volume added together in equal hourly increments over 48 hours.

Phase 3—Early Recovery

After eight hours many patients may take fluids by mouth, and their therapy may be continued with an oral electrolyte-glucose solution containing sodium and potassium salts. Those patients who are more severely ill should remain on the same infusion, now slowed in rate to deliver the rest of the calculated volume by the end of 24 hours. Observed abnormal losses will be added quantitatively to the infusion as 120 mEq/L sodium chloride for gastric drainage and 40 mEq/L sodium chloride plus 40 mEq/L of potassium acetate for intestinal loss. Several interim weighings will give valuable information about success of therapy. The example given and the use of solutions described in the preceding text are summarized in Table 4–3.

Ideally, the patient should show a seven to nine per cent gain in weight at 24 hours. Too little or too much weight gain suggests an error in appraisal or technique. Except as previously noted for hypernatremic dehydration, the next 24 hours will, in most instances, be calculated as maintenance plus any continuing abnormal losses; the deficit usually will have been overcome. The same five-point analysis (volume, osmolality, hydrogen ion status, ICF deficits and calcium ion homeostasis) should be repeated, and individual variation should be managed accordingly. In most patients recovery from the critical phases of the illness will be indicated by the ability to take fluid and solute by mouth. On the second day, whether oral feeding containing calories as carbohydrate and protein may be added or whether high-caloric parenteral feedings should be used depends upon the state of nutrition, the etiology and duration of the disorder, and a number of other factors. These matters have become increasingly more important as the problem of hydration has yielded to better understanding and techniques.

CASE 1—INFANT WITH ENTERITIS AND ISOTONIC DEHYDRATION*

History. A 3-month-old infant has had loose, watery stools for three days, followed by marked anorexia with vomiting four times during the last 12 hours. No urine has been seen for ten hours.

Physical Examination. The weight is 5.0 kg. Temperature is 37.2°C, pulse is 160 per minute, respirations are 60 per minute, and blood pressure is 90/58 mmHg.

His fontanelle and eyes are sunken. Extremities are cold and skin over them is mottled. Abdominal skin stands in folds when pinched (loss of elasticity). Color returns to skin poorly after pinching (loss of

*This and the next three case histories are modified from Finberg L, Kravath RE and Fleischman AR. *In*: Water and Electrolytes in Pediatrics. Philadelphia: WB Saunders, 1982: Chapters 16 and 17.

turgor). No tears. Cry is weak. Reflexes are normal, sensorium is good. Muscle tone is less than normal. Bladder is not palpable. He is not observed to void. Few bowel sounds.

Assessment

Volume

DEFICIT. On the basis of clinical signs and early shock—ten per cent of body weight (100 mg/kg) or 500 ml.

OBLIGATORY WATER LOSSES FOR 24 HOURS. Basal expenditure × 1½ = 5.0 × 60 × 1½ = 450 ml. Note that the dehydrated weight has been used, a small "error" offset for clinical purposes by not taking into account the water of metabolic oxidation (12 ml/100 cal), which is a small amount of "error" in the opposite direction.

ABNORMAL LOSSES. To be observed with the expectation that the fasting state will minimize them.

TOTAL ESTIMATED VOLUME FOR 24 HOURS. 500 + 450 = 950 ml.

Osmolality. The illness is of several days' duration, which suggests loss of electrolytes and water. Physical examination shows circulatory deficit and no signs of CNS dysfunction. Isotonic constriction of body fluids with predominant loss from the ECF is concluded.

How much Na^+ should be in the replacement fluid? Enough to give a concentration of 150 mEq/L in the deficit fraction of therapy (500 ml) or 75 mEq/L of sodium.

Why not include electrolyte in the "maintenance" portion of therapy? With a large Na^+ deficit being replaced, there is no need to add the very small amount of Na^+ for normal maintenance. The sodium salts scheduled to be given, plus glucose, will protect red blood cells from hemolysis.

Hydrogen Ion. In enteritis, a mild to moderate acidemia may be assumed to be present because of loss of base, acid production secondary to starvation, poor tissue perfusion, and, especially, oliguria. Blood gas determination shows P_{O_2} to be 90 mmHg, P_{CO_2} 20 mmHg, pH 7.28, and CO_2 content (HCO_3^-) 8 mEq/L.

Should IV hypertonic bicarbonate be given stat? No. Restoration of volume, especially plasma volume, will enable the kidney and lung to compensate and will correct acidemia of this degree. Give one-quarter to one-third of anion in therapy as base (HCO_3^-, lactate, or acetate). Patient is sick enough without risking cerebral hemorrhage!

ICF Ion Losses (K^+). In any case of enteritis, K^+ losses are of the order of 3 to 10 mEq/kg. Here, the suggestion of hypoactive bowel and poor muscle tone indicates K^+ deficiency.

Add K^+ as chloride or acetate to IV solution, 3 mEq/kg/day or 20 mEq/L as soon as patient voids or has detectable urine in bladder.

Calcium Homeostasis. No special problem is anticipated unless PO_4^- retention is unusual. A high SUN may prove to be a marker for PO_4^- retention.

What laboratory data should be obtained for additional analysis and confirmation? (Weight [mass] and blood gases have already been measured.) Order serum analysis for Na^+, Cl^-, K^+, SUN, and CO_2 content (direct analysis to confirm derived values from blood gas) as a minimum. Save some of the sample for Ca, P, Mg, protein, and glucose analyses if additional problems arise. If you automatically receive 18 or more analyses from an autoanalyzer, dividing the sample will not achieve the intended parsimony accomplished by ordering only what is necessary, as someday health care economists may insist.

Laboratory Results

Na^+	138 mEq/L
Cl^-	116 mEq/L
HCO_3^-	8 mEq/L
K^+	4.6 mEq/L
SUN	50 mg/100 ml

Therapeutic Implementation

Phase 1 (Emergency). Duration: 40 minutes. Two-hundred ml (40 ml/kg) to be given. Step 1 (20 minutes): Plasma (modified) or five per cent albumin—20 ml/kg or 100 ml. Step 2 (20 minutes): Ten per cent glucose solution—20 ml/kg or 100 ml. After Step 2, patient voids 25 ml of urine.

Total volume for Phase 1: 40 ml/kg (200 ml)—one-half for deficit, one-half for "maintenance" water.

Why Step 2 in Phase 1? The glucose solution was given to stop ketosis, provide calories, add water to plasma, and provide water for urine formation.

Alternative Phase 1. Ten per cent glucose with Na^+ 80 mEq/L, Cl^- 60 mEq/L, and HCO_3^- 20 mEq/L over 40 minutes. As before, patient would void 25 ml of urine—easy to specify here, but sometimes missing in real life.

Phase 2 (Repletion). Duration: 7 hours. Intravenous therapy begun to complete administration of 475 ml (one-half of total estimated volume for 24 hours or 950 ml), of which 200 ml has been given. Solution is five per cent glucose with Na^+ 75 to 80 mEq/L, K^+ 20 mEq/L, Cl^- 75 to 80 mEq/L, and

Table 4–3. SUMMARY OF THERAPEUTIC MEASURES USED IN INFANT (5 KG) WITH A 10% BODY WEIGHT LOSS

Phase	Time	Water (ml)	Na^+ (mEq)	K^+ (mEq)	Cl (mEq)	Base (mEq)	Glucose (gm)
1	0–20 min	200	15	0.0	11.0	4.0	20
2	20 min–8 hr	300	15	5.6	16.5	4.1	15
3	8–24 hr	500	30	9.4	27.5	11.9	25
Total	24 hr	1000	60	15.0	55.0	20.0	60

acetate 20 mEq/L. If the patient had not produced urine, the potassium acetate would have been temporarily withheld, and sodium bicarbonate would have been given, 20 mEq/L, with the Cl^- 55 to 60 mEq/L. Rate of administration is 275 ml in 7 hours = 39 ml/hr = 0.66 ml/min.

Phase 3 (Early Recovery). Duration: 16 hours. Continue administration of Phase 2 solution at slower rate: 475 ml in 16 hours = 28 ml/hr = 0.5 ml/min. Alternatively, Phase 3 could be carried out per os, if patient's condition permits or if the IV line falls out.

Phase 4 (Full Recovery). Resumption of oral intake with gradual introduction of infant formula, adding 20 per cent of volume each day with an electrolyte-glucose mixture as the remainder of intake (150 ml/kg/day).

CASE 2—INFANT WITH HYPONATREMIC DEHYDRATION

History. A 6-week-old infant developed a watery diarrhea (6–8 loose stools per day), which has persisted for a week. For the first four days, normal feedings supplemented with plain water were maintained. For the next three days, milk feedings were taken poorly, but weak tea and flavored sugar-water were accepted. Since the onset of vomiting 6 hours ago, there has been no fluid or food intake. The last urination that wet the diaper was noted 12 hours ago.

Physical Examination. Weight is 4.0 kg. Temperature is 36.8°C, pulse is 180/min, respirations are 60/minute, blood pressure is 80/50 mmHg.

Her fontanelle and eyes are sunken. Skin is cold and mottled, showing loss of elasticity and turgor. No tears. Cry is weak. Heart tones are of poor quality. She responds poorly to examiner and to stimuli generally. Tendon reflexes normal. No irritability and patient is very apathetic.

Assessment

Volume

DEFICIT. At least ten per cent of body weight (100 ml/kg) or 400 ml.

OBLIGATORY WATER LOSSES FOR 24 HOURS. Basal expenditure × 1½ = 4.0 × 60 × 1½ = 360 ml.

ABNORMAL LOSSES. To be observed.

TOTAL ESTIMATED VOLUME FOR 24 HOURS. 760 ml.

Osmolality. The history suggests loss of water and sodium salts with partial replacement of water only. Circulatory signs are marked. The change in sensorium is more likely the result of shock than of hypernatremia. Suspect hyponatremic or isonatremic state with greater than ten per cent weight loss. Plan to give more sodium than for isonatremic dehydration. Obtain laboratory analysis as quickly as possible.

Hydrogen Ion. In a very young patient, anticipate acidosis or acidemia from enteric losses and circulatory deficit. Do not anticipate ketonuria in a patient of this age.

ICF Ion Losses (K^+). After a long period of stool loss; K^+ deficit will be high. Replace K^+ as soon as possible after urine formation becomes apparent.

Calcium Homeostasis. Not an anticipated problem but young age of patient makes hypocalcemia a possibility, especially during therapy with base. Watch for high phosphate level in serum despite fasting, if SUN is high.

Laboratory Results

Na^+	128 mEq/L
Cl^-	99 mEq/L
HCO_3^-	12 mEq/L
K^+	3.9 mEq/L
SUN	85 mg/100 ml

Therapeutic Implementation

Phase 1 (Emergency). Duration: 40 to 60 minutes. Step 1: Plasma (modified) or five per cent albumin—20 ml/kg or 80 ml. Step 2: 10 per cent glucose with Na^+ 75 mEq/L, Cl^- 55 mEq/L, and HCO_3^- 20 mEq/L—20 ml/kg or 80 ml.

If laboratory data had not been available, the solution in Step 2 might have been given without added sodium salts. No harm would likely have occurred so long as the next phase was compensatory.

Alternative Phase 1. Assuming laboratory values were known, ten per cent glucose with Na^+ 120 mEq/L, Cl^- 110 mEq/L, and HCO_3^- 30 mEq/L—40 ml/kg or 160 ml.

Total volume for Phase 1 = 160 ml.

Phase 2 (Repletion). Duration six to seven hours assuming urine formation during or after Phase 1. (If no urine appears withhold potassium and revise maintenance volume to one-half of previous allotment.) Five per cent glucose with Na^+ 120 mEq/L, K^+ 20 mEq/L, Cl^- 100 mEq/L, and HCO_3^- lactate, or acetate, singly or combined, 40 mEq/L in 220 ml. The sodium level could range from 100 to 130 mEq/L.

Total volume for Phase 2: 220 ml (one-half of total estimated volume for 24 hours or 760/2, minus volume already administered in Phase 1).

Phase 3 (Early Recovery). Duration: 16 hours. Use the same solution as in Phase 2—380 ml—but administer at a slower rate.

CASE 3—INFANT WITH HYPERNATREMIC DEHYDRATION OF MODERATE SEVERITY

History. A 2-month-old infant has had a high fever for four days. She took milk feedings until 6 hours ago when she vomited, and she has vomited twice since then. She seems thirsty. Loose stools began eight hours ago. The milk feedings were of whole cow's milk.

Physical Examination. The weight is 4 kg. Temperature is 39.5°C, pulse rate is 150 per minute, respirations are 70 per minute, and blood pressure is 100/65 mmHg.

The infant is markedly lethargic, but when stimulated she is over-responsive and very irritable. Her skin is warm and feels velvety smooth but thickened (doughy). Turgor and elasticity are good. Muscle tone is increased; reflexes are very brisk. Neck is slightly resistant to flexion. Fontanelle is normal. Patient voided 30 ml of urine during the examination.

Clinical Analysis. A high solute diet, a prolonged high grade fever, and the abrupt cessation of intake without much stool loss, plus classic examination findings, suggest hypernatremic dehydration as the probable physiologic disturbance.

What should be done in the emergency phase (Phase 1)? Skip Phase 1. Circulation is good, no physiologic emergency exists, and urine formation has been observed. If patient is not so obliging, start administration of IV solution (described later) without K^+ and at an increased rate for 20 to 30 minutes. That will usually result in urine production. If not, withhold the K^+ and confer with a consultant if necessary.

Proceed with assessment after drawing blood for laboratory analyses. Calculate fluid requirement in the usual way.

Assessment

Volume

DEFICIT. 100 ml/kg (10%) of body weight or 400 ml.

ONGOING LOSSES. 4 × 65 × 1½ × 2 (days) = 780 ml.

TOTAL ESTIMATED VOLUME FOR 48 HOURS. Round off to 1180 to 1200 ml, which is to be given over 48 hours.

Osmolality. There is cellular dehydration. Sodium chloride needs are probably small—2 to 4 mEq/kg, or 8 to 15 mEq total. Use as low a concentration of NaCl as is consistent with the avoidance of water intoxication. Patient may be hyperglycemic.

Hydrogen Ion. Hypernatremic patients are often acidemic at this age. Blood gas levels in this patient are now as follows: P_{O_2} 95 mmHg, P_{CO_2} 30 mmHg, pH 7.32, and CO_2 content (HCO_3^-) 12 mEq/L. Give one-half of anion as base.

ICF Ion Losses (K^+). Administration of K^+ salts enables water to be given with low Na^+ concentration and yet avoids water intoxication.

Calcium Homeostasis. Young hypernatremic patients frequently have low calcium levels. Plan to add calcium gluconate to the IV solution. This procedure interdicts the use of bicarbonate as an anion because of possible concretions in the tubing. Use lactate or acetate as base.

Laboratory Results

Na^+	160 mEq/L
Cl^-	130 mEq/L
HCO_3^-	12 mEq/L
K^+	4.1 mEq/L
SUN	15 mg/100 ml
Glucose	250 mg/100 ml
Calcium	8.0 mg/100 ml
Ca^{++}	3.9 mg/100 ml

Therapeutic Implementation

Phase 2 (Repletion). IV solution: 1200 ml of water (2–3% glucose) to which has been added, for example, Na^+ 30 mEq/L (20–40 mEq/L), Cl^- 30 mEq/L (20–40 mEq/L), K^+ 40 mEq/L (30–40 mEq/L), and acetate 40 mEq/L (30–40 mEq/L), with calcium gluconate, 20 ml of ten per cent solution (180 mg of calcium). Rate of administration is 1200 ml in 48 hours or 25 ml/hr.*

Why not supply 2½ per cent glucose, 50 ml/kg, over six hours, since water is what the patient really needs? A convulsion would probably occur because of brain swelling (water intoxication). We have avoided this complication for 15 years, after years of almost weekly occurrence, by the technique described earlier.

Why not achieve expansion with isotonic or one-half isotonic sodium salt solution (75–150 mEq/L)? This will not cause the hypernatremia to worsen or the brain to swell. True, but the patient will probably become edematous and, if high insensible water losses continue, her hypernatremia may worsen and hemorrhage may occur. The early observation of this special difficulty in such patients led to systemic studies of hypernatremic dehydration in the early 1950s. Frequently, one may give such therapy without apparent damage, but it involves a small risk of mortality and a risk of the morbidity of CNS damage a few years later, which are best avoided.

If the patient had a more extreme hyperglycemia, should she have been given insulin? No. Rapid reduction of ECF glucose to physiologic levels is tantamount to rapid water infusion, which causes brain swelling and convulsions. The "diabetic state" is transient and will disappear over a 36-hour period.

CASE 4—INFANT WITH HYPERNATREMIC DEHYDRATION PLUS SHOCK

History. A 3-month-old infant fed whole cow's milk became ill with high fever during the winter. After one day of fever, profuse watery diarrhea began (2–3 stools/hr) along with vomiting; the last time he vomited coffee-grounds–like material. The patient was hospitalized after 16 hours of these symptoms. Urine was last observed 6 hours prior to admission.

Physical Examination. Weight is 5.3 kg. Temperature is 39.1°C, pulse is 160/minute, respirations are 55/minute, blood pressure is 60/30 mmHg.

This infant is very sick, and unaware of his surroundings, but he has increased muscle tone including nuchal resistance to flexion and very brisk deep tendon reflexes. Facies is anxious—starting and unresponsive. Skin shows some loss of elasticity, feels thick or doughy; turgor is fair to poor. Acrocyanosis is present. Pulse is rapid, moderate in strength. Heart tones are good.

*Ranges are given in parentheses.

I. Diagnose the physiologic disturbance using five criteria.
   A. Volume—test for circulatory insufficiency; note pulse rate, skin color, temperature, and turgor. Check skin elasticity. From these data estimate the volume deficit.
   B. Osmolality—review history for evidence of unusual water or salt intake or loss. Assess duration of illness and the type and amount of oral intake. Look for CNS dysfunction and note state of consciousness.
   C. H^+ ion status—presence or absence of hyperventilation; review history.
   D. ICF ion loss—estimate the volume of stool losses semiquantitatively from history, including amount and duration.
   E. ECF—skeleton homeostasis; small or young infants and suspected hypernatremic patients.

II. Estimate 24- or 48-hour total therapy.
   A. Volume.
      1. Deficit.
      2. Estimated 24- to 48-hour maintenance.
      3. Continuing loss.
   B. Composition—for deficit volume (isonatremia).
      1. Give sodium of 150 mEq/L, or 90–110 mEq/L for hypernatremic patients.
      2. Chloride and base anions distributed from I C above.
      3. Potassium supplement—3 mEq/kg/24 hours for diarrheal disease and most other dehydrating illnesses.
      4. Calcium—for symptoms or prophylaxis in hypernatremia.
      5. For maintenance volume—no sodium salts required.
      6. Special solution for hypernatremia—sodium 25–30 mEq/L, chloride 30–40 mEq/L, potassium 40 mEq/L, base (lactate, acetate 25–40 mEq/L, + 10 ml of 10% calcium gluconate/500 ml).

III. Implement therapy.
   A. Emergency (1 hour); skip phase if no circulatory deficit present.
      1. 20 ml/kg plasma (5% albumin) for 20 minutes and 20 ml/kg 10% glucose in H_2O for 20–40 minutes.
      2. 40 ml/kg 10% glucose with sodium 75 mEq/L, chloride 55 mEq, base (HCO_3, lactate) 20 mEq/L, or
      3. 50 ml/kg lactated Ringer's.
   B. Repletion (5–7 hours)—one-half of estimated 24-hour volume (deficit + maintenance/2) as 5 per cent glucose with sodium 50–75 mEq/L, chloride 30–60 mEq, base 20–40 mEq/L. Potassium, if urine present, 20 mEq/L.
   C. For hypernatremia—following emergency phase, if any, special solution given in equal hourly increments over 48 hours (including 48-hour maintenance volume).

IV. Recovery—16–18 hours, continue solution from III, adding potassium if not already added, assuming urine formation is occurring.

Figure 4–1. Protocol for the treatment of severe dehydration.

Clinical Analysis. History and findings are suggestive of both hypernatremia and shock; both are probably present. Give immediate emergency infusion of albumin solution, 20 ml/kg, after drawing blood for analyses.

Assessment

Volume

DEFICIT. More than ten per cent of body weight. Tentatively assume 12 per cent—12 ml/kg × 5.3 kg = 640 ml.

ONGOING LOSSES. 5.3 × 65 × 1½ × 2 (days) = 1040 ml.

ABNORMAL LOSSES. To be observed.

TOTAL ESTIMATED VOLUME FOR 48 HOURS. 640 + 1040 = 1680 ml.

Osmolality. Hypernatremic state.

Hydrogen Ion. Acidemia likely.

ICF Ion Losses (K^+). Liberal K^+ administration needed.

Calcium Homeostasis. Mild hypocalcemia probable. Laboratory data confirm that hyperglycemia is also present.

Laboratory Results

Na^+	168 mEq/L
Cl^-	139 mEq/L
K^+	5.6 mEq/L
HCO_3^-	8.0 mEq/L
SUN	75 mg/100 ml
Glucose	420 mg/100 ml
Calcium	7.8 mg/100 ml

Therapeutic Implementation

Phase 1 (Emergency). Five per cent albumin (20 ml/kg)—110 ml in 20 minutes. Patient improved; acrocyanosis gone, turgor good and urine produced.

Phase 2 (Repletion). Start hypernatremic regimen with 1570 ml over 48 hours. Solution: 2½ per cent glucose with Na^+ 25 mEq/L, K^+ 40 mEq/L, Cl^- 25 mEq/L, and acetate 40 mEq/L, to which has been added calcium gluconate, 30 ml of ten per cent solution. Rate of administration is 33 ml/hr.

This infant is desperately ill and will not survive if treatment is mishandled; and he might easily have CNS complications unless managed very carefully.

REFERENCES

1. Finberg L, Kravath RE, Fleischman AR. *In*: Water and Electrolytes in Pediatrics. Philadelphia: WB Saunders, 1982:5–135, 147–157.
2. Darrow DC. The significance of body size. Am J Dis Child 1959; *98*:416.
3. Taitz LS, Byers HD. High caloric osmolar feedings and hypertonic dehydration. Arch Dis Child 1972; *47*:257.
4. Darrow DC, Pratt EL, Flett J Jr, et al. Disturbances of water and electrolytes in infantile diarrhea. Pediatrics 1949; *3*:429.
5. Govan CD, Darrow DC. The use of potassium chloride in the treatment of diarrhea in infants. J Pediatr 1946; *28*:544.
6. Sperrotto G, Carrazza FR, Marcondes E. Treatment of diarrheal dehydration. Am J Clin Nutr 1977; *30*:1947.

CHAPTER

5

Acute Poisoning

Pierre Gaudreault, M.D.
Frederick H. Lovejoy, Jr., M.D.

Ingestion of toxic materials by children is a common occurrence. It is estimated that annually about 6,000,000 children will ingest toxic products. Children under the age of 5 years represent 80 per cent of these poisonings. Fortunately, the majority of episodes result in low morbidity and mortality. Plants, household products, cosmetics, and over-the-counter preparations are the most frequently ingested substances in children less than 5 years. Intoxication in a child of less than 5 years is the result of accidental ingestion. In adolescents and young adults, it is the result of a suicide attempt, usually with prescription or non-prescription drugs. Intoxication resulting from recreational drug use will not be discussed in this chapter.[1]

Poisonings occur as a result of the ingestion, inhalation, or exposure (rectal, dermal, parenteral) to foreign products. Chemicals, medications, and biologic materials of animal or plant origin are the most common.[2, 3]

DIAGNOSIS

Optimal management of a patient with acute poisoning requires an accurate diagnosis as suggested by the clinical history and physical examination findings and confirmed by laboratory test results.

Clinical History

Following exposure to a toxic agent, initial information the physician obtains should include: (1) identification of the toxic agent, (2) determination of the time and route of exposure, and (3) estimation of the amount ingested. The accuracy of the clinical history is often difficult to ascertain following an acute poisoning, especially when the episode is the result of a suicide gesture or street drug abuse. The history given by a suicidal patient is frequently incorrect. In addition, the contents of street drugs are often misidentified, e.g., drugs sold as amphetamines frequently contain phenolpropanolamine, caffeine, or ephedrine. The physician's awareness of medicine present in the patient's house or current knowledge of drugs locally abused will assist in the identification of the ingested agent. In the case of accidental ingestion, the history is usually more reliable. Determination of the exact name of the ingested product is essential because products with similar names often contain different chemical constituents. For example, Anacin contains aspirin and caffeine, whereas Anacin 3 contains acetaminophen and caffeine. Turpentine and paint thinner are also problematic. Both can be used as paint thinner; turpentine has a greater risk for systemic toxicity, whereas aspiration is the major hazard with paint thinners.

Determination of the time of ingestion is useful. Most patients will develop symptoms within two to four hours of ingestion. The majority of patients who do not show signs or symptoms within six to eight hours of ingestion will remain asymptomatic. However, toxins such as acetaminophen, diphenoxylate hydrochloride, and paraquat, and toxins from the mushroom *Amanita phalloides,* produce symptoms that may be delayed from 12 hours to a few days.[4] The determination of the time of ingestion is of special importance for acetaminophen overdose because the risk of developing hepatotoxicity and the need for Mucomyst (*N*-acetylcysteine) therapy are based mainly on acetaminophen serum concentration at different times after ingestion.[5]

Another important factor is the amount ingested. Although an accurate estimate is difficult to obtain following a suicidal gesture, the amount accidentally ingested by young children can often be determined with the assistance of the parent. In the child, one swallow is equivalent to 5 ml, and in the adolescent it is equal to 10 to 15 ml. When determining therapy, it is important to use the largest estimated amount. If more than one child has taken the poison, it should be assumed that each child has taken the total amount of ingested substance.

Median lethal doses (LD_{50}) are of relatively limited use in clinical toxicology. The LD_{50} can give a rough estimate of the potential toxicity of a given toxin, but it must be remembered that LD_{50}s have been determined in animals or, in some cases, derived from previous case reports in humans. Data from animal investigations are applied only with difficulty to humans, and the accuracy of the reported ingested amount is often of questionable reliability.

Physical Examination

Signs and symptoms are often nonspecific, but in certain instances they may suggest potential toxic agents. For example, miosis is generally seen in patients who have taken narcotics, cholinergic agents, phenothiazines, barbiturates, and alcohols,[6] whereas sympathomimetic agents such as amphetamines or cocaine, psychotropic drugs, and anticholinergic drugs such as tricyclic antidepressants will produce mydriasis. A list of substances with their most frequently associated clinical manifestations, given by system, is presented in Table 5–1.

Assessing and monitoring the patient's respiratory rate, pulse, blood pressure, and state of consciousness are of primary importance. Frequent reappraisals of the heart and respiratory rate, blood pressure, reflexes, response to verbal or painful stimuli, and pupillary signs will help define the severity and progression of clinical illness. These measurements may be also useful in assessing the response to antidotal therapy.

Laboratory Findings

Laboratory analysis should be performed to confirm the substance ingested and to evaluate the biochemical status of the patient. Several

Table 5–1. CLINICAL MANIFESTATION BY SYSTEM WITH ASSOCIATED TOXIC SUBSTANCES

Manifestation	Substances
Central Nervous System	
Depression and coma	Sedatives-hypnotics, narcotics, anticonvulsants, tranquilizers, tricyclic antidepressants, phenothiazines, antimuscarinic agents, hypoglycemic agents, alcohols, aromatic hydrocarbons, carbon monoxide, lead, mercury, lithium, cyanide, gases, solvents.
Stimulation and/or seizures	Amphetamines, xanthines, sympathomimetic agents, psychotropic drugs (phencyclidine, lysergic acid diethylamide, mescaline), cocaine, nicotine, salicylates, ergot, camphor, lead, strychnine, organophosphates, carbamates, chlorinated insecticides.
Hallucinations	Psychotropic drugs, amphetamines, alcohol withdrawal, antihistamines, antimuscarinic agents, cocaine, camphor, tricyclic antidepressants.
Hyperpyrexia	Salicylates, atropine.
Ocular System	
Mydriasis	Antimuscarinic agents, sympathomimetic agents, psychotropic drugs, cocaine, amphetamines.
Miosis	Narcotics, organophosphate insecticides, parasympathomimetic drugs.
Blurred vision	Antimuscarinic agents, alcohols.
Colored vision	Digitalis, quinine.
Scotomas	Quinine, salicylates.
Red eye	Marijuana.
Nystagmus	Dilantin, phencyclidine.
Auditory System	
Tinnitus	Salicylates, streptomycin, ergot, quinine.

Table continued on following page.

Table 5–1. CLINICAL MANIFESTATION BY SYSTEM WITH ASSOCIATED TOXIC SUBSTANCES (*Continued*)

Manifestation	Substances
Cardiovascular System	
Arrhythmias	Digitalis, quinidine, tricyclic antidepressants, phenothiazines.
Tachycardia	Amphetamines, sympathomimetic agents, xanthines, cocaine, tricyclic antidepressants.
Bradycardia	Beta blockers, cardiac glycosides, quinidine.
Hypotension	Narcotics, phenothiazines, antihypertensive agents, tricyclic antidepressants.
Hypertension	Cocaine, amphetamines.
Respiratory System	
Hypoventilation	CNS depressants.
Hyperventilation	Salicylates, cocaine, nicotine, carbon dioxide.
Abnormal odor on breath of:	
Alcohol	Alcohols, phenols, chloral hydrate.
Acetone	Alcohol, acetone, lacquer.
Wintergreen	Methyl salicylate.
Garlic	Phosphorus, arsenic.
Bitter almonds	Cyanide.
Pears	Chloral hydrate, turpentine, camphor.
Gastrointestinal System	
Nausea, vomiting, and diarrhea	Almost any toxic substance can produce these signs or symptoms.
Increased salivation	Organophosphate insecticides, mushrooms.
Decreased salivation	Antimuscarinic agents, antihistamines.
Genitourinary System	
Urine retention	Tricyclic antidepressants, anticholinergic agents.
Dark green urine	Phenol, resorcinol.
Skin and Teguments	
Cyanosis	Nitrites, nitrobenzene, aniline dyes.
Jaundice	Carbon tetrachloride, benzene, aniline dyes, chromates, phenothiazines, quinacrine.
Staining	
Black	Bismuth.
Flushed face	Atropine.
Discoloration of gums	Lead, bismuth, arsenic.
Hematologic System	
Pink blood	Carbon monoxide or cyanide.
Brown blood	Methemoglobinemia.

techniques such as rapid screening tests and the toxic screen may be used to identify the toxic agents.

There are a limited number of rapid screening tests. A flat plate of the abdomen may reveal the presence of radiopaque substances such as heavy metals (lead, mercury, arsenic, etc.), iron-containing capsules and tablets, and less consistently, phenothiazine and chloral hydrate capsules. An x-ray film taken following gastric emptying demonstrates the effectiveness of the removal procedure. A ferric chloride test detects the presence of salicylates or phenothiazines in serum or urine. The test consists of boiling 10 ml of urine and then adding five to ten drops of 10 per cent ferric chloride solution to the urine. A change to green-purple indicates the presence of phenothiazines; a change to burgundy indicates the presence of salicylates. Several substances produce color changes in the plasma. Patients suffering from carbon monoxide poisoning may have bright red blood. Chocolate-colored blood that does not change on exposure to air suggests the presence of methemoglobinemia. Measurement of the anion gap or serum osmolality may also be useful. An elevated anion gap ($Na^+ + K^+ = HCO_3^- + Cl^- + 12$) suggests methanol, ethylene glycol, salicylate, or paraldehyde poisoning. Ethanol, isopropyl alcohol, ethylene glycol, and methanol ingestion may increase serum osmolality (osmolality is 2 × serum Na^+ + BUN/2.8 + blood glucose/ 18).

The response to several pharmacologic agents can assist in the identification of ingested toxins, including naloxone hydrochloride for narcotics, physostigmine for anticholinergic agents, diphenhydramine for phenothiazines which induce extrapyramidal signs, atropine for organophosphate insecticides, deferoxamine for iron, and pyridoxine for isoniazid. Recommended dosages for these agents are given in Table 5–2.

Identification of the specific toxin usually depends on qualitative tests performed on blood or urine or a quantitative measurement using blood. Qualitative identification of an ingested product does not quantify the severity of an intoxication. When qualitative and quantitative tests are used in conjunction with clinical assessment and pharmacologic data on the ingested substance, a logical approach to management is possible. Quantitative measurement does determine the severity of a poisoning. A direct correlation between the blood concentration and the severity of the intoxication must exist for quantification of an ingested substance to be useful. Serum concentrations of aspirin, acetaminophen, barbiturates, carbon monoxide, digoxin, ethanol, iron, lead, lithium, methanol, and theophylline are useful in determining clinical management.

The reliability of a toxic screen in identifying

Table 5–2. AGENTS AND DOSAGES USEFUL IN THE TREATMENT OF POISONING

Agent	Use	Dosage
Activated charcoal	Intestinal decontamination	1 gm/kg PO (can be repeated every 4 hours for 24 hours for tricyclic antidepressants, phenobarbital, and theophylline overdoses).
Ammonium chloride	Acidification of urine	15 mg/kg q6h IV or PO.
Amyl nitrite	Cyanide poisoning	Inhalation of 15 to 30 seconds/minute, until sodium nitrite is prepared.
Apomorphine	Induction of emesis	0.07 mg/kg SC.
Atropine	Cholinergic poisoning (organophosphate poisoning)	0.01 mg per dose IV (repeated until full atropinization).
Calcium disodium edetate ($CaNa_2EDTA$)	Lead poisoning	50–75 mg/kg/day divided in 4–6 doses, IM or IV for 5 days.
Chlorpromazine	Sedation	0.5–1.0 mg/kg PO or IM (maximum 50 mg per dose).
Deferoxamine	Iron poisoning	Test dose: 50 mg/kg IM (maximum 1 gm) Treatment: 50 mg/kg q4h IM or IV (IV rate not to exceed 15 mg/kg/hour), (maximum 6 gm/day).
Diazepam	Seizures or sedation	0.1–0.3 mg/kg IV (PO for sedation).
Dimercaprol (BAL)	Lead poisoning	4 mg/kg q8h IM for 3 days (usually in combination with $CaNa_2EDTA$).
Diphenhydramine	Extrapyramidal tract manifestations of phenothiazines	1 mg/kg IV (maximum 50 mg per dose).
Dobutamine	Hypotension	5–20 μg/kg/min IV
Dopamine	Hypotension	5–20 μg/kg/min IV
Ethanol	Methanol and ethylene glycol poisoning	Oral or intravenous therapy. Loading dose: 1 gm/kg. Maintenance dose: 100–150 mg/kg/hr (as 5–10% solution for IV therapy).
Furosemide	Forced diuresis	1 mg/kg per dose IV.
Ipecac syrup	Induction of emesis	9–12 months: 10 ml PO. 1–12 years: 15 ml PO. 12 years and older: 30 ml PO. (Doses for 1–12 years and 12 years and older may be repeated once if patient does not vomit within 20 minutes.)

Table continued on following page.

Table 5–2. AGENTS AND DOSAGES USEFUL IN THE TREATMENT OF POISONING (*Continued*)

Agent	Use	Dosage
Lidocaine	Ventricular arrhythmias	Loading dose: 1 mg/kg IV Maintenance dose: 30–90 μg/kg/min IV.
Magnesium sulfate	Catharsis	250 mg/kg PO (maximum 30 gm)
Magnesium citrate	Catharsis	5 ml/kg PO.
Methylene blue	Methemoglobinemia	1 mg/kg IV (1 dose).
N-acetylcysteine (Mucomyst)	Acetaminophen poisoning	Loading dose: 140 mg/kg PO. Maintenance dose: 70 mg/kg q4h for 17 doses (give as a 5% solution).
Naloxone hydrochloride	Narcotic poisoning	0.03 mg/kg per dose IV if no response in 2 minutes, 0.03 mg/kg per dose IV.
Nitroprusside	Hypertension	0.5–8 μg/kg/min IV.
Norepinephrine	Hypotension	0.02–0.1 μg/kg/min IV.
Oxygen	Carbon monoxide, cyanide poisoning	FiO_2 100%
Penicillamine	Lead, copper, mercury poisoning	6–12 mg/kg q6h PO (maximum 1 gm/day).
Phenobarbital	Seizures	Loading dose:10–15 mg/kg IV.
Phentolamine	Hypertension	0.1 mg/kg IV slowly.
Phenytoin	Seizures, cardiac arrhythmias	Loading dose: 10–15 mg/kg IV (infusion rate less than 50 mg/min).
Physostigmine salicylate	Anticholinergic poisoning	0.1–0.5 mg IV over 3–5 minutes (maximum 2 mg).
Pyridoxine	Isoniazid poisoning	1 gm for each gram of isoniazid ingested.
Sodium bicarbonate	Alkalization of urine	Loading dose: 1–2 mEq/kg IV (infusion to maintain urine pH of 8).
Sodium nitrite	Cyanide poisoning	0.2 ml/kg of 3% solution IV (maximum: 15 ml).
Sodium thiosulfate	Cyanide poisoning	1 ml/kg of 25% solution IV (maximum 50 ml).
Vitamin K	Warfarin poisoning	2–5 mg IM, or IV

toxic substances is variable. In one study, a false-negative rate of 30 to 50 per cent was determined with a false-positive rate of less than 7 per cent.[7] These data demonstrate the limitation of the toxic screen and emphasize the importance of a good clinical history and physical examination in the identification of the toxic agent.

GENERAL PRINCIPLES OF TREATMENT

The treatment of an acute intoxication includes prevention of absorption of the toxic substance, enhancement of excretion, administration of specific antidotes, and institution of adequate supportive care.

Prevention of Absorption

Poisoning occurs generally through ingestion but may occur through respiration (petroleum distillate hydrocarbon, carbon monoxide). Other routes are rectal (intoxication from aminophylline or aspirin suppository), cutaneous (insecticide poisoning), and parenteral (drug abuse).

Following an acute oral intoxication, gastrointestinal decontamination should be instituted. The removal of the gastric contents can be achieved by either chemical (ipecac syrup and apomorphine) or mechanical (gastric lavage) methods.[8] Chemical methods are the most effective.[9] Ipecac syrup induces emesis in 15 to 20 minutes in 85 per cent of the patients who take one dose and in 30 to 40 minutes in 96 per cent of the patients who take two doses. Three to four episodes of vomiting occur over 30 to 60 minutes following the administration of ipecac syrup.[10] Cephalin and emetine, the two alkaloids of ipecac syrup, exert their effect locally on the gastric mucosa and centrally on the vomiting center in the medulla. Ipecac syrup effectively induces emesis of all ingested toxins, including antiemetic drugs such as the phenothiazines.[10]

The dose of ipecac syrup for children 1 to

12 years of age is 15 ml followed by liberal administration of clear fluids.[8] Milk should not be used because it delays by 20 minutes the time to onset of emesis. If vomiting does not occur within 20 minutes, the same dose may be repeated once. If emesis does not occur within 20 minutes of the administration of the second dose, removal of the ingested product by gastric lavage may be indicated. In patients 12 years and older, 30 ml of ipecac syrup should be administered and may be repeated once. In children between the ages of 9 and 12 months, a single dose of 10 ml ipecac syrup may be given but should not be repeated.[8] The efficacy and safety of ipecac syrup in children less than 9 months of age is unknown and therefore it should not be used in this age group. Ipecac syrup is safe when administered in the recommended dosage. Central nervous system (CNS) and cardiac toxicity occur only when the recommended doses have been significantly exceeded. The fluid extract of ipecac, which is 14 times more concentrated than the syrup, should not be used.

Apomorphine induces emesis in 100 per cent of patients within 2 to 5 minutes. The recommended dose is 0.07 mg/kg subcutaneously. Since apomorphine has to be prepared every three weeks, owing to its instability, and because it may induce CNS depression, *ipecac syrup is the emetic of choice.*

The induction of emesis is contraindicated in patients who ingest a caustic product, are comatose, or have seizures. Relative contraindications include pregnancy, prior myocardial infarction, and the ingestion of a petroleum distillate hydrocarbon.

Gastric emptying is most effective when conducted shortly after ingestion. Thirty to 40 per cent of a marker substance given to animals was removed when emesis was induced within an hour of ingestion. Although under normal circumstances absorption of the majority of medicines tested occurs within four hours of ingestion, it has been demonstrated that the ingestion of large amounts of drugs or of slow-release preparations can result in delayed absorption.[11, 12] Absorption also may be delayed in situations in which the ingested substance may form *concretions*, as seen with meprobamate or salicylate overdose, and when gastric motility is depressed, as seen with anticholinergic intoxication. Despite the alleged time of ingestion, in those instances mentioned previously, emesis or lavage may be indicated for as long as 12 to 24 hours following ingestion.

Gastric lavage is less effective than ipecac syrup–induced emesis, especially for the removal of whole or partially dissolved tablets or capsules. Therefore, gastric lavage should be reserved for the obtunded or comatose patient. The patient's airway should be protected during gastric lavage. The largest tube possible should be used. The patient should be in the head-down position. Lavage should be performed with one-half normal or normal saline and continued until the return is clear. Constant nasogastric suction is effective in removing drugs such as phencyclidine, which are secreted into the stomach.[13]

After gastric emptying, efforts should be directed at preventing the absorption of the remaining toxic product in the intestine. Activated charcoal, a residue from the distillation of wood pulp, forms a stable complex with many ingested toxins and prevents further absorption.[14] A list of drugs and chemicals that are adsorbed by activated charcoal is presented in Table 5–3. Activated charcoal is probably indicated in almost all serious oral overdoses except those of cyanides, alcohols, caustic substances, heavy metals, and aliphatic hydrocarbons. The administration of activated charcoal should be postponed if an oral antidote such as *N*-acetylcysteine is to be administered in the next hour. Activated charcoal should be given in an amount equal to ten times the weight of the ingested product to achieve optimal binding. Clinically, a dose of 1 gm/kg is recommended. Although it should be given as soon as possible after ingestion, the physician should wait 30 to 60 minutes following ipecac syrup–induced emesis. It may be administered via a nasogastric tube after gastric lavage. Activated charcoal is mixed with water (50 ml for a 1 year old to 300 ml for an adolescent) or with an ionic cathartic such as magnesium citrate to form a slurry. Because charcoal is black it may serve as an indicator of gastrointestinal motility. If the toxic substance has an enterohepatic cycle (tricyclic antidepressant, digitoxin), demonstrates prolonged absorption (phenytoin, slow-release theophylline preparations), or exhibits anticholinergic properties (tricyclic antidepressants), administration of activated charcoal every four to six hours for 24 to 36 hours may be indicated. Recently, activated charcoal has been shown to decrease the half-life and enhance the clearance of intravenously administered phenobarbital and theophylline.[15] Although the exact mechanism has not been elucidated, it appears that the drugs are removed from blood across the intestinal mucosa and adsorbed by activated charcoal in the gastrointestinal tract.

Magnesium citrate (5 ml/kg) or sulfate (250

Table 5–3. DRUGS AND CHEMICALS ADSORBED BY ACTIVATED CHARCOAL

Analgesic and Anti-Inflammatory Agents	Acetaminophen Aspirin Indomethacin Mefenamic acid Morphine Opium Propoxyphene Phenylbutazone
Anticonvulsants and Sedatives	Barbiturates Carbamazepine Chlordiazepoxide Diazepam Glutethimide Ethchlorvynol Phenytoin Sodium valproate
Other Drugs	Amphetamines Atropine Chlorpheniramine Cocaine Colchicine Digitalis glycosides Iodine Ipecac *N*-acetylcysteine (Mucomyst) Penicillin Phenolphthalein Phenylpropanolamine Promazine Quinine Tetracycline Theophylline Tolbutamide Tricyclic antidepressants
Other Chemicals	Camphor Mercuric chloride Methylene blue Muscarine Nicotine Oxalates Paraquat Parathion Phenol Strychnine

mg/kg) is effective in increasing the rate of transit of a toxic product through the gastrointestinal tract and thereby reducing its absorption. These cathartics can be mixed with the activated charcoal without reducing the binding capacity of the activated charcoal.

Some toxic substances, such as the insecticides, are well absorbed through the skin. Careful washing of all exposed parts with soap and water following exposure prevents further absorption. In cases of ocular expcsure, the eye should be washed immediately with lukewarm water with the *lids held open*, for *at least* 15 minutes. In cases of corrosive substances, or if ocular pain or irritation persists an ophthalmologist should be consulted. Patients exposed to toxic vapors or particles should be removed from the contaminated area and given oxygen. An enema is a simple and effective method of decontamination for toxic substances given rectally. In the case of substances administered intradermally or subcutaneously, a tourniquet and ice can be applied to decrease the rate of absorption.

Enhancement of Elimination

The severity and duration of an intoxication are determined by the toxin's maximal serum concentration and its rate of elimination, respectively. Once absorption of the toxic substance is prevented, enhancement of its elimination from the body is necessary. Such enhancement of a toxin's elimination can be achieved either by endogenous or external methods.

Endogenous Elimination

Once absorbed into the body, toxins may be eliminated by the kidney, lung, or liver.

The majority of toxins are metabolized predominantly by the liver and then excreted in the bile or urine. Although some drugs such as phenobarbital can increase liver metabolism through enhancement of the P450 system, the time (4–5 days) necessary to achieve this effect renders their use impractical. In some intoxications, the metabolites are more toxic than the parent compound. In these instances, treatment should be directed toward the interruption of the production of toxic metabolites. The administration of ethanol blocks methanol production of formic acid,[16] the administration of an antidote binds postulated toxic intermediates (*N*-acetylcysteine for P450-generated *N*-hydroxylated toxic metabolites), or repetitive charcoal installation binds metabolically active products excreted in the bowel (demethylated by-products of imipramine metabolism).

Several methods can be used to increase urinary elimination of toxic substances, but these techniques involve some risk and should be reserved for the severely intoxicated patient. Fluid diuresis enhances renal elimination by increasing glomerular filtration so that the resorptive sites in the distal tubules have a shorter period of exposure to the toxin. Maintenance of two to three times normal urinary flow is recommended. Ionized diuresis is based on the principle that ionized drugs are less effectively reabsorbed and, as a result, excretion is enhanced. It has been demonstrated that urinary excretion of salicylates and long-acting barbiturates are increased by alkalinization of the urine.[17] Alternatively, the excretion of basic compounds such as amphetamines and phencyclidine is enhanced by acidification of the urine. Intravenous sodium bicarbonate, 1–2 mEq/kg, may be administered every six hours to alkalinize the urine. The urinary and blood pH should be monitored and additional sodium bicarbonate given to maintain a urinary pH of 8. Acidification of the urine can be achieved through the intravenous administration of ammonium chloride, 15 mg/kg every six hours, and ascorbic acid, 1 to 2 gm orally every six hours, to maintain urinary pH of 5. A diuretic such as furosemide, 1 mg/kg, has been used to increase glomerular filtration, thereby enhancing the excretion of toxic compounds. Finally, osmotic diuresis is occasionally instituted to prevent reabsorption of the toxic drug in the proximal and distal tubules. Intravenous mannitol, 0.5 mg/kg, as a 25 per cent solution, may be given every four to six hours.

EXTERNAL METHODS

In certain situations toxins require more rapid removal than can be achieved by endogenous clearance or enhanced renal or hepatic clearance. Exchange transfusion, peritoneal dialysis, hemodialysis, and hemoperfusion have all been used to achieve this aim.[18–20]

These techniques should be considered only for the severely intoxicated patient who is unresponsive to adequate supportive care or whose normal pathways of elimination are compromised. Several pharmacokinetic parameters for a given toxin (volume of distribution [Vd], protein binding, and total body clearance) should be considered prior to institution of these procedures.[21, 22] Only drugs that exist predominantly in the central compartment (blood) are removed by these methods. The amount of drugs absorbed that will remain in the blood compartment can be estimated by the volume of distribution of these drugs. Drugs with a small volume of distribution (<1 L/kg) remain predominantly in the blood compartment, whereas drugs with a large volume of distribution (>1 L/kg) diffuse largely in the extravascular compartment. For example, a significant amount of salicylates (Vd = 0.24 L/kg) can be removed by these procedures, whereas only a small fraction of the total body burden of tricyclic antidepressants (Vd = 20–40 L/kg) can be removed. Drugs that are largely protein-bound have only a small free fraction available for dialysis. Finally, the clearance of toxin achieved by dialysis must be greater than the total body endogenous clearance of the toxin.

Exchange transfusion is usually reserved for infants in whom dialysis cannot be performed (owing to their small size) and for patients in whom the toxin is tightly bound to protein and has a low volume of distribution.

Of the dialysis and hemoperfusion techniques, peritoneal dialysis has the lowest rate of clearance. It has the advantage of achieving correction of electrolyte and chemical imbalances, however. In contrast, hemodialysis is a very effective technique to remove toxins that have low volume distribution, low protein binding, and low intrinsic body clearance. Since the chemical toxin must cross a dialysis membrane, molecule size must be small for hemodialysis to be effective. Hemodialysis also corrects electrolyte and acid-base imbalances.

Hemoperfusion achieves the highest rate of clearance. The major difference between dialysis and hemoperfusion is that in hemoperfusion the blood passes over a perfusion column that contains binding substances (coated activated charcoal, resins, etc.) instead of passing over a dialysis membrane. For this reason the molecular size of the particles is not a limiting factor. Greatest clearance is achieved with toxins of low volume of distribution and low endogenous clearance.

The decision regarding the use of these techniques should be based on the patient's clinical status, the intrinsic toxicity of the toxin, and the effectiveness of the procedure in removing a clinically significant amount of the toxin (Table 5–4).

Systemic Antidotes

Optimal characteristics of a systemic antidote are high specificity and efficacy and a low incidence of adverse effects. The number of antidotes of proven efficacy are limited and include: naloxone hydrochloride for narcotics, sodium nitrite and thiosulfate for cyanide, atropine and pralidoxime for organophosphate insecticides, oxygen for carbon monoxide, methylene blue for methemoglobinemia, deferoxamine for iron, calcium EDTA and dimercaprol for heavy metals, *N*-acetylcysteine for acetaminophen, ethanol for methanol and

Table 5–4. CLINICAL EFFECTIVENESS OF HEMODIALYSIS AND HEMOPERFUSION FOR SELECTED TOXINS

Toxin	Hemodialysis	Hemoperfusion
Acetaminophen	–	–
Amanita phalloides	+	+
Aminophylline	+	+
Amphetamine	–	?
Arsenic	+	?
Atropine	0	?
Barbiturates		
Short and intermediate-acting	–	–
Long-acting	+	+
Boric acid	+	?
Camphor	–	?
Chlordiazepoxide	0	?
Chloroquine	0	?
Chlorpromazine	0	?
Copper	–	?
Diazepam	0	0
Digoxin	0	0
Diphenhydramine	?	?
Ethyl alcohol	+	+
Ethylene glycol	+	+
Fluoride	+	?
Glutethimide	0	0
Heroin	–	?
Iron	0	0
Isoniazid	+	?
Isopropyl alcohol	+	+
Lithium	+	?
Meprobamate	–	?
Methaqualone	–	?
Methyl alcohol	+	+
Methyldopa	–	?
Methyprylon	0	?
Monoamine oxidase inhibitors	?	?
Paraldehyde	?	?
Paraquat	+	?
Phenytoin	–	–
Primidone	–	?
Propoxyphene	0	?
Salicylates	+	+
Thallium	–	–
Theophylline	+	+
Trichlorethanol	+	?
Tricyclic antidepressants	0	0

0 = ineffective.
– = not clinically effective.
\+ = clinically effective.
? = effectiveness unknown.

ethylene glycol, physostigmine salicylate for anticholinergic drugs, diphenhydramine for phenothiazines that produce extrapyramidal tract signs, vitamin K for dicumerol and warfarin, and pyridoxine for isoniazid (see Table 5–2).[23] The efficacy of thioctic acid for *Amanita phalloides* mushroom poisoning and diethyldithiocarbamate for thallium poisoning has not been clearly demonstrated. A number of antisera are also available for spider, snake, and scorpion envenomations.

Supportive Care

Supportive care is necessary in most poisonings to maintain the patient until the liver and kidney have eliminated the toxins.

CNS depression requires close monitoring of vital functions and institution of ventilatory support for respiratory failure. Analeptics should not be used because they have not been shown to improve clinical outcome, their effect is unpredictable, and their use may induce excitation and seizures. Several poisons may cause convulsions by excitation (strychnine, isoniazid, camphor) or by induced metabolic derangement (ethanol-induced hypoglycemia or carbon monoxide–induced hypoxia). Regardless of the cause, anticonvulsant drugs should be administered to terminate seizures; intravenous diazepam is the agent of choice, followed by phenytoin or phenobarbital if necessary. Recommended dosages are listed in Table 5–2. Hyperventilation, hypothermia, steroids, and mannitol are all used in the treatment of cerebral edema accompanying lead and carbon monoxide poisoning.

Drug overdoses often produce hypotension and cardiac arrhythmias.[24] The causes of hypotension are depression of the medullary vasomotor center, blockade of the autonomic ganglia, and reduction of myocardial contractility. In patients with low central venous pressure, fluid and colloid replacement should be instituted. Vasopressors such as dopamine and dobutamine should be used if the patient remains hypotensive. Cardiac arrhythmias should be treated with specific antiarrhythmics as indicated by the nature of the arrhythmia.

Pulmonary edema and tissue hypoxia may result from poisoning. A therapeutic modality indicated in the treatment of pulmonary edema secondary to alveolar injury consists of ventilatory support with positive end expiratory pressure. Inadequate ventilation, impaired alveolar capillary diffusion, impaired oxygen transport (methemoglobin and carboxyhemoglobin), and inhibited cellular oxygenation (cyanide) are all mechanisms responsible for tissue hypoxia. The administration of 100 per cent oxygen is indicated in these instances.

Fluid and electrolyte imbalance may result from the toxic effects of the agent, e.g., metabolic acidosis from methanol or salicylate intoxication, or from therapeutic maneuvers, e.g., catharsis, fluid diuresis, and dialysis. Therefore, serum electrolyte, blood glucose, blood gas, blood urea nitrogen, and serum creatinine levels and urinary output all require close monitoring.

PREVENTION

Poisonings in children usually result from the interaction of a susceptible host, an available poison, and a temporarily unstable environment. The majority of poisonings in children occurs between the ages of 18 months and 3 years. The accessibility of the agent is important. Substances involved in a poisoning incident are frequently improperly stored at the time of the incident. The child's psychosocial environment may also contribute to the poisoning. Factors frequently encountered in families in which a poisoning occurs are: they have moved in the last three months, someone is unemployed, one parent is away from home, the mother is pregnant, someone has had a serious illness in the last month, one or both parents are suffering from depression.[25]

During well-child visits or visits following an episode of intoxication, the physician can help prevent future accidental poisoning by alerting the parents to potential risk situations in the home.[26] The physician should provide anticipatory guidance related to the child's stage of development. For example, parents should be reminded that household products in lower cabinets are a risk for the crawling child (aged 6 to 12 months),[26] and that products such as baby powder may be grabbed by a 4- to 6-month-old child during diaper changing.[27]

When prescribing medications, the physician should encourage parents to use safety containers[28] and should instruct them in the proper storage of medicines and toxic substances.

Besides poison prevention, the physician should discuss the appropriate measures to be taken when a poisoning occurs. Regional poison control centers provide the most accurate information concerning the evaluation and treatment of poisonings.[29] Therefore, after a poisoning, parents and physicians should contact their regional poison center immediately. The physician should recommend that parents keep a bottle of ipecac syrup in the home.

In summary, the physician should educate parents concerning potentially hazardous situations that can lead to a poisoning during the child's development and should provide anticipatory guidance.

ACETAMINOPHEN

Acetaminophen is an effective analgesic and antipyretic medication available in over 200 preparations in its pure form or combined with other drugs. Acetaminophen is a popular substitute for aspirin. Its efficacy, safety, and absence of side effects when taken in therapeutic doses account for its increasing usage.

CLINICAL SUMMARY—Acetaminophen

Pharmacokinetics

Volume of distribution (L/kg)	0.8–1.0
Protein binding (%)	25
Half-life (hours)	1–2
pKa	9.5
Probable hepatotoxic levels (μg/ml)	≥200 (4 hours post-ingestion) ≥50 (12 hours post-ingestion)

Clinical Presentation

Nausea, vomiting, anorexia, and epigastric or right upper quadrant pain are present. Hepatic transaminase levels are elevated after 24–36 hours. Hypoglycemia and hepatic coma may occur.

Treatment

Emesis or lavage: Indicated.

Activated charcoal: Relatively contraindicated.

Catharsis: Relatively contraindicated.

Increased renal elimination: Not indicated.

Hemodialysis or hemoperfusion: Not indicated.

Antidote: *N*-acetylcysteine (Mucomyst): loading dose, 140 mg/kg po; maintenance dose, 70 mg/kg q4hr × 17 doses po

Pathophysiology

At therapeutic doses, acetaminophen is metabolized principally by sulfation and glucuronidation of its parahydroxyl group. The metabolites and the parent compound are not toxic. In contrast, a small fraction of acetaminophen is converted to a reactive metabolite by the cytochrome P450–dependent, mixed-function oxidase enzymes in the hepatic cells. Following normal doses of acetaminophen, the reactive metabolite is detoxified by preferential conjugation with hepatic glutathione and excreted as cysteine and mercapturic acid metabolites.[30] After an acetaminophen overdose (>150 mg/kg in children; 7.5 gm in adults), the sulfate and glucuronide conjugation routes become saturated, resulting in an increased formation of the reactive metabolite. When this amount is sufficient to deplete glutathione by 70 per cent or more, the reactive metabolite binds covalently to cellular protein macromolecules resulting in hepatocellular necrosis.[31]

Clinical Presentation

Clinical manifestations following the ingestion of large amounts of acetaminophen are nonspecific, not predictive of hepatotoxicity, and frequently delayed. Although the patient may experience nausea, vomiting, anorexia, and diaphoresis within two to four hours of ingestion, these signs or symptoms may be delayed for 12 to 24 hours. At that time the patient may also experience right-sided abdominal tenderness and hepatomegaly. Later manifestations include jaundice, clotting disorders, and hepatic encephalopathy. Hypersensitivity reaction, cardiac injury, acute tubular necrosis, and hypoglycemia occur rarely.

Laboratory Findings

The liver is the major target organ of toxicity following an acute overdose of acetaminophen. The hepatic serum transaminase levels (glutamic oxaloacetic and glutamic pyruvic) rise 24–48 hours after ingestion. These enzymes reach their peak levels in the serum three to four days after ingestion. Elevation of serum transaminase levels correlates with the severity of the hepatic injury.[32] A prolongation of the prothrombin time and an increase of the serum bilirubin level above 4 mg/100 ml on the third to the fifth day after ingestion are also indicative of severe hepatotoxicity.[32] Histologic stud-

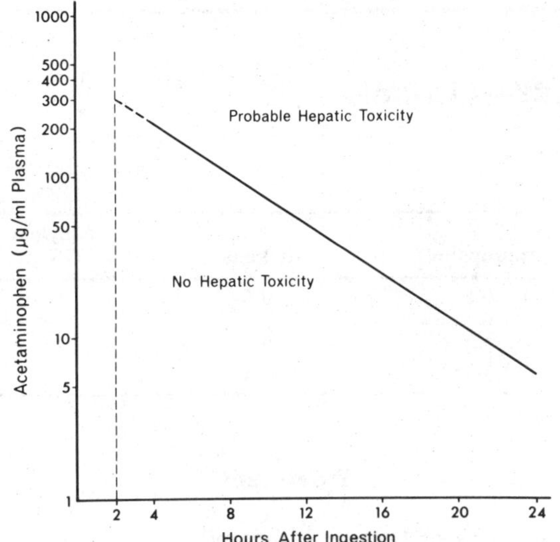

Figure 5–1. Semi-logarithmic plot of plasma acetaminophen levels vs. time. (From Rumack, B. H. and Matthew, H.: Acetaminophen poisoning and toxicity. Pediatrics, *55*:871–876, 1975.)

ies of the liver, following an acetaminophen overdose, have demonstrated damage ranging from cytolysis in mild cases to centrilobular necrosis in severe cases. These histopathologic changes are reversible in survivors, and the liver tissue returns to normal within three months of ingestion.

The determination of the concentration of acetaminophen in the serum is essential to assess the risk of hepatotoxicity.[33] Acetaminophen concentrations in the serum greater than 200 μg/ml, 100 μg/ml, and 50 μg/ml, at 4, 8, and 12 hour post-ingestion, respectively, or any concentrations above the values depicted on the Rumack-Matthew nomogram (Fig. 5–1) indicate a potential risk for hepatotoxicity.[5] The normal acetaminophen serum half-life of one to two hours may be prolonged to more than three to four hours in patients who develop liver damage.

Treatment

The treatment of acetaminophen overdose should include measures to lessen its absorption from the gastrointestinal tract, the administration of compounds containing sulfhydryl groups (*N*-acetylcysteine) to prevent hepatotoxicity, and provision of adequate supportive care.

In the alert patient gastric emptying should be conducted by inducing emesis with ipecac syrup. Activated charcoal effectively adsorbs acetaminophen. However, it should probably not be given if oral *N*-acetylcysteine is to be given within four to six hours. Activated charcoal binds the antidote and may reduce its effectiveness.

The sulfhydryl-containing products used for the prevention of acetaminophen hepatotoxicity include methionine, cysteamine, and *N*-acetylcysteine. *N*-acetylcysteine, administered orally, effectively reduces or prevents hepatotoxicity as demonstrated by prevention of elevation of serum transaminase level, hyperbilirubinemia, and prolongation prothrombin time. Its efficacy and absence of adverse reactions make it the antidote of choice.

N-acetylcysteine (Mucomyst) should be administered by mouth preferably within 8 to 12 hours of ingestion.[33] The patient should be given a loading dose of 140 mg/kg followed by a maintenance dosage of 70 mg/kg every four hours for 17 doses.[33] The available 10 or 20 per cent solutions should be diluted to a 5 per cent solution. The patient may experience nausea, vomiting, or epigastric discomfort following the administration of *N*-acetylcysteine. If an *N*-acetylcysteine dose is vomited within an hour of administration, the dose should be repeated. The 10 and 20 per cent solutions of *N*-acetylcysteine available in the United States are sterile but not pyrogen-free.[34] These solutions have not been approved for intravenous administration.

Fluid diuresis is of no therapeutic value. Hemodialysis or charcoal hemoperfusion enhances the elimination of acetaminophen but not the toxic intermediate. Furthermore, the effectiveness of antidotal therapy has rendered these procedures unnecessary.

ALCOHOLS

Ethanol, isopropanol, methanol, and ethylene glycol share similar pharmacologic and toxicologic characteristics and will be discussed together. Besides alcoholic beverages, sources of ethanol include cough syrups, antiseptics, mouthwashes, and colognes. Isopropanol, a colorless liquid with a slightly bitter taste, is used as a solvent, rubbing alcohol, and disinfectant. It is included also in de-icing and anti-freeze products. Methanol is found in anti-freeze and windshield-washer solutions and is frequently used as a solvent in varnishes and paint removers. Ethylene glycol is mainly encountered in anti-freeze solutions.

CLINICAL SUMMARY—Alcohols

Pharmacokinetics

	Ethanol	Isopropanol	Methanol	Ethylene Glycol
Volume of distribution (L/kg)	0.6	0.6	0.6	0.6
Protein binding (%)	0	0	0	0
Half-life (hours)	2–24	2–3	2–24	3
Toxic concentration (mg/100 ml)	>150	>150	>10	–

Clinical Presentation

Ethanol and isopropanol may cause ataxia, slurred speech, visual disturbances, incoordination, agitation, somnolence, coma, and respiratory depression. Hypoglycemia may occur in a young child.

Methanol may cause metabolic acidosis and visual impairment variably progressing to permanent blindness.

Ethylene glycol may cause metabolic acidosis and acute tubular necrosis.

Treatment

Emesis or lavage: Indicated.
Activated charcoal: Ineffective.
Catharsis: Ineffective.
Increased renal elimination: Not indicated.
Hemodialysis or hemoperfusion: Indicated (see p. 91).
Antidote Ethanol for methanol and ethylene glycol intoxication: loading dose 1 gm/kg po or IV (see p. 91); maintenance dose 100–150 mg/kg/hr po or IV (see p. 91).

Pharmacology

Alcohols are rapidly and completely absorbed following ingestion. Peak serum concentrations occur within one to two hours after ingestion. The concomitant ingestion of a drug (anticholinergic or narcotic) and the presence of food in the stomach may delay absorption of the alcohols. Once absorbed, they are distributed throughout the body water with an apparent volume of distribution of 0.6 L/kg. Alcohols are primarily metabolized in the liver and excreted in the urine.[35–38] Although they are all metabolized by the enzyme alcohol dehydrogenase, they have various degrees of affinity for the enzyme. Ethanol has a greater affinity than isopropanol, methanol, and ethylene glycol. Ethanol and methanol appear to follow zero-order kinetics, whereas isopropanol and ethylene glycol follow first-order kinetics. Isopropanol is metabolized to acetone.[36] Methanol is metabolized to formic acid and formaldehyde, whereas ethylene glycol is metabolized to oxalate, glycolic acid, hippuric acid, or glycoaldehyde.[35–37] These last metabolites are more toxic than the parent compound and are responsible for methanol and ethylene glycol toxicity.

Clinical Presentation

Ethanol,[39] isopropanol,[36] methanol,[40] and ethylene glycol[38] all act as CNS depressants. The onset of symptoms is usually rapid but delayed clinical effects are observed in the case of methanol and ethylene glycol.[38, 40] Blood concentrations of ethyl, isopropyl, and methyl alcohol generally correlate with clinical symptoms. At low concentrations (ethanol, 100–300 mg/100 ml, isopropanol, 50–150 mg/100 ml, and methanol, 20–30 mg/100 ml) the patient manifests visual impairment, slowed reaction time, ataxia, and various degrees of CNS depression. Patients with serum levels greater than 500, 500, and 100 mg/100 ml for ethanol, isopropanol, and methanol, respectively, may exhibit coma, seizures, and cardiovascular or respiratory compromise.[36, 38–40] Currently, ethylene glycol is not measured routinely in blood specimens.

Alcohols irritate the gastrointestinal tract and cause nausea, vomiting, hematemesis, and abdominal pain. Isopropanol is the most irritating of the four alcohols.

Alcohols can cause a number of metabolic aberrations. The severity of these metabolic disturbances is determined by the toxicity of the product and the amount ingested; methanol and ethylene glycol are the most toxic (Table 5–5). Severe metabolic acidosis and an elevated anion gap occur in methanol and ethylene glycol intoxication. All four alcohols increase the serum osmolality.[36] Acetonemia and acetonuria are seen only with isopropanol intoxication. Hypocalcemia and crystalluria (oxalate with casts) are encountered with ethylene glycol poisoning. Hypoglycemia occurs in young children who ingest ethanol or isopropanol.[36]

Formic acid accumulation is responsible for the metabolic acidosis and ocular toxicity of methanol poisoning. Ophthalmologic findings, which appear 16 to 24 hours after ingestion, may progress from hyperemia of the disk, retinal edema, dilated and fixed pupils to permanent blindness.[41]

Renal failure of ethylene glycol intoxication is secondary to acute tubular necrosis induced by the oxalates. Oliguria or anuria may be prolonged but is usually reversible.[42]

Treatment

The rapid absorption of ethanol, isopropanol, methanol, and ethylene glycol makes the decision to institute gastrointestinal tract decontamination difficult. Emptying of the stomach probably should be performed in patients within two to four hours of ingestion.

The aim of treatment of methanol and ethylene glycol intoxication is the prevention of the formation of the toxic metabolites with subsequent removal of these metabolites and the parent compound by dialysis. Ethanol, methanol, and ethylene glycol compete for the oxidative enzyme, alcohol dehydrogenase. The administration of ethanol, which has a greater affinity for the enzyme, will prevent the metabolism of methanol and ethylene glycol.[37, 38, 41] Ethanol should be given orally as a 40 to 50 per cent solution or intravenously as a five to ten per cent solution to patients who have methanol serum levels greater than 15–20 mg/100 ml or to those who have ingested more than 2 mg/kg of ethylene glycol. The loading dose of ethanol is 1 gm/kg. This dose should be followed by the administration intravenously of ethanol at a rate of 100–150 mg/kg/hour, diluted to a 5–10 per cent solution. If ethanol is administered orally, 400–500 mg/kg may be given every four hours. The goal of therapy is to maintain serum ethanol concentration between 100 and 150 mg/100 ml. Therapy should be continued for four to five days in the case of ethylene glycol and until serum concentrations of methanol are less than 5–10 mg/100 ml.

Hemodialysis and hemoperfusion effectively remove ethanol, isopropanol, methanol, and ethylene glycol.[18, 37, 38] These procedures should be considered for patients who fail to respond to adequate supportive care, who have

Table 5–5. DIFFERENTIAL DIAGNOSIS

Criteria	Ethanol	Isopropanol	Methanol	Ethylene Glycol
Metabolic	+ +	+	+ + +	+ + +
acidosis	Lactic acid	Lactic acid	Lactic and formic acid	Lactic, glycolic, and oxalic acid.
Increased anion gap[1]	+ +	+	+ + +	+ + +
Increased serum osmolality[2]	Each 350 mg/100 ml adds 80 mOsm to calculated value.	Each 340 mg/100 ml adds 60 mOsm to calculated value.	Each 350 mg/100 ml adds 80 mOsm to calculated value.	Each 21 mg/100 ml adds 3.5 mOsm to calculated value.
Characteristic features	Hypoglycemia (in young children).	Acetonemia Acetonuria	Congested edema of retina, blindness	Hypocalcemia, crystalluria (oxalate, hippurate), renal failure.
Delayed toxicity	–	–	Ocular (24 hours)	Renal (48 hours)
Major toxic compound	Parent	Parent	Metabolites	Metabolites

Adapted from Lacouture, P. G., Wason, S., Abrams, A., Lovejoy, F. H. Jr.: A review of acute isopropyl alcohol intoxication: diagnosis and management. Am J Med 75:680–686, 1983.

[1]Anion gap: $Na+$ (mEq/L) + K^+ (mEq/L) = CL^- (mEq/L) + HCO_3^- (mEq/L) + 12

[2]Serum osmolality (mOsm/kg H_2O) $= 1.86\ Na^+\ (mEq/L) + \frac{\text{glucose (mg/100 ml)}}{18} + \frac{\text{BUN (mg/100 ml)}}{2.8}$

refractory acidosis or renal failure, and/or have serum levels greater than 50 mg/100 ml for methanol, 500 mg/100 ml for isopropanol, and 500 mg/100 ml for ethanol. The ethanol block should be continued during the dialysis procedures. The maintenance dose of ethanol should be doubled during dialysis. Although peritoneal dialysis can remove alcohols, it should be reserved for patients in whom hemodialysis and hemoperfusion cannot be performed.[43]

Metabolic acidosis should be treated aggressively with sodium bicarbonate. Calcium gluconate should be given to patients with hypocalcemia. Adequate supportive care and close monitoring of cardiorespiratory function should be provided to the comatose patient.

CLINICAL SUMMARY—Carbon Monoxide

Pharmacokinetics

Half-life (hours)	6 (FiO_2:21%)
	1½ (FiO_2:100%)
Toxic concentration	COHb>20%

Clinical Presentation

COHb concentration (%)	*Signs and Symptoms*
20–30	Headache
30–40	Severe headache, vomiting, weakness
40–50	Visual disturbance, tachycardia, syncope
50–60	Coma, seizures
>60	Compromised cardiorespiratory function

Treatment

Emesis or lavage: Not indicated.
Activated charcoal: Not indicated.
Catharsis: Not indicated.
Increased renal elimination: Not indicated.
Hemodialysis or hemoperfusion: Not indicated.
Antidote: FiO_2(100%).

CARBON MONOXIDE

Carbon monoxide (CO) is an odorless, tasteless, non-irritating gas that has approximately the same density as air. It represents the most abundant air pollutant in the lower atmosphere. Cigarette smoke contains about four per cent carbon monoxide, whereas automobile exhaust contains 0.5 to 10 per cent. Persons who die in fires frequently succumb as a result of the carbon monoxide produced during the combustion process. Other common sources of carbon monoxide include sterno, hibachis, and charcoal stoves.

Pathophysiology

Carbon monoxide is generated from the incomplete combustion of carbonaceous materials. Carbon monoxide toxicity results mainly from its propensity to combine with hemoglobin to form carboxyhemoglobin. Carbon monoxide competes with oxygen for binding sites on hemoglobin and decreases the oxyhemoglobin saturation level. In the presence of carbon monoxide the oxygen carried by the red blood cell is bound more tightly to the hemoglobin, and therefore, the amount of oxygen released to the tissue is reduced. Carbon monoxide can also enter cells and inhibit the cytochrome oxidase system.[44]

Clinical Presentation

The severity of carbon monoxide poisoning is determined by (1) the concentration of CO in the inspired air, (2) the length of time of the exposure, (3) the basal metabolic rate of the patient (young children are at higher risk), (4) cardiac or pulmonary status of the patient prior to the incident (those suffering from chronic pulmonary or cardiac insufficiency are at higher risk), and (5) the hemoglobin level (patients suffering from anemia are at higher risk).

The brain and the heart are the most sensitive organs to hypoxia and account for the major toxic manifestations. Cardiovascular signs include tachycardia, arrhythmia, angina, and hypotension. Myocardial insult is reflected by electrocardiographic and echocardiographic abnormalities. Electrocardiographic changes include sinus tachycardia, ST depression, T-wave flattening or inversion, premature ventricular contractions, and various conduction system disturbances. Echocardiographic results have demonstrated abnormal left ventricular motion.[45] Headache is frequently the first sign of carbon monoxide poisoning. Other CNS symptoms include emotional lability, agitation, impaired judgment, and dizziness. The patient may have increasing degrees of CNS depression and seizures. Cerebral edema with increased intracranial pressure may occur. Electroencephalographic tracings may show diffuse slow waves of low voltage.[46] The neurologic sequelae are the result of hypoxia. These sequelae seem to correlate better with the patient's level of consciousness on admission to the hospital than with the amount or length of exposure to carbon monoxide or with the carboxyhemoglobin concentration.[47]

The patient may experience visual disturbances such as decreases in light sensitivity and dark adaptation. Eye examination may reveal visual field defects, venous engorgement and hemorrhages on the retina, and papilledema.[48]

Other signs and symptoms encountered include nausea, vomiting, shortness of breath, and, infrequently, hearing loss.

Laboratory Findings

The severity of the clinical presentation usually correlates with the concentration of carboxyhemoglobin. Concentrations of 20 to 30 per cent are associated with headache; 30 to 40 per cent with severe headache, vomiting, and weakness; 40 to 50 per cent with visual disturbance, tachycardia, and syncope; and 50 to 60 per cent with coma and seizures. Concentrations greater than 60 per cent can be fatal. The classic cherry red or pink color of the blood is seen only with high carboxyhemoglobin concentrations.

Serum creatine phosphokinase and lactate dehydrogenase levels may be elevated transiently.

Treatment

The patient should be removed immediately from the contaminated area and, if the vital signs are stable, should be given moist 100 per cent oxygen. The 100 per cent FiO_2 reduces the half-life from 6 hours to 1½ hours.[49] This treatment should be continued until the carboxyhemoglobin is less than 15 per cent. Hyperbaric oxygen therapy reduces the elimination half-time to approximately one-half hour, but hyperbaric chambers are not widely available.[49, 50]

Supportive care should include careful monitoring of respiratory and cardiac status, the correcting of acid-base disturbances (acidosis), and the treating of seizures and cerebral edema if present.

CORROSIVES

The ingestion of liquid or solid caustic substances may cause severe esophageal or gastric injury resulting in perforation or stricture. Alkali agents frequently involved in caustic ingestion are drain cleaners (sodium hydroxide, potassium hydroxide), laundry and dishwasher detergents (phosphate, carbonate), surface cleaners (ammonia), denture cleaners (bicarbonate, phosphate), and Clinitest tablets (sodium hydroxide). The pH of these alkaline compounds ranges from 7 to 12. Acidic compounds are toilet bowl cleaners (hydrochloric, phosphoric, and sulfuric acids), anti-rust compounds (hydrofluoric and oxalic acids), automobile battery fluids (sulfuric acid), and slate cleaners (hydrofluoric acid). Their pH is less than 7 and may be as low as 2.

Pathophysiology

Alkali agents usually destroy tissue by partially dissolving the tissue protein and fat-forming proteinate. This destruction of the mucous membrane integrity permits rapid penetration of the agents to deeper tissues. The characteristic histopathologic changes are referred to as liquefaction necrosis. Alkali burns mainly involve the esophagus.[51] In contrast to alkali agents, acids produce coagulation necrosis and involve primarily the stomach.[51] Acids are potent dessicants and coagulate tissues. This coagulum prevents the acid's deeper penetration. Household bleach products that contain sodium hypochlorite are frequently ingested. Because of their neutral pH of 6, they rarely cause tissue necrosis.[52]

Additional factors that increase the severity of the tissue destruction and the development of complications include concentration and

CLINICAL SUMMARY—Corrosives

Clinical Presentation

Burns present on oropharyngeal mucosa, possibly extending to esophageal or gastric mucosa. Oral or abdominal pain may be present. Drooling, vomiting, difficulty swallowing, and signs of perforation, may occur.

Treatment

Emesis or lavage: Contraindicated.
Activated charcoal: Contraindicated.
Catharsis: Contraindicated.
Increased renal elimination: Not indicated.
Hemodialysis or hemoperfusion: Not indicated.
Antidote: Dilute with water.

quantity of the product, length of contact with the mucosa, and relative tonicity of the pyloric sphincter.[53] Alkali or acid burns usually evolve through three stages. The acute phase is characterized by an initial vascular thrombosis, followed by cell death and necrotic tissue accumulation, ending in four to seven days with the formation of an ulcer. This phase is followed by a latent phase during which granulation takes place. It occurs between the second and fourth week post-ingestion. The esophageal wall is at its weakest at this time. The last phase, the chronic phase, begins with fibroblast proliferation and connective tissue formation. This scar tissue can then result in stricture formation.

Clinical Presentation

The ingestion of caustic substances may produce burns of the oropharyngeal cavity. Excess salivation, drooling, dysphagia, painful swallowing, and retrosternal pain may indicate injury to the oral or esophageal mucosa. Vomiting, epigastric pain, or tenderness also may be experienced. It has been demonstrated that the presence or absence of signs and symptoms does not predict the presence or severity of esophageal injury.[54] The presence of respiratory distress may indicate tracheal or pulmonary involvement secondary to aspiration.

During the first 72 hours following ingestion the patient is at the highest risk for perforation and circulatory collapse. Delayed complications such as stricture formation and chronic malnutrition may occur after three or four weeks but may take months to appear.

Laboratory Findings

Esophagoscopy is the most accurate way to evaluate the involvement of the esophagus following the ingestion of a caustic substance.[54–56] Esophagoscopy should be performed within 48 hours post-ingestion, the time when the risk of perforation is low. Steroids should be instituted within 48 hours of ingestion if they are to be used. Several classifications of esophageal injury noted during esophagoscopy have been proposed.[57, 58] These classifications are based on the depth of burn and range from a superficial involvement of the mucosal layer (grade 1) to transmural involvement and perforation of the tissue (grade 3) (Table 5–6).

The esophagoscope should not be advanced beyond the first area of ulceration.[56] When performed by an experienced endoscopist using a flexible fiberoptic endoscope, this procedure carries a low risk of morbidity.

Table 5–6. CLASSIFICATION OF ENDOSCOPIC FINDINGS

Grade 0	Absence of esophageal injury.
Grade 1	Burn limited to the mucosa and characterized by the presence of edema and/or erythema.
Grade 2	Burn penetrating beyond the mucosa characterized by the presence of ulceration and/or whitish membrane.
Grade 3	Presence of perforation.

Adapted from Hawkins, D. B., Demeter, M. J.: Caustic ingestion: controversies in management. A review of 214 cases. Laryngoscope *90*:98–109, 1980.

A barium swallow (esophagogram) should be used to document a perforation or to observe the progress of a stricture. No clear correlation can be demonstrated between the esophagographic findings during the acute stage and the final outcome.[59]

Treatment

Initial treatment should consist of the immediate washing with water of the caustic agent off the esophagus. The use of neutralizing agents, such as vinegar to neutralize alkali or sodium bicarbonate to neutralize acid burns, is no longer recommended. Chemical neutralization is an exothermic reaction that produces heat that may increase the esophageal injury.[60]

Ipecac syrup–induced emesis subjects the esophageal mucosa to repeated exposure to the caustic agents and therefore *is contraindicated.* The passage of a nasogastric tube for gastric lavage may cause iatrogenic esophageal perforation and therefore *lavage should not be attempted.* If a nasogastric tube is necessary for nutritional support it should be positioned under direct visualization during the esophagoscopy.

The use of antibiotics is controversial. Broad spectrum antibiotics have been recommended prophylactically when steriod therapy was instituted. However, becase of the low incidence of infection in uncomplicated esophageal burns, *prophylactic antibiotics should be avoided,* and antibiotics should be instituted only at the first sign of infection.

The role and efficacy of steroids in the prevention of stricture following a corrosive agent remains unclear. Experimental studies have shown that steroids delay the formation of connective tissue, but clear evidence that steroids reduce stricture formation is lacking. Furthermore, data suggest that only injuries of moderate severity benefit from steroid therapy.[57] In order to benefit from the antifibroblast action of steroids, treatment should be initiated within 48 hours of injury. Prednisone, 2 mg/kg/day orally or parenterally, should be given to patients with grade 2 esophageal burns for three to four weeks (see Algorithm for the Emergency Room Management of Caustic Ingestion). After that period the status of the esophageal burns should be reassessed.

The treatment of patients who have caustic burns includes the provision of adequate supportive care and careful monitoring for signs of gastric or esophageal perforation or stricture. Depending on the severity of the burn, the patient may require total or partial parenteral nutrition followed by a progressive diet. Patients who develop esophageal stricture may require dilatations, and sometimes, esophageal replacement with colon.

CLINICAL SUMMARY—Hydrocarbons

Clinical Presentation

Aspiration may produce coughing, tachypnea, fever, and rales. CNS depression and seizures also occur. Cardiac arrhythmias, hemolysis, albuminuria, glycosuria, hematuria, pyuria, hepatomegaly, and liver dysfunction, are less frequent.

Treatment

Emesis or lavage: See indications on page 97.

Activated charcoal: Not indicated.

Catharsis: Not indicated.

Increased renal elimination: Not indicated.

Hemodialysis or hemoperfusion: Not indicated.

Antidote: None.

HYDROCARBONS

Hydrocarbon ingestion represents approximately 5 per cent of all reported accidental ingestions in children under the age of 5 years. The hydrocarbons most frequently involved in an acute poisoning are fuels (gasoline, kerosene), furniture polishes (mineral seal oil), lubricants, solvents (xylene, toluene, benzene, turpentine), charcoal lighter fluids, and paint thinners or removers. These products are mixtures of aliphatic and aromatic hydrocarbons

Table 5–7. RELATIVE RISK OF SYSTEMIC TOXICITY VERSUS ASPIRATION HAZARDS OF SELECTED HYDROCARBONS

Hydrocardon	Use	Systemic Toxicity	Aspiration Hazard
Toluene, benzene, xylene	Solvents in paints, lacquers, cleaning agents	+ + +	+
Carbon tetrachloride	Grain fumigant, solvent	+ + +	+
Turpentine	Paint thinner, textile cleaner, shoe polish	+ + +	+
Naphtha	Paint and glue thinner	+	+ + +
Gasoline	Fuel	+	+ + +
Kerosene	Heating, cooking fuel	+	+ + +
Mineral seal oil	Furniture polish	+	+ + +
Diesel oil	Fuel	+	+ +
Petrolatum	Ointments, creams	–	–
Lubricating oil	Machine lubricant	–	–
Paraffin wax	Emollients, candles, dental molds	–	–

+ + + = High risk
+ + = Moderate risk
+ = Low risk
– = No risk

and their different physical and chemical properties determine their toxicity.

Pathophysiology

The toxicity of ingested hydrocarbons results primarily either from their systemic toxicity following gastrointestinal absorption in the case of aromatic (benzene, toluene, xylene) or halogenated (carbon tetrachloride, chloroform) hydrocarbons or from their pulmonary toxicity following aspiration in the case of aliphatic hydrocarbons (gasoline, naphtha, kerosene). The relative risk of aspiration *versus* systemic toxicity for the most frequently ingested hydrocarbons is presented in Table 5–7.

The lungs, CNS, and gastrointestinal tract are most frequently affected following an acute hydrocarbon ingestion.

Pulmonary toxicity is seen principally with the aspiration of aliphatic hydrocarbons into the respiratory tract.[61, 62] Products with low viscosity (gasoline, petroleum, ether) have a high aspiration hazard. Following aspiration, an intense local irritation ensues, followed by the development of chemical pneumonitis, hemorrhagic bronchopneumonia, and atelectasis. Pneumatoceles, pleural effusion, pneumothorax, and pulmonary edema may also occur.

The aliphatic and aromatic hydrocarbons affect the CNS through different mechanisms. Evidence suggests that aliphatic hydrocarbons directly stimulate or depress the CNS without necessarily causing hypoxia.

Irritation of the gastric and intestinal mucosa, resulting in vomiting and diarrhea, is encountered mainly with aliphatic hydrocarbons. Aliphatic and aromatic hydrocarbons can affect the cardiac, hepatic, renal, and hematopoietic systems.

Clinical Presentation

Coughing, tachypnea, respiratory distress, rales, and cyanosis are seen in patients who have aspirated hydrocarbons. Fever is associated with the development of chemical pneumonitis.[63, 64]

CNS symptoms following a hydrocarbon poisoning include lethargy, obtundation or agitation, seizures, and coma. Coma seen with alipathic hydrocarbons is associated with decreased deep tendon reflexes, whereas coma due to aromatic hydrocarbons is associated with increased deep tendon reflexes.[63, 64]

Vomiting and diarrhea are encountered in up to 50 per cent of aliphatic hydrocarbon ingestions. Other complications such as myocarditis, cardiomegaly, cardiac arrhythmia, hemolysis, albuminuria, glycosuria, hematuria, pyuria, hepatomegaly, and liver dysfunction are infrequently encountered following an acute ingestion.[64]

Hydrocarbons are also abused by adolescents. The most common method consists of placing hydrocarbons in a plastic bag, shaking the bag to induce vaporization, and inhaling the hydrocarbon directly from the bag. The patient experiences a pleasurable sensation and CNS excitation. Patients may also have hypercapnea and relative hypoxia, leading to cardiac arrhythmias and CNS depression. Products that contain hydrocarbons most frequently abused through inhalation include airplane glue and model cement (acetone, toluene, naphtha), nail polish remover (acetone), and liquid shoe polish (toluene and chlorinated hydrocarbon).

Laboratory Findings

There is no good correlation between radiologic findings and the patient's clinical status. Furthermore, a time lag may exist between the appearance of symptoms and the appearance of radiologic abnormalities. Radiographic changes may be seen within 30 minutes but may be delayed up to 12 hours following ingestion.[63]

Patients who develop chemical pneumonitis demonstrate an elevated white blood cell count with a shift to the left. Other laboratory test results that may be abnormal are blood gas levels, urinalysis results, and kidney and liver function tests.

Treatment

A rational approach to the management of hydrocarbon poisoning requires the accurate identification of the hydrocarbon, which allows for the determination of the relative risk of aspiration *versus* systemic toxicity.

Patients in whom the risk of systemic toxicity outweighs the risk of aspiration, and in whom gastric emptying should be instituted, are those who have ingested: (1) a large amount of aliphatic hydrocarbon (probably 10–12 ml/kg), (2) an aromatic (toluene, xylene) or halogenated (carbon tetrachloride, trichlorethane) hydrocarbon, and (3) a hydrocarbon used as a vehicle for more toxic substances such as pesticides and heavy metals.[65, 66] Emesis induced by ipecac syrup probably is the most effective and safest method for emptying the stomach.[66] Gastric lavage should be reserved for the patients in coma or having seizures. Activated charcoal does not effectively bind aliphatic hydrocarbons.

The mainstay of therapy following an aliphatic hydrocarbon ingestion is adequate supportive care. The physician should monitor carefully for the appearance of signs or symptoms of pulmonary toxicity. *Corticosteroids and prophylactic antibiotics do not decrease the morbidity or mortality associated with aliphatic hydrocarbon pneumonitis and therefore are not indicated.*[67, 68] Antibiotics should be administered only to patients who develop bacterial superinfection. Fever and elevated leukocytosis are present in patients who develop chemical pneumonitis and are not necessarily an indication of infection the first 48 hours following aspiration.[65] Other measures should include the close monitoring of neurologic, renal, hepatic, and cardiac status of the patient.

Recent data demonstrate that the majority of children brought for medical evaluation following the ingestion of hydrocarbons do not experience pulmonary complications.[69] It is suggested that only patients who are symptomatic at the time of the initial evaluation, or who become symptomatic during a six- to 8-hour observation period, should be hospitalized.[69]

IRON

Iron is contained in a large number of over-the-counter medications. More than 100 products containing iron are listed in the *Physicians' Desk Reference.* Iron preparations usually are dispensed as ferrous sulfate, fumarate, or gluconate. The severity of the poisoning is determined by the amount of elemental iron ingested. The percentage varies with each salt, i.e., 33 per cent for the fumarate, 20 per cent for the sulfate, and 12 per cent for the gluconate. The majority of iron poisonings result from the ingestion of multi-vitamin preparations or prenatal vitamins containing iron.

Pathophysiology

Ferrous iron is absorbed primarily by the duodenum and jejunum, oxidized to its ferric state, and bound to ferritin, an iron-storage protein.[70] The ferric iron is then released from ferritin into the plasma, where it is bound to transferrin. Transferrin becomes attached to sites in the bone marrow and releases the iron necessary for erythropoiesis. The iron content of the body is regulated by absorptive mechanisms because there is no specific mechanism for excretion of iron. Approximately one milligram of iron is lost each day from the intestine, skin, or urinary tract. Following an overdose, the absence of an effective excretory mechanism leads to the accumulation of iron

CLINICAL SUMMARY—Iron

Pharmacokinetics

Protein binding (%)	99
Toxic concentration (μg/100 ml)	Concentration more than the total iron binding capacity (>350).

Clinical Presentation

Nausea, vomiting, bloody diarrhea, abdominal cramps, lethargy, hypotension, metabolic acidosis, shock, coma, and seizures may be present.

Treatment

Emesis or lavage: Indicated.
Activated charcoal: Not indicated.
Catharsis: Not indicated.
Increased renal elimination: Not indicated.
Hemodialysis or hemoperfusion: Indicated in renal failure for iron-deferoxamine complex.
Antidote: Deferoxamine; test dose 50 mg/kg IM, (Maximum 1 gm; maintenance dose 50 mg/kg IM, or IV, q4h. IV infusion should not exceed 15 mg/kg/hr) (see p. 99).

in target organs. If the transferrin's binding capacity is exceeded, the remainder of the iron circulates in its free form. It is the unbound iron that causes systemic toxicity.[70, 71]

The gastrointestinal tract and the liver are the two major organs affected by an acute iron overload. Iron produces hemorrhagic, necrotic lesions of the stomach and proximal small bowel, and the distal small bowel suffers segmental infarction characterized by marked mucosal congestion and submucosal venous thrombosis. The mucosa, submucosa, basement membrane, cytoplasm, and nuclear tissue show heavy iron staining.[71]

In the liver, histopathologic studies demonstrate parenchymal cellular necrosis with leukocytic infiltration and fatty degeneration. The periportal hepatocytes are affected to a greater degree than the central cells. In animals, toxic doses of iron produce a marked decrease of glycogen in the liver with an increase of stainable iron. In severe intoxication, hemorrhage in the lungs and kidneys has been reported. In addition, the lung may exhibit focal atelectasis, emphysema, and vascular congestion. The heart and the renal tubules may undergo fatty degeneration. The absence of staining for iron in specimens from the lungs, heart, and kidneys suggests that changes in these organs may be secondary to other events such as hypotension, acidosis, and coagulopathy.[71]

Clinical Presentation

The clinical presentation of the acutely poisoned child can evolve through three phases.

First Phase. The ingestion of more than 20 mg/kg of elemental iron may lead to toxicity; the severity of the clinical presentation is proportional to the amount of elemental iron ingested. Signs or symptoms of iron poisoning usually appear one-half to six hours after ingestion and are secondary to gastrointestinal mucosal irritation. Nausea, vomiting, hematemesis, abdominal pain, melena, and bloody diarrhea may be seen. Lethargy and hypotonia secondary to decreased cerebral perfusion or a direct effect of iron on the CNS may occur. In severe cases, intestinal bleeding and shift of fluid from the vascular compartment to the extracellular space may lead to a decrease in plasma and blood volume, resulting in decreased cardiac output with reflex tachycardia. Direct injury to the vessels by iron, the release of vasodilatating agents such as ferritin, serotonin, and histamine, and fluid losses all contribute to hypotension.[71] Metabolic acidosis encountered in severe poisoning is primarily due to the converison of ferrous to ferric iron with the release of hydrogen ions, the accumulation of organic acids as a result of the inhibition of the Krebs cycle, and hypoperfusion.[71]

Second Phase. The patient may experience a period of relative stability.[72] The appearance and duration of this period is probably related to the severity of the ingestion. Therefore, it is imperative to pursue adequate treatment and supervision because the patient's status may deteriorate again. Hypotension may progress to shock and vascular collapse. Several hematologic and metabolic disturbances such as leukocytosis, bleeding disorders, hyperglycemia or hypoglycemia,[72] and acidosis may occur. The patient can develop coma and seizures. Hepatic and renal failure may occur.

Third Phase. Intestinal scarring may result in pyloric or antral stricture two to five weeks after ingestion.[73] Diffuse fibrosis with fatty degeneration of the liver also has been noted.

Table 5–8. CORRELATION BETWEEN SERUM IRON CONCENTRATION AND CLINICAL PRESENTATION WITHIN SIX HOURS OF INGESTION

Serum Concentration (μg/100 ml)	Clinical Presentation
<125	No symptoms.
125–300	No symptoms or nausea, vomiting, or melana.
300–500	Vomiting, abdominal cramps, bloody diarrhea, lethargy.
500–1000	Gastrointestinal symptoms, decreased blood pressure.
>1000	Hypotension, shock, metabolic acidosis, coagulopathy, coma.

Laboratory Findings

The severity of the intoxication correlates with the serum iron concentration. Normal serum iron concentrations range from 100–125 μg/100 ml. Concentrations less than 300 μg/100 ml are associated usually with no or mild symptoms. Those between 300–500 μg/100 ml are associated with mild manifestations of toxicity. Patients with concentrations above 500 μg/100 ml levels may manifest moderate signs of toxicity. Levels of more than 750–1000 μg/100 ml are associated with severe intoxication (Table 5–8). Hematocrit, hemoglobin level, white blood cell count, and blood glucose and serum electrolyte levels should be monitored. Leukocytosis greater than 15,000 mm^3 and blood glucose level more than 150 mg/100 ml correlate with serum iron concentrations of more than 300 μg/100 ml and are indicative of a potentially serious intoxication.[74] A flat plate of the abdomen may reveal the presence of ingested iron (prenatal iron preparations, but usually not other vitamin preparations with iron) and document the success or failure of the gastrointestinal decontamination.

Treatment

Patients who have ingested more than 20 mg/kg of elemental iron are at risk for developing signs of toxicity. The severity of the poisoning is proportional to the amount of iron ingested. Measures to prevent gastrointestinal absorption should be taken. The removal of iron from the stomach in an alert patient is accomplished best by induced emesis with ipecac syrup. If the patient is obtunded, a gastric lavage is performed with a large-bore tube. A flat plate of the abdomen may help determine the efficacy of the gastric emptying. The procedures should be repeated when evidence of radiopaque material persists in the stomach. Iron pills will rarely form a mass of concretions requiring surgical removal. In patients who have ingested a larger amount of iron (50 mg/kg) the instillation of 50 to 100 ml of a one per cent solution of bicarbonate should follow the aforementioned procedures.[75] This solution will promote the formation of a ferrous carbonate salt, which is poorly absorbed. Deferoxamine administered orally also forms a complex with the iron and prevents its absorption; 5 to 10 gm may be given in cases of severe intoxication.[76] Phosphate-containing preparations have been associated with complications and are not recommended.[75]

Deferoxamine, isolated from *Streptomyces pilosus* and treated chemically to obtain the metal-free ligand, is the chelating agent of choice.[76, 77] It will bind the free iron and will compete for the iron with ferritin and transferrin. Deferoxamine removes only a small amount of the iron from transferrin[78] and does not bind the iron in the cytochrome systems or hemoglobin.[78] Deferoxamine may be administered orally to prevent further absorption of iron from the gastrointestinal tract in severe intoxication or may be given intramuscularly or intravenously to chelate the absorbed iron. Patients with a history of a large ingestion of iron (50 mg/kg), signs or symptoms of more than mild gastrointestinal upset, leukocytosis greater than 15,000/mm,[3] blood glucose levels higher than 150 mg/100 ml, or a serum iron concentration more than 300 μg/100 ml, should receive a provocative chelation challenge. The dose of deferoxamine is 50 mg/kg intramuscularly (maxium of 1 gm). Passing of a vin rose–colored urine signifies free iron chelated to deferoxamine, and therapy should be continued. The patient should be given 50 mg/kg every 4 hours intramuscularly or as a constant intravenous infusion until signs of toxicity have subsided, serum iron level is less than the total iron binding capacity, and the vin rose–colored urine has stopped for four to six hours. The intravenous infusion rate should not exceed 15 mg/kg/hr owing to the risk of inducing hypotension. The intravenous route is preferred to the intramuscular route in severely intoxicated patients. Such patients may benefit from an oral administration of deferoxamine to prevent further absorption of iron.

Adequate supportive care directed to the correction of fluid loss, hypotension, metabolic acidosis, and hemostasis disturbance is essential. Dialysis can remove only a small portion (1–4%) of the iron-chelate complex, and should be used only in patients with renal failure.

CLINICAL SUMMARY—Lead

Pharmacokinetics

Location of distribution	Blood, soft tissue, bone
Half-life	35 days (blood) 40 days (soft tissue) 20 years (bone)
Toxic concentration	>30 μg/100 ml

Clinical Presentation

Increased irritability, anorexia, lethargy, vomiting, abdominal pain, and ataxia may occur. In more severe cases coma and seizures are present.

Treatment

Emesis or lavage: Indicated.
Activated charcoal: Not indicated.
Catharsis: Indicated.
Increased renal elimination: Not indicated.
Hemodialysis or hemoperfusion: Not indicated.
Antidote: Ca EDTA at 50–75 mg/kg/24 hrs IM or IV; dimercaprol (BAL) at 12–24 mg/kg/24 hrs IM (see pp. 101–102).

LEAD

Lead is a malleable metal with a low melting point that is found in paints, plastics, storage batteries, bearing alloys, insecticides, and ceramics. It is not significantly altered by normal chemical interaction and therefore remains toxic throughout all phases of its processing. The children of lead workers and children who live in old, dilapidated housing, near major bridges, freeways, or lead smelters are at greater risk for developing lead poisoning. Automobile exhaust is an important source of lead fumes in cities.

Pathophysiology

Lead poisoning results from the ingestion of products saturated with lead or from the inhalation of lead vapor or fumes. Approximately 10 per cent of ingested lead is absorbed.[79] However, children with severe iron deficiency can absorb as much as 50 per cent.[80] Lead salts are absorbed in the small intestine by active and passive transport. In contrast to the intestinally absorbed lead, 30 to 50 per cent of the inhaled lead can be absorbed.

Once absorbed, 90 per cent of the lead is deposited in dense bone and the remainder enters soft tissues such as the kidneys, liver, and brain. The half-life of lead in the blood and soft tissue is about 35 and 40 days, respectively. In the bone, the half-life may be as long as 20 years. In humans, lead is slowly accumulated over the years, with a total body burden of 50–350 mg of lead by the age of 60 years. Men have a higher concentration of lead in nearly all tissues than women. Lead is mainly excreted by the kidneys and small amounts are found in the bile, nails, and hair.

Urinary excretion occurs principally by glomerular filtration, but some active transport at the tubules may occur.[81] Urinary excretion is dependent on renal flow and glomerular filtration rate.

Lead interacts with sulfhydryl groups and decreases the enzyme activity necessary for heme synthesis and for hemoglobin and cytochrome production. Lead diminishes the conversion of δ-aminolevulinic acid (d-ALA) to porphobilinogen and the conversion of protoporphyrin IX to heme, resulting in the accumulation of d-ALA and free erythrocyte protoporphyrin in the blood.[82] The increase of these substances becomes a sensitive and early indicator of greater body-lead burden. Lead also affects the CNS; however, the exact mechanism responsible for the functional disturbance is poorly understood. In the CNS lead causes edema and has a direct, cytoxic effect, whereas in the peripheral nervous system it causes segmental demyelination and axonal degeneration. Functionally, there is a decrease in nerve conduction velocity. In the kidney, lead may damage the proximal tubules, resulting in a lessening of reabsorption of glucose, amino acids, and phosphates. These changes are reversible with chelation. Prolonged exposure of high concentrations of lead may lead to more serious damage characterized by interstitial fibrosis, sclerosis of vessels, and glomerular atrophy leading to renal failure. Lead can also induce colic, but the exact pathogenesis remains unclear.[83]

Clinical Presentation

Lead poisoning can be difficult to diagnose and is frequently unrecognized because its symptoms are often nonspecific and subtle.[83, 84] The presence and severity of the symptomatology is related to the amount and length of exposure to lead. The signs and symptoms encountered are anorexia, constipation, vomiting, abdominal pain, and hepatosplenomegaly. Parents may have noticed a change in the child's behavior or the presence of irritability, hyperactivity, or lethargy. If the exposure is severe the patient may develop coma with increased intracranial pressure and seizures. Patients without overt signs of intoxication but exposed to prolonged blood lead concentrations, ranging from 30 to 50 μg/100 ml, may develop decreased nerve conduction, greater psychomotor activity, learning disorders, and fine motor dysfunctions.[85]

Laboratory Findings

Hematologic changes are usually the first laboratory abnormalities noticed. Chronic lead exposure produces a microcytic, hypochromic anemia with expanded reticulocytosis, basophilic stippling, and eosinophilia. Free erythrocyte protoporphyrin levels in whole blood are greater than 150 μg/100 ml. The d-ALA concentration is higher in urine and serum. These changes of chronic lead exposure may not be seen following an acute exposure. Lead concentrations between 30 to 60 μg/100 ml result in biochemical disturbances, but symptoms are noticed usually when concentrations exceed 60 μg/100 ml. Serum lead values greater than 100–125 μg/100 ml represent a medical emergency.[83, 84]

Radiographs may reveal augmented deposition of calcium in metaphyseal areas of long bones. A plain film of the abdomen may show radiopaque material in the intestine.

Other laboratory abnormalities may include an abnormal electroencephalogram, pleocytosis in the cerebrospinal fluid, leukocyturia, glycosuria, and aminoaciduria.

Treatment

The therapy of lead poisoning is based upon the degree of the lead body burden and the severity of the clinical presentation.[83, 84, 86, 87]

Children without symptoms but with lead blood concentrations between 30 and 60 μg/100 ml and free erythrocyte protoporphyrin greater than 50 μg/100 ml with or without positive findings on x-rays of the abdomen or knees should have a lead mobilization test to evaluate their lead body burden. This test consists of the administration of a single 50 mg/kg dose of calcium disodium edetate (EDTA) intramuscularly and collection of urine for 24 hours. If the ratio of micromoles of lead excreted in the urine per 24 hours to millimoles of calcium EDTA administered exceeds 1:0, there is an excessive lead burden and a large mobilizable pool of lead. Such patients should receive additional chelation.

Patients who have blood lead concentrations greater than 60 μg/100 ml, with or without symptoms, should be given chelating agents.[83, 84, 86, 87] Calcium EDTA and dimercaprol are the two agents used in the acute phase. Calcium EDTA, which forms a stable complex with lead drawn from the soft tissue pool, is administered at dosages of 50–75 mg/

kg/24 hours intramuscularly or intravenously divided in four doses. If, after the administration of calcium EDTA for five days, further chelation is required, a two to three day rest period should be observed before reinstituting therapy. The toxicity of calcium EDTA is mainly renal and usually occurs when doses greater than 75 mg/kg/day are administered for prolonged periods. Dimercaprol (BAL) removes lead directly from the erythrocyte, thereby producing a rapid fall in blood lead concentration. The dosage is 12–24 mg/kg/24 hours intramuscularly given in three divided doses. Dimercaprol is usually administered in conjunction with calcium EDTA to patients with blood lead levels exceeding 80–100 μg/100 ml or showing signs or symptoms of encephalopathy. Penicillamine is usually reserved for the long-term treatment of lead poisoning.[83, 84, 86, 87]

In addition to the potential nephrotoxicity of these chelating agents, the greater quantity of lead excreted through the kidneys may lead to renal damage. Therefore, careful monitoring of the kidney function is mandatory. Maintenance of an adequate urinary flow reduces the risk of renal toxicity.

Additional complications such as seizures and cerebral edema require prompt treatment. Diazepam is the agent of choice to stop seizures, followed by phenytoin or phenobarbital. Fluid restriction, steroids, and hypertonic solutions such as mannitol are the mainstays of anti-cerebral edema therapy.

Patients suffering from lead poisoning frequently exhibit anemia. Iron supplementation should follow chelation therapy.

Finally, before the child returns to his or her environment, measures should be taken to eliminate the lead source.

CLINICAL SUMMARY—Salicylic Acid

Pharmacokinetics

Volume of distribution (L/kg)	0.13
Protein binding (%)	40–80
Half-life (hours)	3–6
pKa	3.5
Toxic concentration (mg/100 ml)	30

Clinical Presentation

Vomiting, tinnitus, hyperventilation, respiratory alkalosis, metabolic acidosis (in a young child), hypoglycemia, dehydration, agitation or obtundation, coma, and seizures may be present.

Treatment

Emesis or lavage: Indicated.
Activated charcoal: Indicated.
Catharsis: Indicated.
Increased renal elimination: Alkalization of urine (see p. 104).
Hemodialysis or hemoperfusion: Indicated (see p. 104).
Antidote: None.

SALICYLIC ACID

Aspirin remains one of the most common accidentally ingested drugs especially in the child less than the age of 5 years.[88] The pattern of poisoning has changed over recent years. The percentage of accidental poisoning due to salicylates in children less than 5 years old, when compared with poisonings due to all drugs as reported to the National Clearinghouse for Poison Control Centers, has decreased from 21.7 per cent in 1968 to 3.4 per cent in 1977. However, the number of children presenting with therapeutic aspirin overdose has increased. The decrease in the incidence and severity of acute salicylate poisoning in children may be attributed, in part, to the introduction of child resistant containers and limitation of aspirin of 1.25 grains to 36 tablets per bottle.[89]

Pathophysiology

Aspirin is rapidly and completely absorbed when administered at therapeutic doses. Aspirin absorption may be delayed by the ingestion of an excessive amount of the drug, enteric-coated preparations, or the concomitant ingestion of other medications (anticholinergics, narcotics, etc.) or food.[90] Once absorbed, acetylsalicylic acid is rapidly hydrolyzed to salicylic acid, which is responsible for most of the pharmacologic activities of aspirin. Salicylic acid is partly metabolized in the liver and partly excreted unchanged in the urine. Salicylic acid is excreted in the urine as salicyluric acid (75%), salicyl phenolic glucoronide (10%), salicyl acyl glucuronide (4%), gentisic acid (1%), and free salicylic acid (10%). The excretion of the free salicylic acid is variable and depends on the urinary pH. In an alkaline urine (pH 7.5–8) up to 85 per cent of an ingested dose of aspirin is eliminated as free salicylate.

Hepatic biotransformation of salicylic acid to salicyluric acid and the phenolic glucuronide is limited. Saturation of these metabolic pathways is responsible for the prolongation of the half-life of salicylic acid from three to six hours in therapeutic doses and from 15 to 30 hours in overdoses. Approximately 40 to 80 per cent of salicylic acid is bound to albumin and its volume of distribution is 0.13 L/kg. Acidosis in overdose increases the volume of distribution.

Salicylic acid induces several metabolic alterations. By uncoupling oxidative phosphorylation, it increases oxygen consumption and the production of carbon dioxide with a subsequent increase in the depth of respiration. Direct stimulation of the respiratory center in the medulla by salicylic acid is responsible for the rise in respiratory rate. The respiratory alkalosis produced is compensated by the renal excretion of bicarbonate, sodium, and potassium. Salicylic acid inhibition of the Krebs cycle and carbohydrate and lipid metabolism results in the production of lactic acid and ketone bodies, which produce metabolic acidosis. Salicylic acid in overdose is hepatotoxic, producing an elevation of liver enzyme levels (serum glutamic oxaloacetic transaminase, serum glutamic pyruvic transaminase, and alkaline phosphatase) in the plasma and a prolongation of the prothrombin time. Salicylic acid inhibits platelet aggregation, which prolongs the bleeding time.

Clinical Presentation

Clinical manifestations of mild salicylate intoxication include nausea, vomiting, tachypnea, hyperpnea, tachycardia, tinnitus, and lethargy. Greater insensible water loss, vomiting, and poor fluid intake, especially in young children, may lead to severe dehydration. Coma, seizures, cerebral edema, hyperthermia, and respiratory or cardiovascular failure may occur in severe poisoning. Coma, seizures, and dehydration occur more frequently in salicylate intoxication resulting from the administration of excessive amounts of aspirin over time than in acute overdose.[91] Pulmonary edema, myocardial, renal, and hepatic failure are seen infrequently.

Laboratory Findings

Following an acute overdose the Done nomogram may be used to estimate the severity of the intoxication (Fig. 5–2).[92] Serum concentrations of salicylate less than 30 mg/100 ml are associated with no symptoms. Levels between 30 and 70 mg/100 ml are associated with mild to moderate symptoms, and concentrations between 70 and 100 mg/100 ml are associated with severe symptoms. Serum levels above 100 mg/100 ml represent a potentially lethal intoxication. It is difficult to establish a correlation in chronic salicylate poisoning between the serum concentration and severity of clinical presentation. Factors such as the underlying

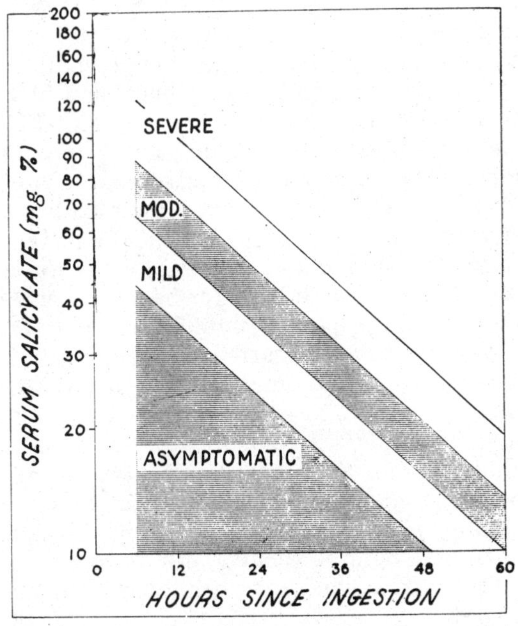

Figure 5–2. Done nomogram for salicylate poisoning. (From Done, A. K.: Salicylate intoxication. Significance of measurements of salicylate in blood in cases of acute ingestion. Pediatrics, *26*:800–807, 1960.)

disease, dehydration, and acidosis influence the severity of the intoxication.

In young children metabolic acidosis prevails, whereas in adults respiratory alkalosis is more frequent. Metabolic acidosis increases the non-ionized fraction of salicylic acid and favors further penetration of salicylates into the tissue.[93] The increase of salicylic acid in the brain is responsible for the severe clinical picture seen in pediatric overdose.[94]

Other metabolic disturbances encountered include hyperglycemia or hypoglycemia, ketonemia, lactic acidemia, prolonged bleeding time, elevated serum glutamic oxaloacetic transaminase and glutamic pyruvic transaminase levels, and prolonged prothrombin time.

Treatment

An amount of ingested aspirin greater than 150 mg/kg should be removed by emesis with ipecac syrup in the alert patient and gastric lavage in the comatose patient. Activated charcoal adsorbs aspirin, reduces its absorption, and should be administered after gastric emptying. Magnesium citrate or sulfate is given to increase gastrointestinal transit.

Alkalizing the urine and increasing renal flow will enhance the excretion of free salicylic acid.[95] Intravenous sodium bicarbonate, 1–3 mEq/kg q4–6h, should be administered to maintain a urinary pH of 7.5–8. To assure alkalization of the urine and to prevent paradoxic aciduria, sufficient potassium should be given (3–4 mEq/kg/daily). Urinary and blood pH should be monitored closely. Metabolic acidosis should be corrected promptly with the administration of sodium bicarbonate. Parenteral fluids are given to correct the fluid losses, to meet daily requirements, and to increase urine flow to two or three times the normal rate. The goal of therapy for hepatic injury is to support the patient until liver repair and regeneration have occurred. This support consists of an adequate maintenance of fluid balance, control of bleeding, correction of hypoglycemia, and treatment of any other complications that may occur. The protein intake should be restricted and neomycin or lactulose administered if hepatic failure occurs. Seizures should be treated with diazepam followed by phenytoin or phenobarbital if necessary.

Peritoneal dialysis, exchange transfusion, hemodialysis, and hemoperfusion remove salicylates from the blood.[18] Hemodialysis and hemoperfusion achieve the highest clearance of aspirin and are the techniques of choice. Hemodialysis will also correct acid-base imbalance. These techniques present risks and should be reserved for patients who have renal failure, who are unresponsive to adequate supportive care, or who have a salicylic acid concentration greater than 100–150 mg/100 ml.

THEOPHYLLINE

Theophylline and aminophylline, two methylxanthine derivatives, are used commonly for the treatment of apnea in the premature infant and reactive airway disease in children and adults. Methylxanthines inhibit the phosphodiesterase enzyme, leading to an increase of adenosine 3′,5′-cyclic monophosphate (cyclic AMP) in the smooth muscle of the bronchioles that results in bronchodilatation.

Pathophysiology

Theophylline is a potent stimulant of the CNS. Nervousness, restlessness, insomnia, tremors, and hyperesthesia can be seen after an overdose. These symptoms are followed by seizures and coma with higher theophylline concentrations. Theophylline also stimulates the medullary respiratory center. It produces nausea and vomiting through an irritating effect on the gastric mucosa and through a CNS effect. Theophylline raises the heart rate. As the serum concentration of theophylline increases, the incidence of serious arrhythmias rises. In animals, theophylline infusion lowers the threshold for electrically induced ventricular fibrillation, and this threshold may be reduced further by hypoxia, hypercapnea, and acidosis.[96] Theophylline produces a lower peripheral vascular resistance and raises cerebrovascular resistance, resulting in a lessening of the cerebral blood flow and the oxygen tension.

Theophylline is rapidly absorbed from the stomach and upper small bowel at therapeutic doses. However, its absorption may be delayed if a large amount of regular or sustained-released preparations is ingested. The peak serum level may be delayed up to 17 hours following an overdose.[12] Sixty per cent of absorbed theophylline is bound to albumin in blood. Its volume of distribution is 0.5 L/kg.[97] Theophylline is metabolized to 1,3 β-dimethyl uric acid, 1 methyl uric acid, and 3 methyl uric

CLINICAL SUMMARY—Theophylline

Pharmacokinetics

Volume of distribution (L/kg)	0.3–0.7
Protein binding (%)	53–65
Half-life	Age dependent (see p. 105)
pKa	8.6
Toxic concentration (μg/ml)	20

Clinical Presentation

Nausea, vomiting, hematemesis, tachycardia, agitation or obtundation may be present. In severe cases there are life-threatening arrhythmias, seizures, coma, and neurologic sequelae.

Treatment

Emesis or lavage: Indicated.
Activated charcoal: Indicated.
Catharsis: Indicated.
Increased renal elimination: Not indicated.
Hemodialysis or hemoperfusion: Indicated (see p. 106).
Antidote: None.

acid. These pathways are saturable.[98] Only 5 per cent of a theophylline dose is excreted unchanged through the kidneys.

Several factors influence the clearance rate and half-life of theophylline. Clearance rate increases from approximately 30 ml/kg/hour in newborns to 100 ml/kg/hour in 1-year-old children. Adolescents have a clearance rate of about 75 ml/kg/hour. The clearance rate decreases to 50 ml/kg/hour in adults. The half-life is influenced also by age. The newborn demonstrates a theophylline half-life of 20 hours. The half-life is 6 to 7 hours in a 6-month-old child and 3.5 to 4 hours for children between 1 and 9 years of age. Cigarette smoking, phenobarbital, acute viral illness, and high protein diet increase the clearance rate and shorten the half-life. In contrast, hepatic cirrhosis, congestive heart failure, and drugs such as cimetidine, propranolol, erythromycin, tetracycline, and cephalexin shorten the clearance rate and prolong the half-life. In overdose, the decay curve is prolonged.[12]

Clinical Presentation

The gastrointestinal tract, the cardiovascular and central nervous systems are the most frequently affected following a theophylline overdose.

Nausea, vomiting, and hematemesis are more frequently encountered when serum concentrations exceed 20 μg/ml but can occur at therapeutic doses (10–20 μg/ml).

Signs and symptoms of CNS toxicity include restlessness, irritability, agitation, and obtundation. Generalized tonic-clonic seizures usually occur in severe intoxication. Following an acute overdose, the incidence of convulsions increases with rising serum levels (Table 5–9). However, seizures have been recorded in pa-

Table 5–9. INCIDENCE OF SIGNS OR SYMPTOMS OF THEOPHYLLINE INGESTION WITH SERUM CONCENTRATION

Serum Concentration (μg/ml)	Vomiting		Seizures		Tachycardia		Other Arrhythmias	
	N	%	*N*	%	*N*	%	*N*	%
0–49	7/10	70	0/10	0	4/10	40	0/10	0
50–99	14/16	88	0/16	0	11/16	69	1/16	6
≥100	2/2	100	1/2	50	2/2	100	1/2	50

Adapted from Gaudreault, P., Wason, S., Lovejoy, F. H., Jr.: Acute pediatric theophylline overdose: a summary of 28 cases. J Pediatrics *102*:474–476, 1983.
N = case ratio.

tients with serum concentrations in the range of 20–40 μg/ml. Seizures may be protracted, repetitive, and at times resistant to anticonvulsant therapy.

Tachycardia is the most frequent clinical manifestation of cardiovascular toxicity. Life-threatening arrhythmias such as premature ventricular contractions, ventricular tachycardia or fibrillation, idioventricular rhythms, and asystole appear to be less frequent in children than adults.[99] The incidence of these arrhythmias rises with greater theophylline serum concentrations (see Table 5–9).

The presence of hypoxia, acidosis, or concomitant cardiopulmonary disease appears to increase the frequency of the cardiac or neurologic manifestations.

Treatment

Initial therapy following an acute oral overdose includes the removal of theophylline from the stomach by emesis with ipecac syrup in the alert patient or by gastric lavage in the obtunded patient. Because of a possible delay in absorption following the ingestion of large amounts of regular or sustained release theophylline, these measures should be instituted regardless of the alleged time of ingestion. Emesis or gastric lavage should be followed by the administration of activated charcoal and an ionic cathartic such as magnesium citrate. Repetitive activated charcoal increases the clearance of theophylline. Therefore, administration of activated charcoal should be repeated every four hours until the serum concentration falls below 30 μg/ml.[100] At least two blood specimens for the determination of theophylline concentrations should be drawn four hours apart to ascertain that the theophylline serum level has reached its peak and that no further absorption is occurring.

Hemodialysis and hemoperfusion can significantly increase the clearance of theophylline. However, following an acute overdose in healthy adolescents, protracted seizures and life-threatening arrhythmias occur rarely when serum concentrations are less than 80 μg/ml (see Table 5–9). Therefore, hemodialysis or hemoperfusion should be reserved for those pediatric patients who fail to respond to adequate supportive care or who have serum concentrations greater than 80 to 100 μg/ml.

Vigorous gastrointestinal tract decontamination and supportive care remain the treatment of choice for the majority of patients.

Seizures should be treated with diazepam, phenytoin, and/or phenobarbital. In case of severe intoxication the patient's cardiac status should be monitored and arrhythmias treated appropriately.

CLINICAL SUMMARY—Tricyclic Antidepressants

Pharmacokinetics

Volume of distribution (L/kg)	6–30
Protein binding (%)	85–98
Half-life (hours)	25–81
pKa	9.5
Toxic concentration (ng/ml)	>500

Clinical Presentation

Mydriasis, dry mucous membrane, tachycardia, and decreased peristalsis may occur. Hallucinations, coma, and seizures may be present. Hypotension, heart conduction defects, and ventricular arrhythmias are possible.

Treatment

Emesis or lavage: Indicated.

Activated charcoal: Indicated (repeat q4–6h for 24 hours).

Catharsis: Indicated.

Increased renal elimination: Not indicated.

Hemodialysis or hemoperfusion: Not indicated.

Antidote: None.

TRICYCLIC ANTIDEPRESSANT

Tricyclic antidepressants were first introduced in the early 1960s. These drugs are used primarily in the treatment of depression in adults and in the treatment of enuresis in children. Tricyclic antidepressants are becoming one of the most frequently used drugs in suicide attempts. The tricyclic antidepressants possess various degrees of anticholinergic, adrenergic, and α-blocking properties. Although the antidepressant potency, cardiac toxicity, and pharmacokinetics vary among tricyclic antidepressants, no significant differences in their general toxicity are found in overdoses.

Clinical Pharmacology

In therapeutic doses, tricyclic antidepressants are rapidly absorbed. However, following an overdose their absorption is slowed by their ionization in the stomach and by their reduction of gastrointestinal peristalsis. Once absorbed, the tricyclic antidepressants are 85 to 98 per cent bound to plasma proteins. Protein binding is increased by alkalization and decreased by acidosis. Tricyclic antidepressants are distributed to tissues, especially the myocardium.[101, 102] Myocardial concentrations have been reported at 40 to 200 times the plasma concentrations. The tricyclic antidepressants are metabolized in the liver by demethylation, hydroxylation, and glucoronization and then excreted by the kidneys. The tricyclic antidepressants are also secreted into the stomach (5–16%) and into the hepatobiliary circulation (5%). Some of the metabolites such as desipramine and nortriptyline, the metabolites of imipramine and amitriptyline respectively, are pharmacologically active. The half-life of tricyclic antidepressants varies, ranging from 25 to 81 hours.[101, 102]

Pathophysiology

Although the quantity of tricyclic antidepressant necessary to induce clinical manifestations varies, amounts less than 20 mg/kg usually produce a low mortality rate, whereas amounts greater than 50 mg/kg are associated with a high incidence of death.[103]

Confusion, agitation, or hallucinations, attributed to the anticholinergic effects of tricyclic antidepressants, occur in mild to moderate overdose. In severe overdose, the patient may develop coma, generally within six hours of the ingestion and lasting, on the average, 24 hours. Generalized tonic-clonic seizures are encountered also. The patient's pupils are usually dilated.[103]

The mortality related to tricyclic antidepressants is secondary to their cardiac toxicity. The effects of tricyclic antidepressants on the heart are due to three major pharmacologic actions. First, their anticholinergic activity induces tachycardia and mild elevation of the blood pressure. Second, the tricyclic antidepressants block the re-uptake of norepinephrine at the adrenergic synapse. This increased adrenergic stimulation results in tachycardia, mild hypertension, and mildly elevated cardiac output. Severe adrenergic stimulation results in ventricular tachycardia and ectopies. Finally, tricyclic antidepressants have "quinidine-like" effects, which produce a prolongation of the refractory period and a rise in the stimulation threshold, along with a lowering of the cardiac conduction velocity and ventricular automaticity. These effects can result in profound bradycardia, prolongation to the QRS interval of more than 100 milliseconds on the electrocardiogram, idioventricular rhythm, and asystole. The "quinidine-like" effects of tricyclic antidepressants may predispose the patient to re-entry arrhythmias such as ventricular tachycardia. Decreased myocardial contractility and the α-adrenergic blocking action of tricyclic antidepressants on the vessels are responsible for hypotension.[104]

Other anticholinergic signs are dry mucous membranes, diminished peristalsis, and urinary retention.

Laboratory Findings

There is no direct correlation between serum concentrations and clinical manifestations.[105] However, serum concentrations greater than 1000 ng/ml are indicative of a severe intoxication with serious risk of cardiac arrhythmias and CNS manifestations. The serum concentrations of the active metabolites, as well as of the parent compound, are necessary for interpreting the blood data.

A QRS interval equal to or greater than 100 milliseconds also indicates a serious intoxication with possible development of seizures, life-threatening arrhythmias, cardiac arrest, and death.[105] The conduction defect is dose dependent. A QRS interval prolongation to more than 100 milliseconds is encountered

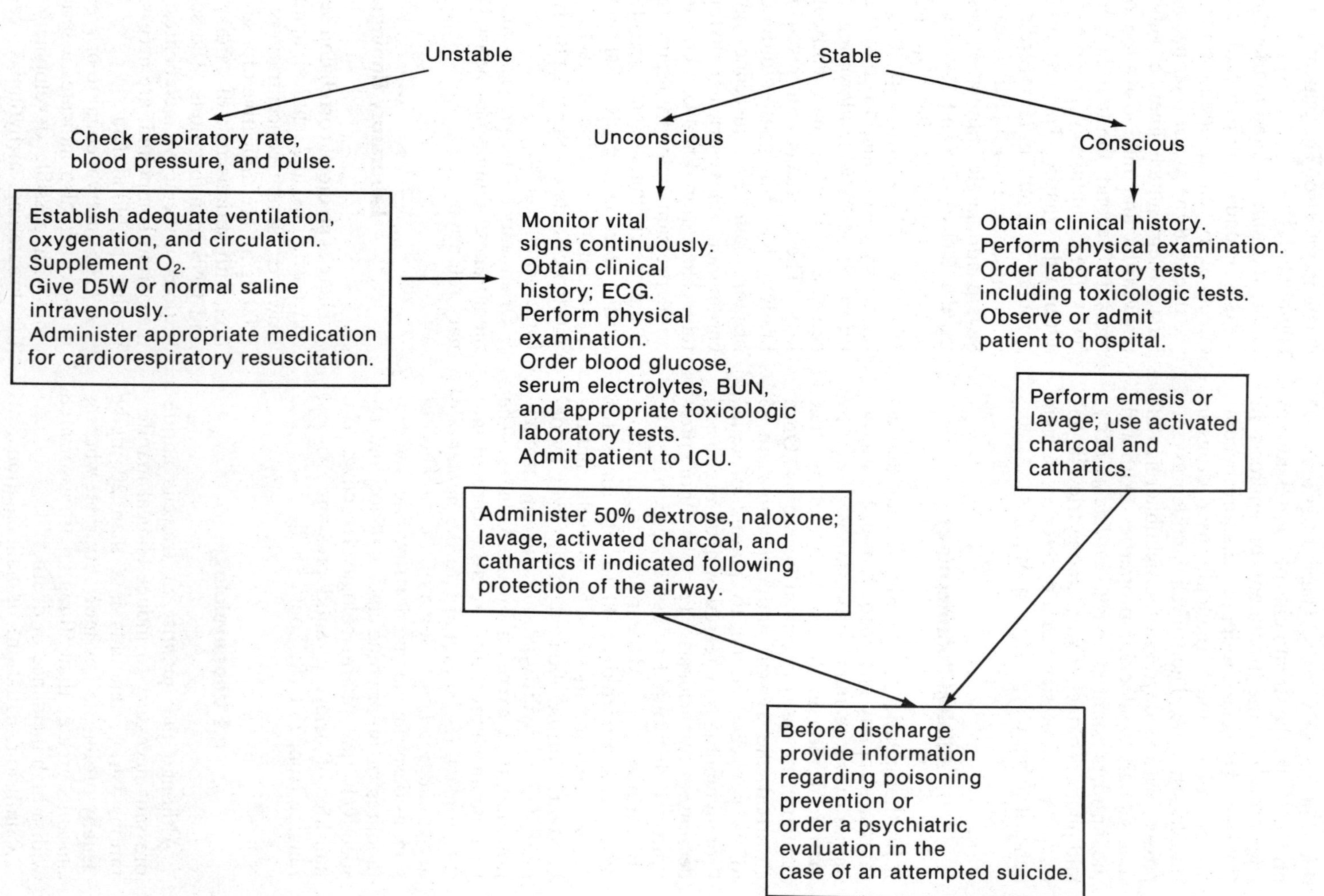
ALGORITHM FOR THE GENERAL MANAGEMENT OF ACUTE POISONING
PATIENT'S VITAL SIGNS
Unstable
Stable
Check respiratory rate, blood pressure, and pulse.
Unconscious
Conscious
Establish adequate ventilation, oxygenation, and circulation. Supplement O_2. Give D5W or normal saline intravenously. Administer appropriate medication for cardiorespiratory resuscitation.
Monitor vital signs continuously. Obtain clinical history; ECG. Perform physical examination. Order blood glucose, serum electrolytes, BUN, and appropriate toxicologic laboratory tests. Admit patient to ICU.
Obtain clinical history. Perform physical examination. Order laboratory tests, including toxicologic tests. Observe or admit patient to hospital.
Perform emesis or lavage; use activated charcoal and cathartics.
Administer 50% dextrose, naloxone; lavage, activated charcoal, and cathartics if indicated following protection of the airway.
Before discharge provide information regarding poisoning prevention or order a psychiatric evaluation in the case of an attempted suicide.

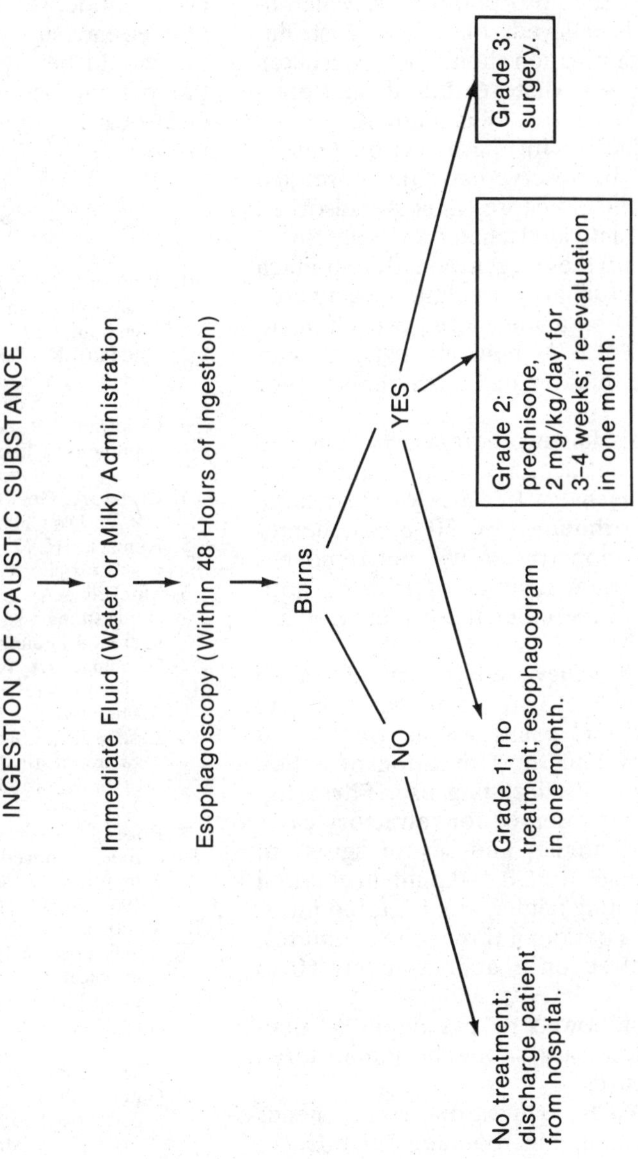
ALGORITHM FOR THE EMERGENCY ROOM MANAGEMENT
OF CAUSTIC INGESTION
INGESTION OF CAUSTIC SUBSTANCE
Immediate Fluid (Water or Milk) Administration
Esophagoscopy (Within 48 Hours of Ingestion)
Burns
NO
YES
No treatment; discharge patient from hospital.
Grade 1; no treatment; esophagogram in one month.
Grade 2; prednisone, 2 mg/kg/day for 3–4 weeks; re-evaluation in one month.
Grade 3; surgery.

usually when tricyclic antidepressant serum levels are greater than 1000 ng/ml. Other common electrocardiographic changes include right bundle branch block, first degree heart block, and Q-T interval prolongation.

Treatment

In overdose, the absorption of tricyclic antidepressants is delayed; therefore, gastrointestinal decontamination should be undertaken in almost all cases whatever the alleged post-ingestion time. In the alert patient, emesis should be induced with ipecac syrup. Gastric lavage should be reserved for the obtunded patient. Tricyclic antidepressants are adsorbed effectively by activated charcoal. Because of the secretion of these agents in the stomach and the hepatobiliary circulation, activated charcoal should be administered every four to six hours for 24 to 48 hours to patients with seizures, life-threatening arrhythmias, or coma.

Fluid diuresis has no therapeutic value because tricyclic antidepressants are mainly metabolized in the liver. Because of their large volume of distribution (>6–30 L/kg), hemodialysis and hemoperfusion will not remove a clinically significant amount of tricyclic antidepressants and therefore these measures are not indicated.[103]

Physostigmine salicylate has been advocated for the treatment of cardiac arrhythmias and seizures. However, its intrinsic neurologic and cardiac toxicity and short duration of action have resulted in its declining use. Physostigmine salicylate is reserved for refractory cases of cardiac arrhythmia, and severe agitation. The dosage ranges from 0.1–0.5 mg in children to 1–2 mg in young adults, administered intravenously over a period of three to five minutes. Its duration of action is approximately 60 to 120 minutes.

Diazepam, followed by phenytoin or phenobarbital if necessary, should be administered to control seizures.

Supraventricular tachycardia rarely needs treatment. Sodium bicarbonate, 1.0 mEq/kg administered intravenously as a bolus, has abolished ventricular arrhythmias in children.[106] If successful, bicarbonate should be given to maintain blood pH between 7.4 to 7.5. Sodium bicarbonate can correct hypotension, especially in patients with acidosis, and can also restore normal conduction.[104] If bicarbonate does not eliminate ventricular arrhythmias, phenytoin or lidocaine should be tried. For hypotension, Trendelenburg positioning and crystalloid administration followed, if necessary, by vasopressors such as norepinephrine or dopamine should be used. First degree block does not require therapy. Severe bradycardia secondary to heartblock and unresponsive to atropine necessitates the insertion of a transvenous pacemaker.[104]

One of the most important aspects of tricyclic antidepressant overdose is the provision of adequate supportive care. Cardiac monitoring should be continued for 6–12 hours after the patient becomes symptom free and the electrocardiogram is normal.

REFERENCES

1. Wilford BB, ed. Drug abuse, a guide for the primary care physician. Chicago: American Medical Association, 1981.
2. Haddad LM, Winchester JF, eds. Clinical management of poisoning and drug overdose. Philadelphia: WB Saunders, 1983.
3. Goldfrank LR, ed. Toxicologic emergencies. A comprehensive handbook in problem solving. 2nd ed. New York: Appleton-Century-Crofts, 1982.
4. Curtis JA, Goel KM. Lomotil poisoning in children. Arch Dis Child 1979; *54*:222–225.
5. Rumack BH, Matthew H. Acetaminophen poisoning and toxicity. Pediatrics 1975; *55*:871–876.
6. Mitchell AA, Lovejoy FH Jr, Goldman P. Drug ingestions associated with miosis in comatose children. J Pediatr 1976; *89*:303–305.
7. Ingelfinger JA, Isakson G, Shine D, et al. Reliability of toxic screen in drug overdose. Clin Pharmacol Ther 1981; *29*:570–575.
8. Easom JM, Lovejoy FH Jr. Efficacy and safety of gastrointestinal decontamination in the treatment of oral poisoning. Pediatr Clin North Am 1979; *26*:827–836.
9. Boxer L, Anderson FP, Rowe DS. Comparison of Ipecac-induced emesis with gastric lavage in the treatment of acute salicylate ingestion. J Pediatr 1969; *74*:800–803.
10. Manoguerra AS, Krenzelok EP. Rapid emesis from high dose of Ipecac syrup in adults and children intoxicated with antiemetics or other drugs. Am J Hosp Pharm 1978; *35*:1360–1362.
11. Jung D, Powell JR, Walson P, Perrier D. Effect of dose on phenytoin absorption. Clin Pharmacol Ther 1980; *28*:479–485.
12. Gaudreault P, Wason S, Lovejoy FH Jr. Acute pediatric theophylline overdose: a summary of 28 cases. J Pediatr 1983; *102*:474–476.
13. Aronow R, Done AK. Phencyclidine overdose: an emerging concept of management. JACEP 1978; *7*:56–59.
14. Neuvonen PJ. Clinical pharmacokinetics of oral activated charcoal in acute intoxications. Clin Pharmacokinet 1982; *7*:465–489.
15. Berg MJ, Berlinger WJ, Goldberg MJ, et al. Acceleration of the body clearance of phenobarbital by oral activated charcoal. N Engl J Med 1982; *307*:642–644.
16. McMartin KE, Ambre JJ, Tephly TR. Methanol

poisoning in human subjects. Role for formic acid accumulation in the metabolic acidosis. Am J Med 1980; *68*:414–418.
17. Berg KJ. Acute acetylsalicylic acid poisoning: treatment with forced alkaline diuresis and diuretics. Eur J Clin Pharmacol 1977; *12*:111–116.
18. Winchester JF, Gelfand MC, Knepshield JH, Schreiner GE. Dialysis and hemoperfusion of poisons and drugs—update. Trans Am Soc Artif Intern Organs 1977; *23*:762–842.
19. Pond S, Rosenberg J, Benowitz NL, Takki S. Pharmacokinetics of haemoperfusion for drug overdose. Clin Pharmacokinet 1979; *4*:329–354.
20. Bennet WM, Muther RS, Parker PA, et al. Drug therapy in renal failure: dosing guidelines for adults. Ann Intern Med 1980; *93*:62–89, 286–325.
21. Rane A, Wilson JT. Clinical pharmacokinetics in infants and children. Clin Pharmacokinet 1976; *1*:2–24.
22. Tilstone WJ, Winchester JF, Reavey PC. The use of pharmacokinetic principles in determining the effectiveness of removal of toxins from blood. Clin Pharmacokinet 1979; *4*:23–37.
23. Spoerke DG Jr. Guide to acquisition, storage and uses of antidotes. Am J Hosp Pharm 1981; *38*:498–506.
24. Benowitz NL, Rosenberg J, Becker CE. Cardiopulmonary catastrophes in drug-overdosed patients. Med Clin North Am 1979; *63*:267–296.
25. Silbert R. Stress in families of children who have ingested poisons. Br Med J 1975; *3*:87–89.
26. Lovejoy FH Jr, Chafee-Bahamon C. The physician's role in accident prevention. Pediatr Rev 1982; *4*:53–60.
27. McCormick MA, Lacouture PG, Gaudreault P, Lovejoy FH Jr. Hazards associated with diaper changing. JAMA 1982; *248*:2159–2160.
28. Walton WW. An evaluation of the poison prevention packaging act. Pediatrics 1982; *69*:363–370.
29. Thompson DF, Trammel HL, Robertson NJ, Reigart JR. Evaluation of regional and non-regional poison centers. N Engl J Med 1983; *308*:191–194.
30. Jollow DJ, Thorgeirsson SS, Potter WZ, et al. Acetaminophen-induced hepatic necrosis. Metabolic disposition of toxic and nontoxic doses of acetaminophen. Pharmacology 1974; *12*:251–271.
31. Mitchell JR, Thorgeirrson SS, Potter WZ, et al. Acetaminophen-induced hepatic injury: protective role of glutathione in man and rationale for therapy. Clin Pharmacol Ther 1974; *16*:676–684.
32. James O, Lesna M, Roberts SH, et al. Liver damage after paracetamol overdose. Comparison of liver function tests, fasting serum bile acids, and liver histology. Lancet 1975; *2*:579–581.
33. Rumack BH, Peterson RC, Koch GG, Amara IA. Acetaminophen overdose. 662 cases with evaluation of oral acetylcysteine treatment. Arch Intern Med 1981; *141*:380–385.
34. Prescott LF, Illingworth RN, Critchley JA et al. Intravenous *N*-acetylcysteine: the treatment of choice for paracetamol poisoning. Br Med J 1979; *2*:1097–1100.
35. Mendelson JH. Biologic concomitants of alcoholism. N Engl J Med 1970; *283*:24–32.
36. Lacouture PG, Wason S, Abrams A, Lovejoy FH Jr. A review of acute isopropyl alcohol intoxication: diagnosis and management. Am J Med 1983; *75*:680–686.
37. Gonda A, Gault H, Churchill D, Hollomby D. Hemodialysis for methanol intoxication. Am J Med 1978; *64*:749–758.
38. Peterson CD, Collins AJ, Himes JM, et al. Ethylene glycol poisoning: pharmacokinetics during therapy with ethanol and hemodialysis. N Engl J Med 1981; *304*:21–23.
39. Sellers EM, Kalant H. Alcohol intoxication and withdrawal. N Engl J Med 1976; *294*:757–762.
40. Kaplan K. Methyl alcohol poisoning. Am J Med Sci 1982; *244*:170–177.
41. Erlanson P, Fritz H, Hagstam KE, et al. Severe methanol intoxication. Acta Med Scand 1965; *1177*:393–408.
42. Collins JM, Hennes DM, Holzgang CR, et al. Recovery after prolonged oliguria due to ethylene glycol intoxication. Arch Intern Med 1970; *125*:1059–1062.
43. Dickerman JD, Bishop W, Marks JF. Acute ethanol intoxication in a child. Pediatrics 1968; *42*:837–840.
44. Stewart RD. The effect of carbon monoxide on humans. Ann Rev Pharmacol 1975; *15*:409–423.
45. Corya BC, Black MJ, McHenry PL. Echocardiographic findings after acute carbon monoxide poisoning. Br Heart J 1976; *38*:712–717.
46. Garland H, Pearce J. Neurological complications of carbon monoxide poisoning. Q J Med 1967; *36*:445–455.
47. Smith JS, Brandon S. Morbidity from acute carbon monoxide poisoning at three-year follow-up. Br Med J 1973; *1*:318–321.
48. Kelley JS, Sophocleus GJ. Retinal hemorrhages in subacute carbon monoxide poisoning. Exposures in homes with blocked furnace flues. JAMA 1978; *239*:1515–1517.
49. Myers RA, Linberg SE, Cowley RA. Carbon monoxide poisoning: the injury and its treatment. JACEP 1979; *8*:479–484.
50. Anderson GK. Treatment of carbon monoxide poisoning with hyperbaric oxygen. Milit Med 1978; *143*:538–541.
51. Muhlendahl KE, Oberdisse U, Krienke EG. Local injuries by accidental ingestion of corrosive substances by children. Arch Toxicol 1978; *39*:299–314.
52. Landau GD, Saunders WH. The effect of chlorine bleach on the esophagus. Arch Otolaryngol 1961; *80*:174–176.
53. Knopp R. Caustic ingestions. JACEP 1979; *8*:329–336.
54. Gaudreault P, Parent M, McGuigan MA, et al. Predictability of esophageal injury from signs and symptoms. A study of caustic ingestion in 378 children. Pediatrics 1983; *71*:767–769.
55. Cello JP, Fogel RP, Boland RC. Liquid caustic ingestion. Spectrum of injury. Arch Intern Med 1980; *140*:501–504.
56. Middlekamp JN, Cone AJ, Ogura JH, et al. Endoscopic diagnosis and steroid and antibiotic therapy of acute lye burns of the esophagus. Laryngoscope 1961; *71*:1354–1362.
57. Hawkins DB, Demeter MJ, Barnett TE. Caustic ingestion: controversies in management. A review of 214 cases. Laryngoscope 1980; *90*:98–109.
58. Holinger P. Management of esophageal lesions caused by chemical burns. Ann Otol Rhinol Laryngol 1980; *77*:819–829.
59. Stannard MW. Corrosive esophagitis in children. Assessment by the esophagogram. Am J Dis Child 1978; *132*:596–599.
60. Rumack BH, Burrington JD. Caustic ingestions: a rational look at diluents. Clin Toxicol 1977; *11*:27–34.
61. Gerarde HW. Toxicological studies on hydrocarbons.

IX. The aspiration hazard and toxicity of hydrocarbons and hydrocarbon mixtures. Arch Environ Health 1963; *6*:329–341.
62. Bratton L, Haddow JE. Ingestion of charcoal lighter fluid. J Pediatr 1975; *87*:633–636.
63. Eade NR, Taussig LM, Marks MI: Hydrocarbon pneumonitis. Pediatrics 1974; *54*:351–356.
64. Zieserl E. Hydrocarbon ingestion and poisoning. Compr Ther 1979; *5*:35–42.
65. Beamon RF, Siegel CJ, Landers G, Green V. Hydrocarbon ingestion in children: a six year retrospective study. JACEP 1976; *5*:771–775.
66. Ng RC, Darwish H, Stewart DA. Emergency treatment of petroleum distillates and turpentine ingestion. Can Med Assoc J 1974; *111*:537–538.
67. Marks MI, Chicoine L, Legere G, Hillman, E. Adrenocorticosteroid treatment of hydrocarbon pneumonia in children—a cooperative study. J Pediatr 1972; *81*:366–369.
68. Steele RW, Conklin RH, Mark HM. Corticosteroids and antibiotics for the treatment of fulminant hydrocarbon aspiration. JAMA 1972; *219*:1434–1437.
69. Anas N, Namasonthi V, Ginsburg CM. Criteria for hospitalizing children who have ingested products containing hydrocarbons. JAMA 1981; *246*:840–843.
70. Murray MJ. Iron absorption. Clin Toxicol 1971; *4*:545–558.
71. Whiten CF, Brough AJ. The pathophysiology of acute iron poisoning. Clin Toxicol 1971; *4*:585–595.
72. Jacobs J, Greene H, Gendel BR. Acute iron intoxication. N Engl J Med 1965; *273*:1124–1127.
73. Gandhi RK, Robarts FH. Hour-glass stricture of the stomach and pyloric stenosis due to ferrous sulfate poisoning. Br J Surg 1962; *49*:613–617.
74. Lacouture PG, Wason S, Temple AC, et al. Emergency assessment of severity in iron overdose by clinical and laboratory methods. J Pediatr 1981; *99*:89–91.
75. Bachrach L, Correa A, Levin R, Grossman M. Iron poisoning: complications of hypertonic phosphate lavage therapy. J Pediatr 1979; *94*:147–149.
76. Robotham JL, Lietman PS. Acute iron poisoning: a review. Am J Dis Child 1980; *134*:875–879.
77. Whitten CF, Gibson GW, Good MH, et al. Studies in acute iron poisoning. I. Desferrioxamine in the treatment of acute iron poisoning: clinical observations, experimental studies and theoretical considerations. Pediatrics 1965; *36*:322–335.
78. Lovejoy FH Jr. Chelation therapy in iron poisoning. J Toxicol Clin Toxicol 1982–1983; *19*:871–874.
79. Moore MR. Diet and lead toxicity. Proc Nutr Soc 1979; *38*:243–250.
80. Ziegler EE. Absorption and retention of lead by infants. Pediatr Res 1978; *12*:29–34.
81. Rabinowitz MB, Wetherill GW, Koppe JD. Lead metabolism in the normal human: stable isotope studies. Science 1973; *182*:725–727.
82. Chisolm JJ Jr. Heme metabolites in blood and urine in relation to lead toxicity and their determination. Adv Clin Chem 1978; *20*:225–265.
83. Klein R. Lead poisoning. Adv Pediatr 1977; *24*:103–132.
84. Chisolm JJ Jr, Barltrop D. Recognition and management of children with increased lead absorption. Arch Dis Child 1979; *54*:249–262.
85. Needleman HL, Gunnoe C, Leviton A. Deficits in psychological and classroom performance of children with elevated dentine lead levels. N Engl J Med 1979; *300*:689–695.
86. Centers for Disease Control. Preventing Lead Poisoning in Young Children. U.S.D.H.E.W. (Report 00–2629) Atlanta, GA: Bureau of State Services, Environmental Health Services, April 1978.
87. Chisolm JJ Jr. Treatment of acute lead intoxication—choice of chelating agents and supportive therapeutic measures. Clin Toxicol 1970; *3*:527–540.
88. Saracino M, Flowers J, Lovejoy FH Jr. The epidemiology of poisoning from drug products. Am J Dis Child 1980; *134*:763–765.
89. Done AK. Aspirin overdosage: incidence, diagnosis and management. Pediatrics 1978; *62*:890–897.
90. Todd PJ, Sills JA, Harris F, Cowen JM. Problems with overdoses of sustained-release aspirin. Lancet 1981; *1*:777.
91. Gaudreault P, Temple AR, Lovejoy FH Jr. The relative severity of acute versus chronic salicylate poisoning in children: a clinical comparison. Pediatrics 1982; *70*:566–569.
92. Done AK. Salicylate intoxication: significance of measurements of salicylate in blood in cases of acute ingestion. Pediatrics 1960; *26*:800–807.
93. Hill JB. Experimental salicylate poisoning: observations on the effects of altering blood pH on the tissue and plasma salicylate concentrations. Pediatrics 1971; *47*:658–665.
94. Buchanan N, Kundig H, Eyberg C. Experimental salicylate intoxication in young baboons: a preliminary report. J Pediatr 1975; *86*:225–232.
95. Berg KJ. Acute acetylsalicylic acid poisoning: treatment with forced alkaline diuresis and diuretics. Eur J Clin Pharmacol 1977; *12*:111–116.
96. Horowitz LN, Spear JF, Moore EN, Rogers R. Effects of aminophylline on the threshold for initiating ventricular fibrillation during respiratory failure. Am J Cardiol 1975; *35*:376–379.
97. Ogilvie RI. Clinical pharmacokinetics of theophylline. Clin Pharmacokinet 1978; *3*:267–293.
98. Weinberger M, Ginchansky E. Dose-dependent kinetics of theophylline disposition in asthmatic children. J Pediatr 1977; *91*:820–824.
99. Helliwell M, Berry D. Theophylline poisoning in adults. Br Med J 1979; *2*:1114.
100. Berlinger WG, Spector R, Goldberg MJ, et al. Enhancement of theophylline clearance by oral activated charcoal. Clin Pharmacol Ther 1983; *333*:351–354.
101. Hollister LE. Tricyclic antidepressants. N Engl J Med 1978; *299*:1106–1109.
102. Hollister LE. Tricyclic antidepressants. N Engl J Med 1978; *299*:1168–1172.
103. Callaham M. Tricyclic antidepressant overdose. JACEP 1979; *8*:413–425.
104. Marshall JB, Forker AD. Cardiovascular effects of tricyclic antidepressant drugs: therapeutic usage, overdose, and management of complications. Am Heart J 1982; *103*:401–414.
105. Petit JM, Spiker DJ, Ruwitch JF, et al. Tricyclic antidepressant plasma levels and adverse effects after overdose. Clin Pharmacol Ther 1977; *21*:47–51.
106. Brown TC. Sodium bicarbonate treatment for tricyclic antidepressant arrhythmias in children. Med J Aust 1976; *2*:380–382.

CHAPTER

6

Diabetic Ketoacidosis

Dorothy J. Becker, M.B., B.Ch., F.C.P. (Paed)
Allan L. Drash, M.D.

Diabetic ketoacidosis (DKA) is a potential complication in every patient with insulin-dependent diabetes mellitus (IDDM). It is an inevitable consequence of untreated or inadequately controlled IDDM. DKA may be part of the initial presentation of IDDM. Ketoacidosis is the most common cause of re-hospitalization in the child with known IDDM.

DKA is a serious, life-threatening metabolic complication of IDDM. It is our impression that the frequency of DKA is declining, both as the presenting feature of IDDM and as a later-recurring problem. There appears to be considerable variation in the frequency of DKA in children and adults in different geographic areas of the world. Although these data are poorly documented and scanty, physicians from Israel and southern Europe report that DKA is uncommon in their countries.[1] The incidence of DKA appears to be slightly higher in central Europe, and even higher in Scandinavia and the United States,[1] where DKA remains a major problem in diabetic children. From our experience at Children's Hospital of Pittsburgh, DKA (defined as a serum bicarbonate level of 15 mEq/L or less), as the presenting feature of newly diagnosed patients, has declined from approximately 80 per cent of cases in the 1950s to 50 per cent currently. The severity of DKA in these children also appears to have lessened. Only 25 per cent of our patients over the past two years had a pH less than 7.2. Severe acidosis with dehydration is more common in our newly diagnosed girls than boys, and it is associated with higher mean glycosylated hemoglobin and serum cholesterol levels in the girls. They also have a greater frequency of evidence of infection or pre-existing infection. The reason for sex differences in DKA is not apparent.

Despite improvement in therapy, DKA remains a major cause of death in IDDM. It is the most common cause of death in the diabetic under 20 years of age.[2] However, with prompt therapy and constant vigilance, the mortality rate in our patients appears to have declined over the past ten years.[2] The overall mortality rate due to DKA is approximately 7 per cent in the United States and United Kingdom, with reports ranging from 1 to 19 per cent.[3] Approximately 65 per cent of all the DKA admissions reported in this study occur in children and adolescents. The mortality is far higher in adults, with death mostly resulting from the complications of myocardial infarction and cerebral vascular accident.

It is hoped that with increasing understanding of the pathogenesis of this disorder and careful therapy, together with education of the physician and patient population, the overall morbidity and mortality rates of this acute complication can be appreciably lessened in the future.

PRESENTATION AND CLINICAL FEATURES

Insulin deficiency results in a series of understandable and predictable metabolic events, which have associated clinical concomitants. The pathogenesis of these events is described later. In patients with new-onset diabetes, presumably there is a gradual drop in the release of insulin from B-cells with an associated impairment in the metabolism of energy intermediates, including carbohydrate, fat, and protein. The first recognizable symptoms are associated with postprandial hyperglycemia and glycosuria because the concomitant hyperlipidemia and alterations in protein metabolism are not yet clinically evident.[4] Thus, the classic initial clinical features of IDDM include polyuria, polydipsia, polyphagia, and visual disturbances, all associated with hyperglycemia. This condition progresses to a catabolic state with fatigue and weight loss due to altered muscle metabolism. Abnormal fat metabolism results in hypercholesterolemia and ketosis. If the diagnosis of IDDM or of poor control of IDDM is not made at this phase, the symptoms progress to vomiting, abdominal pain, anorexia, dehydration, "sighing" respiration, and, later, impairment of the central nervous system (CNS) or coma. In our experience, most patients have a clinical course of approximately four weeks before development of DKA. In some cases, the symptoms have been identified for only a few days and, in previously diagnosed patients, often for only a few hours prior to their presentation with severe metabolic derangement.

In our experience, very severe DKA is seen most commonly in the infant and toddler. It declines in frequency as the presentation of IDDM in the older child.[4] Similarly, hyperosmolar diabetic coma (severe hyperglycemia with no ketosis) also occurs more often in the younger child.[5] The degree of metabolic derangement in DKA can vary widely from severe uncompensated metabolic acidosis to diabetic ketosis in which there is hyperglycemia and ketonemia with ketonuria and normal acid-base balance. Diabetic ketosis occurs in approximately 50 per cent of our patients.[4] Although the clinical presentation of the patient usually parallels the severity of the biochemical changes, one frequently sees patients who are in surprisingly good clinical condition relative to the severity of their metabolic derangement. One also sees patients who are in poor clinical condition relative to the mildness of metabolic derangement.

The biochemical alterations of DKA are hyperglycemia, dehydration, ketosis, acidosis, and electrolyte disturbance. Often, a linear relationship exists between the concentration of glucose in the blood and the severity of the metabolic acidosis. Exceptions at either extreme occur frequently. Thus, patients may have severe hyperglycemia and hypernatremia with resultant hyperosmolarity and minimal or no ketosis. Hyperosmolar diabetic coma, a rare complication of diabetes in childhood, is at one extreme of this biochemical derangement with marked hyperglycemia but no ketosis and little acidosis. Conversely, we have seen a number of children with severe metabolic acidosis and only mild to moderate hyperglycemia with blood glucose levels in the range of 200–300 mg/100 ml. These patients usually have an acute onset with severe vomiting and frequently have previously diagnosed diabetes. We consider any patient to have DKA whose serum bicarbonate level is less than 16 mEq/L, irrespective of serum pH, i.e., whether or not the acidosis is compensated. We define a serum pH of less than 7.2 in a diabetic as severe ketoacidosis. Hyperlipidemia is almost invariably present in patients with DKA with elevations in both serum cholesterol and triglyceride concentrations. Increases in the serum levels of electrolytes, BUN, and creatinine also occur, depending upon the degree of dehydration. Similarly, the hemoglobin value, hematocrit, and white blood count may be high.

Although the serum sodium concentration is usually high, when associated with severe dehydration, it may be mildly or moderately depressed. The depressed sodium level results from excessive urinary losses and some movement of sodium from the extracellular space into the intracellular space, secondary to the hyperosmolarity associated with hyperglycemia. Serum sodium levels may also be spuriously low in association with the concomitant hyperlipidemia with increased fat displacing plasma water.[6] Some clinical laboratories first extract these circulating lipids, and it is important to determine whether or not hyperlipidemia has been allowed for in each laboratory.[7] Serum potassium levels are usually initially normal or even elevated, depending upon the degree of acidosis and dehydration. This occurs despite severe total body potassium deficit with markedly diminished intracellular concentrations of potassium. During therapy, even with adequate replacement of potassium, there is usually a decline in the serum concentrations of potassium.[8] Like potassium concentration, the concentration of phosphorus in the blood is variable at presentation but usually drops markedly during therapy because of excessive urinary losses with an associated total body phosphorus deficit.[8] Reduction of the intracellular phosphate content is associated with a loss of 2,3-diphosphoglycerate (2,3-DPG), which is probably most important in the red blood cells. Thus, 2,3-DPG, which controls the oxygen affinity of hemoglobin, may be important in oxygen transfer at the tissue level.[9] However, this subject is highly controversial. Although severe hypophosphatemia frequently occurs during therapy in DKA, identifiable associated complications have not been reported in this condition. The importance of hypophosphatemia is therefore not yet clear in DKA.[10]

The glycosylated hemoglobin concentrations

in DKA are variable and probably depend on both the prior duration and severity of hyperglycemia.[4] Routine urinary test findings in DKA indicate glycosuria and ketonuria. Proteinuria and hyaline casts are frequently found at presentation. Both findings depend on the degree of dehydration.

PATHOGENESIS

Insulin Deficiency

The pathophysiology and presenting features of DKA are the subject of a number of recent reviews.[11–13] Ketoacidosis in the newly diagnosed diabetic patient may have a fairly extensive prodrome consisting of the classic symptoms of polydipsia, polyuria, and polyphagia, or it may develop within a few hours in an insulin-treated diabetic child who had otherwise previously been in good health. The first case appears associated with absolute insulin deficiency due to failure of insulin secretion by the pancreatic B-cells, although circulating levels may be detectable in the low-normal range at the time of presentation.[4, 14] In the insulin-treated diabetic child, the cause apparently is relative insulin deficiency with fairly normal circulating insulin levels that are lower than the body's requirement at that time. In both cases, insulin deficiency may only be relative to the high ambient plasma glucose concentration.[11] Reasons for the apparently greater requirement for insulin may be (1) infection, (2) dehydration, (3) physical or emotional stress with overproduction of counter-regulatory hormones, (4) insulin antagonism by elevation of free fatty acid levels, (5) diminished number of insulin receptors associated with acidosis, and (6) circulating insulin antibodies in previously treated patients. Circulating insulin antibodies are usually of low affinity and must be a rare cause of an acute reduction of insulin action.

The absolute or relative insulin deficiency produces a situation of acute intracellular starvation in most of the cells of the body. The accompanying metabolic changes in diabetic ketoacidosis are thus very similar to those found in prolonged starvation. The major effects are those of insulin deficiency, which is accompanied by an acute elevation of the counter-regulatory hormones, presumably stimulated by the insulin deficit and its metabolic consequences.[15]

The metabolic consequences of the insulin deficit are enhanced glycogenolysis and gluconeogenesis resulting in greater hepatic glucose output, increased lipolysis, and reduction of peripheral glucose utilization, lipogenesis, and protein synthesis.

Counter-regulatory Hormones

As suggested previously, absolute insulin deficiency, *per se,* does not account for the development of ketoacidosis in the majority of patients. Even when insulin therapy is omitted, ketoacidosis is not precipitated without the concomitant increment of some, if not all, the counter-regulatory hormones.[11] These hormones, glucagon, catecholamines, cortisol, and growth hormone, which are also known as the stress hormones, antagonize the action of insulin on carbohydrate, protein, and fat metabolism. In DKA of both adults and children there is almost invariably an elevation of at least three, if not all, of the counter-regulatory hormones. The most important for the development of ketogenesis appear to be glucagon and catecholamines because of the rapid onset of their metabolic effect.[11, 16] The actions of glucagon include the following: (1) glycogenolysis, (2) elevated gluconeogenesis, (3) enhanced ketogenesis, probably by suppression of malonyl CoA, which regulates the carnitine acyl transferase enzymes, and (4) possible proteolysis.[17, 18] Catecholamine actions are as follows: (1) lipolysis by stimulation of lipase, (2) gluconeogenesis, (3) possible ketogenesis, and (4) reduction of peripheral glucose utilization.[17]

Cortisol and growth hormone excesses, both of which occur in DKA, have much slower actions but play an important role in the pathogenesis of DKA after a number of hours.[11, 17] The actions of increased circulating cortisol are the catabolism of protein, reduction of peripheral utilization of glucose, augmentation of both gluconeogenesis and ketogenesis along with weak lipolysis. The effects of growth hormone elevation are lipolysis, gluconeogenesis (by an undefined mechanism), augmentation of ketogenesis, and reduction of peripheral glucose utilization.

The Mechanism of Hyperglycemia

The degree of hyperglycemia in DKA varies and does not necessarily correlate with the severity of acidosis. The major source of blood glucose elevation is the continued hepatic glucose output due initially to glycogenolysis and due later to continued gluconeogenesis stimulated by the combination of insulin deficiency and glucagon and catecholamine excess, augumented by the action of cortisol and growth hormone.[19, 20] Superimposed on the elevated glucose output is the reduction of peripheral glucose utilization caused by the absolute or relative insulin deficiency as well as the catecholamine action on muscle and adipose tissue.[21] Most of the glucose formed is excreted in the urine, resulting in a major caloric loss. As long as there is normal renal function, the circulating blood glucose does not increase much above 300–400 mg/100 ml. However, once severe dehydration ensues owing to osmotic diuresis, the diminished glomerular filtration rate prevents further excretion of glucose, and the serum glucose level increases markedly. The more dehydrated the patient, the higher the serum glucose level.[22]

The Mechanism of Hyperlipidemia

DKA is associated almost invariably with hypertriglyceridemia and elevated circulating non-esterified fatty acids (NEFA). The major source of these lipids is lipolysis of the adipose tissue due to stimulation of lipase caused by a combination of insulin deficiency and catecholamine, cortisol, and growth hormone excess.[23] A minor source of serum triglycerides and NEFA may be the hepatocytes.[24] As a result of extensive lipolysis, the serum in DKA may be extremely turbid, with increased viscosity and the danger of sludging in small blood vessels. A major complicating factor caused by severe hyperlipidemia is the spuriously low measurement of plasma electrolytes due to displacement of plasma water by the lipids. Thus, severe hyponatremia may be an artifact of hyperlipidemia unless the lipid is extracted prior to analysis or the true electrolyte concentrations are calculated.[6, 7]

Aminoacidemia

Because DKA is a catabolic condition, with reduced protein synthesis and continued proteolysis associated with both insulin deficiency and cortisol and glucagon excess, it causes increased concentrations of circulating branch-chain amino acids, i.e., leucine, isoleucine, and valine. By contrast, the gluconeogenic amino acid concentrations, particularly those of alanine and glutamine, are diminished because of greater hepatic uptake.[25, 26]

The Mechanism of Ketogenesis[23]

The liver is the sole source of ketone-body production. Acetoacetate and β-hydroxybutrate are metabolized from the increased circulating NEFA delivered from the adipose cells. The liver is set in the ketogenic mode by a combination of insulin deficiency and glucagon excess. The higher ketone body production is controlled by the rate of lipolysis and thus by the substrate availability, and to a minor extent by the supply of ketogenic amino acids, which are leucine and isoleucine. Continued gluconeogenesis, stimulated by glucagon with possibly an additive action of catecholamines and cortisol, produces sufficient NAD for ketone production. The long-chain fatty acids are transported into the mitochondria after combining with carnitine by the action of two carnitine acyl transferase enzymes. Sequential β-oxidation results in the formation of acetoacetate which is in equilibrium with β-hydroxybutyrate. Acetone may be formed by spontaneous decarboxylation of acetoacetate and may be excreted through the lungs or kidneys. Under the condition of severe acidosis, particularly that associated with hypoxia or lactic acidosis, most of the ketone bodies exist as β-hydroxybutyrate. This finding is important because β-hydroxybutyrate does not react with nitroprusside when the serum and urine are tested for ketones. Only acetoacetate will give the classic purple color. As the acidosis resolves, β-hydroxybutyrate is converted to acetoacetate and may give the impression of an increasing production of ketones if one is not aware of this so-called fictitious ketosis. This production of acetoacetate occurs at a time when there is an actual reduction in the total plasma ketone body concentration.[27]

Two studies have shown that the hepatic overproduction of ketone bodies alone cannot account for the huge increase in the circulating ketone concentration in DKA.[28, 29] It is suggested that a reduction in ketone body clearance and utilization is also necessary to explain the severe ketoacidosis. Insulin deficiency and catecholamine excess have been shown to lessen peripheral ketone body utilization, particularly by muscle. Excretion of ketone bodies through the lungs and kidneys is not sufficient to compensate for the greater hepatic production and lesser muscle utilization, particularly when glomerular filtration is diminished due to dehydration.

Mechanism of the Metabolic Acidosis

In children with DKA, the major cause of acidosis is the accumulation of ketone bodies. β-Hydroxybutyrate and acetoacetate both are strong acids and contribute to the classic anion gap found in DKA.[30] When severe dehydration is found with peripheral vascular shutdown and anoxia, an accumulation of lactic acid with lactic acidosis occurs, contributing to the general metabolic acidosis.[31] Patients with DKA usually have a normochloremic acidosis with an elevated anion gap. However, during therapy, despite continued excretion of the ketone bodies, acidosis frequently persists with the appearance of hyperchloremia and disappearance of the anion gap. Excretion of ketone bodies is not associated with a rise in the serum bicarbonate concentration, suggesting the loss of a great deal of alkali together with the ketones in the urine. However, it is likely that the apparent loss of bicarbonate may also occur on a dilutional basis or may be associated with alterations in anion distribution. It is thought that the administration of chlorides during rehydration can only partially account for the hyperchloremia, and the lack of adequate amounts of alkali causes the persistent metabolic acidosis. Serum electrolyte balance is maintained by elevated chloride concentration.[32]

Effects on Renal Function

Water Loss

A major effect of uncontrolled diabetes is osmotic diuresis associated with glycosuria. This water loss results in severe dehydration and, eventually, reduced glomerular filtration. If the decrease in plasma volume is severe, diminished peripheral circulation, shock, and, occasionally, renal tubular necrosis can result.

Electrolyte Loss

The glycosuria of DKA classically is accompanied by a loss of sodium, potassium, calcium, phosphate, and magnesium in the urine. The loss of sodium, calcium, and phosphate is apparently related to both insulin deficiency and glucagon excess, which have a direct effect on the renal tubules. The contraction of the intravascular circulating volume together with the sodium loss stimulates aldosterone secretion. Aldosterone's action on the tubules may account for some of the potassium loss. However, most of the potassium and phosphate loss is due to movement of these cations from the intracellular space into the intravascular space and into the urine due to insulin deficiency. Glucagon excess may induce resistance to the sodium-retaining actions of mineralocorticoids so that circulating aldosterone does not exert its sodium-retaining action.[33, 34] As mentioned previously, the alkali loss through the kidney associated with the excretion of ketone bodies can result in a total body bicarbonate deficit which must be replenished.

Effects on the Brain

Changes in the level of consciousness are a hallmark of severe DKA. These changes can vary from lethargy to stupor and coma. Even when there is no clinical change in the level of consciousness, DKA, particularly when associated with severe hyperosmolarity, is associated with major electroencephalographic (EEG) abnormalities that are usually reversible.[35] Alterations in the level of consciousness appear to be most closely associated with hyperosmolarity due to hyperglycemia, with or without hypernatremia. If there is severe ketoacidosis and dehydration, there may be relative cerebral anoxia, which can also contribute to changes in the level of consciousness. Severe phosphate loss will result in deficiency of 2,3-DPG. This loss results in increased oxygen affinity of hemoglobin and relatively decreased delivery of oxygen to the tissues, i.e., a shift of the Bohr curve to the left.[9] When a patient is severely acidotic, the Bohr curve is effectively shifted to the right. Thus, acidosis and 2,3-DPG reduction counterbalance each other. Severe phosphate depletion without severe acidosis shifts the Bohr curve to the left and, theoretically, is associated with tissue anoxia. However, measurements of oxygen partial pressure were not abnormal in a number of studies.

Hyperosmolar Non-ketotic Coma

In pediatric practice, hyperosmolar non-ketotic coma is an unusual condition that occurs mainly in very young or mentally retarded children.[5] Presumably, these patients are unable to obtain access to sufficient water to prevent severe dehydration. This condition occurs in the presence of a relative insulin deficiency, resulting in excessive glucose production and an osmotic diuresis. However, there appears to be enough insulin to suppress lipolysis and thus prevent an excess production of ketone bodies. Presumably, there is an unexplained limitation to the output of counter-regulatory hormones that would usually occur in a stress situation and stimulate ketogenesis. Coma in these patients is associated with severe hyperosmolarity, metabolic acidosis, and a high incidence of death associated with cerebral edema. It should be remembered that an equal degree of hyperosmolarity can occur in the presence of ketoacidosis.

CAUSES OF DIABETIC KETOACIDOSIS

In both newly diagnosed patients and insulin-treated patients with diabetes, DKA usually is associated with a precipitating factor, making the relative insulin deficiency functionally absolute. The most common precipitating cause is an acute infection, which carries with it an increase in the insulin requirement. Relatively routine pediatric illnesses such as flu, otitis media, and gastroenteritis may rapidly induce ketosis and subsequent acidosis in a previously apparently healthy child or one with well-controlled diabetes. The progression to DKA usually suggests that prompt intervention at home was not accomplished, often because of failure to recognize the early deterioration. DKA is usually associated with rise in the counter-regulatory hormones, particularly cortisol. Insulin withdrawal is probably an unusual cause of acute DKA. Presumably, this is not because insulin is never withheld. It is more likely that most patients have insulin antibodies, and thus have a store of circulating insulin to protect them. The mild insulin deficiency that is induced would result in acute DKA only if it is accompanied by an increase of the counter-regulatory hormones. In most diabetic children the occurrence of DKA after diagnosis is not common. Probably the second most common precipitating causes of DKA after diagnosis are physical and mental stress. There is a small group of patients who have recurrent DKA in response to emotional stress. This response seems related to an acute rise in catecholamine secretion with an accompanying rise in free fatty acid (FFA) production due to lipolysis and subsequent ketogenesis. This response can occur within hours in a previously healthy person with perfectly normal circulating insulin levels. Although this phenomenon is rare in the majority of children with IDDM, it accounts for a large proportion of episodes of DKA, occurring frequently in a small subset of patients. These children appear to have an excessive biochemical response to stress or a defect in the clearance rates of related hormones or substrates. Such patients are referred to as "psychogenic diabetics" and are often adolescent girls from disorganized homes. Our recent experience has shown a similar incidence in pre- and post-adolescent boys. The onset of DKA in these children is usually rapid and the response to medical therapy is prompt. However, the problem will recur unless underlying behavioral problems are identified and resolved. Exercise can also precipitate acute ketoacidosis in a patient who is already partially decompensated. Again, this is presumed to be related to an elevation of catecholamines and glucagon levels in excess of available insulin. Finally, the Somogyi effect may precipitate DKA with insulin excess, causing hypoglycemia with subsequent hyperglycemia induced by an excess production of counter-regulatory hormones. The Somogyi effect classically is associated with the production of ketones and may be severe enough to cause ketoacidosis.

DIFFERENTIAL DIAGNOSIS

If the patient has a known history of diabetes, the differential diagnosis of alterations in consciousness is between DKA and hypoglycemia. Measurement of blood glucose levels by one of the more accurate reagent strips (Chemstrip bG, Visidex, and Dextrostix [with a monitor]) and of serum or urine ketones with Acetest (rather than Keto-Diastix) should give the accurate diagnosis.

Because patients with ketoacidosis often have abominal pain with vomiting, an acute abdomen must enter the differential diagnosis. A patient with diabetes may have an acute abdomen, most commonly from appendicitis.

Severe gastroenteritis is rarely associated with ketoacidosis due to inhibition of insulin secretion with accompanying hyperglycemia and ketosis. Such patients have temporary diabetes and sometimes may require very small amounts of insulin. Lastly, some drugs induce non-diabetic ketoacidosis, the most common being salicylate intoxication in children. In addition, large doses of diazoxide or salbutamol have been reported to induce non-diabetic ketoacidosis. Chronic alcoholism associated with reduced food intake can cause severe hyperketonemia with acidosis. However, alcoholism is usually associated with hypoglycemia.

CLINICAL ASSESSMENT

Most of the diagnostic signs and symptoms of DKA are sequelae of the metabolic disorder. The only feature that is not readily explained is the devastating effect of DKA on the CNS. Patients will almost always present with polyuria and polydipsia of variable duration. These symptoms eventually result in dehydration with consequent hypovolemia, tachycardia, and shock. Metabolic acidosis is usually accompanied by abdominal pain and vomiting—the mechanism of which is not totally clear. DKA typically causes hyperventilation (Kussmaul breathing), which is deep sighing ventilation with a long air column. If the patient is extremely acidotic ($pH < 7$), CNS depression often occurs and the respiratory rate may fall in association with carbon dioxide retention. When acidosis is severe, the serum potassium level may be high. However, because of insulin deficiency there is a great deal of intracellular potassium loss due mainly to potassium diuresis, which accounts for gastric stasis, ileus, muscle weakness and cramps, and the risk of cardiac arrhythmia. The loss of intracellular magnesium and phosphate may add to these symptoms.

The presenting abdominal symptoms and signs may be similar to those of an acute abdomen. Because of the frequent increase in serum amylase levels in DKA, a number of workers have suggested an association of DKA with acute pancreatitis in some of these patients. However, serum amylase levels increase in approximately 70 per cent of patients with DKA, most of whom have no clinical evidence of acute pancreatitis. The raised serum amylase levels are usually associated with severe hyperglycemia, and the origin of the enzyme is likely to be the salivary glands.[36] Reports indicate that approximately 10 per cent of patients with DKA are comatose and coma is associated with a greater mortality risk. Our impression is that the incidence of coma is diminishing at our center because of earlier recognition of decompensating diabetes. Disturbances in the level of consciousness are common, varying from disorientation to agitation, lethargy, stupor, and coma. Cerebral edema at presentation is unusual, and the mechanism of CNS abnormalities appears to be related mainly to the degree of hyperosmolarity. Because DKA is often precipitated by infection, accompanying signs and symptoms should be sought. It is important to note that even in the presence of infection, pyrexia is rare in association with DKA, and leukocytosis frequently occurs despite the absence of infection.

Initial clinical assessment of the patient should be made rapidly and should include: (1) state of hydration, (2) blood pressure and cardiac output, (3) renal function (polyuria or anuria), (4) cerebral function, including a very careful evaluation of the optic discs for papilledema, and (5) complicating and precipitating factors.

Immediately after the clinical assessment, baseline biochemical evaluation of the patient should be made prior to initiation of insulin therapy. This evaluation should include:

1. Urinalysis for glucose and ketones preferably with more sensitive indicators such as Clinitest and Acetest tablets or Chemstrips bG, rather than Keto-Diastix or other strips that are insensitive to the degree of glycosuria and possibly give false-negative results for acetonuria.[37]
2. Serum glucose level using a sensitive laboratory technique after screening with one of the paper strip methods such as Chemstrips bG, Visidex, or Dextrostix (with a monitor).
3. Serum electrolyte levels.
4. Values of arterial or venous gases. In our experience, we have not found values of arterial gases necessary for monitoring patients, and we have used venous blood unless there is peripheral vascular collapse. The measurement of blood gases should include pH, P_{CO_2}, and bicarbonate.
5. Plasma osmolarity should be measured directly or calculated using the formula:

$$2 \times \text{Na mEq/L} + \frac{\text{glucose mg/100 ml}}{18} + \frac{\text{BUN mg/100 ml}}{2.8}$$

6. Serum or plasma ketones levels should be measured using an Acetest tablet.
7. BUN and creatinine levels.
8. Serum calcium and phosphorus values.
9. Serum amylase level (if indicated).
10. Hemoglobin value, hematocrit, and white blood cell count.
11. Microscopic examination of urine.

THERAPY

The development of DKA is usually relatively slow and should be corrected relatively slowly. The only indication for very rapid correction is impending or actual shock. This maxim is probably even more important in treatment of children than of adults.

Rehydration

Because a major feature of DKA is water loss associated with loss of electrolytes, rehydration is the cornerstone of therapy. It is probably more important in the early stages of therapy than insulin delivery. We routinely rehydrate our patients for approximately one hour prior to the administration of insulin while awaiting report of laboratory results. The fluid used is normal saline without the addition of potassium until urine excretion has been confirmed and a serum potassium level is available. The advantage of this initial hour of rehydration is that it allows one to assess the degree of dehydration and rate of blood glucose decrement associated with volume expansion rather than insulin action. Rehydration is very useful in the child in whom the degree of dehydration is not apparent from clinical assessment. Some of the plasma glucose reduction during this period is probably caused by improved insulin action in previously treated patients. The fluid deficit is then calculated according to body weight, and the deficit is corrected over 24 hours with one-half the correction over the first eight hours. It is extremely important to assess continually water balance in the patient with an actual measurement of the total fluid infused or taken orally and the total urine volume lost. The initial fluid rate should be between 10 and 20 ml/kg/hr. Excessive infusion should be avoided unless it is needed for correction of hypotension and shock. Unless severe hyperosmolarity persists after the first hour, the rehydration fluid is changed to half-normal saline in order to supply maintenance fluid, correct the deficit, and replace continual losses. It is mandatory to reassess the fluid status on a regular basis and not to calculate the fluid requirements based on the initial status without re-evaluation.

Maintenance and replacement fluid volumes can be calculated on a weight or surface area basis with allowances being made for age. Most of the rehydration treatment should be administered intravenously and oral fluids should be avoided in the very ill patient, particularly if there has been prior vomiting. Even when oral fluids are tolerated, gastric stasis and ileus may prevent rapid absorption of fluids and make it difficult to calculate actual delivery to the intravascular space. The composition of the rehydration fluid depends on the patient's serum sodium and potassium levels and the serum osmolarity. In general, one should attempt to rehydrate, at least initially, with iso-osmolar solutions, and as the serum osmolarity diminishes, some free water should be administered. Only very rarely is there an indication for the administration of intravenous fluids that do not contain sodium. The aim should be to reduce the serum osmolarity slowly by constant administration of solutions containing sodium (unless the serum sodium levels rise), and later to add glucose (see following section). The concentration of K^+ should not exceed 40 mEq/L except in rare circumstances. Maintenance and replacement fluid volumes can be calculated according to body weight in kilograms (Fig. 6–1).

Insulin Therapy[12, 38]

For many years, the conventional mode of insulin therapy in DKA has been intermittent subcutaneous injections of crystalline insulin. Fairly high doses (100–200 units) were recommended, particularly in adults.[39] In children, the tendency was to use slightly lower doses, although these doses would still be considered high compared with the low doses currently shown to be effective. Since the mid-1970s, a number of studies in both adult and pediatric populations have shown that low-dose intravenous or intramuscular insulin delivery corrects the hyperglycemia and ketoacidosis in DKA equally as rapidly and effectively as the previously used high doses. With lower insulin doses, more physiologic circulating insulin levels are achieved, and hypoglycemia, hypokalemia, and hypophosphatemia have been shown to occur less frequently in comparative studies.[40, 45] Thus, low-dose insulin therapy is the treatment of choice in children with DKA because it appears this level of insulin delivery achieves its goal in the majority of cases.[38, 46] Occasionally, a patient appears to have a greater than usual degree of insulin resistance, requiring slightly higher insulin doses for reversal of the ketoacidotic state. The choice of insulin delivery route should depend on the condition of the patient and the facilities available. If DKA is very mild with minimal acidosis and dehydration, the subcutaneous route of insulin delivery is convenient and effective, especially if the patient does not require intravenous rehydration. The dosage regimen is approximately 0.25 units/kg given every 4–6 hours prior to meals. It should be remembered that crystalline insulin given subcutaneously has a half-life of approximately four hours with the duration of action being six hours at the most. Therefore, patients must receive insulin at least every six hours, even during the night if they are not eating, in order to prevent recurrent ketosis. The dose given during the night can be decreased slightly if ketosis is nearly cleared and should always be accompanied by a small meal.

If the patient is significantly dehydrated, subcutaneous insulin is poorly and irregularly absorbed. Under these circumstances, the use of the intravenous route is preferred for insulin delivery by means of a continuous infusion of 0.1 units/kg/hr after an initial loading bolus of 0.1 units/kg. Although some investigators believe that a loading dose is not necessary,[47] it seems logical to achieve physiologic insulin levels immediately, particularly in the patient who has not had prior insulin therapy. The insulin is delivered in a fairly concentrated solution (approximately 1 unit/ml in normal saline) with the infusion controlled by a syringe pump or IVAC Pediatric Pump through a line, which is connected piggyback to the rehydration intravenous infusion set. A change of the syringe or infusion bag every four to five hours and the use of a concentrated solution of insulin minimize the problems of insulin adherence to the plastic of the infusion system. Thus, the use of albumin has not been necessary.[48] *The mixing of insulin in the rehydration fluid directly is dangerous* because the delivery rate will depend on the rate of rehydration rather than on insulin need. In addition, these dilute solutions of insulin have a greater propensity for loss of insulin onto the surface of the infusion apparatus. The advantage of the intravenous delivery of insulin is the smooth pattern of circulating insulin levels achieved. The physician is able to increase or decrease the amount of insulin delivered with immediate effect since intravenous insulin has a half-life of three to eight minutes. Contrary to popular belief, the patient does not require greater vigilance from a biochemical standpoint when insulin is infused intravenously. The same care is needed irrespective of the route of insulin delivery. However, greater care is required to ensure that the intravenous delivery system and the pump are working effectively. A number of investigators believe that constant intravenous infusion of insulin should not be used in community hospitals that do not have adequate facilities, particularly the use of some type of pump system. The use of intravenous insulin boluses should be discouraged, as it results in supraphysiologic insulin levels being achieved followed immediately by subphysiologic levels with a rapid decline, possibly stimulating an enhanced secretion of counter-regulatory hormones.[38, 49]

Intramuscular insulin delivery with a loading dose of 0.25 units/kg followed by 0.1 units /kg/

	Maintenance Fluid		Deficit (10% dehydration)
Fluid	100 ml/kg	for first 10 kg	100 ml/kg
	50 ml/kg	for second 10 kg	
	20 ml/kg	for >20 kg	
Na	3 mEq/kg		6 mEq/kg
K	2 mEq/kg		5 mEq/kg

Thus, a 30-kg patient with 10 per cent dehydration would need:

	Maintenance	Deficit	Total
Fluids	1700 ml	3000 ml	4700 ml
Na	90 mEq	180 mEq	270 mEq
K	60 mEq	150 mEq	210 mEq

Fluids could be given according to the following procedure:

Hour	ml/kg/hr	Fluid Composition	
1st	15	Normal saline	
2nd	10	Half-normal saline plus 40 mEq KCL/L	Add 5% glucose when necessary
9th–8th	8	Half/normal saline plus 30 mEq KCL/L	
9th–24th	5	Quarter-normal saline plus 20 to 30 mEq KCL/L	

Figure 6–1. Calculation of maintenance fluid.

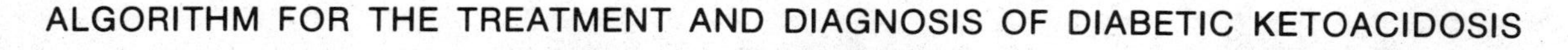

ALGORITHM FOR THE TREATMENT AND DIAGNOSIS OF DIABETIC KETOACIDOSIS

DIFFERENTIAL DIAGNOSIS

↓

Clinical Evaluation
(Hydration, shock, CNS, renal output, and precipitating cause).

↓

Biochemical Evaluation
(Glucose, Na, K, Cl, pH, P_{CO_2}, HCO_3, osmolality, acetone, BUN, Ca, P, Hb, Hct, WBC).

↓

Therapy

- Fluids: First hour normal saline; then half-normal saline and potassium. ? Phosphorus
- Insulin: 0.1 units/kg bolus IV, then 0.1 units/kg/hr continuous IV OR 0.25 units/kg bolus IM, then 0.1 units/kg/hr IM; then SC insulin, 0.25 units/kg q 4–6 hr.
- Bicarbonate: if pH <7.2.
- Glucose: D5W after blood glucose <300 mg/100 ml.

↓

Continue monitoring
(Hourly samples of blood and urine; glucose and acetone; serum Na, K, Cl, osmolality, pH, HCO_3; Ca, Pi every 3 hours; accurate I and O.

↓

Possible complications
(Hypoglycemia, hypokalemia, cerebral edema, hypocalcemia, persistent acidosis, and vascular thrombosis).

hr has been used with the same success as the continuous intravenous routes.[43] The disadvantage of this mode of therapy is the repeated pain of an intramuscular injection, which is avoided with the use of intravenous routes. The amount of insulin given initially should be tailored so that the drop in blood glucose level is approximately, but no more than, 100 mg/100 ml/hr. If the blood glucose level drops more rapidly than this rate the insulin dose should be reduced, and if it drops to less than 75 mg/100 ml/hr, the insulin dose should be increased. We have not found that the dose required varies with age.

Continuous intravenous insulin or hourly muscular insulin delivery is continued until the acidosis is corrected, the hyperglycemia is under control, and ketonemia is virtually absent. Ketonuria will persist for some time after correction of the metabolic acidosis. If a patient is able to eat meals prior to the achievement of these goals, a small increment of insulin should be given to cover the anticipated hyperglycemia. A dose of subcutaneous insulin (0.1–0.25 units/kg, depending on the ambient blood glucose level and appetite) should be given approximately one-half hour prior to the discontinuation of intravenous insulin. The patient should then be given subcutaneous insulin, approximately 0.25 units/kg every 4–6 hours. The next 24 hours should be used to evaluate the patient's total dose requirements. Thereafter, a regimen of intermediate-acting plus short-acting insulin can be started, with the total long-acting insulin dose requirement approximately two-third to three-fourths of the previous day's total crystalline insulin dose. This regimen should be given with approximately the same dose of crystalline insulin as had been used in a single injection on the prior day.

Potassium

Potassium should be given together with the initial insulin dose unless severe hyperkalemia is present ($K^+ > 6$ mEq/L). Potassium is given prophylactically to prevent dangerous hypokalemia from occurring with the movement of serum potassium back into the cells or into the urine. Electrocardiographic (ECG) monitoring is very useful in indicating hyperkalemia and hypokalemia, by demonstrating peaked T-waves in the former and U-waves in the latter. Intracellular potassium deficiency, even when it occurs without accompanying hypokalemia, can result in gastric stasis, ileus, and arrhythmia. Failure to replace potassium is an important cause of death in DKA. Potassium should be administered even when low-dose insulin therapy is used. If bicarbonate is administered, a greater amount of potassium may be needed. In all dehydrated patients, potassium should be given at a rate of 20–40 mEq/L with the intravenous rehydration fluid. If, despite this therapy, the plasma potassium levels drop into the hypokalemic range ($K^+ < 3.5$ mEq/L), a higher concentration may be necessary. Under most circumstances, it is safe to give the potassium in the form of potassium chloride because it is unlikely that the additional chloride administration will significantly contribute to the degree of hyperchloremia that is sometimes seen. If necessary, half the potassium can be given as potassium chloride and the other one-half as potassium phosphate (see later discussion). It should be remembered that 80 per cent of the administered potassium can be lost in the urine during the first 24 hours, and continued oral potassium supplementation in the diet is recommended after an episode of ketoacidosis. Most normal diets contain enough potassium to replenish the body's store.

Phosphate Therapy

Phosphate is lost from the intracellular space by the same mechanism as that causing potassium depletion. The institution of insulin therapy causes a drop in serum phosphate in the majority of patients, resulting occasionally in severe hypophosphatemia. The inclusion of phosphate in the rehydration solution is a subject of continued controversy. The administration of phosphate supplements in the treatment of DKA can prevent early but not late hypophosphatemia and has been reported to maintain normal 2,3-DPG levels, although this has not been shown to be associated with improved peripheral oxygen delivery.[9] Although there is one report of phosphate therapy's improving the level of consciousness in patients with DKA,[50] such is not the case in our experience.[10] High-dose phosphorus supplementation, in children particularly, is associated with the development of severe hypocalcemia and tetany.[51] By contrast, low dose therapy in our studies, does not prevent late hypophosphatemia because most of the supplement is lost in the urine, particularly in patients with severe initial acidosis who require bicarbonate therapy.[10] Total serum calcium, but not ionized serum calcium is diminished in many ill patients with DKA even without the use of phosphate supplements.[10] Because the severe complications of hypophosphatemia are rarely if ever described in children with DKA, and because the benefits of phosphate therapy are not demonstrated conclusively, many pediatricians believe that there is, at present, no indication for phosphate therapy because of the concomitant risk of hypocalcemia. However, others hold that severe hypophosphatemia, *per se,* may be dangerous and that careful supplementation with phosphate with continued monitoring of serum calcium levels and clinical signs of hypocalcemia is a logical form of therapy. We now add phosphate therapy only for the severely ill patient with DKA. The most common mode of administration is half the potassium as potassium chloride and the other half as potassium phosphate. Preferably, phosphate should be given independent of potassium needs as a sodium phosphate solution in a dosage of approximately 4 mM/kg over a 12-hour period. Dietary phosphate supplements should be continued after intravenous rehydration has stopped, in order to correct the total body phosphate deficit and maintain normal intracellular levels of 2,3-DPG.

Magnesium

Although magnesium loss in the urine with intracellar depletion has been documented in DKA, its clinical effects are not clear. Thus, the replacement of magnesium in the rehydration fluid is not commonly carried out. However, severe magnesium depletion can be associated with transient hypoparathyroidism and hypocalcemia. Improvement in resistant hypocalcemia and carpopedal spasm has been reported in one child with DKA after magnesium supplementation.[51]

Bicarbonate Administration

Bicarbonate administration is, perhaps, one of the most controversial areas in the therapy of DKA.[52] It is agreed that severe acidosis should be treated with bicarbonate because of the risk of arrhythmia, reduced cardiac contractility, and possible contribution to circulatory collapse and insulin resistance. The most important danger is impaired ventilatory capacity. There is debate about the definition of severe acidosis. The reason for avoiding the use of bicarbonate is its potential effect on the cerebrospinal fluid pH,[53] the production of severe hypokalemia,[52] the possibility of hypophosphatemia,[10] and the excessively rapid shift of the oxygen dissociation curve to the left that would result in reduced tissue oxygenation, particularly in the presence of diminished 2,3-DPG.[52] Because it has been shown that the paradoxic drop in CNS pH occurs in patients given bicarbonate and in those not given bicarbonate,[54] this danger has been de-emphasized recently. However, the effect of bicarbonate administration on CNS oxygen tension and its possible role in the production of cerebral edema in dogs have made a number of physicians very cautious about its use.[55] Our current recommendation is to add bicarbonate to the rehydration fluid when the serum pH is less than 7.2 or the serum bicarbonate level is less than 12 mEq/L. The amount to be replaced is calculated to correct the serum bicarbonate to a level of 15 mEq/L, and it is given over four to six hours without any bolus administration. Bicarbonate therapy is discontinued as soon as the venous bicarbonate level has reached the 15 mEq/L, even when the calculated amount has not yet been delivered. To calculate the amount of bicarbonate needed, one subtracts the actual serum bicarbonate level from 15, multiplies that value by the weight in kilograms and a correction factor of 0.6.

Glucose Delivery

As the patient's serum glucose level approaches 250–300 mg/100 ml, or possibly when the serum glucose level falls at a rate greater than 100 mg/100 ml/hr, glucose is added to the intravenous fluid, usually as 5 per cent dextrose water and half-normal saline. If the serum glucose level continues to fall rapidly, 10 per cent dextrose water is given to provide calories to the patient who has had a major caloric loss over the past few weeks. The reason for preventing the drop in blood glucose level below 250 mg/100 ml is the result of studies by Arieff and Kleeman, showing that cerebral edema can be induced in rabbits if the blood glucose level drops rapidly below this level from hyperglycemic levels.[56] Thus glucose is added to prevent both a blood glucose decrement of more than 100 mg/100 ml from high levels and to allow the development of normoglycemia from 250 mg/100 ml slowly.

Other Therapeutic Considerations

If the patient is extremely acidotic and in shock, the administration of oxygen for a short time may improve peripheral oxygen delivery. The catheterization of the bladder is rarely necessary and carries with it the risk of infection. If the patient is unconscious, nasogastric suction is necessary to prevent the inhalation of vomitus. Under all circumstances, the precipitating event of the episode of DKA should be sought and treated accordingly. During therapy continuous clinical and biochemical monitoring is mandatory. Initially, hourly measurements should be made of plasma glucose level, electrolyte levels, osmolarity, and blood gas values. Serum calcium and phosphorus concentrations should be measured intermittently. The frequency of electrolyte measurements can be decreased as the patient improves, although blood glucose levels should be obtained every one or two hours. Accurate measurements of fluid intake and output should be made along with appropriate changes in the therapeutic regimen. If possible, the patient should be treated in a metabolic ward or intensive care unit, where the staff is fully conversant with the therapy of DKA. Careful watch for the complications of DKA should be maintained throughout the first 12–24 hours of therapy.

COMPLICATIONS OF DKA

Persistent Acidosis

Persistent acidosis may or may not be accompanied by continued hyperglycemia and may be related to insulin resistance, requiring a higher insulin dose regimen. However, the usual cause is unrecognized or untreated infection or inadequate fluid replacement.

Overhydration

Overhydration results from overestimation of the initial fluid deficit or failure to monitor the patient's fluid balance during the course of therapy. Overhydration may result in peripheral edema or even cardiac failure in the very young child. Peripheral edema may also be caused by hypoalbuminemia, which is frequently seen during the correction of DKA.[10]

Hypoglycemia

Often, hypoglycemia occurs 8–12 hours after the initiation of therapy if serum glucose levels are not monitored regularly. This complication is less likely to occur with the use of low-dose insulin regimens.[57] Hypoglycemia is a possible cause of lethargy, disorientation, and recurrence of coma or seizures. It can be prevented by increasing glucose delivery or reducing the insulin dose as soon as low serum glucose levels are obtained.

Hypokalemia

Low serum potassium levels reflect even lower intracellular concentrations. These intracellular potassium deficits account for some of the symptoms accompanying DKA such as gastric stasis and ileus. If sufficient potassium supplements are not given, classic ECG changes of hypokalemia are observed. Hypokalemia is potentially lethal owing to cardiac arrhythmia. Serum potassium levels should be monitored carefully even if insulin is given subcutaneously and oral hydration is possible.

Cerebral Edema

Cerebral edema is the most feared complication of DKA, occurring more frequently in children than in adults, and has very high mortality and morbidity rates. It most commonly occurs after three to twelve hours of therapy, even in patients who did not have significant hyperosmolarity. After initial improvement in clinical, biochemical, and CNS signs, patients develop greater irritability, CNS depression, and, later, seizures and coma. These conditions may occur even without obvious papilledema. The pathogenesis remains an enigma. There are a number of theories attempting to explain cerebral edema, none of which is entirely satisfactory or proven.[58] These theories are as follows:

1. A rapid drop of the blood glucose levels below 250 mg/100 ml. However, of the 17 patients reported in the medical literature, only nine had blood glucose levels that reached this range.[58]

2. A rapid drop of serum osmolarity or hyponatremia below 125 mEq/L. It is difficult to assess accurate serum sodium levels because of the associated hyperlipidemia in these patients. Despite this difficulty, the serum sodium

levels were not lower than 130 mEq/L in seven of the reported cases. Also, rapid changes in serum osmolarity could not be documented.[58, 59]

3. Overhydration or rapid fluid administration. Again, the theory is difficult to prove because many patients who receive the same amount of intravenous fluid as those who develop cerebral edema do not have any adverse effects. In the patients reported, the amounts and rates of fluid administration were variable. In addition, two patients had received only oral fluids prior to the development of cerebral edema.[58]

4. An increased polyol activity in the brain. It is postulated that the accumulation of osmotically active sorbitol in the brain can account for the elevated CNS pressure that is documented in the majority of patients with DKA who were studied. However, it seems that the osmotic contribution of sorbitol is not sufficient to cause cerebral edema.[60, 61]

5. Cerebral anoxia associated with decreased 2,3-DPG levels. Such an event could be precipitated by rapid bicarbonate infusion or change in pH.[55] This treatment was not unusual in the patients reported in the medical literature. However, cause and effect have not been proven.

A patient who develops any signs of cerebral edema should be referred to a neurologist immediately and treated with mannitol or glycerol with appropriate cerebrospinal fluid pressure monitoring.

PREVENTIVE THERAPY OF DKA

The development of DKA in the child or adolescent with previously diagnosed diabetes mellitus is caused by a failure of therapy, the responsibility for which must be borne by the patient, the family, the physician, and the entire therapeutic team. DKA certainly should be preventable in the known diabetic. Proper daily blood or urine monitoring or both by the patient or family should identify metabolic alterations that may lead to DKA and thus allow initiation of therapeutic intervention, which should prevent the progression of the metabolic problem. We require our patients to check three to four urine or blood specimens daily for glucose content as well as to check the initial morning urine specimen for acetone. The presence of acetone necessitates that each voiding thereafter be checked for acetone. The persistence of acetonuria for more than six hours is an indication to contact the physician for specific directions.

The general principles of preventive management include an increase in oral fluid intake and the administration of additional regular insulin at a dose of 0.1–0.25 units/kg every 4–6 hours in the presence of persistent acetonuria. The development of nausea and continuous vomiting requires examination by a physician and, frequently, hospitalization. Temperature elevation should also be reason for direct observation by the physician. The usual childhood illnesses, such as "flu," laryngitis, tonsillitis, and otitis media, which may be tolerated by the average child with little or no major disability, may rapidly lead to serious metabolic disorder in the child with diabetes. The parents must understand that early contact with their physician is essential to prevent DKA. The availability of a 24-hour "hotline" is most important in ensuring that the families of diabetic children receive prompt and accurate direction for management of impending illness.

A particular problem has arisen since the widespread acceptance of home blood glucose monitoring. It is the position of most patients and many physicians that the utilization of blood glucose level observations makes urine testing superfluous. This is not true. Observations of blood glucose concentration provide no information on the presence or absence of ketonemia or ketonuria. Although it is true that DKA rarely occurs in the presence of normal or modestly elevated blood glucose values, it is also true that many children and adolescents do not perform accurate measurements of blood glucose concentrations. Persistent or episodic hyperglycemia may not be recorded by the child who is performing one or two blood glucose determinations daily. In the past year, we have admitted several patients with previously diagnosed diabetes mellitus for treatment of ketoacidosis who were supposedly monitoring blood glucose concentration carefully. Almost certainly, if these children had been doing at least one urinalysis daily for acetone, the family would have been alerted earlier about a change in metabolic status and would have responded to it. We now insist that all of our patients on routine home blood glucose monitoring assess at least one urine specimen daily (preferably the first void) for both glucose and acetone content. The presence of acetonuria necessitates more attention from the parents.

Despite the best intentions and careful observation and intervention by the family, a small number of cases of DKA in individuals with known diabetes mellitus will almost inevitably continue to occur. Most of these cases will be the result of emotional stress in children whose physiologic response to stress is excessive. The long-term approach to these patients must be based on psychiatric evaluation and family counseling. The other major group of patients who may develop acute onset of DKA are those with acute infections, usually viral and associated with gastroenteritis. A preventive approach to DKA is essential if the mortality associated with IDDM in children is to be reduced. Education about diabetes and its complications is the cornerstone upon which this approach must be constructed. The utilization of a therapeutic team, including physician, diabetes nurse–educator, dietician, and social worker–behaviorist, will enhance the likelihood that adequate education will be delivered and continuing needs met. Prompt attention to intercurrent illnesses, even minor ones, is essential.

The beginning of ketosis should lead to greater fluid intake and additional doses of regular insulin after hypoglycemia has been excluded as a cause of the acetonuria. Recurrent vomiting necessitates intravenous fluid therapy to prevent or to treat dehydration.

DKA in the child can and should be prevented. An important objective for the next decade is to eliminate the morbidity and mortality associated with this metabolic derangement.

REFERENCES

1. International Study Group for Diabetes in Childhood & Adolescence. Personal communication.
2. Dorman J, Laporte R, Kuller LH, et al. The Pittsburgh Insulin Dependent Diabetes Registries: the Mortality Experience. Diabetes 1984: *33*:271.
3. Schade, DS, Eaton RP, Alberti KGMM, Johnston DG. The Importance of Diabetic Coma. *In* Diabetic Coma. Albuquerque; University of New Mexico Press, 1981:3–9.
4. Children's Hospital of Pittsburgh Diabetes Registry (unpublished observations).
5. Rubin HM, Kramer, R, Drash A. Hyperosmolality complicating diabetes mellitus in childhood. J Pediatr 1969; *74*:177–186.
6. Frier BM, Steer CR, Baird JD, Bloomfield, S. Misleading plasma electrolytes in diabetic children with severe hyperlipidemia. Arch Dis Child 1980; *55*:771–775.
7. Steffes MW, Freier EF. A simple and precise method of determining true sodium, potassium, and chloride concentrations in hyperlipemia. J Lab Clin Med 1976; *88*:683–688.
8. Bradley RF. Diabetic ketoacidosis and coma. *In*: Marble A, White P, Bradley RF eds. Joslin Diabetes Mellitus. Philadelphia: Lea & Febiger, 1971: 361–416.
9. Gibby OM, Veale KE, Hayes TM, et al. Oxygen availability from the blood and effect of phosphate replacement of erythrocyte 2,3–diphosphoglycerate and hemoglobin oxygen affinity in diabetic ketoacidosis. Diabetologia 1978; *15*:381–385.
10. Becker DJ, Brown DR, Steranka BH, Drash AL. Comparison of the effects of potassium phosphate and potassium chloride on calcium and phosphorus homeostasis during the treatment of diabetic ketoacidosis. Am J Dis Child 1983; *137*:241–246.
11. Schade DS, Eaton RP: Pathogenesis of diabetic ketoacidosis: a reappraisal. Diabetes Care 1979; *2*:269–306.
12. Alberti KGMM, Hockaday TDR. Diabetic Coma: a reappraisal after 5 years. Clin Endocrinol Metab 1977; *6*:421–455.
13. MacGillivray MH, Brock E, Voorhess ML. Acute diabetic ketoacidosis in children: role of the stress hormones. Pediatr Res 1981; *15*:99–106.
14. Parker ML, Pildes RS, Chaok L, et al. Juvenile diabetes mellitus: a deficiency of insulin. Diabetes 1968; *17*:27–32.
15. Levine, R., Goldstein MS. On the mechanism of action of insulin. Recent Prog Horm Res 1955; *11*:343–380.
16. Gerich JE, Lorenzi M, Bier DM, et al. Effects of physiological levels of glucagon and growth hormone on human carbohydrate and lipid metabolism. J Clin Invest 1976; *57*:875–884.
17. Schade DS, Eaton RP, Alberti KGMM, Johnston DG. Regulation of Intermediary Metabolism in Normal Man. *In*: Diabetic Coma. Albuquerque: University of New Mexico Press, 1981:10–19.
18. Unger RH. Glucagon physiology and pathophysiology. N Engl J Med 1971; *285*:443–448.
19. Bearn AG, Billing BH, Sherlock S.The response of the liver to insulin in normal subjects and in diabetes mellitus. Hepatic vein catheterization studies. Clin Sci 1952; *11*:151–165.
20. Owen OE, Block BSP, Patel M, et al.: Human splanchnic metabolism during diabetic ketoacidosis. Metabolism 1977, *26*:381–398.
21. Forbath N, Hetenyi G Jr. Glucose dynamics in normal subjects and diabetic patients before and after a glucose load. Diabetes 1966; *15*:778–789.
22. Clements, RS Jr, Vourganti B. Fatal diabetic ketoacidosis: major causes and approaches to their prevention. Diabetes Care 1978; *1*:314–325.
23. McGarry JD, Foster DW. Hormonal control in ketogenesis. Arch Intern Med 1977; *137*:495–501.
24. McGarry JD, Foster DW. Regulation of hepatic fatty acid oxidation and ketone body production. Ann Rev Biochem 1980; *49*:395–420.
25. Felig P, Marliss E. Ohman JL, Cahill GE. Plasma amino acid levels in diabetic ketoacidosis. Diabetes 1970; *19*:727–729.
26. Blackshear PJ, Alberti KGMM. Sequential amino acid measurements during experimental diabetic ketoacidosis. Am J Physiol 1975; *228*:205–211.
27. Stephens JM, Sulway MJ, Watkins PJ. Relationship of blood acetoacetate and 3-hydroxybutyrate in diabetes. Diabetes 1971; *20*:485–489.
28. Balasse EO, Havel RJ. Evidence for an effect of insulin on the peripheral utilization of ketone bodies in dogs. J Clin Invest 1971; *40*:801–803.
29. Miles JM, Rizza RA, Haymond MW, Gerich JE.

Effects of acute insulin deficiency on glucose and ketone body turnover in man: evidence for the primacy of overproduction of glucose and ketone bodies in the genesis of diabetic ketoacidos. Diabetes 1980; *29*:926–930.
30. Adrogue HJ, Wilson H, Boyd AE, et al. Plasma acid-base patterns in diabetic ketoacidosis. N Engl J Med 1982; *307*:1603–1610.
31. Hockaday TDR, Alberti KGMM. Diabetic coma. Clin Endocrinol Metab 1972; *1*:751–788.
32. Oh MS, Banerji MA, Carroll HJ. The mechanism of hyperchloremic acidosis during the recovery phase of diabetic ketoacidosis. Diabetes 1981; *30*:310–313.
33. DeFronzo R, Cooke CR, Andres R, et al. The effect of insulin on renal handling of sodium, potassium, calcium, and phosphate in man. J Clin Invest 1975; *55*:845–855.
34. Saudek CD, Boulier PR, Arky RA. The natriuretic effect of glucagon and its role in starvation. J Clin Endocrinol Metab 1975; *36*:761–765.
35. Tsalikian E, Becker DJ, Crumrine PK, et al. Electroencephalographic changes in diabetic ketoacidosis in children. J Pediatr 1981; *99*:355–359.
36. Knight AH, Williams DN, Ellis G, Goldberg DM. Significance of hyperamylasemia and abdominal pain in diabetic ketoacidosis. Br J Med 1973; *3*:128–131.
37. Rosenbloom AL and Malone J. 1. Recognition of impending ketoacidosis delayed by ketone reagent strip failure. JAMA 1978; *240*:2462–2464.
38. Schade DS, Eaton RP, Alberti KGMM, Johnston D. Insulin Dosage. *In*: Diabetic Coma. Albuquerque: University of New Mexico Press, 1981:144–160.
39. Arky RA, Hurwitz D. Management of emergencies: VII. The therapy of diabetic ketoacidosis. N Engl J Med 1966; *274*:1135–1137.
40. Alberti KGMM, Nattrass M. Severe diabetic ketoacidosis. Med Clin North Am 1978; *62*:799–814.
41. Alberti KGMM, Hockaday TDR, Turner RC. Small doses of intramuscular insulin in the treatment of diabetic coma. Lancet 1973; *2*:515–522.
42. Kitabchi AE, Ayyagari V, Guerra SMO. The efficacy of low-dose versus conventional therapy of insulin for treatment of diabetic ketoacidosis. Ann Intern Med 1976; *84*:633–638.
43. Moseley J. Diabetic crises in children treated with small doses of intramuscular insulin. Br Med J 1975; *1*:59–61.
44. Martin MM, Martin ALA. Continuous low-dose infusion of insulin in the treatment of diabetic ketoacidosis in children. J Pediatr 1976; *89*:560–564.
45. Drop SLS, Duval-Arnauld BJM, Gober AE, et al. Low-dose intravenous insulin infusion versus subcutaneous insulin injection: a controlled comparative study of diabetic ketoacidosis. Pediatrics 1977; *59*:733–738.
46. Drash AL. The treatment of diabetic ketoacidosis. J Pediatr 1977; *91*:858–860.
47. Fort P, Waters SM, Lifshitz F. Low-dose insulin infusion in the treatment of diabetic ketoacidosis: bolus versus non-bolus. J Pediatr 1980; *96*:36–40.
48. Page M, Alberti KGMM, Greenwood R. Treatment of diabetic coma with continuous low dose infusion of insulin. Br Med J 1974; *2*:687–690.
49. Clumeck N, DeTroyer A, Naeije R. Treatment of diabetic coma with small intravenous boluses. Br Med J 1976; *11*:394–396.
50. Martin HE, Smith K, Wilson MI. The fluid and electrolyte therapy of severe diabetic acidosis and ketosis. Am J Med 1958; *24*:376–389.
51. Zipf WB, Bacon GF, Spencer ML, et al. Hypocalcemia, hypomagnesemia, and transient hypoparathyroidism during therapy with potassium phosphate in diabetic ketoacidosis. Diabetes Care 1979; *2*:265–268.
52. Schade DS, Eaten RP, Alberti KGMM, Johnston DG. Bicarbonate Administration. *In*: Diabetic Coma, Albuquerque: University of New Mexico Press, 1981: 171–183.
53. Posner JB, Plum F. Spinal fluid pH and neurologic symptoms in systemic acidosis. N Engl J Med 1967; *277*:605–613.
54. Assal JP, Aoko TT, Manzano FM, Kozak GP, Metabolic effects of sodium bicarbonate in the management of diabetic ketoacidosis. Diabetes 1974; *23*:405–411.
55. Bureau MA, Begin R, Berthiaume Y, et al. Cerebral anoxia from bicarbonate infusion in diabetic acidosis. J Pediatr 1980; *96*:968–973.
56. Arieff AL, Kleeman CR. Cerebral edema in diabetic comas. 2. Effects of hyperosmolality, hyperglycemia and insulin in diabetic rabbits. Clin Endocrinol Metab 1974; *38*:1057–1067.
57. Kitabchi AE. Treatment of diabetic ketoacidosis with low-dose insulin. Adv Intern Med 1978; *23*:115–135.
58. Rosenbloom AL, Riley WJ, Weber FT. Cerebral edema complicating diabetic ketoacidosis in childhood. J Pediatr 1980; *96*:357–361.
59. Duck SC, Weldon VV, Pagliara AS, Haymond MW. Cerebral edema complicating therapy for diabetic ketoacidosis. Diabetes 1976; *25*:111–115.
60. Clements RR, Blumenthal SA, Morrison AD, Winegrad AI. Increased cerebrospinal fluid pressure during treatment of diabetic ketosis. Lancet 1971; *2*:671–678.
61. Arieff AI, Kleeman CR. Studies on mechanisms of cerebral edema in diabetic comas: effects of hyperglycemia and rapid lowering of plasma glucose in normal rabbits. J Clin Invest 1973; *52*:571–583.

CHAPTER

7

Drowning

John Pearn, M.D., Ph.D.

Drowning and near-drowning are inescapable themes for all physicians, whether emphasis is placed on emergency-room care of the potential survivor or on preventive aspects. An understanding of the management of clinical aspects of the near-drowned child has become increasingly necessary in recent decades. The field is a rapidly evolving one.

In Western countries, trauma has become the biggest killer of children from 1 to 14 years of age,[1] and of all forms of trauma drowning ranks either first, second, or third in importance, depending on the age and domicile of the child.[2–4] This "distressing and major component of child trauma"[5] now is the biggest killer of pre-school children in some tropical and temperate countries[3] and in some colder climes as well.[6] In Africa and in Western countries bordering the Pacific, the rate of childhood immersion accidents has increased dramatically in the last decade.[7, 8] Each year, of the 100,000 or more persons who drown,[9] more than 8000 children die from accidental immersion.[10] Delayed death due to near-drowning still claims a significant percentage of those extracted from the water with a salvageable heart beat.[11, 12–15]

For every child who drowns in fresh water, another is rescued (albeit unconscious and apneic) who eventually survives. Survival rates approximate 50 per cent[3] and vary with age and sex, and with temperature and osmolality (salt *versus* fresh) of the water involved.[16] In serious salt-water immersions, survival rates for children are as high as or higher than those encountered in fresh-water immersions and approach 70 per cent.[4, 17] This difference probably relates to duration of immersion before rescue or extraction rather than to differences resulting from any pathophysiologic dynamics relating to water osmolality. A significant current challenge to the emergency-room specialist and pediatrician is to effect an increase in these overall survival rates yet at the same time not to increase chronic morbidity rates (from hypoxic brain damage) among the survivors. Debate concerning this potential danger remains current.[12–14, 18–20] With better rescue-site resuscitation and paramedic support during transport to hospital, more potential survivors are now reaching the hospital with residual vital signs. With better immediate care in emergency rooms and casualty departments, more children are technically alive and therefore are included among case series of the near-drowned. This phenomenon has given rise to an apparent paradox, in that post-rescue mortality rates have risen. Although there is no doubt that modern approaches (barbiturate rescue, modified ventilatory approaches, hypothermia, etc.) carry their own potential iatrogenic risk, the observed increase is probably due to the fact that recent aggressive approaches have meant that many attempt the resuscitation and treatment of all patients, no matter how apparently hopeless.[12]

The causes, survival rates, and prognosis of immersion accidents all differ when children are compared with adults.[2, 16, 18, 20–23] Alcohol use,[15] suicide,[24] and boating accidents are important factors inescapable in the management of many near-drowned adults,[25] but they are of little relevance to the great problem of near-drowning as it is presently encountered with children.[26] The prognosis of childhood survivors is also relatively better,[13, 23, 27] probably because of a combination of factors including (1) the nonspecific resilience of the tissues of the young subjects, together with (2) the brain-protecting effect of the diving reflex, which is most active in infants and young children.[28, 29]

Secular trends occur in all forms of childhood trauma. A disturbing feature is that while the rate of childhood accidents generally is decreasing,[22] that for drowning is not. Sea drownings have been with us always; but recent sociologic changes relating to the home ownership of swimming pools, changes towards more casual family lifestyles, and the emancipation of children have been important factors in the current epidemic of fresh-water drownings. Salt-water immersions involving children are now less common than fresh-water immersions, even in littoral regions.[13, 19, 20] In the United States alone there are now over 10 million plastic wading pools and over 4 million surface swimming pools,[5] of which at least 1.6 million are of the more dangerous in-ground variety.[30] Estimates of the number of U.S. pool users are as high as 45 million, and the proportion of pool owners and users (relative to the general population) may well be as high or higher in other countries. Most recent case series of childhood drownings now include a predominance of victims from swimming-pool immersions.[14] In-ground pools cause 80 per cent of child swimming-pool fatalities.[30] Motel, hotel, and caravan and trailer park pools are a particular hazard in all reported series. In affluent communities in tropical and subtropical countries, pool to house ratios are between 1:40 and 1:13.[8] Even in temperate climates, where winters may be freezing, pool to house ratios are as high as 1:10.[31] In Finland, as many near-drownings take place in swimming pools as in lakes, and twice as many in swimming pools as in the sea.[19] Family doctors and emergency-room specialists who work in cities and counties where there is no safety legislation for the fencing of pools can expect to treat a significant number of gravely ill toddlers who have survived near-drowning episodes. Those clinicians working in areas where there is effective safety legislation treat predominantly older children or children who have survived salt-water near-drowning.

Studies from the United States,[10] Europe,[32] Australia,[3] and New Zealand[33] report two age peaks for child drownings—one involving preschool children especially in the 1- to 2-year age range,[3, 4] and a later peak (8–12 years)[33] that involves boys almost exclusively and is often associated with a scenario of disobedience or trespassing.[30] Young teenagers are also at risk from alcohol use during boating and swimming outings and from the relatively common, but dangerously underrated practice of hyperventilating before diving and underwater swimming.[10]

Besides drowning in pools and in the sea, children drown in the family bathtub, in creeks and rivers, in flumes and irrigation and construction trenches, in dams and fishponds, and in buckets.[3, 19, 34–36] Children also drown secondary to child abuse.[37] Epileptic children are at increased risk from drowning,[38] but surprisingly, the realized risks (that is, cases of children who actually succumb) are low.[39, 40]

To be meaningful, risks rates for drowning must specify the osmolality of the water involved (salt *versus* fresh) and be age-corrected. Crude national and world figures for all types of drowning in both salt and fresh water combined suggest an overall rate of 5.6 deaths per 100,000 annually.[9, 25, 41, 42] These statistics are helpful in drawing broad comparisons but from the preventive point of view do not place special "at risk" groups of children in perspective. Annual risk rates for fresh-water drowning and near-drowning alone may vary from as high as 50 per 100,000 for toddlers during their second year of life[3] to rates of less than 1.5 per 100,000 for female teenagers.

Besides the special vulnerability of the 1- to 2-year-old child, groups of children classified by certain factors other than age are also overrepresented in the cases seen in emergency rooms and hospital casualty departments.[43]* Children from families of high socio-economic status are particularly vulnerable to the risks of fresh-water drowning in home in-ground swimming pools; by contrast, children from homes of low socio-economic status are more vulnerable to the risks of accidental bathtub immersions causing fatality or near-fatality.[21, 35, 37, 44] Experienced emergency-room physicians agree that the general clientele who require life support measures do not represent the population in general but are from subgroups within society who are at special risk both from trauma and from potentially life-threatening non-traumatic illness.

The emergency-room or casualty physicians will see near-drowned children who manifest a whole spectrum of clinical severity. At one end of the spectrum is the child who has been rescued apparently lifeless from the water but in the ensuing 30 minutes to 2 hours (the average time it takes to reach the emergency room) has recovered well. In many cases the child is fully conscious (with the triage approach to classification, this group is classified as category A or awake).[12, 27] Of all near-drowning accidents involving children, the fully-conscious child is the most common patient local and casualty room physicians will see. At the other end of the spectrum is the

*"Emergency room," "casualty department," "triage bay," and "reception room" are synonymous terms used in various countries.

child with fixed, dilated pupils, the only vital sign being some electrical cardiac activity unrecognizable as a normal electrocardiographic (ECG) complex. The last five years have seen a vigorous approach to therapy in an attempt to salvage the patients in this very severely affected group.[27] The principal, current problem is how to interpret the results of vigorous intervention therapy because there are a number of variable baseline factors relating to the pathogenesis of the damaged brain and lung. Such variables, of course, operate before the child reaches the hospital and combine to produce a complex of variables that is often not only unquantifiable, but also unknowable. Scientific evaluation has been difficult either because the patients have been considered as one group, or because they have been classified on a pulmonary basis using such classifications as wet *versus* dry drowning, primary *versus* secondary drowning, fresh-water *versus* salt-water drowning, cold water *versus* warm water drowning,[27] with the most important variable—immersion time—always unknowable in a real-life situation involving humans. The natural history of near-drowning with the more severe degrees of hypoxic insult is still debated.[14]

There are few more rewarding experiences for the emergency-room physician than saving the near-drowned child.

PATHOPHYSIOLOGY

Water

In approximately 90 per cent of drowning fatalities death is believed to be due to the inhalation of water into the alveoli. The fluid in which children drown is a water mixture of inorganic substances, gases, dissolved organic matter, and particulate matter, including bacteria, fungi, diatoms,[42] zooplankton, and phytoplankton.

Sea water contains a mixture of salts, of which total concentration varies from place to place but of which proportions remain constant.[45, 46] Salinity is defined as the total mass of solids (in grams) in solution in one kilogram of water and is expressed as parts per thousand (ppt) or gm/kg. In case series of children who drown in inland seas or in delta regions, the salinity may be very low, approaching that of fresh water. In oceanic sea water, a typical salt-ion profile is as follows: sodium, 10.5 gm/kg; magnesium, 1.3 gm/kg; calcium, 0.4 gm/kg; chloride, 18.9 gm/kg; and sulfate, 2.6 gm/kg. Oceanic sea water thus typically contains 34.48 gm/kg of dissolved salts, of which 29.54 gm/kg is sodium chloride. Sea water contains 2.9 per cent sodium chloride compared with 0.87 per cent sodium chloride for human plasma.

Fresh water contains variable amounts of organic material, dissolved salts, and free and nascent gases. Most young children who drown do so in chlorinated fresh water pools or in bathtubs with variable concentrations of soap; however, the chemical effects of chlorine and soap in fresh water are currently believed not to be of consequence in the pathophysiology of lung syndromes in survivors. Experimental studies with dogs have not demonstrated big differences in the effects on the surface tension of lung surfactant between chlorinated water and simple fresh water.[47] However, when compared with the effects observed following salt water aspiration, both types of fresh water elevate the minimal surface tensions of tracheal and lung aspirates significantly. In experimental studies using dogs, the test subjects survive total immersion marginally longer if the drowning medium is salt water (or even normal saline) than if it is fresh water, but the reasons are unclear.

Although children drown in vessels filled with paint, fertilizer, and agricultural and industrial and domestic chemicals,[36] such occurrences are rare. When they occur, specific problems of management (particularly with respect to the treatment of tracheal and bronchial epithelial burns) must be addressed.

The Submerged Child

Although death comes quickly and very unsubtly, one of the complications inherent in drowning is that there are several ways in which subjects die while in the water.[42] Brain death is the end result, but the first link in the chain leading to death may be cerebral hypoxia, carbon dioxide narcosis, laryngeal spasm, vagal cardiac inhibition, or ventricular fibrillation. In a pedantic sense, some investigators define "true drowning" as death due to the aspiration of fluid into the air passages; and death due to laryngeal spasm or vagal cardiac effects might be more correctly termed "death from submersion" rather than drowning.

Irrespective of the osmolality of the inhaled water, it is now known that relatively large volumes of water may move from alveoli into the blood stream. Various osmotic effects act on alveolar and bronchial epithelium differently, with secondary accumulation of fluid and pink froth, particularly in sea-water victims. In fresh-water victims, it has been known since the pioneering experiments of Swann in 1951[48, 49] that large volumes of water can pass across the alveolar-capillary interphase.[50]

How much fluid is needed to drown a child is unknown. Certainly depth is no guide, because children can drown in less than 20 centimeters of water in the family bathtub and in ornamental ponds. Intoxicated and epileptic subjects and persons with cervical and head injuries can drown in very shallow water. As little as 1 ml/kg of fresh water instilled into the trachea causes gross physiologic responses in the lungs. In studies using a simulated aspiration of 11 ml/kg of fresh water or less, gross lung changes result; however, the increase in blood volume is not greater than the capacity of the heart and kidney to compensate for this potential fluid overload.[51] The heart compensates by using the basic reflexes described by Starling's law, the Bainbridge reflex, and the Anrep effect.

Experimental studies in dogs show that the anesthetized animal continues to breathe spontaneously (albeit with grossly altered ventilatory patterns) after aspiration of 22 ml/kg, if the water is inhaled as a single event, and the animal is in effect then rescued from the water.[52] The implication is that in the case of a typical childhood drowning (of a 13 kg, 2-year-old toddler) the amount of inhaled water needed to drown the child probably exceeds 0.3 liters, if a true "wet drowning" occurs.

A considerable amount of informed opinion holds to the belief in "dry drowning" in humans, a condition of fatal cerebral hypoxia due to inadequate ventilation. It is not caused by water aspiration and is secondary to laryngeal spasm or mechanical blockage by mucus and froth. The frequency of dry drowning is variously estimated at 10 to 20 per cent.[53] Good experimental evidence supports the phenomenon of "dry drowning."[51] In experimental drowning with diatom monitoring[42] of minks, muskrats, and beavers, it was shown that not all animals that are trapped fully submerged and "drown" actually take water into the lungs.[54] When dry drowning occurs, it appears that when a small amount of water enters the larynx or trachea, immediate laryngeal spasm (as a vagal reflex) occurs. An immediate outpouring of thick mucus occurs, foam and froth develop, and in some cases a physical mucous plug may form. It seems likely that when the spasm relaxes pre-terminally, more water is prevented from entering the trachea and lungs by the foam and froth, which act as a physical barrier. In these cases, loss of consciousness is caused by anoxia or carbon dioxide narcosis, and death due to brain anoxia follows.

The Drowning Episode (Figure 7–1)

When an unsupervised child gets into difficulty in the water, an initial period of voluntary apnea takes place. From personal observations on infants and toddlers in so-called drown-proofing classes, which are well-meaning but misguided in my view, I was struck by how little the infant and young child struggle as their heads go below the surface—usually they simply hold their breath, make automatic but ineffective paddling type movements, and go calmly to the bottom.

At the age of peak drowning risk (1 to 2-years), it is certain that the diving reflex still operates atavistically to some degree. Its presence can be demonstrated in adult volunteers.[65] Before the drowning child loses consciousness, this reflex occurs within seconds; the submerged child manifests bradycardia and shunting of blood from the cutaneous and splanchnic vascular beds to the cerebral and coronary circulation.[56] Blood pressure starts to rise immediately.[57] These reflex changes are independent of baroreceptor and chemoreceptor input, but depend on both sensory afferents in the trigeminal nerve and reflexive voluntary inhibition of the medullary respiratory centers.[58] Water temperatures above 20°C (the most common temperature in the case of real-life drownings)[59] do not influence the brain-protecting diving reflex,[28] but progressively lower temperatures augment it.[60] The hypothermic brain-sparing effects of near-drowning in cold water may be mediated through an augmented diving reflex as much as through physical chilling of the body core.[12]

In experimental situations using animals, reflex bradycardia is more intense in the frightened or startled animal than in those diving or submerging voluntarily.[54] If this response is the same in humans, a case can be made on physiologic grounds against the practice, condemned by most pediatric groups throughout the world, of so-called drown-proofing of young infants.

The breath can be held voluntarily until a

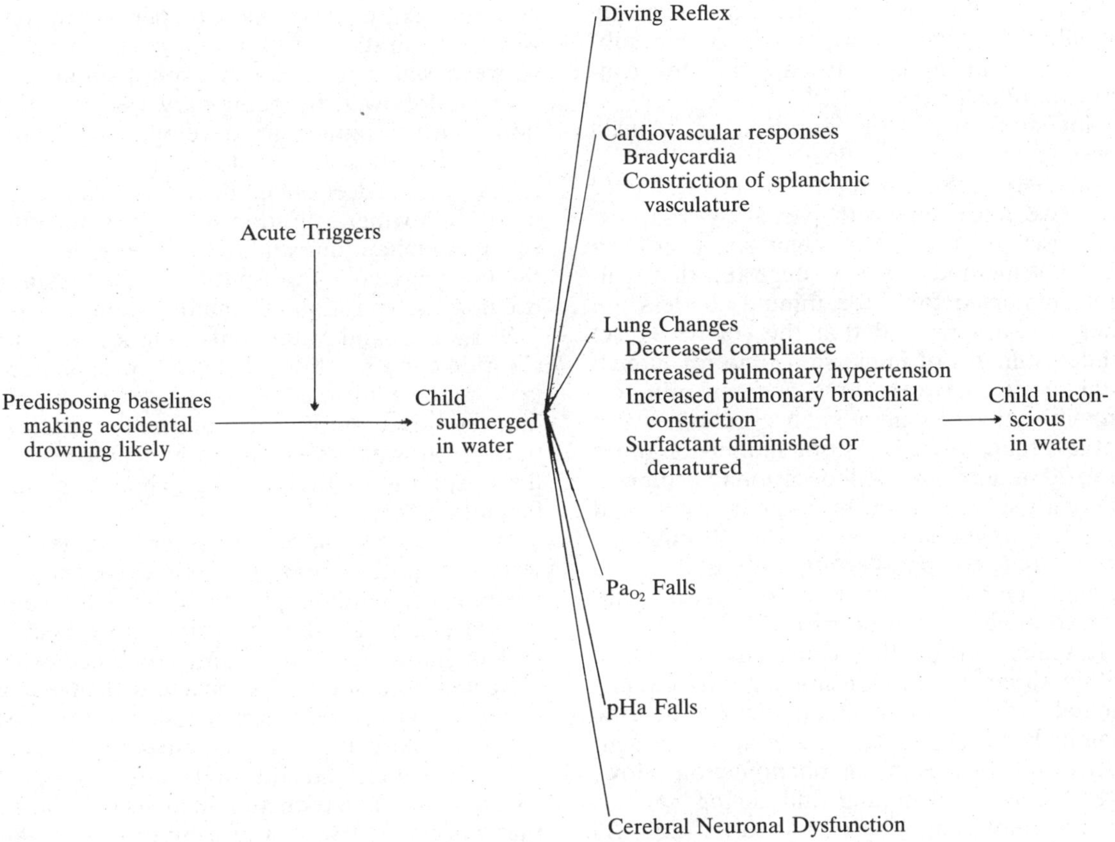

Figure 7–1. The Drowning Chain.

"breaking point" (when a breath must be taken) is reached. The period of breath-holding may be divided into two parts, the first characterized by voluntary inhibition of respiratory muscle activity, and the second in which involuntary diaphragmatic movements occur with reduction of intrathoracic pressure and during which inspiration is prevented only by the voluntary closure of the upper airways.[61] The breaking point is determined by both the hypercarbic and hypoxic drives. The influence of high carbon dioxide or low oxygen concentrations is synergistic; the breaking point occurs at Pa_{CO_2} levels below 55 mmHg if there is associated hypoxia, and at Pa_{O_2} levels below 100 mmHg if the Pa_{CO_2} exceeds 45mm Hg.

When the submerged child reaches the breaking point and an inspiration has to be made, arterial hypoxemia has already developed, and tachycardia, tissue hypoxia, and acidosis occur. Gasping follows. Glottal spasm may then occur. Experimental animal studies,[47] human autopsy studies, clinical series,[51] and case series in which the resuscitators were interviewed all indicate that occluding laryngeal spasm occurs in between 10 and 15 per cent of cases.

Besides gasping, large quantities of water are usually swallowed.[36] Even before consciousness is lost, emesis with aspiration of gastric contents is likely.[62]

In older children, the dangerous practice of hyperventilation before underwater endurance games or dives can change the dynamics of the breath-holding breaking point. If the hypercarbic drive to breathe is lost, unconsciousness (from cerebral hypoxia) may occur before the hypoxic breaking point is reached. Under these circumstances, breathing with fluid aspiration will occur after the patient is unconscious.[63] Whenever the first submerged breaths are taken, a period of secondary apnea follows. In experimental animals, apnea occurs within 10 seconds of fluid aspiration.[47]

Involuntary gasping under water may continue for minutes before respiratory arrest occurs. Arrhythmias are inevitable in all cases of near-drowning and, with absence of ventilation, lead within minutes to brain death, if rescue and resuscitiation are not effected. The spleens of drowned victims are relatively bloodless,[42] because the hypoxia of the submerged victim apparently causes reflex constriction of splenic vessels.

Not surprisingly, the duration of hypoxia necessary to cause the death of an otherwise fit and well child remains unknown. After extensive interviews with parents, neighbors, and rescuers in an Australian study using a "bracket method," it was suggested that children immersed for three minutes or less are likely to survive; and that the (of necessity) crude estimates of immersion time for human fatalities lie between three and ten minutes, providing that the immersion occurs in water not less than 15–20°C.[20] Long immersion times (5 to 20 minutes) are still occasionally compatible with survival even in warmer water; and very long immersion times (5 to 40 minutes) are certainly compatible with both survival and normal neurologic function in children immersed in very cold water (0–15°C).[12]

It seems certain that consciousness is lost within three minutes of submersion. Experimental work with semi-aquatic fur–bearing mammals has shown that there are significant species differences in this phenomenon. However, even in swimming and diving animals such as mink, consciousness is lost within 2½ minutes, and the electroencephalogram (EEG) becomes flat within 4½ minutes.[54] In practice, when a child loses consciousness, cerebral hypoxia is almost always the cause. In boating accidents, in accidents involving falls through ice, and in cold-water accidents involving children who can swim, immersion hypothermia can occur without primary drowning asphyxia. Consciousness is lost when the core body temperature falls below 34°C.[12]

Events in the Lungs

As soon as water enters the lungs a number of pathophysiologic events occur: (1) peripheral airway resistance increases, (2) variable degrees of laryngeal spasm occur, (3) reflex pulmonary vessel vasoconstriction, leading to pulmonary hypertension takes place, (4) lung compliance decreases, (5) ventilation-perfusion ratios fall, (6) fluid shifts occur across the alveolar membrane, (7) surfactant loss occurs (salt water), or properties alter (fresh water), (8) foam and froth are produced, and (9) anatomical changes take place in alveolar epithelial cells.

Besides producing laryngeal spasm, vagal efferents cause obstruction to peripheral airways.[64] Aspiration of even very small amounts of fresh water (1 ml/kg in experimental animals) is followed by pulmonary vasoconstriction with the immediate development of pulmonary hypertension due to a parasympathetic reflex.[65] This latter phenomenon is seen particularly following aspiration of fresh water into the mammalian lung and, to a lesser extent, in the case of sea-water aspiration but does not occur with aspiration of amniotic fluid.

Sea water, and water containing sodium and chloride concentrations that are approximately iso-osmolar with plasma do not denature pulmonary surfactant but may dilute it or wash it out. Fresh water or significantly hypo-osmolar fluid aspiration causes marked change in surfactant activity.[47]

With the aspiration of larger volumes of water (e.g., 2.5 ml/kg), intrapulmonary reflexes cause shunting of blood through non-ventilated areas both in experimental animals[65] and in humans.[50] This shunt, combined with surfactant loss or inactivation and with alveolar collapse, causes a significant reduction in mechanical compliance,[66] a phenomenon that further compounds and adds to the effective right-to-left shunt. The reduction in lung compliance that occurs following the aspiration of even relatively small amounts of fluid can be partly prevented by inhibition of vagal acitivity in experimental animals, implying that its genesis is primarily due to a tenth nerve reflex.[66] A mechanical blockage of the bronchial tree is caused by a combination of bronchial spasm, changes in the elastic properties of lung tissue, and increases in the non-elastic resistance due to physical blockage of the airways by fluid and foam.

The intrapulmonary shunt (i.e., percentage of cardiac output that passes through perfused but unventilated lungs and is therefore unoxygenated) increases dramatically after the aspiration of water; specifically, it increases from the normal range of 5 to 18 per cent to levels approaching 75 per cent within minutes of fresh-water inhalation.[52] Clinical studies in humans have shown that even in children who are conscious, alert, and clinically normal, the shunt takes at least several days to revert fully to pre-accident levels.

The water flux occurs across the alveolar epithelium, through a basement membrane, finally through the endothelial capillary lining into the capillary lumen before hemodilution occurs. This flux causes rapid and severe distortion of pulmonary ultrastructure. Histologic studies show damage to both Type 1 and Type 2 epithelial cells (pneumonocytes). Type 1 pneumonocytes are affected earlier and more severely than Type 2, although the functional effects of surfactant loss, which is believed to be produced by the latter cells, is perhaps the more severe. Endothelial changes consist of cell swelling, micro-vesicle formation, cell detachment from the basement membrane, and cell disruption.[67] The disruption of cells causes release of plasminogen activator, which increases the fibrinolytic activity of blood in the emergent pulmonary vein.

The loss or denaturization of surfactant can develop progressively, even after an apparent successful initial resuscitation. This phenomenon is known as "secondary drowning" and is potentially fatal if not recognized and treated. Although clinically evident secondary drowning occurs in only about five per cent of all cases,[68] it is probable that some degree of hyaline membrane formation occurs in most cases of near-drowning. An outpouring of proteinaceous exudate occurs, which is relatively cell free and may take a number of days to resolve.

Hypoxic March

The cause of death in the acute drowning victim is irreversible cerebral anoxia brought about by (1) cessation of ventilation, due to water in the lungs, or to glottic spasm; and/or (2) ventricular fibrillation or cardiac asystole.

The chain of cardiorespiratory events follows an inexorable sequence: (1) voluntary apnea, (2) diving reflex (with shunting of blood from the cutaneous and splanchnic beds) to a variable degree, (3) arterial hypoxemia, (4) tachycardia and hypertension, (5) tissue hypoxia, (6) tissue acidosis, (7) inhalation with aspiration of water or glottic spasm leading to secondary apnea; consciousness lost at variable places in the sequence, (8) involuntary respiratory movements, continuing under water until respiratory arrest occurs, (9) bradycardia, (10) arrhythmias, (11) hypotension and loss of cerebral and coronary perfusion, (12) cardiac arrest, and (13) brain death. Although cardiac changes may occur from one of several causes, there is no doubt that respiration fails as a result of hypoxia.[66]

Even with only moderate inhalation volumes (i.e., 22 ml/kg body weight) there is good experimental evidence that the heart decompensates temporarily and does not handle the acute increase in blood volume well, particularly that occurring following fresh water inhalation.[52] However, if some oxygenation can be effected during rescue, or if the heart can be mechanically helped by external cardiac compression, cardiac recovery at least can occur with adequate redistribution of the transudated fluid.[52]

Brain Death

The significant link in the pathophysiologic chain occurring in the drowning child is brain death, and it may occur either before or after cardiac asystole. There are four links in the final sequence of brain death in immersion accidents:

State of Decreased Neuronal Metabolism. This state is the so-called cytotoxic stage.[69] After consciousness is lost a short period of reversibility of the altered neuronal metabolism occurs, before intracellular hypoxia and acidosis cause permanent damage. Not all neurons are equally vulnerable, and those associated with more subtle forms of intellectual activity are affected first. In survivors of childhood fresh-water–immersion accidents, formal psychometric studies have shown that skills requiring visual-motor coordination are particularly affected.[23] The EEG becomes flat during this stage but this condition is reversible. Oxygen depletion arrests neuronal activity, and it is probable that the depletion of oxygen stores progresses more rapidly and is more responsible for these early changes than the effect of the accumulation of potentially lethal quantities of hydrogen ion.[70] It is also probable that the order of deleterious influence is hypoxia, acidosis, and hypercarbia.

Vasogenic Stage[71]**.** This stage is a short period during which extravasation of large molecules from cerebral vessels occurs. The blood-brain barrier breaks down, with both fluid and macromolecules passing into parenchyma.

Stage of Edema.[72] Dissolution of vascular and cell wall integrity (functional if not anatomical) leads to both intracellular and intercellular increases in osmotic pressure. If the patient survives, edema develops. It is thought that cerebral edema caused by ischemia is harmful only in that it may cause sufficient hemispheric swelling to result in mass effect and herniation. There is no evidence to date to indicate that edema, *per se,* increases the extent of neuronal death.[73] In survivors, the speed with which significant cerebral edema develops remains uncertain, and in several recent studies this phenomenon has been reported as not being a real problem in the first 24 hours after rescue.[15, 74, 75]

Stage of Permanent Cerebral Death. This condition occurs either within minutes of submersion, and the child is taken to the mortuary rather than the emergency room of the hospital, or is an iatrogenic clinical state created by therapeutic technology.[76] It is important to appreciate that early (up to several hours) post-rescue signs of apparent brain death (flat EEG, fixed and dilated pupils, no vital signs except the ECG trace) are not fully interpretable with our current knowledge as they apply to children, and some 20 per cent or so will eventually survive with neurologic salvage. In cases of true brain death there is, of course, no recovery,[76] although patients can exist with ventilator support in a state of true brain death for 12 weeks or longer.[77]

Survivors and Potential Survivors

The child who is still alive when rescued or who has (at least) some cardiac activity when in the emergency room or casualty department will be at a finite pathophysiologic point along the brain death sequence. If a child has a residual heart beat when rescued or if cardiac circulation can be restored by resuscitation, death may still occur owing to a combination of cerebral hypoxia, cardiac decompensation, acute lung damage,[68, 78] and septicemia.[45, 79]

"A clear understanding of the biologic changes that occur after near-drowning is important for successful therapy."[51]

RESCUE AND FIRST AID MANAGEMENT

In virtually every case of child drowning and near-drowning, the child is near to the shore, and rescue of the child, or extraction of the body from the water, is theoretically easy. Although special techniques have been developed for the cardiopulmonary resuscitation of an adult while a trained rescuer and victim are still in the water,[80] these techniques have no general place in the attempted resuscitation of the child immersion victim. Exceptions, of couse, may occur but are rare. The child, once located, can be brought out of the water within seconds. In a number of instances of childhood drownings in dams or neglected green algae–filled swimming pools, a frantic period occurs during which the child, known to be in the water, cannot be found. Occasionally, an hysterical parent will see the child floating on the surface or lying on the bottom of the pool and will rush off and telephone a spouse or call for help. In my experience, some 10 per cent of parents are ineffective in a practical rescue or extraction of their child from the water.

There is no substitute for a well-trained resuscitator.[81] First aid of the apparently drowned is standard, whether it is pursued at the rescue site or in the casualty department while intubations, monitors, defibrillators, and related hardware are being coordinated. The airway must be cleared, initial breaths given, carotid pulse checked and, if it is absent, combined external cardiac compression (ECC) and expired air resuscitation (EAR) administered. In experimental studies using drowned dogs, the heart can be restarted by mechanical stimulation, and provided that submersion has not occurred for extreme lengths of time (e.g., longer than 10 minutes) it is possible to restore circulation.[82] Even in children who are truly dead when extracted from the water, correctly administered cardiopulmonary resuscitation (CPR) should cause some lessening of pupillary dilatation, and the body should become pink to some degree.

Approximately 80 per cent of victims who do survive will make their first respiratory gasp within five minutes of rescue. Many do so within the first minute after extraction from the water.

The mechanics of EAR may be difficult because of the reduced compliance of the water-containing mechanically altered lungs.[50] The pressure used to inflate the lungs of the near-drowned subject has to be greater than that used for victims who are apneic from other causes; the reduced pulmonary compliance follows tracheal aspiration of both salt and fresh water. The usual danger of overinflation during EAR remains, however, and in experimental studies with near-drowned dogs interstitial emphysema and air embolism can be produced relatively easily by overinflation.[66]

It is very important that an unconscious but breathing near-drowned child be managed (both at the rescue site and during transport to hospital) in the coma position, i.e., the semi-prone position with the head to one side. This general rule of first aid is crucial in the case of a near-drowned child, because regurgitation of large amounts of water from the stomach is very common.[83]

Of all patients pulled unconscious from the water who do survive, less than five per cent will be brain damaged.[23, 84] All such children extracted from the water must be given the benefit of skilled resuscitation in spite of the apparent hopelessness of the situation or fears about possible prognosis.[12]

A small but unknown percentage of children who are unconscious and apneic when rescued from the water nevertheless make a successful recovery in spite of the absence of skillful resuscitation. However, poor technical CPR and effective CPR not commenced within at least ten minutes after rescue are two unfavorable prognostic factors.[13] There is usually no need to be concerned about rewarming at the rescue site when children are rescued from very cold water (<15°C). Ventricular fibrillation due to hypothermia is not a problem until the body temperature falls to approximately 28°C.[12] It is known from both experimental[85] and clinical evidence[86] that if technically good resuscitation is applied, the hypothermic brain can withstand long periods of hypoxia, in extreme cases up to one hour.[87] There is good clinical evidence that the hypoxic brain of the near-drowned child suffers less permanent damage if the body core temperature is reduced until adequate ventilation in the emergency room can be re-established.[88]

All emergency-room physicians have a responsibility to promote the teaching of CPR, and example is the first step. In the United States for the last decade, 66 per cent of general practitioners stated, in reply to a questionnaire, that they were not required to take a practical course in CPR at their medical schools.[89] There is good evidence that trained "first aiders" can turn potential fatalities into survivors. A trained person is also more likely to start resuscitation earlier, giving the victim a better chance of absolute survival and less residual neurologic damage.[90, 91] In a retrospective analysis of childhood survivors of near-drowning, undertaken as part of the Brisbane Drowning Study, the survival rate in the presence of a trained resuscitator was 70 per cent, and in the absence of a trained resuscitator the survival rate was 40 per cent. It seems inescapable that this difference is not simply due to chance, and that trained resuscitators do in fact turn potential fatalities into survivors in a significant number of cases.

All near-drowning victims must be admitted to the hospital for observation because of the risk of secondary drowning.[68, 92] Secondary drowning can occur after both salt-water and fresh-water inhalation, but the pathophysiology differs in each case. The surfactant is not denatured by salt water but is washed out of alveoli.[92] The return of consciousness to normal, or almost normal (after rescue or resuscitation), does not necessarily mean that all danger has passed because deaths are still reported in this group.[50, 93] The question is often asked, "How long should one persist with first aid cardiopulmonary resuscitation efforts in the apparently drowned?" Forty-five minutes to one hour is the best time according to current guidelines developed from a synthesis of published work taking into account both consecutive, unselected series and reports of the outcome of severe, prolonged immersions.[2, 12–15, 18–20] In the case of cold-water immersions, or when the victim is hypothermic or possibly intoxicated, one must press on indefinitely until a positive diagnosis can be made in the emergency room. In a number of cases amazing survivals are reported after immersions of more than 20 minutes in ice-cold water, with excellent recovery.[94–96]

MANAGEMENT

Clinical History

In the emergency room or casualty department, while the child is being assessed and life support instituted and maintained, it is important that as complete a history as possible is obtained. Key factors of the history include: (1) documented or estimated time of accident, (2) type of water (salt, fresh) and degree of contamination, (3) approximated or estimated temperature of water, (4) estimated duration of the immersion or estimated bracket of time during which the child is believed to have been immersed,[23] (5) details of the rescue, (6) documentation of resuscitation attempts, time before CPR was attemped after extraction from the water, and the presence of vomiting during resuscitation, (7) time to the first spontaneous gasp after apnea, (8) details of transport to hospital and maintenance of CPR (or otherwise) during transport, (9) specific features surrounding the immersion incident.[97–100]

An estimate of the time when the submersion occurred is obviously important, and questions about the water osmolality are now believed to be of relative inconsequence. A scientific debate that started some 30 years ago has persisted in clinical circles about whether or not water osmolality is of relevance in the practical context of decisions concerning emergency care of the near-drowned child.[48, 49, 101] Modell's work in the 1960s indicated that if the individual survived near-drowning, the electrolyte changes were likely to be transient and to revert spontaneously to normal.[102] This work and a number of subsequent case series have shown that initial management of the critically ill survivor can discount whether salt or fresh water was involved.[103] Management is governed by clinical assessment and by the results of tests performed on the child after arrival at the emergency room and initial CPR.[50, 104]

In a small percentage of children there will be other coincidental illnesses (epilepsy, asthma, etc.)[38, 40] It is important that the admission history documents these illnesses, as subsequent management may be influenced by them; alerting the emergency-room physician to such coincidental diseases may allow him or her to better anticipate complications. The history should also indicate whether medicine or alcohol (in the case of the younger teenager) is related to the drowning incident.[24, 97, 98] The history should also state whether or not physical injuries have been sustained. Although uncommon, injuries nevertheless occur in most case series, and it is essential when the near-drowning is precipitated by a closed head injury (e.g., from a fall at the edge of a swimming pool) that the medical team be aware of this complication. The possibility of a cervical spine dislocation caused by a diving accident is included in this category.[21, 26]

The admission history should also contain details of the health of other members of the family because they can sometimes provide information about the current drowning accident.[37] The usual social history is also particularly important in this type of case, because certain families are more likely to be represented in such case series. The drowning accident itself is caused by one or more acute triggers, which are superimposed on a vulnerable baseline predisposition. It is known that accidents in general can be attributed to a lowering of a particular threshold because of identifiable intra-familial factors.[100] Finally, as in any pediatric clinical history, it is essential to document the prior developmental history of the child. There is good evidence to indicate that, at least with respect to toddlers (who form the major group of drowning victims in children), it is particularly the bright and adventurous 1- and 2-year-olds who get themselves into potential drowning situations.[23] If questions of subsequent neurologic damage arise, it is desirable to have documented the pre-accident developmental history as a baseline.

Clinical Examination

It is important that the examination be thorough and *systematic,* because from time to time unexpected disease is present that may be related to the cause of drowning itself. Such an unexpected condition (e.g., subarachnoid hemorrhage) might prevent recovery, which might reasonably be expected in other situations.[110] Special attention must be paid to respiratory, cardiovascular, and neurologic systems,[105] to body temperature, and to the elucidation and documentation of baseline states of relevant signs of all body systems, irrespective of the degree of clinical recovery that is present or of the apparent satisfactory recovery of the patient. Initial documentation of pulse, blood pressure, and cardiac signs, as soon as the child reaches the casualty department, is important, because observations of potential myocardial damage and its recovery in the first 30 to 60 minutes after admission may be important when decisions about the use of barbiturates are being made. When a decision is made to attempt a barbiturate rescue in a victim who is comatose or worse (e.g., decerebrate, decorticate, etc.), it may have to be delayed because of potential myocardial toxicity.

In the respiratory system, clinical examination for the presence of pneumothorax is important; subcutaneous air crepitation may reveal the presence of pneumomediastinum. It is important also to seek clinical evidence of aspiration of gastric contents. A number of acute phenomena are seen in the examination of the central nervous system (CNS) during the post-rescue phase. They include spasms,[20, 111, 112] epileptic seizures,[18, 106] opisthotonic stiffening, and progressive neurologic deterioration (which may lead rapidly to coma), which is secondary to pulmonary surfactant inactivation or loss. It is important also to document the clinical appearance of the optic fundi. If fundal hemorrhages are present at the time of admission, they must be recorded so that they are not misinterpreted as having developed during management. If formal monitoring of intracranial pressure (ICP) is not undertaken, the appearance of changes in the optic fundi is a help. However, changes in the fundi are a very crude index because they lag many hours, and sometimes days, behind changes in the ICP.

Grading of the level of consciousness must be done accurately, so it can be used as a baseline for those patients in whom deterioration may occur later and as an essential guide for triage classification, which determines the intensity of treatment in some centers.[105] If the child is awake but cold (it is common for a child to be admitted with a temperature of approximately 35°C), it must be realized that blunted sensorium or unusual behavior may be due to hypothermia rather than to the result of post-anoxic effects or hypoxia when this sign is noted. In hypothermic patients, clinical signs may develop in various body systems because of hypoxia; interpretation is difficult under these circumstances.[107, 108]

A significant number of patients are agitated, screaming, disoriented, depersonalized, or occasionally (in older children and younger teenagers), combative.

Some degree of hypothermia is present in the majority of comatose children and in a significant proportion of those who are conscious but with blunted sensoria. However, in some children the temperature may be elevated. A number of near-drowned victims have an elevated body temperature within three hours after rescue.[53] Whether this elevation represents infection or is a nonspecific response to acute anoxia (like leukocytosis) is unknown.

Tests and Investigations

Laboratory and ancillary investigations are required for immediate diagnosis, and establishment of baselines by which improvement can be judged, or against which the rate and severity of deterioration can be compared and documented objectively. For this reason, in near-drowning cases, it is good clinical practice to undertake certain tests and investigations that under other circumstances might be considered unnecessary. In the case of less severely affected children, and particularly those who are conscious and improve prior to arrival in the emergency room, clinical judgment is required concerning the number and type of tests that are appropriate.[84, 105]

Respiratory

Chest X-Rays. A chest x-ray is, of course, an urgent requirement in every case however well the patient may seem at the time of admission. X-rays should be repeated daily in the conscious child until the time of discharge from the hospital; an average of two days is the norm. One final chest x-ray is required at the follow-up outpatient visit. The initial chest x-ray may be of little value by itself, as it is often relatively normal, even in cases that progress to gross lung complications. Its greatest value is as a baseline test.[103] In the unconscious child, especially if rapid clinical changes are occurring, serial chest x-rays may be needed every four to six hours, or more frequently if positive end-expiratory pressure (PEEP) is being used. There is considerable medical literature relating to radiologic changes in the chest, in near-drowning cases,[113–123] dating from Rosenbaum's classic study in 1964.[123] Chest x-rays remain one of the most rapid, simple, and accurate methods of monitoring the status of the patient.[113] In a significant percentage of those children who arrive in the emergency room alive, pneumothorax will be present or will develop. Surgical emphysema may occur following tracheostomy. The appearance of a normal or almost normal chest x-ray on admission does not mean that complications will not ensue within hours or days.[116, 124] X-ray changes of pulmonary edema are seen in about 85 per cent of all near-drowning cases, and there are no reported differences between the radiologic appearances of salt-water and fresh-water[117] cases. The most frequent patterns observed are of diffuse infiltration throughout both lung fields with concentrations in the perihilar and medial basal areas.[117, 123] Thus, there may be no findings, perihilar pulmonary edema, generalized pulmonary edema,[113] pulmonary edema with localized floccular condensates, or any of these patterns with signs of pneumonia and pneumothorax superimposed. The heart changes seen on x-ray are usually not dramatic.[116] In most cases, irrespective of neurological improvement, clearing of the lungs occurs within three to five days (or even quicker[116]), with complete disappearance of infiltrates by seven to ten days.[113] Exceptions occur when pneumonia, lung abscess, or pneumothorax is present. Lung scans are not practical in the assessment of the near-drowned child at present.

Blood Tests. Blood gas levels, pH, and bicarbonate levels are the most important tests for initial evaluation and for the guide to therapy of the near-drowned patient, as Modell wrote over a decade ago[125]; with newer trials of therapeutic intervention (PEEP, hypothermia, etc.) this statement is even more true today. Even if consciousness has not been lost, more than 80 per cent of near-drowned children have superimposed hypoxemia, acidosis, or both. Assessment of the arterial Pa_{O_2}, Pa_{CO_2}, pH, and base excess levels are, of course, mandatory; as with x-rays, an accurate assessment is required both for diagnosis and for the establishment of baseline levels against which clinical improvement or deterioration can be judged. Arterial hypoxemia must be monitored closely.[51] Experimental studies have shown that oxygen levels fall to 25 mmHg within 15 minutes after near-drowning, even if ventilation is maintained after fluid aspiration.[52] Depletion of oxygen stores progresses ten times more rapidly than the accumulation of lethal quantities of hydrogen ion,[70] but Pa_{O_2} levels measured during treatment do not always correlate well with prognosis.[19] Persistent arterial hypoxemia is a sensitive indicator of lung damage, because low levels of arterial oxygen may remain even after post-aspiration intrapulmonary shunts can no longer be demonstrated.[50] As part of the arterial Pa_{O_2} measurements, if 100 per cent oxygen is breathed for a short time, the use of an appropriate nomogram allows one to measure the degree of intrapulmonary shunting.[176]

Acidosis, rather than hypercarbia, is the critical factor causing death.[70] Absolute levels of acidosis, rather than its rate of development, are the important factors. Circulatory arrest is complete when pHa levels fall to 6.5. It is routine to use the Siggaard-Andersen acid-base nomogram to calculate the base deficit; pH and P_{CO_2} are plotted on standard axes, and the base deficit is read from the third axis. In the usual case of acute acidosis following admission, the total base deficit present in the blood can be calculated and corrected with sodium bicarbonate when appropriate. The pH of arterial blood of a near-drowned victim varies widely, with an average of 7.21,[50] 7.23,[117] and 7.3[98] in a three-study series, with an average base deficit of 10 mEq/L. Possibly one-fifth of all patients have an initial pH of 7.0 or less.[2] Experimental studies show that the pH falls to 7.25 within 15 minutes after a near-drowning episode, even if ventilation is maintained.[52] The degree of acidosis that can be observed is no different in salt-water and fresh-water near-drownings.[78] Acidosis and hypoxia become additive in producing circulatory collapse at a Pa_{O_2} below 25 mmHg and at a pHa level below 6.80.[70] Corrections for temperature have to be made in hypothermic patients.[79, 126, 127] The acidosis is mixed initially, but the respiratory component is usually transient in survivors, leaving a more subacute metabolic acidosis, which is the result of tissue hypoxia and usually requires correction with bicarbonate. The degree of acidosis does not always correspond with the level of consciousness, and conscious patients with pHa below 6.9 are reported.[117] The antithesis may also hold true; Modell and co-workers[84] have described two victims with admission pHa's of 7.43 and 7.41 who subsequently had severe brain damage or died. Frates found that an initial pHa of 7.1 or less did not discriminate well between those who survived and those who died.[4] Oakes reported a neurologically sound survivor who had an admission pHa of 6.67.[15] In general, however, a pHa of <7.0 (measured when the patient has reached the emergency room and is being stabilized for ventilation), is a poor prognostic sign.[2, 13, 15, 19] Except in cases of respiratory complications in which hypoxemia may take days to be corrected, acidosis should be corrected and stabilized within six hours.[78]

Tracheal Swabs. Tracheal swabs are important, both at the time of admission and daily thereafter in all but those patients who are improving dramatically, and whose discharge from the hospital is imminent. The medical literature concerning bacterial infections that may follow near-drowning is impressive, and fatal fungal and protozoal infections can also occur.[13, 128–132]

Respiratory Function Tests. Respiratory function tests (RFTs) should be undertaken as early as practical in children over the age of 6 years. RFTs are possible as soon as the child is awake, and the clinical situation is stabilized. It is important to document baseline respiratory function values before the child is discharged from the hospital, as they form a valuable method of serial documentation of convalescence. Respiratory function values may not necessarily return to normal for up to four months and in some cases not at all.[115]

BLOOD

The usual tests for hemoglobin, white blood cell, and electrolytes are required, although significant changes in electrolytes (requiring correction in survivors) are rarely encountered.[50, 98] Blood culture is appropriate at the first sign of pneumonia and in the case of children manifesting fresh or novel neurologic signs after a refractory period.[128, 132] Serum osmolality is appropriate in all cases initially and as a monitor of the degree of dehydration produced if furosemide and fluid deprivation are being used to prevent an increased ICP.[105] In appropriate cases, plasma levels of anticonvulsants should also be measured.[39,40] Finally, blood alcohol level should be measured in all patients over the age of 12 years, as its correlation with approximately 60 per cent of adult drownings and near-drownings is irrefutable.[133, 134]

Cardiovascular System

Myocardial irritability occurs as a result of hypoxia, and ventricular fibrillation is likely to occur as a consequence.[70] An admission ECG is required in all patients, irrespective of the clinical state, and continual ECG monitoring is required in all comatose patients. The ECG will aid in diagnosis of asystole and will distinguish it from other arrhythmias and from the situation in which a hypothermic heart is beating in sinus bradycardia with low output. Many arrhythmias are caused by hypothermia, and some will resolve spontaneously on warming to 32°C.[135] In the case of myocardial damage from hypoxia or acidosis with a resulting low cardiac output, monitoring by ECG is mandatory if barbiturate rescue (especially with pentobarbitone) is being attemped.[136]

Central Nervous System

In the case of comatose children, an EEG is essential, particularly for establishing a baseline. The place of ICP monitoring still remains unresolved, but many centers have now instituted it, and its usefulness should become obvious in the next few years. The underlying theory is that brain damage is due not only to the primary anoxic insult, but to subsequent events relating to suboptimal cerebral perfusion. Intracerebral shunts and "squeezes" may certainly develop in the post-anoxic brain. Several recent reports have noted that increased ICP, if it does occur, is not an acute phenomenon in the first 12 to 24 hours after rescue. Computerized axial tomography (CAT) scans should be undertaken in comatose patients not responding to treatment within the first few hours after admission. Cerebral atrophy is likely to develop in those patients who develop a permanent vegetative existence. Uncommon but occasionally encountered cases of subarachnoid hemorrhage may be detected by CAT scan. Although formal psychometry is not appropriate while the child is in the hospital, it is essential that an IQ measurement be made after discharge. In patients without permanent neurologic signs, the overall IQ is not reduced, although disparities in performance on subscales may occur.[20, 23]

Other Systems

Organs other than the brain and lungs are very resistant to hypoxia. Renal complications are almost never encountered, and when they do appear they are caused by other secondary complications such as pneumonia.[53] Although hemoglobinuria occurs occasionally after both fresh-water and salt-water near–drowning, in practice it almost never has any effect on the kidney.

It is estimated that about 10 per cent of children in bathtub drownings may be involved in a syndrome of child abuse or neglect (SCAN), the battered child syndrome.[37] For this reason, in all but the most straightforward cases of bathtub drownings, it is appropriate to undertake a radiologic skeletal survey.

Skull and cervical injuries can occur as a precipitating factor in a near-drowning episode. For this reason, particularly in children other than toddlers, if there is any doubt about exactly what happened at the time of the drowning accident, and if serial clinical review in the intensive care unit (ICU) poses questions about damage to the spinal cord, it is essential that a comprehensive radiologic neck series be performed.

Admission and Nursing Care

Because of the potential for secondary complications,[68] all survivors should be admitted to the hospital. In cases of children who are conscious (Modell-Conn categories A and B) (see section on Prognostic Indicators), it is ideal to admit a parent with the child. This is a particularly stressful time. Arterial and venous punctures for various tests and investigations are painful. The child may have a blunted sensorium, a severe post-hypoxic headache, and fear caused by the subjective sensation of inadequate ventilation.

Nursing care in ICUs is very sophisticated. Several areas however require special mention:

1. Because of ventilation-perfusion (V/Q) abnormalities in the child's lung while mechanical ventilation is being undertaken, routine positional and turning changes are necessary.[137]

2. Tracheal toilet and suctioning must be done very carefully and gently because of the tendency for ICP to increase dramatically during this procedure.

3. The child's head cannot be left dependent during turning, positional changes, or suction, because it raises cerebral venous pressure and hence ICP.[12]

4. Temperature control is particularly challenging.[105, 106] If the child is recovering spontaneously but is hypothermic at admission and is conscious, it is appropriate to let the child warm spontaneously. If controlled hypothermia is going to be induced as part of a neurologic treatment procedure, then temperature should be maintained between 30 and 32°C.

Fluid Management

The role of the administration of fluids, or their retention, has gone through several stages in the last two decades. During the last five years, several centers have used a regimen of fluid deprivation and even the withdrawal of fluid to prevent rises in post-anoxic ICP. It has been done by giving furosemide, intravenously (1 mg/kg) and monitoring diuresis. This treatment is combined with an active policy of no intravenous fluids. Recent Canadian reports have suggested that fluid withdrawal may be effective in improving the neurologic quality of recovery[105] but Modell's group has not confirmed this point, which remains unresolved. Some workers believe that the use of plasma may be required if a satisfactory circulating volume cannot be maintained.[138] At this stage of knowledge, it seems prudent to monitor ICP by using an intracranial pressure switch. The extradural bolt is the most widely used instrument for this purpose. It should be used in comatose patients in whom clinical improvement has not occurred after 12 hours or more of intensive care management. If an increase occurs, it should be treated with a combination of barbiturates and hypothermia with fluid restriction. Elevated ICP, if it occurs, is not usually a sudden phenomenon and urgent reduction using mannitol is inappropriate. The problem is best managed with hyperventilation, hypothermia, barbiturates, and dexamethasone. An adjunct to fluid management is the problem of nutrition. It is ideal to commence feeding in the unconscious patient by an intragastric tube with a guarded airway.

A significant volume of water may be absorbed from the stomach in near-drowning, and it is essential that a stomach tube be passed early when the child arrives in the casualty department or the ICU.[106, 139] Aspiration of stomach contents can cause significant lung problems.[140–144] The tube can be left *in situ* and used to supply milk or fortified liquids, which may help reduce the incidence of gastrointestinal bleeding.

Drugs

Sympathomimetic drugs may be required during the ongoing resuscitation. They are often started at the rescue site or at the time of admission. In extreme cases intravenous or intracardiac adrenaline is required, although in some centers experience with intratracheal installation of 1:1000 adrenaline acid tartrate seems effective. Dopamine is less effective in severe acidotic states. Acidosis should be corrected by the use of intravenous bicarbonate used empirically in resuscitation and subsequently on a planned dosage basis if the pH falls below 7.2.

In desperate situations when drugs (e.g., isoprenaline and bicarbonate) are being administered during external cardiac compression, they must be given in the largest central vein available. Reduction in concentration and significant delay in the time-curve of injected agents occur if these drugs are introduced by peripheral injection (e.g., into the antecubital vein).[145]

Although its use is still championed by some workers, the efficacy of dexamethasone has not been confirmed. However, its use to reduce intracanial pressure, in a dosage of 0.1 mg/kg every eight hours for up to two days with appropriate ICP monitoring, would be considered current reasonable practice. Serum potassium levels should be watched closely during this time and supplements given if they fall too low.

Most workers now advocate the use of prophylactic antibiotics because of potential infection in both salt-water[128, 130] and fresh-water cases.[131, 132] Infection with exotic organisms such as amoeba[13] and marine fungi[132] is also reported but is very unusual in childhood near-drowning. Whether or not to use antibiotics prophylactically has not been determined scientifically. Some physicians do not use them routinely in the near-drowned. However, as immune functions are depressed in hypothermic patients, and as there are a considerable number of case reports of patients who die from septicemia,[108] it seems prudent to use them, because their complication rates are low. Septicemia caused by gram-positive and gram-negative organisms may occur. Infection may also be caused by the trans-pulmonary spread from inhaled water of *Vibrio* and fungi. Ampicillin, 500 mg every 6 hours, is an appropriate antibiotic. The subsequent use of ampicillin depends upon the results of daily, routine serial blood cultures. In a Dutch series of nine patients with secondary drowning, three victims who were submerged in contaminated and muddy water (as opposed to salt water or clean fresh water) all died from sepsis.[108] Necrotizing pneumonitis caused by inhaled impurities of mud, sand, and sewage is a potentially fatal complication, and for this reason prophylactic antibiotics seem justified.[126] An appropriate stratagem is to keep a close clinical and microbiologic watch for other potential exotic organisms that are encountered from time to time, and then to treat these appropriately once a specific diagnosis is made from laboratory findings.

Ventilation

Mechanical ventilation is required when children are unable to maintain arterial oxygen and carbon dioxide levels within normal limits by their own efforts.

A Pa_{O_2} of less than 60 mmHg (8.0 kPa) breathing air or less than 80 mmHg (10.6 kPa) breathing oxygen is an indication that mechanical ventilation is required.[126] An arterial CO_2 tension of about 56 mmHg (7.5 kPa) is also an indication.

Mechanical ventilation has always been required for a small proportion of near-drowned children and for a very large proportion of those who are admitted to sophisticated ICUs. However, since the more widespread use of barbiturate coma, mechanical ventilation has been used in the majority of children still comatose after arrival in the ICU. Tidal volume, rate, and peak flow have to be set individually, depending on the age and size of the child. Tidal volumes of 12 to 15 ml/kg are usually appropriate. Questions about optimal wave form, delivered by modern ventilating machines, remain unanswered, although there is experimental evidence in infant pigs that the use of a pressure platform (square wave) may lead to less ventilator-induced reduction in compliance.[126, 140] Ventilator mode should be CPAP/PEEP (constant-positive airway pressure/positive end-expiratory pressure). Although all near-drowned comatose children should be intubated and PEEP used, a percentage of victims (especially among those who are older) will tolerate a mask and will benefit from CPAP rather than the simple breathing of atmospheric air or the simple breathing of oxygen-enriched mixtures in a face box or tent.

The discovery and use of PEEP generally has been hailed as one of the significant therapeutic milestones in medicine,[141] and its use in near-drowning survivors has now been well established for over a decade.[119, 121] Its value lies not only in its ability to increase Pa_{O_2} but also in its optimal ability to minimize lung damage.[140] Constant positive pressure, throughout and between the respiratory cycles, "does not, as may be thought, drive the fluid out of the alveoli and keep it at bay purely by hydrostatic pressure."[126] Rather, it spreads the edemic fluid more thinly owing to an increase in alveolar size, reducing the barrier to gas diffusion and promoting more efficient gas exchange.[142] PEEP acts by preventing alveolar microatelectasis.[105] In theory, its early use in the near-drowned victim may have a prophylactic effect on the development of pulmonary edema.[126] PEEP and CPAP are used in both fresh-water and salt-water cases of near-drowning.[119, 120, 122]

PEEP is usually started at 2.5 cm H_2O and the effect on pulse and blood pressure noted.[138] A PEEP of 5 to 10 cmH_2O (0.67–1.33 kPa) is usually required,[105] although the level must be determined individually. There is a balance between ensuring adequate oxygenation and not causing too great a reduction in cardiac output. Patients who develop progressive signs of secondary drowning[68] may need a PEEP of 10 to 15 cmH_2O.[108] PEEP is required for various periods often ranging between 12 and 60 hours, 24 hours being the average in one reported series.[108] Weaning to IPPV (intermittent positive pressure ventilation) with ZEEP (zero end-expiratory pressure) should take place as soon as possible to reduce the risk of pneumothorax and tracheomalacia. The rate of pneumothorax, occurring as a complication of PEEP, is not greater than 5 per cent in all cases of PEEP used for non-traumatic chest injury; good evidence exists to suggest that when it occurs, the pneumothorax is more closely linked to the primary lesion than due to PEEP ventilation.[121]

Some evidence suggests that Pa_{CO_2} should not be reduced below normal levels, as post-anoxic cerebral perfusion may be reduced,[143] although specific studies with other variables controlled in near-drowned children have not yet been reported. Although oxygen toxicity should not occur, its specific effects on the near-drowned lung have not been studied experimentally.[144] Suctioning of the trachea and attention to bronchial toilet are very important, especially in view of the high incidence of aspiration of gastric contents at the time of the initial accident.[83]

When the arterial blood gases are stable and no progressive changes are seen on chest x-ray, attempts are made to wean the patient from PEEP. By trial and errror (very short interruptions of PEEP) the physician interprets when PEEP can be reduced and then withdrawn.[121] A phase of ZEEP then ensues before weaning from the ventilator finally occurs.

Barbiturate Rescue

The concept of barbiturate rescue arose two decades ago from human case reports followed by experimental primate studies.[146–149] The effects of acute cerebral hypoxia (ischemia caused by carotid artery ligation) could be dramatically reduced if the subject was treated with intravenous barbiturates. Although the most protection was observed when the experimental subject was primed with barbiturate before anoxia, some improvement was still obtained when the drug was administered after the event. Clinical series quickly followed.[150, 151] The results were quickly extended to some open heart surgery and head injury cases,[152, 153] and recently trials have been reported in the case of a near-drowning.[105]

The theory behind the use of barbiturate rescue has been strengthened by the experimental findings that impaired *reperfusion* of the post-anoxic brain may be responsible for ultimate neuronal death, rather than the period of global hypoxia *per se,* at least for five minutes of total brain ischemia.[154] Initial studies were undertaken with phenobarbital in a dose of 3 to 5 mg/kg, with a total infusion dosage of 15 mg/kg for the first 90 minutes. Subsequent studies and trials on near-drowned children have used the longer-acting drug phenobarbital, in a total dosage of 50 mg/kg/day on the first day, and 25 mg/kg/day for days two to four inclusive.[105] At one recommended phenobarbital plasma level of 75 to 100 mg/L (in the presence of hypothermia), the patient will remain comatose, and provided that body core temperature is not less than 30°C, at these blood levels the EEG will not be flat unless brain death is present.[105]

Barbiturate coma may act by reducing ICP, by altering brain metabolism, by changing cerebral blood flow in the microcirculation, or (it is speculated) by a direct pharmacologic effect on the toxic products of hypoxic metabolism. Other drugs exist that have an effect on raised ICP. Lidocaine, for example, may be just as effective as barbiturates and causes less cardiovascular depression.[155] Further studies may be expected to cast better light on this question.

In desperate cases (patients still comatose in the ICU, and certainly those with fixed, dilated pupils), it would seem that nothing is lost by trying barbiturate rescue. Its true value (and optimal duration and minimal dosage if it is proved to be of value) must await future work.

Controlling Raised ICP

Experimental and clinical studies on head injuries have demonstrated that raised ICP is deleterious. Because of this demonstration and the strong suggestion that barbiturate-rescue techniques may operate, at least in part, through lowering ICP, it is current good practice to control raised ICP when it is demonstrated. Experimental studies on cerebral blood flow after five minutes of total ischemia in dogs have shown that ICP is not raised in the first hours after rescue. There is a stage of persistent hypoperfusion after such an hypoxic insult owing to an increase in cerebral vascular resistance, rather than blockages due to microemboli and increased blood viscosity.[143] The smooth-muscle cells of the cerebral vasculature remain responsive to Pa_{CO_2} levels even in the case of permanent neuronal damage with a flat EEG.

Increased ICP can be controlled by both short- and long-acting barbiturates, by lidocaine,[155] by gentle nursing techniques, and by reduction of handling and painful stimuli to a minimum, by hypothermia (with or without chlorpromazine), and by external cooling. Although it takes a number of hours to act, perhaps the most effective method is intramuscular dexamethasone in a loading dose of

0.2 mg/kg, with a maintenance dosage of 0.1 mg/kg, every 8 hours thereafter.

Hypothermia

The role of hypothermia is difficult to evaluate, and its individual effect with combined aggressive therapy of the near-drowned remains unknown.[84] In the child who is awake, albeit with blunted consciousness, there is no point in rewarming rapidly. Rewarming should be allowed to progress over the next six to eight hours after rescue. In the victim who remains comatose for 30 to 60 minutes after extraction from the water, significant core hypothermia is the rule, with temperatures usually in the range of 34 to 35°C if water temperature was not low. In practice, temperature usually falls further in an air-conditioned intensive care room, unless steps are taken to actively rewarm the child. If a decision is made to induce hypothermia actively (by ice packs, barbiturate coma, intravenous chlorpromazine, etc.) it should be done under ECG monitoring as soon as the respiratory and cardiovascular systems are stabilized.

The role of hypothermia is difficult to evaluate. Its presence can be the result of two diametrically opposed features: it can be the result of chilling from cold water in which the child was immersed, with the implication of brain sparing, and there are an increasing number of anecdotal case reports to support this role; and it can be a measure of long immersion time, or of absent or poor vital signs post-rescue, and thus may be a poor prognostic sign.[19]

Complications in the Post-Rescue Period

Besides the over-riding importance of neurologic deficit, a number of other complications may develop in individual cases.

In children who drown or nearly drown in fluids other than water, questions of acute poisoning may arise. Poisoning is seen particularly in children who drown in buckets,[36] in chemical disposal trenches and pits, in sewage ponds and pits, and in ditches used as effluent for industrial or agricultural chemicals. These cases, fortunately uncommon, must be treated individually. Chemical necrosis of the trachea and larynx is encountered in some such cases and is treated by debridement with humidity control and by broad antibiotic coverage.

Septicemia sometimes ensues in near-drowning cases,[45] and aquatic and marine fungi, protozoa, and bacteria cross the alveolar walls with great speed. The incidence and importance of viral infections following near-drowning remain undetermined.

Pneumothorax and pneumomediastinum are occasionally encountered and are not uncommon in young children following inappropriate or unskilled attempts at CPR.

Gastrointestinal bleeding has been reported in up to one-third of all near-drowned children requiring mechanical ventilation.[2] A good case can be made for prophylactic cimetidine in all such cases.

The phenomenon of secondary drowning is one of the most feared complications.[68] The condition is potentially fatal unless anticipated and treated accordingly. Symptoms vary considerably. In the conscious patient the development of tachypnea, the inability to take a deep breath, a burning retrosternal pain, a pleuritic pain with a hoarse rasping cough, and expectoration of large amounts of frothy pink sputum herald the presence of this condition.[53] Cyanosis may develop if it is not already present, and respiratory failure may occur rapidly.[126] The single most important sign, and one of the very serious prognostic concerns, is the return of coma in a patient who has had a lucid period. Before the full implication of secondary drowning was realized, return of coma had a uniformly fatal outcome.[53]

Why some children develop seconary drowning and others do not is still unknown. Fresh water inactivates surfactant more than salt water,[47] but anoxic damage to the Type II pneumonocytes is also probably important. In clinical series of cases of fresh-water drowning, water osmolality does not seem to be of significance in the genesis of this complication.[68, 108]

Physiologic studies have shown that immersion of the body up to the neck for even one hour or less produces significant pulmonary-capillary engorgement.[156] It may be that in children who have sustained a near-drowning accident after swimming for some time, the alveolar collapse and wall damage is aggravated if the capillary bed is "pre-engorged."

In patients who are conscious and breathing well but in whom subsequent deterioration heralds the development of the respiratory distress syndrome, a mask and CPAP or intubation with PEEP results in very significant improvement in blood gas values. PEEP ventilation should never be discontinued during the pulmonary edema phase.[108] Some experimental studies have shown that if PEEP is given immediately after rescue (by manually operated resuscitators with a PEEP valve), arterial oxygen levels return to normal much more quickly than if standard (ZEEP) ventilation is used (10 minutes to return to normal, *versus* 2 hours).[157] With the more widespread practical implementation of this finding, it is probable that the incidence of secondary drowning in survivors will be reduced.

There is one other complication concerning the critically ill child in the ICU. It relates to the parents of the child and it is a psychological phenomenon known to all pediatricians who care for desperately ill children. Parents often project guilt-induced hostility onto the staff.[2] It is probable that some degree of this hostility will be present in every case, particularly in those parents whose child does not show a good therapeutic response in the first 24 hours after admission. The main aspect of managing this phenomenon is to recognize that it is a constant potential problem and that it can be minimized by early sensitive handling and good communication.

The Child Who Dies in the Emergency Room or Intensive Care Unit

Some children die in the emergency room within the first hour after arrival at the hospital. The exact percentage who do depends on the efficiency of ambulance transport and paramedic services, local demographic and population distributions, and the size and sophistication of hospitals in the practice of caring for near-drowned children. In practice, up to 30 per cent of children who are comatose when they arrive at the emergency room may die.[84] Children who die in emergency rooms and ICUs, like children who are already dead when extracted from the water, become coroner's cases. Debate continues about osmolality of body fluids (particularly blood, cerebrospinal fluids [CSF], and vitreous humor) in the forensic literature,[158] and some simple tests on these fluids may produce new information on the pathophysiology of drowning. In appropriate cases, a telephone call to the coroner may result in permission to perform a lumbar puncture with CSF examination to be performed soon after death. This subject, of course, requires sensitive handling.

When a desperately ill near-drowned child is admitted to the emergency room, the parents are routinely excluded while resuscitation and the initial establishment of mechanical ventilation and other life support systems are institued. This is a terrible period for parents, especially because in the majority of cases deep guilt and often recrimination are present. If it is certain that the child is dying, it is good medical practice to give the parents some warning, so that if death does occur they can prepare themselves.

Stopping Therapy in the Intensive Care Unit

In the emergency room, if there is still no cardiac activity after arrival and ECG assessment shows the heart to be in asystole unresponsive to electrical or sympathomimetic stimulation, if the pupils are fixed and dilated, and if there are no other unusual circumstances (hypothermia, history of epilepsy, etc.) it would be wise to discontinue resuscitation attempts after one hour from the time of extraction from the water.

In patients who are flaccid or decerebrate and who have fixed, dilated pupils but who have an adequate or salvageable cardiac output, questions always arise about the appropriateness of continuing resuscitation attempts. Although there is a high incidence of neurologic damage and death in this type of near-drowning (42 per cent in Oakes' series[15]), one is still unable "to predict survival accurately, and therefore one cannot withhold treatment for fear of the consequences."[15] Studies from Florida[84] and Canada[105] support this view, irrespective of the type of therapeutic management planned for the patient. Even when a child has been extracted from cold water or has become hypothermic since rescue appears dead, it is absolutely essential to press on with resuscitative efforts until the core temperature is at least 31°C, and to persist with resuscitative efforts for at least one hour after this temperature has been reached.

With modern therapy using barbiturate rescue with or without hypothermia, the decision to stop treatment is not appropriate in the first three to four days after rescue, as it may take this time for even a neurologically saved child to recover after such iatrogenic obtundation. It is absolutely wrong to consider stopping therapy unless the criteria of true brain death are present. There are cases on record in which an initial decerebrate state of several days was followed by neurologic recovery, with the ultimate intellect well within the normal range.[159]

If a decision is made to stop therapy in the ICU, it is essential that brain death be documented. A completely flat EEG from a patient at normal body temperature not receiving hypnotic drugs; and a decision obtained by two independent physicians, at least one of whom is not involved with the case directly, are needed for documentation. Auditory brainstem responses are of great value in the diagnosis of brain death; Wave I may be preserved if lower brainstem function is still intact, even when true cortical death has occurred.[160, 161] If brain scans are available, the demonstration of "no flow" is valuable confirmatory evidence of brain death.

PROGNOSIS

Fatalities

The drowning and death of a child from the family's point of view is, in a sense, the beginning of a new era.[162] A typically affected family is one, often of middle or upper social class, who had a bright, intelligent toddler one minute and a suddenly and unexpectedly dead one the next.[23, 44] By contrast with the situation in which a child dies after a medical illness,[163] the very suddenness of the drowning accident gives the family no time to anticipate the tragedy, and the normal ego-defense mechanisms of anticipatory grieving cannot occur.[164] In many respects, the intrafamily dynamics in a "drowning" family resemble those encountered in "sudden infant death" families in which it is widely recognized that post-death problems can be immense.[165]

Also, many such accidents are interpreted by one or both parents as having been preventable. Usually, one parent was close to the scene of the accident.[2] Guilt often occurs within the family because one parent may have promised to fence the swimming pool or one parent may have been left alone with the children at the time of the evening meal, and the baby drowned in the family bathtub while under the parent's supposed supervision. Under these types of circumstances, the prognosis for the family is not good. Studies have shown that there is an increased risk of family dissolution after the drowning of a young child; over half such families move from the physical scene of the house and endeavor to start a new life elsewhere.[162] Families of drowned children are more likely to be "new" to a particular society in which such accidents are more common because of climatic or sociologic reasons.[44] Under such circumstances, a significant part of the cause can be attributed to the fact that parents who did not grow up in a high-risk environment did not appreciate the threat to their child.[21] When these conditions exist, there is another potential complication: the bereft and grieving parents are at higher risk for psychiatric sequelae, because the traditional support of an extended family and its ties are not usually present.

All forms of childhood trauma occur more frequently when family routine is broken, the so-called vulnerable period. Childhood drowning accidents are no exception in this regard, and one study has shown that a parental vulnerable period was one cause (of several often acting simultaneously) in about 40 per cent of accidental child drownings.[21] One common cause is marital strife. If a child is drowned or almost drowned because of inadequate parental supervision caused by marital strife, the prognosis for the family (already strained) is not good. As a counsel of perfection, if close support and sensitive case work can be instituted, one might hope that the high risk of post-accident family dissolution can be reduced. In the staff comprising a highly trained and sophisticated team, which is the norm for modern ICUs, it is not always traditional for emphasis to be placed on the social work follow-up of families whose child dies in the emergency room or ICU. With increasing awareness of potential problems that occur when children succumb within the first few hours or days after extraction from the water, it is hoped that vulnerable families can be helped.

Survivors

If a child is alive when extracted from the water, or if a heart beat commences after rescue owing to resuscitative efforts, one of several prognostic outcomes is possible:

1. Rapid recovery without physical or intellectual sequelae. If one considers all patients who survive, this is the most common outcome, and occurring in some 90 per cent or more of all cases of near-drowning in childhood. The average duration of hospital inpatient stay varies between one and two days.[13–15, 19, 20, 23, 84, 88, 98, 105]

2. Rapid partial recovery without physical sequelae but with minimal, definite evidence of neurologic impairment.[19, 23] This clinical syn-

drome, called by some workers minimal cerebral dysfunction (MCD), is caused by the fact that particular islands of mental functioning are "picked out" by the hypoxic insult. Such children often appear clumsy, and may develop secondary behavior problems because of inconsistency in their mental abilities for different types of school tasks.[23]

3. Rapid partial recovery without physical sequelae but with significant intellectual deficit.[19]

4. Rapid partial physical recovery with initial intellectual deficit that shows improvement over a long period.[88, 106, 159] There are several case reports of children who have shown signs of very severe mental retardation but in whom intellect improves four to eight weeks after discharge from the hospital.[106, 159]

5. Incomplete recovery with permanent neurologic signs and very significant intellectual deficit.[2, 18, 23, 79, 166] Cerebral palsy manifested as spastic quadriplegia or paraplegia is the most common outcome. Neuropathies and extrapyramidal syndromes are also described. Epilepsy may also be a feature.

6. Physical survival but with spastic quadriplegia and a vegetative existence.[2, 14, 18–20, 23, 53, 105, 167] Of all children pulled from the water apparently dead, the incidence of this feared outcome in survivors is not greater than three per cent.[23] However, if one considers the children who are still comatose with fixed, dilated pupils when they reach the ICU or a referral hospital (usually within one to two hours after a rescue), the incidence of gross spastic quadriplegia and amentia is much higher and occurs with a frequency of between 10 and 40 per cent in survivors.[18, 105]

7. Delayed death due to near-drowning.[19, 20, 23, 53, 105, 167] The incidence is approximately 10 per cent of all children who are still alive when extracted from the water, but if one considers those children who are still comatose with fixed and dilated pupils on arrival at the ICU, the incidence of death is between 50 and 100 per cent, provided that the water was not freezing and hypothermia is not present.

No comparative studies of survivors of salt-water opposed to fresh-water immersions have yet been undertaken, but most workers believe that the prognosis of salt-water near-drowning is no worse than that of fresh water near-drowning and may be better.[9, 20, 23, 92] Clinical practice indicates that it is the presumed period of cerebral hypoxia and to a lesser but significant extent water temperature that are important. The last words on prognostic indicators of the near-drowned child have not yet been written, but at this stage of knowledge practical questions of prognosis depend on the manifestations of acute hypoxia more than any other factor. For this reason, prognoses can be made solely by an assessment of what happens clinically from the moment of rescue up until the end of the first 12 hours or more in the emergency room.

For practical purposes *prognosis* means neurologic prognosis. Significant chest complications can develop in the convalescent period (especially if the water was polluted).[115] Studies of large series have shown that permanent lung sequelae are very common.[62] Reported complications include peripheral airway disease and bronchial hyper-reactivity.

In the last decade there has been some minor divergence of views about the prognosis of children who have suffered near-drowning accidents. It is now realized by all workers in this field that different degrees of optimism and pessimism really depend on the selection of cases that form the series. General practitioners and pediatricians are more interested in knowing the per cent chance of mortality or neurologic damage when they are involved with the initial drowning episode or when they are treating a child during the happier stages of convalescence. Anesthetists and emergency-room physicians in some parts of the world deal principally with children who are very ill indeed, *ab initio,* and in whom the prognosis is obviously going to be worse, as a group. Of the children who are extracted from the water and survive, figures from a Florida series have shown that at least 83 per cent will be neurologically normal,[84] and from the Brisbane Drowning Study it is known that this percentage will exceed 90 per cent.[23] For those children requiring mechanical resuscitation in the ICU, the prognosis is more grave. The survival of this group of select cases may be as low as 50 per cent.[2] Studies on an unselected case series (total population study) from Brisbane indicated that, in general, these survivors fell into an "all or none" type of classification,[23] and this result has been obtained elsewhere.[53, 168, 169] If patients are breathing spontaneously when they reach the ICU (usually within two hours of rescue) they usually do very well.[138] In the small percentage of children who manifest long-term sequelae, mental retardation and cerebral palsy are significant. Neuropathies have been reported but are rare in child survivors.

Table 7–1. PROGNOSTIC INDICATORS, IN CHRONOLOGIC AND PATHOPHYSIOLOGIC SEQUENCE, DETERMINING SURVIVAL AND MORBIDITY IN THE NEAR-DROWNED CHILD

1. Water temperature
2. Time to the first spontaneous respiratory gasp
3. Whether CPR was administered, and whether administered by a trained operator
4. The presence or absence of coma on arrival at the hospital (1–2 hours after rescue)
5. The presence of fixed, dilated pupils on arrival at the hospital
6. Medical therapy
7. An arterial pH below 7.00
8. Arterial oxygenation value when first measured in the ICU, below 60 mmHg (8.0 kPa) in air

Prognostic Indicators

At least ten different prognostic indicators have been used by various workers that might give an indication of prognosis during the period of crucial medical intervention in the first two to three hours after rescue. Some of these, such as the estimate of immersion time, are not of value.[23] Some workers believed that the victim's age might be a good prognostic sign, but recent studies have shown that this variable is not helpful. The remaining eight criteria that can be used for prognosis are shown in Table 7–1. Naturally, each of these criteria can be used additively or cumulatively, but the relative importance of each as a prognostic indicator has not yet been scored quantitatively.

At this stage of knowledge, two systematic approaches to the prediction of outcome appear to give the best prognostic score. One approach is based on the time to the first respiratory gasp (from the Brisbane Drowning Study), and the other is based on the neurologic state of the child in the ICU. These two approaches are, of course, quite separate from the observer's point of view, are not mutually exclusive, and correlate well. The approach that uses the estimated time to the first respiratory gasp can be employed for all patients, irrespective of severity. One simply obtains an estimate of the time that the child took to make an initial respiratory heave, and this heave occurs in about 70 per cent of cases within the first three to five minutes after extraction from the water, usually in the context of frantic resuscitative efforts by rescuers or bystanders. This method has the advantage of giving confidence early in an otherwise worrisome situation; although its power has not been studied in detail, it is probably not a fine discriminator for varying degrees of neurologic damage in those with delayed onset (after 30 minutes) of a spontaneous respiratory effort. This method is negated for the child who is very cold.

The time or latency to the onset of respiratory activity is of great benefit as shown by the interviewing of 60 or so sets of parents, resuscitators, and neighbors as part of the Brisbane Drowning Study. Animal experiments in Moscow found, independently, that the re-establishment of respiration after post-anoxic coma was a reliable and valuable indicator of the degree of reversiblity of damage.[168]

Approximately one-third of childhood survivors of near-drowning accidents in warm water will manifest minimal cerebral dysfunction.[23] Quantitative estimates of risks in childhood near-drowning, using the "time to first gasp" concept, are shown in Table 7–2.

The second type of prognostic approach focuses on neurologic signs and classification at the time of the admission to the emergency room. It has the advantage that it can be scored exactly by an objective observer and does not require estimates but has the disadvantage that the times when it should be applied have not yet been finalized. At this stage one uses the time as "time of arrival at the emergency facility," which in practice is usually between one and two hours but varies considerably.

Table 7–2. TIME TO FIRST GASP AFTER RESCUE AND ITS CORRELATION WITH SURVIVAL

Time to First Gasp (minutes)	Deaths (%)	Survivors with Minimal Cerebral Dysfunction or Worse (%)	Survivors with Mental Retardation and Cerebral Palsy (%)
1	0	0	0
1–5	0	<5	0
5–15	<5	5–10	0
15–30	5–30	30–50	<10
30–60	50	100	30
60–120 or later	60–100	100	50–80

This approach, the Modell-Conn Triage system,[12, 27, 84, 105] is being used in a number of centers, and is one powerful tool that can be used to answer crucial questions. It has the advantage that it can predict broad categories of outcome in a critically ill near-drowned child (the child who is still comatose one to two hours after rescue).

If one uses the Modell-Conn prognostic system, patients are classified into three categories: A (awake), B (blunted consciousness), and C (comatose). In a retrospective analysis of Conn's Toronto series using HYPER therapy (i.e., therapy directed against hyper-hydration, hyper-excitability, and hyper-rigidity), patients in category C (comatose when admitted to the emergency unit, in practice one to two hours post-anoxia) who had not been treated with barbiturates and hypothermia had a mortality rate of 33 per cent, with 25 per cent showing permanent neurologic sequelae and 62 per cent showing normal recovery.[105] In patients who were comatose and apneic and quite flaccid one to two hours after the accident (but with a heartbeat), in spite of very aggressive HYPER therapy, the mortality rate was still greater than 80 per cent.[105]

It is likely that both prognostic systems (time to first gasp and the ABC-Triage system) provide additive information that should be helpful. Prognostic estimates should be based on a combination of both approaches. No prospective studies have yet been published for either system, and it is certain that refinements will be forthcoming to give even better predictors than those currently available.

Besides these two broad approaches, other prognostic indicators are obviously valuable. All of them should be used, as they can shade the prognosis either optimistically or pessimistically.

Water temperature should be taken into account if it is very cold, because of the undoubted series of otherwise impossible "saves" who were immersed in very cold water.[170–172]

Whether or not the child is still comatose on arrival at the hospital is in itself a valuable prognostic indicator. Although studies that have separated the feature "duration of coma" from other neurologic signs are not available, it is known from studies of childhood head-injury cases that the duration of coma is a valuable prognostic indicator. Few children who are comatose for more than seven days regain their pre-injury personality.[173]

The presence of fixed and dilated pupils by the time the child arrives at the ICU, is also a valuable prognostic sign. It is a bad sign as regards survival, and as an indication for the potential of catastrophic brain damage in survivors.[13, 14, 18, 105] The mortality rate among those in coma with fixed and dilated pupils in the ICU remains between 50 and 100 per cent, unless special cases of hypothermia can be excluded.[88]

It must be stressed that all investigators of this problem have encountered occasional exceptions to these gloomy prognostic indicators, but they are very unusual and for this reason tend to be published.[159, 174]

Approximately one to two per cent of all near-drowning survivors, and perhaps 20 to 30 per cent of those requiring prolonged artificial ventilation (not as a consequence of HYPER therapy), exist in a permanent vegetative state. All pediatricians and neurologists know of these cases, and all case series report them.[2, 20, 23, 169] Some investigators believe that to save life at the price of a surviving but vegetative brain is a tragedy worse than death.[12] However, because at this stage there seems to be a better than 40 per cent chance of achieving neurologic salvage in these desperately ill children, there is no alternative but to press on with all the resources available to those caring for the critically ill child.

The Survivor Who Is Normal

Over 70 per cent of those children rescued will survive and function normally in every way. Full recovery, without any pulmonary or neurologic or intellectual sequelae will occur in over 60 per cent of those who are unconscious and apneic when pulled from the water. Such children who make a complete recovery, are back to normal within two days or so. This group of children usually manifest the typical post-hospitalization syndrome for days or several weeks after discharge, but apart from this, there are no long-term personality effects. What is very important is that such survivors do not have any fear of water, and they remain at the same risk of drowning as they did prior to the accident. Sociologic studies as part of the Brisbane Drowning Study showed that only 10 per cent of parents take effective action to prevent the same tragedy from happening again after the child returns home.

Although objective testing has shown that pulmonary function abnormalities may persist for up to 16 weeks after the accident, lung function generally returns to normal, and on routine testing FVC and FEV_1/FVC ratios are normal.[115] Some studies have shown that more sophisticated testing of lung function in freshwater survivors may reveal that over half have asymptomatic peripheral airways disease with increased bronchial hyperreactivity.[62] It is likely that such damage is caused by the aspiration of gastric contents at the time of the accident. As a counsel of perfection, because of the relatively rapid deterioration in pulmonary function following cigarette smoking that occurs in individuals with bronchial hyperreactivity, it may be wise to counsel parents against future smoking by the child.

Prospective Studies and the Need for Objectivity

All workers agree that the value of vigorous therapeutic techniques (barbiturate coma and its consequent mechanical ventilation, hypothermia, etc.) cannot yet be fully assessed. Two retrospective studies published in 1980 from two major centers dealing with the near-drowned (Modell's group in Florida,[84] and Conn's group in Toronto[105]) have given conflicting answers for the use of these techniques, and the question remains open whether such therapy is necessary.[84] Oakes' study in 1982, from San Jose, also found that there was still no unequivocal evidence for the validity of hypothermia, barbiturate coma, and steroids, although cases were not randomized for the respective treatments.[15] The answer must, of course, come from prospective studies. There will be an iatrogenic price to pay for this type of therapy, and this price is as yet unknown. Prolonged induced paralysis may lead to lung abnormalities, and barbiturate coma and hypothermia increase the potential hazards to the patient.[84] Some degree of lung damage from the use of ventilation is to be expected; in the case of immature lungs, and possibly the immature lungs damaged by osmotic and anoxic insult, every known technique of resuscitation, irrespective of the type of respirator used, will result in some degree of "respirator lung."[40] Pulmonary interstitial fibrosis has been recorded following near-drowning also. At this exciting time of therapy for the near-drowned child, there is a great need for as much work as possible in this important area, so that these uncertain questions can be resolved.

ALGORITHM FOR ACCIDENTAL DROWNING IN CHILDHOOD

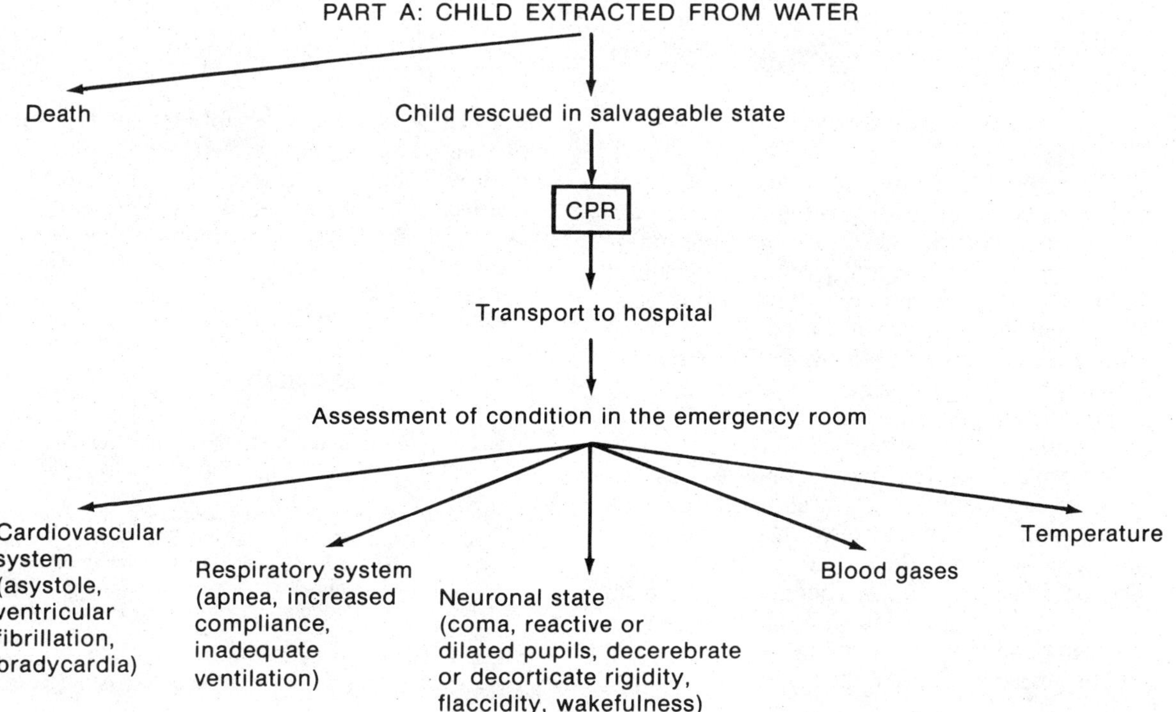

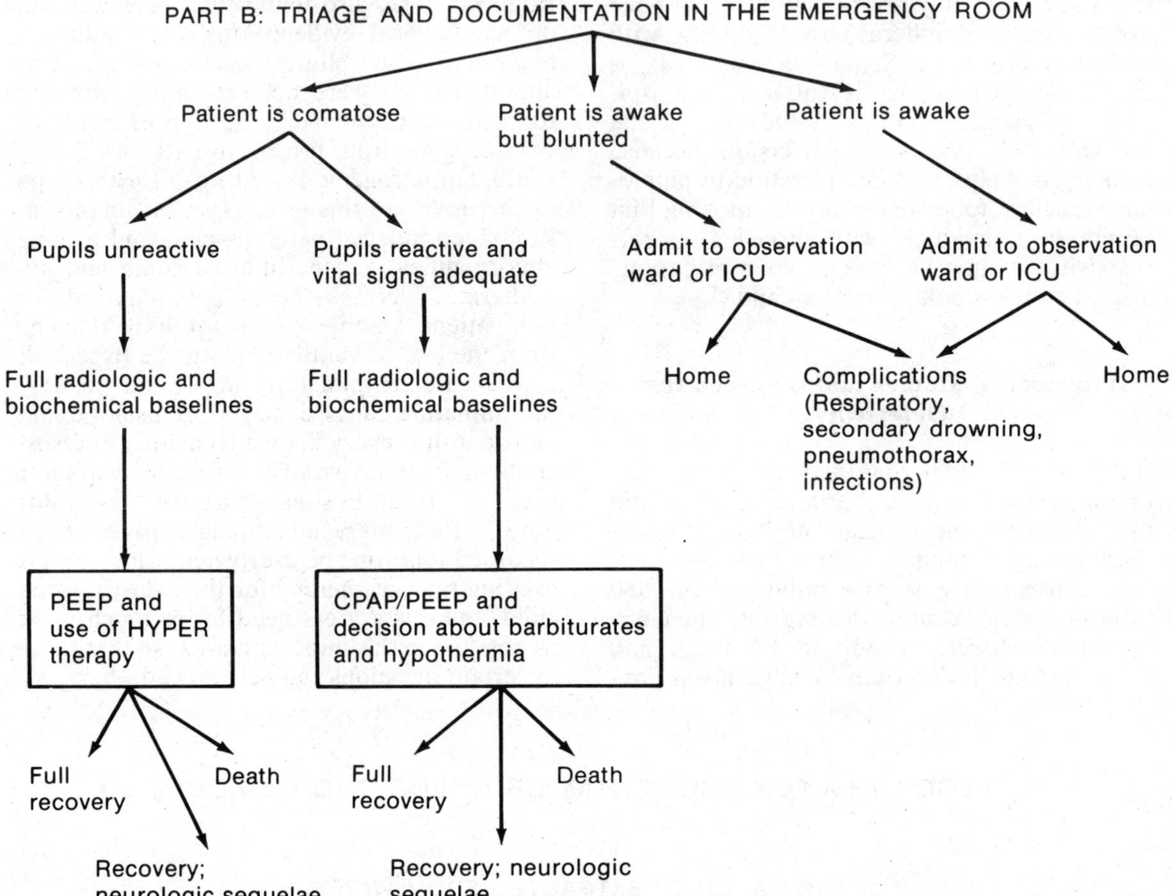

SUMMARY

From the perspective of public health, the key consideration in drownings is prevention of such accidents in the future, and the emergency-room physician and pediatrician cannot ignore it.[10] Children who suffer serious accidents may be involved in another accident if causal factors are not removed. The situation is well known in the case of accidental childhood poisoning,[100] and in the Brisbane Drowning Study, of 56 initial survivors from the primary study, three had second serious immersion accidents, one fatal. Although all agree that parents have a responsibility in taking action after the event, in practice they do not. Some results have been achieved from intensively pursued educational programs to prevent childhood drowning accidents, but doubt remains whether the main target population at risk is most amenable to this type of approach. For this reason, it is very important that those who have cared for such critically ill children take an active role in the prevention of drowning in the individual whom they have saved and in those who remain at risk in the wider community.

REFERENCES

1. Simpson JS. Trauma: the leading childhood killer in Canada and elsewhere. Clin Pediatr 1976; *15*:313–316.
2. Fandel IF, Bancalari E. Near-drowning in children: clinical aspects. Pediatrics 1976; *58*:573–579.
3. Pearn JH, Nixon J, Wilkey I. Freshwater drowning and near-drowning accidents involving children. A five year total population study. Med J Aust 1976; 2:942–946.
4. Pearn JH, Wong RYK, Brown J, et al. Drowning and near-drowning involving children. A five-year

total population study from the City and County of Honolulu. Am J Public Health 1979; *69*:450–454.
5. Pearn J, Brown J, Hsia EY. Swimming pool drownings and near-drownings involving children. A total population study from Hawaii. Milit Med 1980; *145*:15–18.
6. Williams HD, Modell JH. Statistics and Public Health Considerations. *In*: Modell JH, ed. The Pathophysiology and Treatment of Drowning and Near-drowning. Springfield, Illinois: Charles C Thomas, 1971; 3–7.
7. Hassall IB. Drownings in private swimming pools. NZ Med J 1982; *95*:129–130.
8. Pearn JH, Nixon J. Are swimming pools becoming more dangerous? Med J Aust 1977; *2*:702–704.
9. Miles S. Drowning. Br Med J 1968; *3*:597–600.
10. Brooks JG. The child who nearly drowns. Am J Dis Child 1981; *135*:998–999.
11. Modell JH. Drown versus near-drown: a discussion of definitions. Crit Care Med 1981; *9*:351–352.
12. Conn AW, Edmonds JF, Barker GA. Cerebral resuscitation in near-drowning. Pediatr Clin North Am 1979; *26*:691–701.
13. Orlowski JP. Prognostic factors in pediatric cases of drowning and near-drowning. JACEP 1979; *8*:176–179.
14. Frates RC. Analysis of predictive factors in the assessment of warm-water near-drowning in children. Am J Dis Child 1981; *135*:1006–1008.
15. Oakes DD, Sherck JP, Maloney JR, Charters AC. Prognosis and management of victims of near-drowning. J Trauma 1982; *22*:544–549.
16. Pearn JH. Survival rates following serious immersion accidents in childhood. Resuscitation 1978; *6*:271–278.
17. Patrick M, Bint M, Pearn J. Salt water drowning and near-drowning accidents involving children. A five-year total population study in South-East Queensland. Med J Aust 1979; *1*:61–64.
18. Peterson B. Morbidity of childhood near-drowning. Pediatrics 1977; *59*:364–370.
19. Kruus S, Bergstrom L, Suutarinen T, Hyvonen R. The prognosis of near-drowned children. Acta Paediatr Scand 1979; *68*:315–322.
20. Pearn JH, Bart RD, Yamaoka R. Neurological sequelae following childhood near-drowning. A total population study from Hawaii. Pediatrics 1978; *64*:187–192.
21. Pearn JH, Nixon J. An analysis of the causes of freshwater immersion accidents involving children. Acc Anal Prev 1979; *11*:173–178.
22. Gustafsson LH. Childhood accidents. Three epidemiological studies on the etiology. Scand J Soc Med 1977; *5*:5–13.
23. Pearn JH. Survivors of childhood freshwater immersion accidents: neurologic and psychometric studies. Lancet 1977; *1*:7–9.
24. Plueckhahn VD. Drowning: community aspects. Med J Aust 1979; *2*:226–228.
25. Dietz PE, Baker SP. Drowning: epidemiology and prevention. Am J Public Health 1974; *64*:303–312.
26. Poyner B. How and when drownings happen. Practitioner 1979; *222*:515–519.
27. Modell JH, Conn AW. Current neurological considerations in near-drowning. Can Anaesth Soc J 1980; *27*:197–198.
28. Gooden BA. Drowning and the diving reflex in man. Med J Aust 1972; *2*:583–586.
29. Hunt PK. Effect and treatment of diving reflex. Can Med Assoc J 1974; *111*:1330–1331.
30. Anonymous. Swimming pool drownings. Metropolitan Life Insurance Co Statistics Bulletin (US) 1977; *58*:4–6.
31. Pearn JH, Thompson J. Drowning and near-drowning in the Australian Capital Territory: a total five-year population study of immersion accidents. Med J Aust 1977; *1*:130–133.
32. Labrune B. La noyade. Soins 1972; *17*:29–31.
33. Horwood LJ, Fergusson DM, Shannon FT. The safety standards of domestic swimming pools. NZ Med J 1981; *94*:417–419.
34. Pearn JH, Nixon J. Bathtub immersion accidents involving children. Med J Aust 1977; *1*:211–213.
35. Pearn JH, Brown J, Wong RY, Bart R. Bathtub drownings: report of seven cases. Pediatrics 1979; *64*:68–70.
36. Scott PH, Eigen H. Immersion accidents involving pails of water in the home. J Pediatr 1980; *96*:282–284.
37. Nixon J, Pearn J. Non-accidental immersion in the bath: another extension to the syndrome of child abuse and neglect. Child Abuse Neglect 1977; *1*:445–448.
38. Sonnen AE. Epilepsy and swimming. Monogr Neurol Sci 1981; *5*:265–270.
39. Pearn JH. Epilepsy and drowning in childhood. Br Med J 1977; *1*:1510–1511.
40. Pearn J, Bart R, Yamaoka R. Drowning risks to epileptic children: a study from Hawaii. Br Med J 1978; *4*:1284–1285.
41. Pearn J. Drowning in Australia: a national appraisal with particular reference to children. Med J Aust 1977; *2*:770–771.
42. Peabody AJ. Diatoms and drowning—a review. Med Sci Law 1980; *20*:254–261.
43. Pearn J. Predisposing factors leading to child trauma. J Epidemiol Community Health 1978; *32*:190–193.
44. Nixon J, Pearn J. An investigation of sociodemographic factors surrounding childhood drowning accidents. Soc Sci Med 1978; *12*:387–390.
45. Kelly MT, Avery DM. Lactose-positive Fibrio in seawater: a cause of pneumonia and septicemia in a drowning victim. J Clin Microbiol 1980; *11*:278–280.
46. Anonymous. Oceans. *In*: Encyclopaedia Britannica. 15th ed. Macropaedia vol. 13. Chicago: Encyclopaedia Britannica 1974: 484–486.
47. Giammona ST, Modell JH. Drowning by total immersion: effects on pulmonary surfactant of distilled water, isotomic saline and sea water. Am J Dis Child 1967; *114*:612–616.
48. Swann HG, Spafford NR. Body salt and water changes during fresh and sea water drowning. Tex Rep Biol Med 1951; *9*:356–382.
49. Swann HG, Brucer M, Moore C, Vezien BL. Fresh and sea water drowning: a study of the terminal cardiac and biochemical events. Tex Rep Biol Med 1967; *5*:423–437.
50. Modell JH, Davis JH, Giammona ST, et al. Blood gas and electrolyte changes in human near-drowning victims. JAMA 1968; *203*:99–105.
51. Modell JH. Biology of drowning. Ann Rev Med 1978; *29*:1–8.
52. Bergquist RE, Vogelhut MM, Modell JH, et al. Comparison of ventilatory patterns in the treatment of freshwater near-drowning in dogs. Anesthesiology 1980; *52*:142–148.

53. Rivers JF, Orr G, Lee HA. Drowning. Its clinical sequelae and management. Br Med J 1970; *1*:157–161.
54. Gilbert FF, Gofton N. Terminal dives in mink, muskrat and beaver. Physiol Behav 1982; *28*:835–840.
55. Campbell LB, Gooden BA, Horowitz JD. Cardiovascular responses to partial and total immersion in man. J Physiol (Lond) 1969; *202*:239.
56. Elsner R, Gooden BA. Reduction in reactive hyperemia in the human forearm by face immersion. J Appl Physiol 1970; *29*:627–630.
57. Elsner R, Gooden BA, Robinson SM. Arterial blood gas changes and the diving response in man. Aust J Exp Biol Med Sci 1971; *49*:435–444.
58. Gooden BA, Lehman RG, Pym J. Role of the face in the cardiovascular responses to total immersion. Aust J Exp Biol Med Sci 1970; *48*:687–690.
59. Pearn JH, Nixon J. Swimming pool immersion accidents. An analysis from the Brisbane Drowning Study. Med J Aust 1977; *1*:432–437.
60. Corriol J, Rohner JJ. Role de température de l'eau dans la bradycardie d'immersion de la face. Arch Sci Physiol 1968; *22*:265–274.
61. Agostoni E. Diaphragm activity during breath holding: factors related to its onset. J Appl Physiol 1963; *18*:30–36.
62. Laughlin JJ, Eigen H. Pulmonary function abnormalities in survivors of near drowning. J Pediatr 1982; *100*:26–30.
63. Craig AB. Causes of loss of consciousness during underwater swimming. J Appl Physiol 1961; *16*:583–586.
64. Colebatch HJH, Halmagyi DFJ. Effect of vagotomy and vagal stimulation on lung mechanics and circulation. J Appl Physiol 1963; *18*:881–887.
65. Colebatch HJH, Halmagyi DFJ. Reflex pulmonary hypotension of fresh-water aspiration. J Appl Physiol 1963; *18*:179–185.
66. Colebatch HJH, Halmagyi DFJ. Lung mechanics and resuscitation after fluid aspiration. J Appl Physiol 1961; *16*:684–696.
67. Nopanitanya W, Gambill TG, Brinkhous KM. Fresh water drowning. Pulmonary ultrastructure and systemic fibrinolysis. Acta Pathol 1974; *98*:361–366.
68. Pearn JH. Secondary drowning involving children. Br Med J 1980; *2*:1103–1105.
69. Kogure K, Busto R, Scheinberg P, et al. Energy metabolites and water content in rat brains during the early stage of development of cerebral infarction. Brain 1974; *97*:103–114.
70. Kristoffersen MB, Rattenborg CC, Holaday DA. Asphyxial death: the roles of acute anoxia, hypercarbia and acidosis. Anesthesiology 1967; *28*: 488–497.
71. Itoh U, Omno K, Nakamura R, et al. Brain edema during ischemia and after restoration of blood flow. Measurement of water, sodium, potassiaum content and plasma protein permeability. Stroke 1979; *10*:542–547.
72. Tomita M, Gotoh F, Sato F, et al. Determination of the osmotic potential for swelling of cat brain in vitro. Exp Neurol 1979; *65*:66–77.
73. Kogure K, Busto R, Scheinberg P. The role of hydrostatic pressure in ischemic brain edema. Ann Neurol 1981; *9*:273–282.
74. Nugent SK, Rogers MC. Resuscitation and intensive care monitoring following immersion hypothermia. J Trauma 1980; *20*:814–815.
75. Rockoff MA, Marshall LF, Shapiro HM. High-dose barbiturate therapy in humans: a clinical review of 60 patients. Ann Neurol 1979; *6*:194–199.
76. Jennett B, Gleave J, Wilson P. Brain death in three neurosurgical units. Br Med J 1981; *282*:533–539.
77. Parisi JE, Kim RC, Collins GH, Hilfinger MF. Brain death with prolonged somatic survival. N Engl J Med 1982; *306*:14–16.
78. Dick AE, Potgieter PD. Secondary drowning in the Cape Peninsula. S Afr Med J 1982; *62*:803–806.
79. Fleetham JA, Munt PW. Near-drowning in Canadian waters. Can Med Assoc J 1978; *118*:914–917.
80. March NF, Matthews RC. New techniques in external cardiac compressions. JAMA 1980; *244*: 1229–1232.
81. Harries MG. Survival after cardiac arrest. Int Med 1979; *1*:13–15.
82. Bowden K. Drowning. Med J Aust 1957; *1*:39–43.
83. Fraser-Darling A. Electrocution, drowning, and burns. Br Med J 1981; *282*:530.
84. Modell JH, Graves SA, Kuck EJ. Near-drowning: correlation of level of consciousness and survival. Can Anaesth Soc J 1980; *27*:211–215.
85. Kopf G, Mirvis D, Meyers R. Central nervous system tolerance to cardiac arrest during profound hypothermia. J Surg Res 1975; *18*:29–34.
86. Stevenson JG, Stone EF, Dillard DH, et al. Intellectual development of children subjected to prolonged circulatory arrest during hypothermic open heart surgery in infancy. Circulation 1974; *50*(suppl 2):54–59.
87. White RJ, Austin PE, Austin JC, et al. Recovery of the subhuman primate after deep cerebral hypothermia and prolonged ischaemia. Resuscitation 1973; *2*:117–122.
88. Young RSK, Zalneraitis EL, Dooling EC. Neurological outcome in cold water drowning. JAMA 1980; *244*:1233–1235.
89. Hoffman E. A review of undergraduate teaching on major trauma and cardiopulmonary resuscitation: data from 74 medical schools in 22 countries. Resuscitation 1973; *2*:123–131.
90. Lund I, Skulberg A. Cardiopulmonary resuscitation by lay people. Lancet 1976; *2*:702–704.
91. Copley DP, Mantle JA, Rogers WJ, et al. Improved outcome for prehospital cardiopulmonary collapse with resuscitation by bystanders. Circulation 1977; *56*:901–905.
92. Donaldson JC, Royall JD. Drowning and near-drowning. Postgrad Med J 1978; *64*:71–79.
93. Wong FM, Grace WJ. Sudden death after near-drowning. JAMA 1963; *186*:724–726.
94. Domiguez de Villota E, Barat J, Peral G, et al. Recovery from profound hypothermia with cardiac arrest after immersion. Br Med J 1973; *4*:394–395.
95. Kvittingen TD, Naess A. Recovery from drowning in fresh water. Br Med J 1963; *1*:1315–1317.
96. Theilade D. The danger of fatal misjudgement in hypothermia after immersion. Anaesthesia 1977; *32*:889–892.
97. Plueckhahn VD. The aetiology of 134 deaths due to "drowning" in Geelong, during the years 1957 to 1971. Med J Aust 1972; *2*:1183–1187.
98. Gilfoil MP, Carvajal HF. Near-drowning in children. Tex Med 1977; *73*:39–44.
99. Sibert R. Stress in families of children who have ingested poisons. Br Med J 1975; *3*:87–89.
100. Sobel R, Margolis JA. Repetitive poisoning in children: a psychological study. Pediatrics 1965; *35*:641–651.
101. Donald KW. Drowning. Br Med J 1955; *2*:155–160.

102. Modell JH. Serum Electrolyte Changes. *In*: The Pathophysiology and Treatment of Drowning and Near-drowning. Springfield, Illinois: Charles C Thomas, 1971: 41–49.
103. Putman CE, Tummillo AM, Myerson DA, Myerson PJ. Drowning: another plunge. Am J Roentgenol Radium Ther Nucl Med 1975; *125*:543–548.
104. Modell JH. The pathophysiology and treatment of drowning. Acta Anaesthesiol Scand 1968; *29*(suppl):263–272.
105. Conn AW, Montes JE, Barker GA, Edmonds JF. Cerebral salvage in near-drowning following neurological classification by triage. Can Anaesth Soc J 1980; *27*:201–299.
106. Wegener FH, Edwards RM. Cerebral support for near-drowned children in a temperature involvement. Med J Aust 1980; *2*:135–137.
107. Wind J. Human drowning: phylogenetic origin. J Hum Evolution 1976; *5*:349–363.
108. Eggink WF, Bruining HA. Respiratory distress syndrome caused by near- or secondary drowning and treatment by positive end-expiratory pressure ventilation. Neth J Med 1977; *20*:162–167.
109. Bowden K. Electrical and drowning accidents: treatment. Med J Aust 1953; *1*:600–603.
110. Harries MG. Drowning and its treatment. Practitioner 1978; *220*:771–773.
111. Edmonds C. A salt water aspiration syndrome. Milit Med 1970; *135*:779–785.
112. Fuller RH. The clinical pathology of near-drowning. Proc Roy Soc Med 1963; *56*:33–38.
113. Hunter TB, Whitehouse WM. Fresh-water near-drowning: radiological aspects. Radiology 1974; *112*:51–56.
114. Gordon I. The anatomical signs in drowning. A critical evaluation. Forensic Sci 1972; *1*:389–395.
115. Jenkinson SG, George RB. Serial pulmonary function studies in survivors of near drowning. Chest 1980; *77*:777–780.
116. Raskin MM. Pulmonary edema of acute overdose reaction and near-drowning. South Med J 1976; *69*:1063–1065.
117. Hasan S, Avery W, Fabian C, Sackner M. Near drowning in humans. A report of 36 patients. Chest 1971; *59*:191–197.
118. Fine NL, Myerson DA, Myerson PJ, Pagliaro JJ. Near-drowning presenting as the adult respiratory distress syndrome. Chest 1974; *65*:347–349.
119. Rutledge RR, Flor RJ. The use of mechanical ventilation with positive end-expiratory pressure in the treatment of near-drowning. Anesthesiology 1973; *38*:194–196.
120. Glasser KL, Civetta JM, Flor RJ. The use of spontaneous ventilation with constant-positive airway pressure in the treatment of salt water near drowning. Chest 1975; *67*:355–357.
121. von Haeringen JR, Blokzijl EJ, van Dyl W, et al. Treatment of the respiratory distress syndrome following nondirect pulmonary trauma with positive end-expiratory pressure with special emphasis on near-drowning. Chest 1974; *66*:305–345.
122. Glauser FL, Smith WR. Pulmonary interstitial fibrosis following near-drowning and exposure to short-term high oxygen concentrations. Chest 1975; *68*:373–375.
123. Rosenbaum HT, Thompson WL, Ruller RH. Radiographic pulmonary changes in near-drowning. Radiology 1964; *83*:306–312.
124. Mullanney PJ. Acute immersion syndrome. Postgrad Med 1970; *48*:89–91.
125. Modell JH. Hospital Therapy. *In*: Modell JH, ed. The Pathophysiology and Treatment of Drowning and Near-drowning. Springfield, Illinois: Charles C Thomas 1971; 95–113.
126. Telfer ABM. Acute respiratory distress and positive end-expiratory pressure. Practitioner 1979. Special Report, 32–36.
127. Kelman GR, Nunn JF. Nomograms for correction of blood P_{O_2}, P_{CO_2}, pH, and base excess for time and temperature. J Appl Physiol 1966; *21*: 1484–1490.
128. Blake PA, Merson MH, Weaver RE, et al. Disease caused by a marine *Vibrio*. Clinical characteristics and epidemiology. New Engl J Med 1979; *300*:1–5.
129. Gluer J, Hall B, Hayes J, Davis G. Coliform status of domestic swimming pools. Med J Aust 1979; *1*:154–155.
130. Rosenthal SL, Zuger JH, Apollo E. Respiratory colonization with *Pseudomonas putrefaciens* after near-drowning in salt water. Am J Clin Pathol 1975; *64*:382–384.
131. Mission C. Hygiene des piscines. Brux Med 1977; *57*:327–334.
132. Fisher JF, Shadomy S, Teabeaut JR, et al. Near-drowning complicated by brain abscess due to *Petriellidium boydii.* Arch Neurol 1982; *39*:511–513.
133. Editorial. Alcohol and drowning. Med J Aust 1981; *1*:157–158.
134. Mackie I. Alcohol and aquatic disasters. Practitioner 1979; *222*:662–665.
135. Golden FS, Rivers JF. The immersion incident. Anesthesia 1975; *30*:364–373.
136. Brophy TO'R. Barbiturate protection for hypoxic brain damage. Med J Aust 1980; *2*:114–115.
137. Forese AB, Bryan AC. Effects of anesthesia and paralysis on diaphragmatic mechanics in man. Anesthesiology 1974; *41*:242–255.
138. Simcock AD. Sequelae of near drowning. Practitioner 1979; *222*:527–530.
139. de Otter G. Low-pressure aspiration of fresh water and sea water in the non-anoxic dog. An experimental study on the pathophysiology of drowning. Forensic Sci 1973; *2*:305–316.
140. Reineke H, Dick W, Ahnefeld FW, et al. Pulmonary compliance and gas exchange in newborn pigs during artificial ventilation. Resuscitation 1974; *3*:69–79.
141. Pontoppian H, Wilson RS, Rie MA, Schneider RC. Respiratory intensive care. Anesthesiology 1977; *47*:96–116.
142. Gilston A. The effects of PEEP on arterial oxygenation. An examination of some possible mechanisms. Intensive Care Med 1977; *3*:267–271.
143. Miller CL, Alexander K, Lampard DG, et al. Local cerebral blood flow following transient cerebral ischemia. II. Effect of arterial P_{CO_2} on reperfusion following global ischemia. Stroke 1980; *11*: 542–548.
144. Morgan AP. The pulmonary toxicity of oxygen. Anesthesiology 1968; *291*:570.
145. Kuhn GJ, White BC, Swetnam RE, et al. Peripheral versus central circulation times during CPR: a pilot study. Ann Emerg Med 1981; *10*:417–419.
146. Wells BA, Keats AS, Cooley DA. Increased tolerance to cerebral ischemia produced by general anesthesia during temporary carotid occlusion. Surgery 1963; *54*:216–223.
147. Wilhjelm BJ, Arnfred I. Protective action of some anaesthetics against anoxia. Acta Pharmacol 1965; *22*:93–98.
148. Hoff JT, Smith AL, Hankinson HL, et al. Barbitu-

rate protection from cerebral infarction in primates. Stroke 1975; *6*:28–33.

149. Nemoto EM, Bleyaert AL, Stezoski SW, et al. Global brain ischemia: a reproducible monkey model. Stroke 1977; *8*:558–564.
150. Smith AL. Barbiturate protection in cerebral hypoxia. Anesthesiology 1977; *47*:285–293.
151. Hagerdal M, Welsh FA, Keykhah M, et al. The protective effects of a combination of hypothermia and barbiturates in cerebral hypoxia. Crit Care Med 1978; *6*:110–111.
152. Marshall LF, Smith RW, Shapiro HM. The outcome with aggressive treatment in severe head injuries. Part I. The significance of intracranial pressure monitoring. J Neurosurg 1979; 50:20–25.
153. Marshall LF, Smith RW, Shapiro HM. The outcome with aggressive treatment in severe head injuries. Part II. Acute and chronic barbiturate administration in the management of head injury. J Neurosurg 1979; *50*:26–30.
154. Miller CL, Lampard DG, Alexander K, Brown WA. Local cerebral blood flow following transient cerebral ischemia. I. Onset of impaired reperfusion within the first hour following global ischemia. Stroke 1980; *11*:534–541.
155. Bedford RF, Persing JA, Pobereskin L, Butler A. Lidocaine or thiopental for rapid control of intracranial hypertension? Anesth Analg 1980; *59*: 435–437.
156. Levinson R, Epstein M, Salkner MA, Begin R. Comparison of the effects of water immersion and saline infusion on central haemodynamics in man. Clin Sci Mol Med 1977; *52*:343–350.
157. Dick W, Lotz P, Milewski P, Schindewolf H. The influence of different ventilatory patterns on oxygenation and gas exchange after near-drowning. Resuscitation 1979; *7*:255–262.
158. Rammer L, Gerdin B. Dilution of blood in fresh water drowning. Post-mortem determination of osmolarity and electrolytes in blood, cerebrospinal fluid and vitreous humor. Forensic Sci 1976; *8*:229–234.
159. Pearn JH, DeBuse P, Mohay H, Golden M. Sequential intellectual recovery after near-drowning. Med J Aust 1979; *1*:463–464.
160. Starr A. Auditory brain-stem responses in brain death. Brain 1976; *99*:543–544.
161. Uziel A, Benezech J. Auditory brain-stem responses in comatose patients: relationship with brain-stem reflexes and levels of coma. Electroencephalogr Clin Neurophysiol 1978; *45*:515–524.
162. Nixon J, Pearn J. Emotional sequelae of parents and sibs following the drowning or near-drowning of a child. Aust NZ J Psychiatry 1977; *11*:265–268.
163. Fischhoff J, O'Brien N. After the child dies. J Pediatr 1976; *88*:140–146.
164. Raphael B. The management of pathological grief. Aust NZ J Psychiatry 1975; *9*:173–180.
165. Toley K. The choice of a surviving sibling as "scapegoat" in some cases of maternal bereavement—a case report. J Child Psychol Psychiatry 1975; *16*:331–339.
166. Dean JM, Kaufman ND. Prognostic indicators in pediatric near-drowning: the Glasgow Coma Scale. Crit Care Med 1981; *9*:536–539.
167. Modell JH. Definitions and Descriptions. *In*: The Pathophysiology and Treatment of Drowning and Near-drowning. Springfield, Illinois: Charles C Thomas, 1971; 9–12.
168. Gurvitch AM. Determination of the depth and reversibility of post-anoxic coma in animals. Resuscitation 1974; *3*:1–26.
169. Eriksson R, Fredin H, Gerdman P, Thorson J. Sequelae of accidental near-drowning in childhood. Scand J Soc Med 1973; *1*:1–6.
170. Kvittingen TD, Naess A. Recovery from drowning in fresh water. Br Med J 1963; *1*:1315–1317.
171. Siebke H, Rod T, Breivik H, Link B. Survival after 40 minutes' submersion without cerebral sequelae. Lancet 1975; *1*:1275–1277.
172. Sluiter HJ. Survival after submersion. Lancet 1975; *2*:513.
173. Stover SL, Zeiger HE. Head injury in children and teenagers: functional recovery correlated with the duration of coma. Arch Phys Med Rehabil 1976; *57*:201–205.
174. Montes JE, Conn AW. Near-drowning: an unusual case. Can Anaesth Soc J 1980; *27*:172–174.
175. Lawson JS, Oliver TI. Domestic swimming pool drowning in children. Positive results of a practical prevention program. Aust Paediatr J 1978; *14*:275–277.
176. Nunn JF. Nomograms and Correction Charts. *In*: Nunn JF. ed. Applied Respiratory Physiology. 2nd ed. London: Butterworth & Co Ltd, 1977: 459.

CHAPTER

8

Diagnosis and Management of the Comatose Child

Bennett A. Shaywitz, M.D.

Coma is one of the most urgent and critical problems of diagnosis and management confronting the pediatrician, and in no small measure, the patient's quality of life, if not survival itself, may hinge upon the care and skill of the physician who is responsible for emergency care. This chapter provides a framework for a rational and efficient approach to the comatose child. In addition to discussing the definition, etiology, pathophysiology, differential diagnosis, examination, management, and prognosis in coma and criteria for death, I detail the management of status epilepticus.

DEFINITION

Coma represents the most severe degree in a continuum of acutely altered states of consciousness, which may begin with *clouding of consciousness,* progress to an acute confusional state, delirium, obtundation, stupor, and, finally, coma.[1–3] Clouding of consciousness represents the earliest and least disturbed of the states. Although a relatively mild disorder characterized by reduced wakefulness, clouding of consciousness may blend into an *acute confusional state,* in which stimuli are frequently misinterpreted, memory is impaired, and drowsiness and agitation alternate. *Delirium* is a closely related condition characterized by confusion, abnormal perception, and loss of attention. Disorientation, particularly for time, is prominent. Its onset is rapid and duration is relatively short, lasting four to seven days. *Obtundation,* still another step in the progression to coma, indicates a mild to moderate reduction in alertness. If the situation deteriorates to the point where only vigorous and persistent stimulation will rouse the patient, I refer to the patient's condition as *stupor.*

Coma is the final step in the progression, and its definition is perhaps the most critical, since numerous outcome studies use the duration of coma as a dependent variable in predicting future neurologic deficit. In clinical situations the most readily applied features are those proposed by Jennett and Teasdale: the patient cannot open the eyes, obey commands, nor utter words.[4] The definition excludes some patients who do not obey commands and do not speak but are able to open their eyes. Such patients are described as in a vegetive state, a term that is used in preference to neocortical death, apallic state, coma vigil, and akinetic mutism.[5] The vegetive state is present when the patient in coma (eyes closed, not obeying commands, not uttering words) begins to open the eyes spontaneously or in response to verbal stimuli. This response occurs within two to four weeks after the onset of coma and is accompanied by the return of sleep-wake cycles. Although their eyes are open, patients do not obey any verbal commands, do not make comprehensible sounds, and do not localize motor responses.

Pathologically, the vegetive state is characterized by profound disruption of the cerebral cortex. Clinically, it must be differentiated from the "locked-in" syndrome, a state produced by selective de-efferentation of motor pathways in the brainstem without disruption of consciousness. Such patients are unable to move, but show their alertness by blinking or moving their eyes vertically. The "locked-in" state is caused most commonly by ischemia in the distribution of the basilar artery and is extremely rare in childhood.

ETIOLOGY

Structural abnormalities of the brain account for between 20 and 30 per cent of coma. For the most part, these abnormalities involve disturbances affecting supratentorial structures and include such processes as traumatic injuries sustained in motor vehicle accidents and falls (acute epidural and subdural hematomas), brain tumors, and abscesses. Disturbances affecting infratentorial structures are very rare in childhood, though traumatic injuries resulting in brainstem ischemia have been reported. *Toxic-metabolic* disturbances are, by far, the principal causes of coma in children, accounting for 70 to 80 per cent of cases. They are classified most reasonably in three general categories: (1) disturbances affecting the transfer of oxygen (hypoxia) or substrate (hypoglycemia) to the brain, (2) exogenous toxins (poison), and (3) endogenous toxins (infections, metabolic disorders).[1–4]

PATHOPHYSIOLOGY

The first and most critical diagnostic decision facing the physician is to determine whether coma is a result of a structural or a toxic-metabolic process. Whereas new diagnostic techniques, particularly computed axial tomography (CAT scan) of the head, have allowed us to make this decision with great reliability, the clinical presentation and course also will enable this decision to be made if CAT scanning is not immediately available.[6]

Structural brain disorders cause coma by one of two mechanisms: First, disease processes may affect the brainstem directly, thus disrupting those mechanisms influencing arousal and consciousness. Second, disease processes may affect one of the cerebral hemispheres focally; the subsequent development of brain edema around this focal cerebral lesion results in a secondary compression and disruption of arousal mechanisms located in the brainstem. If the process occurs relatively slowly, a clinical picture that Plum and Posner have termed the *central syndrome* is observed.[1] The rapid accumulation of an intracerebral mass, as observed in acute epidural hematomas, produces the *uncal syndrome*. Each of these syndromes is discussed in the cases that are decribed later.

In contrast, toxic-metabolic disturbances are characterized by a clinical course that is inconsistent with either central or uncal syndrome but rather presents a picture of neurologic dysfunction that simultaneously affects several different neuroanatomic levels of the neuraxis, a sequence of events that is explicable only on the basis of toxic-metabolic perturbations of diverse portions of the central nervous system (CNS). The clinical expression of these events is a constellation of motor signs indicative of lower brainstem dysfunction and yet intact pupillary responses suggesting an intact midbrain.

EXAMINATION OF THE COMATOSE CHILD

Information obtained through the history is often of great help in the diagnosis of the child in coma. For example, previous history of multiple injuries in an unconscious infant should alert the physician to the possibility of head injury as a result of child abuse. Similarly, a history of siblings or other family members on long-term medications, particularly neuroleptics, suggests the possibility of drug ingestion. A recent history of fever or upper respiratory infection raises the suspicion of encephalitis, whereas a history of sinusitis suggests the possibility of a bacterial infection causing a brain abscess. Recurrent episodes of coma should alert the physician to consider metabolic disorders, particularly hyperammonemias.[7]

In most cases, however, even the most reliable and complete history will not permit the differentiation between structural and toxic-metabolic disturbances that is so critical in planning rational management. Thus, the physician must differentiate these categories on the basis of the delineation and evolution over time of the findings from a focused neurologic examination particularly applicable to the comatose individual. Core components of this examination include the Glasgow Coma Scale (GCS) and specific brainstem reflexes (corneal, pupillary, occulocephalic, and oculovestibular).

Glasgow Coma Scale

The Glasgow Coma Scale (GCS) represents a simple but comprehensive examination that can be repeated frequently and reproducibly (Table 8–1).[8–11] Responsiveness is assessed by scoring three separate facets of consciousness: eye opening, motor response, and verbal response (see Table 8–1). For the most part,

Table 8–1. GLASGOW COMA SCALE

Parameter	Score
Eye Opening (E)	
Spontaneous	4
Responds to speech	3
Responds to pain	2
Nil	1
Best Motor Response (M)	
Obeys commands	6
Localizes pain	5
Withdraws	4
Abnormal flexion	3
Extensor response	2
Nil	1
Verbal Response (V)	
Oriented	5
Confused conversation	4
Inappropriate words	3
Incomprehensible sounds	2
Nil	1

The Glasgow Coma Scale is designed as a standardized assessment of the patient with disturbed consciousness. The tests can be performed serially to determine the patient's progress. The coma scale (E + M + V) = 3 to 15. All combinations equal to 7 or less define coma. Approximately 50 per cent of scores that equal 8 also define coma. Patients achieving a score of 9 or more are non-comatose.

scoring is relatively unambiguous. For example, children with spontaneous eye opening are scored 4 whereas those with eye opening in response to verbal stimuli of any kind is scored as 3. Less responsive individuals open their eyes in response to pain only (scored 2) or not to any stimulus (scored 1). The standard painful stimulus is supraorbital pressure or pressure on the fingernail with a pencil. The motor response is always scored as the best response elicited from the least affected extremity, an important consideration, particularly if paresis is present. Most of the responses are straightforward. Patients who obey simple commands receive a score of 6; less conscious patients who respond to the painful stimulus by moving their hands toward the supraorbital area receive a 5, and those who simply withdraw their extremities but who do not make an effort to move toward the stimulus receive a score of 4. *Abnormal flexion,* which is scored 3, is the most ambiguous of the terms, and refers to one of the following responses: extension then flexion, extreme stereotyped flexion, flexion of the fingers over the thumbs, extreme wrist flexion, and abduction of the upper arm. Extensor responses to pain, without any flexion, are scored 2, and patients who make no response at all to pain receive a score of 1.

Verbal responses are less apt to be confused. Patients who are oriented to time and place receive a score of 5; those who are able to converse but who are not oriented are scored 4, whereas those patients whose speech is inappropriate, i.e., composed of intelligible but isolated words, receive a score of 3. If the patients' response is simply incomprehensible sounds or groans, they are scored 2, and failure to make any verbal response to a painful stimulus results in a verbal score of 1. For the scale as a whole, patients who lie with their eyes closed and make no motor or verbal response to painful stimulation are given the minimal total score of 3. Fully responsive individuals receive the total maximal score of 15.

Brainstem Reflexes

Whereas the Glasgow Coma Scale has proved to be extremely useful in assessing head injuries and coma in adults after cardiac arrest, its role in assessing coma in children from causes other than head trauma remains to be defined. Furthermore, some of the scale items, particularly the verbal responses, are not always applicable in young children. In addition, many patients have an endotracheal tube in place, precluding a reliable estimate of the verbal response. Assessment of corneal, pupillary, oculocephalic, and oculovestibular reflexes provides important information about the function of particular regions within the brainstem and represents the second major core component of the examination of the child in coma.[1, 2, 4]

The corneal reflex is elicited by touching the cornea with a wisp of cotton and observing the reflex closure of the eyelid. It is mediated by sensory (branches of the trigeminal nerve) and motor (branches of the facial nerve) components that have neuroanatomic centers within the pons. Pupillary responses are elicited by shining a bright light into the pupil; they are mediated by components of the optic and oculomotor nerves, reflecting mesencephalic structures. Oculocephalic responses or doll's-eye movements are elicited by rotating the child's head rapidly toward one side and observing the eyes' deviation towards the opposite side. For example, rotation of the head towards the right side results in deviation of the eyes to the left. Caloric oculovestibular responses may be elicited by heat, cold, and electrical stimulation. In clinical practice, ice-water is used to stimulate the horizontal semicircular canals (cold calorics). The procedure is simple: the child's head is elevated approximately 30 degrees from the horizontal and the tympanic membrane is irrigated with 50 ml of ice-water. Tonic deviation of the eyes towards the stimulus indicates an intact response. For example, in a comatose individual, stimulation of the left tympanic membrane results in tonic deviation of the left eye laterally towards the left and of the right eye medially towards the left. The tonic deviation of the eyes represents the slow phase of nystagmus, the quick component having been abolished once the child became comatose.

Both the oculocephalic (doll's-eye movement) and oculovestibular (cold-caloric) reflexes are mediated by similar neural mechanisms—the oculovestibular reflex elicited by a more vigorous stimuli. The afferent component of the reflex is mediated by fibers from the vestibular portion of the eighth nerve with nuclei in the pons. From these pontine centers synapses occur with cells within the nearby sixth-nerve nucleus; these centers control lateral movement of the eye on the same side as the stimulus. Synapses occur within the medial longitudinal fasiculus (MLF) coursing between the pons and mesencephalon and controlling the medial movement of the eye on the side opposite to the stimulus. Thus any disease process that disrupts the region of brainstem between the sixth-nerve nucleus in the pons and the third-nerve nucleus in the mesencephalon will result in an abnormal oculocephalic or oculovestibular response.

Whereas some clinicians have emphasized the utility of respiratory patterns in assessing the depth of coma, in our experience these findings are of limited usefulness. For example, Cheyne-Stokes respiration may be seen in children relatively early in the course of the central syndrome, and central neurogenic hyperventilation may be seen when brain edema has affected pontine structures. However, in practice, most children are intubated and frequently paralyzed with pancuronium, and their respiration is controlled in an effort to better manage such factors as increased intracranial pressure.

DIFFERENTIAL DIAGNOSIS

Although a great variety of disease processes may produce disordered states of consciousness in children (Table 8–2), the most critical emergent issue remains the differentiation between structural and toxic-metabolic disorders of the brain, a discrimination facilitated by the application of the GCS and brainstem reflexes described. This clinical approach is illustrated in the following series of cases.

Table 8–2. DIFFERENTIAL DIAGNOSIS OF COMA

Structural brain disease	Trauma, resulting in intracranial hemorrhage, e.g., epidural, subdural, and intracerebral hematoma
	Neoplasms, e.g., primary brain tumors, rarely, solid CNS tumors associated with lymphoma
	Vascular disease, e.g., infarction, hemorrhage (secondary to arteriovenous malformation)
	Localized cerebral infection (abscess, empyema)
Toxic-metabolic brain disease	Hypoxic-ischemic encephalopathy (strangulation, drowning, carbon-monoxide poisoning, myocarditis with myocardial infarction)
	Exogenous poisoning:
	a. Sedatives (barbiturates, glutethimide)
	b. Neuroleptics (phenothiazines, tricyclic antidepressants, butyrophenones)
	c. Acetylsalicyclic acid
	d. Heavy metals (lead, iron)
	e. Anticonvulsants (phenobarbital, phenytoin)
	Generalized CNS infections (meningitis, encephalitis)
	Metabolic disorders (Reye's syndrome, diabetic ketoacidosis, hypoglycemia, hyperammonemias, organic acidurias)
	Status epilepticus

Case 1: Rapid Evolution of the Uncal Syndrome

An 8-year-old boy was riding in the front seat of his mother's automobile when it was struck from behind by another car. The child was thrown forward with his head striking the dashboard and was unresponsive for almost five minutes. He awoke slowly over the next half hour but then became drowsier and four hours after the initial injury was again unresponsive. At that time he was brought to the emergency room for evaluation. Examination indicated that he lay with his eyes closed but would open them in response to a painful stimulus (score 2 for eyes), would not utter any sounds (score 1 for verbal response), and would try to push the examiner away with his right hand (score 5 for motor response, total GCS = 7). He did not move his left side. His corneal reflex was intact, his left pupil responded briskly to light, but his right pupil was dilated and responded sluggishly. Dysconjugate responses were elicited on both the oculocephalic and oculovestibular reflexes, with the right eye not moving as well medially as the left eye moved laterally. Within two hours he no longer responded to painful stimuli by either movement or by eye opening (GCS = 3), his right pupil became more dilated and now did not respond to light, and the right eye failed to move medially either on the doll's-eye maneuver or after cold-caloric stimulation. Before treatment could be initiated, he died.

Comment

This clinical history, a concussive injury followed by a lucid interval, then a progressive and rapid deterioration, illustrates the classic presentation of an *epidural hematoma.*[12] The initial head injury produces the concussion and a fracture of the parietal bone, resulting in an injury of the middle meningeal artery. When the initial injury is relatively mild the child will regain consciousness, and, in fact, the so-called lucid interval following the concussive injury is observed in 25 per cent of cases. The progressive and rapid evolution in the neurologic condition described is the result of a rapid accumulation of blood following injury to the middle meningeal artery. As the blood accumulates in the epidural space, the cerebral hemisphere is compressed, resulting in paralysis of the limbs contralateral to the injury. Continued accumulation of blood in the epidural space results in a displacement of the uncal portion of the temporal lobe through the tentorial notch with subsequent compression of the third nerve on the side of the hematoma and compression of arterial blood supply to the brainstem. This diagnosis is usually confirmed on CAT scan.

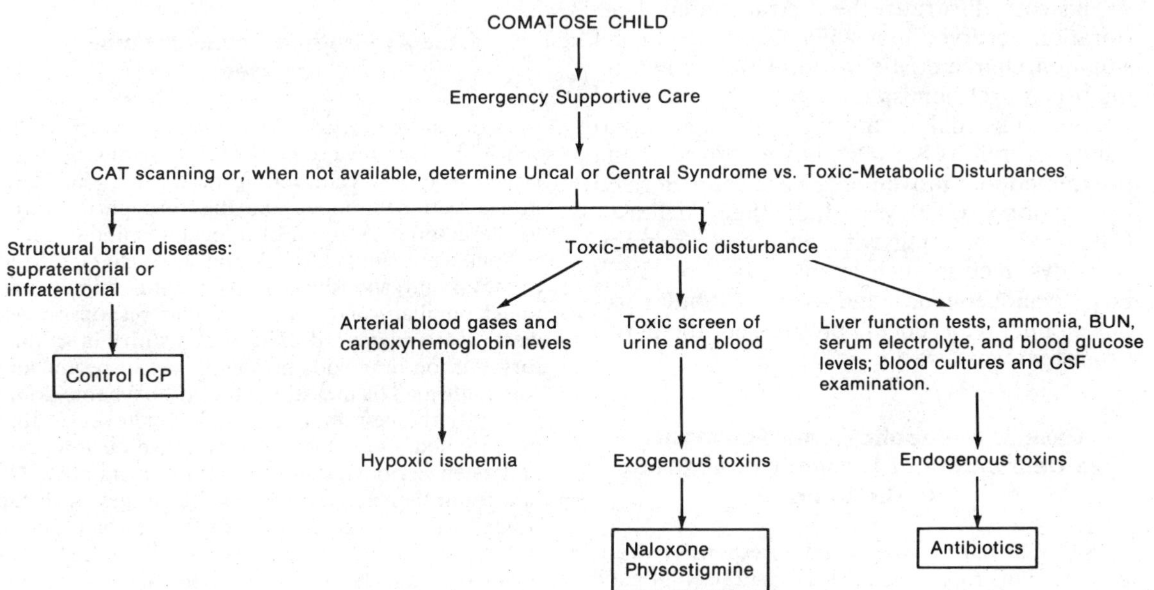

Case 2: Rostral-Caudal Deterioration in the Central Syndrome

A 14-year-old girl was standing on a street corner, talking to a friend, when a car jumped the curb and struck the children. Her friend was killed immediately, but she survived and was brought to the emergency room. She opened her eyes in response to supraorbital pressure (eye-opening score 2), did not utter any words (verbal-response score 1), and tried to push the examiner's hand away (motor-response score 5, total GCS = 8). Brainstem reflexes indicated normal corneal, pupillary, and oculocephalic reflexes. She appeared to have a left hemiparesis as well. Four hours later she no longer opened her eyes to any stimulus (eye-opening score 1), did not utter any sounds (verbal-response score 1), and appeared to exhibit flexion movements of her upper extremities with extensor movements of her lower extremities after painful stimulation (motor-response score 3, total GCS = 5). Her corneal, pupillary, and oculocephalic responses remained intact. Two hours later, however, she began to exhibit extensor responses of both upper and lower extremities in response to pain (motor-response score 2, GCS = 4). At this time her pupils were mid-position and did not respond to light. Dysconjugate movements were elicited on oculovestibular testing. By the following morning she no longer made any response to painful stimuli (GCS = 3). Her pupils were mid-position and fixed and no response was elicited on either doll's-eye maneuver or cold-caloric stimulation. At autopsy, an intracerebral hematoma with marked edema was noted in the right parietal area.

Comment

This case illustrates the rostral-caudal deterioration observed in a slowly evolving clinical situation characteristic of *brain edema* involving a cerebral hemisphere. Initially, the child seemed to be making appropriate responses to painful stimuli (GCS = 8), but as brain edema progressed, her movements were characterized by flexion (GCS = 5) and then extensor (GCS = 4) posturing with evidence of brainstem dysfunction such as disruption of pupillary, oculocephalic, and oculovestibular reflexes. Finally, as edema progressed, the entire brainstem was affected.

Case 3: Metabolic Coma Secondary to Deprivation of Oxygen or Substrate to the Brain

A 14-year-old boy was found unresponsive by his parents in his room at 5 P.M. He had been in good health immediately preceding this incident, and in fact was in school that afternoon. He was a good student and was not known to take any drugs. Everyone in the home was healthy and no drugs, other than aspirin and acetaminophen, were used by his parents. On examination, he would not open his eyes to painful stimuli (eye-opening score 1), would make incomprehensible sounds (verbal-response score 2), and would move all extremities equally, localizing the painful stimulus by pushing the examiner's hand away (motor-response score 5, GCS = 8). Corneal, pupillary, and oculocephalic responses were intact. CAT scan, results of cerebrospinal fluid examination, and electroencephalogram (EEG) were normal, and toxic agents were not identified in his urine or blood. Within four hours he opened his eyes and was lucid. He gave a history of a severe headache with nausea prior to losing consciousness. Follow-up examinations over the next year indicated that he had unilateral headaches associated with nausea, which occurred once each month, but did not become comatose with any of them.

Comment

Coma secondary to *cerebral ischemia* will result in deprivation of both oxygen and substrate to the brain. This case illustrates encephalopathic migraine, an unusual disorder described by Gascon and Barlow.[13] It is believed to represent a type of basilar artery migraine and demonstrates the vasoconstrictive phase of the migraine attack. Coma secondary to anoxia may occur after suffocation and near-drowning in which the causes are obvious. At times, however, the diagnosis of coma secondary to anoxia is less clear, as the following case illustrates.

Case 4: Multiple Family Members Affected

Two children, aged 3 and 7 years, and their 28-year-old mother were found unconscious by their father when he returned from work at 10 P.M. Police were summoned and they brought all three to the emergency room of a local hospital. Examinations were similar for all and were characterized by total unresponsiveness to painful stimuli but intact pupillary and oculovestibular responses. All were beet red, and despite a noncontributory history, carbon-monoxide poisoning was suspected and was confirmed by measuring the carboxyhemoglobin level. By the next morning the father revealed that his wife had a long history of affective disorder and had been seriously depressed for six months. He had found her in their car, in the garage, with the doors to the garage closed and the motor running, but was ashamed to tell anyone about his wife's problems. The children were in bed at the time, but their bedroom was above the garage and fumes apparently seeped into the bedroom and intoxicated them.

COMMENT

Carbon monoxide produces *hypoxia* by competing with oxygen for binding sites on hemoglobin. It should be suspected in any case involving multiple cases of coma in a family.

Case 5: Coma Secondary to Exogenous Toxins

A 2-year-old boy was rushed to the emergency room when he could not be aroused in the morning. Initial questioning of the parents suggested that he might have obtained some of his grandmother's medicine (she was a diabetic with chronic congestive heart disease and a long history of psychiatric difficulties). Examination indicated that the child would not respond to verbal commands (verbal-response score 1) nor would he open his eyes (eye-opening score 1). He did not make any movements with painful stimuli (motor-response score 1, GCS = 3). Coroneal, oculocephalic, and oculovestibular responses were not obtained, but pupils were dilated widely and reacted briskly to light. He was febrile (104°F rectally) and had a tachycardia with a heart rate of 130 beats/minute. Within minutes of administration of 2 mg physostigmine, he began to move spontaneously, and two hours later a tricyclic antidepressant was identified in his urine. Except for supportive care, no further therapy was administered, and the child recovered completely within two days.

COMMENT

This case represents the triad of hyperpyrexia, mydriasis, and tachycardia that are the hallmarks of tricyclic-antidepressant poisoning. Other findings may include urinary retention and decreased secretion, symptoms emphasizing the anticholinergic effects of the tricyclic agents. Treatment is directed at increasing the concentration of acetylcholine at the synaptic cleft, and the most effective strategy employs the drug physostigmine, which inhibits acetylcholinesterase, the enzyme responsible for degradation of the transmitter. Doses of physostigmine, 0.5–2 mg, intravenously, may result in rapid improvement, though this improvement is often short-lived. Physostigmine itself may be dangerous and must be used cautiously (see Chapter 5).[14]

EXOGENOUS TOXINS IN CHILDHOOD COMA

Exogenous toxins are among the most frequent causes of coma in children, and often the most perplexing. Studies, primarily of adult populations, indicate that in 50 per cent of cases the exogenous toxin is self-administered and that 50 per cent of the victims take more than one drug.[15] Both barbiturate and nonbarbiturate sedatives and hypnotics (glutethimide, benzodiazepine, and ethanol) are the most common agents responsible.

Brainstem reflexes may be altered significantly by a variety of exogenous toxins. Opiates characteristically produce pinpoint pupils, whereas anticholinergic agents produce pupillary dilatation. Glutethimide may produce moderately dilated pupils that do not respond to light. Furthermore, barbiturates and other sedatives, tricyclic antidepressants, succinylcholine and other agents affecting the neuromuscular junction, and anticonvulsive agents such as phenytoin may all alter the oculocephalic and oculovestibular responses. Coma secondary to narcotic overdose may be seen in adolescents and may be suspected particularly in the presence of miosis and pulmonary edema. Treatment with naloxone at doses of 0.01 mg/kg may be diagnostic and lifesaving (see Chapter 5).

Alcohol intoxication is a common cause of stupor and coma in adolescents. Stupor occurs with blood alcohol concentrations in the 250–300 μg/100 ml range, and coma with concentrations greater than 300 μg/100 ml. Alcoholic coma has been reported in infants fed a high-protein, high-carbohydrate diet.[16]

Coma due to salicylate intoxication is a common pediatric emergency, and the associated hyperventilation usually provides a clue to the diagnosis. Less commonly appreciated are cases of delayed onset of coma following salicylate ingestion, which is believed to represent unbound, un-ionized salicylate "trapped" in the brain.[17] The anti-diarrheal agent Lomotil has also been reported to cause a delayed onset of coma.[18]

Lead encephalopathy occurs in children under 3 years of age and is usually heralded by ataxia, vomiting, stupor progressing to coma, and severe and protracted convulsions. Laboratory studies indicate increased intracranial pressure with elevation of protein in cerebrospinal fluid (CSF) and blood lead levels greater than 120 μg/100 ml.[19]

Case 6: Coma Secondary to a Presumed Endogenous Toxin

An 11-year-old girl was well until five days prior to admission, when she developed cough, fever, and coryza. She was treated symptomatically with antihistamines and aspirin, and the day before admission she developed vomiting and a progressive deterioration in state of consciousness. On admission to the pediatric Intensive Care Unit she would not utter any sounds (verbal-response score 1), did not open her eyes (eye-opening score 1), and made withdrawal movements with all extremities in response to painful stimuli (motor-response score 4, GCS = 6). Corneal, pupillary, and oculocephalic responses were intact. A diagnosis of *Reye's syndrome (RS)* was suspected and was confirmed when the arterial blood ammonia level was reported to be 624 μg/100 ml (normal up to 150 μg/100 ml). Management for severe RS was immediately instituted, including intracranial pressure (ICP) monitoring via an intraventricular catheter, controlled, assisted ventilation with maintenance of P_{CO_2} at 20–23 mmHg, phenobarbital, and mannitol and furosemide as indicated. Treatment continued for seven days and then was slowly tapered. She was discharged one week later in good condition.

Comment

Since its initial, simultaneous description by Reye and coworkers[20] and Johnson and colleagues,[21] RS has been reported in more than 1000 children and is now the most common metabolic encephalopathy of childhood. This case illustrates the classic presenting symptoms of vomiting and progressive deterioration in consciousness accompanied by evidence of hepatic dysfunction, typically an elevation in blood ammonia concentration. Cerebral edema is the most serious complication of RS, and measures directed at its management have resulted in impressive reductions in mortality and morbidity.[22]

The decision to implement aggressive and invasive measures to combat increased ICP in RS is made on the basis of both clinical and laboratory criteria. We generally begin such measures when there is evidence of a decreasing level of consciousness with a GCS score of 7 or less and blood ammonia concentrations greater than 300 μg/100 ml, as was found in this case. The measures employed are detailed in the section on management of coma in this chapter as well as in Chapter 9. In general, such measures include limiting fluid intake, controlling respirations to maintain P_{CO_2} between 23 and 25 mm Hg, administering phenobarbital to reduce cerebral metabolism, and providing mannitol and furosemide as needed to reduce ICP.

A particularly difficult clinical problem is the timing of the cessation of these invasive management procedures (see page 167). To date, no uniform rules are available, though recent experience with new electrophysiologic procedures suggests that they may be helpful in the future.[23] For a more detailed discussion, please refer to Chapter 9 on Reye's syndrome.

Coma Caused by Other Endogenous Toxins

Whereas RS is the most common metabolic encephalopathy, coma secondary to CNS infections such as meningitis and encephalitis is certainly more frequent. The same techniques used in RS may need to be employed in each of these infectious conditions should elevated ICP complicate the picture, and in fact intracranial pressure monitoring has been useful in cases of elevated ICP accompanying bacterial meningitis.[24] Clearly, specific antibacterial therapy for bacterial meningitis and antiviral treatment of herpes simplex encephalitis are vital in these situations and the reader is referred to other sources for more details.[25, 26]

Coma is also seen in some cases of overwhelming liver disease (hepatic coma) and in renal disease (uremic coma). In infants, coma may be the presenting symptom of an inherited hyperammonemia such as ornithine transcarbamylase or carbamyl phosphate synthetase deficiency. Other inborn errors associated with coma include citrullinemia, hyperprolinemia, maple syrup urine disease, hypervalinemia, and green acyl dehydrogenase deficiency.[27, 28]

Case 7: Coma Secondary to Status Epilepticus

A 4-year-old girl had been ill with a sore throat for 10 days preceding her hospitalization and had received antibiotic therapy. On the day of admission her mother noted that she seemed to "stiffen up." From that time on she continued to make occasional gurgling sounds and to have facial twitching but seemed unresponsive to her mother's voice. She was brought to a local hospital where the physicians who examined her thought they found nuchal rigidity and saw bilateral papilledema. Following antibiotic therapy, the child was transferred to our tertiary care center's pediatric ICU. On admission she was totally unresponsive verbally (score 1) and would not open her eyes (score 1) but withdrew all extremities to painful stimuli (motor-response score 4, GCS = 6). Pupillary, corneal and oculovestibular responses were intact. CAT scan indicated what was believed to be cerebral edema, but ICP was initially normal and remained so. CSF examination showed 2000 per mm^3 red blood cells (RBCs), no white blood cells (WBCs), and normal protein and glucose levels. Her EEG indicated continuous, generalized seizure activity, though no movements were noted clinically. Treatment was initiated as described in the "Management of Status Epilepticus" section. She remained in the hospital for one month and made a slow but steady recovery. At discharge, she was talking and seemed to be on her way to recovery.

COMMENT

Status epilepticus is discussed in the following section.

STATUS EPILEPTICUS

The term status epilepticus generally refers to repeated or persistent generalized or lateralized convulsive seizures of prolonged duration without intermittent periods of consciousness. Exactly what is meant by "prolonged" remains controversial, though most investigators suggest that seizures of 30 minutes or longer represent status epilepticus.[29, 30]

Etiology

The etiology of status epilepticus differs considerably in children and adults. Thus, 40 per cent of status epilepticus in adults results from trauma, neoplasms, and vascular disease, disorders which rarely cause status epilepticus in childhood. In contrast, infectious, toxic-metabolic and chronic encephalopathic disturbances cause 40 per cent of status epilepticus in children but only 20 per cent in adults. In more than half the cases of childhood-onset status epilepticus, no cause is ever found, whereas in adults, less than a third of patients have no demonstrable etiology.[31–35]

Pathophysiology

Convulsive status epilepticus is a medical emergency with mortality and morbidity increasing significantly if status epilepticus lasts longer than 60 to 90 minutes. Evidence from several lines of investigation supports the belief that more than 60 minutes of convulsive status epilepticus produces irreversible neuronal damage in the hippocampus, amygdala, cerebellum, thalamus, and middle cerebral cortical layers even in animals adequately ventilated throughout the convulsion, a pattern of neuronal damage that parallels that observed in children dying after status epilepticus. Such neuronal damage is believed to occur as a consequence of a cascade of metabolic disturbances affecting cellular oxygenation and the accumulation of potentially toxic products such as polyenic fatty acids. In addition, prolonged and continuous generalized seizures may eventually produce hypoglycemia, hypotension, and cardiovascular and respiratory failure.[36]

Management

GENERAL PRINCIPLES[37]

Status epilepticus must always be considered a medical emergency, because as noted above, good evidence suggests that prolonged convulsive seizures may produce neuronal damage. Furthermore, the likelihood of damage is greater if the condition is associated with inadequate ventilation or impaired general circulation. Thus, it is mandatory that any child with this condition be admitted as quickly as possible to a pediatric ICU, where the emergency treatment must be directed towards establishing and maintaining an appropriate airway and providing adequate circulation as well as stopping the seizures. This emergency treatment nearly always necessitates the placement of an endotracheal tube and controlled, assisted ventilation, and may include the administration of agents designed to treat hypotension and cardiac decompensation. Investigations in animals have indicated that the ability of the brain to satisfy the energy expenditure produced by the prolonged seizure state is limited, suggesting that administration of 10 per cent glucose may be helpful. In some cases it is possible that brain edema is a factor in the perpetuation of the seizures. Thus, if the usual agents are not effective in treating the symptoms, some clinicians begin treating the child for brain edema (see Chapter 9).

PHARMACOTHERAPY

More specific therapy is directed at the reduction and elimination of the seizure state using anticonvulsant drugs. As a general principle, the *intravenous route of administration is mandatory*. A number of drugs have been employed in the treatment of status epilepticus, but in recent years diazepam (Valium) has proved to be a rapid and effective anticonvulsant agent. The drug is administered intravenously over a 2-minute interval at the initial dose of 0.25 mg/kg (maximum 10 mg). If seizures continue, a dose of 0.4 mg/kg (maximum 15 mg) is repeated after 10 minutes, and if this is not successful within 30 minutes, still another dose, 0.5 mg/kg (maximum 20 mg), is given. Although the maximum dose in any individual has not been established, doses greater than 45 mg over two hours must be monitored closely. There is a well-documented risk of respiratory arrest with this agent, particularly if the child has received concurrent doses of barbiturates. In addition, high doses of diazepam may be associated with cardiac arrhythmias and hypotension.[38]

Because the duration of anticonvulsant action of diazepam is short-lived, perhaps as brief as 15 minutes, it is necessary to treat concomitantly with another anticonvulsant agent. Although a number of agents have been employed, most clinicians consider either phenobarbital or phenytoin to be the drug of choice.[39]

Phenytoin is less likely to interact with diazepam and produce respiratory difficulties, and thus is the preferred drug in patients older than neonates. It is administered intravenously at a 15 mg/kg loading dose. If seizures continue, a dose of 10 mg/kg is repeated after 1 hour, and again after 4 hours. Subsequent dosages depend on phenytoin serum concentrations, which should approach 25 μg/ml. Phenytoin must be given slowly and heart rate monitored carefully to avoid cardiac arrhythmias.

Phenobarbital is a traditional and effective agent not only when used with diazepam, but also when used by itself in the treatment of status epilepticus in children. Although it may not reach the required concentrations in the brain as rapidly as does diazepam, its wide therapeutic index makes it a useful agent. Phenobarbital is given intravenously over 5 to 10 minutes at a loading dose of 10–15 mg/kg in older children and 15–20 mg/kg in neonates. The daily dose should then be adjusted accordingly to effect a plasma barbiturate concentration of 30–50 μg/ml over the subsequent 48 hours. This adjustment usually necessitates administering 10 mg/kg per day for that period before the dose is reduced to maintenance levels of 5 mg/kg. *Although the combination of diazepam and phenobarbital may result in respiratory depression, such a complication is not a problem with the intubated child.*

Combinations of the three agents should be effective in most cases, but if another agent is necessary, a continuous intravenous infusion of a short-acting barbiturate such as thiopental at a dosage of 3–5 mg/kg/hr should be considered. Such patients must be monitored carefully, since high blood levels of barbiturates may cause cardiovascular depression. If seizures continue, two other anticonvulsant agents may be employed, paraldehyde and lidocaine.[40] Paraldehyde may be given intravenously as a 10 per cent solution at a loading dosage of 200 mg/kg over 5 minutes and then at 20 mg/kg/hr. Complications include pulmonary hemorrhage, pulmonary edema, and metabolic acidosis. Paraldehyde diluted 10-fold with mineral or peanut oil may be administered rectally at a dose of 0.3 ml/kg (maximum dose 5 ml); repeating this procedure after 1 hour and again after 2 hours might be considered. Lidocaine in large doses may actually precipitate seizures, but at dosages of 1 μg/kg/min it may prove an effective anticonvulsant. Finally, if all measures fail, general anesthesia with agents such as halothane and enflurane may be necessary.

If possible, EEG monitoring should be employed, though electrical evidence of seizures may continue despite the effective treatment of any clinically evident convulsion. EEG monitoring is particularly critical in children who are receiving paralytic agents for the treatment of pulmonary disease or increased ICP. In such patients the EEG provides the only objective assessment of cortical seizure activity.

MANAGEMENT OF COMA

Although the management of an individual in coma often assumes the appearance of a technical *tour de force* characterized by an array of drugs and equipment that is intimidating to the novice, the principles of management are not difficult to understand and may be considered as comprising ten points (Table 8–3).

Assure Oxygenation. The provision and maintenance of an adequate airway, along with

Table 8–3. MANAGEMENT OF COMA

1. Assure oxygenation
2. Maintain circulation
3. Administer glucose
4. Reduce increased intracranial pressure
5. Treat seizures
6. Combat infection
7. Correct electrolyte imbalance
8. Adjust body temperature
9. Consider specific antidotes
10. Control agitation

the maintenance of circulation, remains the most important primary responsibility of those ministering to the comatose child. Oxygenation frequently necessitates paralyzing the child with pancuronium in order to insert a nasotracheal or endotracheal tube, or performing a tracheotomy. Tracheal intubation is clearly just the initial step in the process, and constant monitoring of pulmonary status is critical. Monitoring includes not only control of arterial blood gas status but provision of optimum pulmonary toilet (frequent suctioning, postural drainage).

Maintain Circulation. Restoration and maintenance of physiologic blood pressure and cardiac dynamics is as critical as assuring oxygenation. The physician's skill in providing access to the vascular compartment via intravenous and intra-arterial lines remains a most critical facet in overall care. Once vascular access is assured, more specific measures may be employed, such as the correction of hypovolemia via blood or fluid replacement as well as pharmacologic therapy directed at increasing myocardial contractility and peripheral vasoconstriction.

Administer Glucose. In contrast to adults, in whom insulin overdosage and its consequences are a frequent metabolic cause of coma, hypoglycemia in children is unusual. However, once blood has been drawn for the necessary laboratory tests, administration of 25 g of glucose given intravenously as a 50 per cent solution over 5 minutes is recommended.

Reduce Increased Intracranial Pressure (ICP). Increased ICP occurs frequently in coma because of structural disorders such as head trauma[41] and toxic-metabolic disturbances such as Reye's syndrome,[22] meningitis,[24] and near-drowning[42] (Table 8–4).

The first step in the management of increased ICP is the implementation of measures that allow the accurate second-to-second monitoring of ICP. As indicated previously, this measure involves the insertion of a ventricular catheter or subarachnoid bolt as soon as increased ICP is suspected.

Fluid intake is usually limited to two thirds of maintenance requirements, though care must be taken that intravascular volume is not reduced so much that blood pressure is lowered.

Positioning the patient's head 30 degrees above the horizontal will often maintain ICP at a physiologically acceptable pressure.

Sedation of the patient with morphine may reduce agitation that is often associated with

Table 8–4. MANAGEMENT OF INCREASED ICP

1. Monitor ICP
   a. ventricular catheter
   b. subarachnoid bolt
2. Limit fluid intake
3. Control ventilation
   P_{CO_2} 23–25 mmHg
4. Prevent seizures
   phenobarbital, 10 mg/kg
5. If ICP > 20 mmHg
   a. mannitol, 0.25–1 g/kg q3–6h
   b. furosemide, 1 mg/kg q3–6h
6. Sedation
7. Consider pentobarbital, 5 mg/kg
8. Dexamethasone, 0.25 mg/kg q6h

increased ICP. When ICP is elevated (usually above 20 mmHg for more than 2 minutes), more specific measures are employed. These measures include the following:

1. Control of ventilation so that P_{CO_2} is maintained at 23–25 mmHg.

2. Administration of phenobarbital (loading dose 10–15 mg/kg) to maintain phenobarbital level at 15–30 μg/ml. Alternatively, pentobarbital may be administered at a loading dosage of 5 mg/kg with increments of 1–2 mg/kg every 2 to 3 hours to maintain the barbiturate level. Although the results of animal studies suggest that the routine use of barbiturates is not indicated in patients in coma following cardiac arrest,[43] good evidence supports the use of barbiturates in the reduction of increased ICP.

3. Administration of drugs proved to reduce ICP. Traditionally, the most effective agent to reduce ICP has proved to be mannitol, an osmotic diuretic, which when given in as small amounts as 0.25 g/kg will reduce ICP for as long as 4 to 6 hours. If the small dose is ineffective, larger doses, ranging up to 1 g/kg, may be given. More recently, another diuretic has proved to be effective in the reduction of ICP, i.e., furosemide, 1 mg/kg every 3 to 6 hours, is an important adjunct to therapy.

4. A steroid, usually dexamethasone, at a loading dose of 0.5 mg/kg and maintenance dosages of 0.25 mg/kg every 6 hours is effective in reducing ICP from brain tumors and head trauma, *but its efficacy in increased ICP from other causes is not clear.*

One of the most difficult decisions in managing the child in coma with increased ICP is when to stop some of the measures just described. Thus, we are frequently faced with a child who remains paralyzed with pancuronium in order to control respirations with P_{CO_2} maintained at 23–25 mmHg and who has been receiving phenobarbital and perhaps dexamethasone and, intermittently, mannitol or furosemide. If ICP remains below 20 mmHg for 24 hours without our having to administer any mannitol or furosemide, we will eliminate the phenobarbital and begin tapering the dexamethasone and allow the P_{CO_2} to increase toward more physiologic levels. If ICP remains in the normal range we will eliminate the pancuronium and allow the child to respire on his or her own. If ICP should increase again, we reinstitute therapy for at least another 24 hours. Most recently we have used somatic-evoked cortical responses as an index of the degree of recovery in children with increased ICP from Reye's syndrome.[23] Whether such techniques will be helpful in other clinical situations remains to be determined. For more details please see Chapter 9.

Treat Seizures. Coma occurring as a result of status epilepticus has been discussed previously. However, seizures may occur at other times, particularly in children in coma due to an hypoxic insult. If the seizures are generalized tonic-clonic and last for more than 15 minutes they should be treated with the same vigor as status epilepticus. However, if they are infrequent and focal, less aggressive measures are usually employed. Those agents used for the treatment of status epilepticus (see the previous discussion) may be used and consist of phenobarbital administered first as a loading dose of 10 mg/kg, followed by a maintenance dosage of 5 mg/kg/day to maintain blood levels at 15–30μg/ml; or phenytoin given as a 15 mg/kg loading dose, followed by a maintenance dosage of 5 mg/kg/day to maintain blood levels at 10–20 μg/ml.

Combat Infection. If bacterial infection is suspected as the principal etiologic factor in the genesis of coma or if infection has been superimposed on the already comatose child, appropriate and specific antibacterial therapy is necessary.

Correct Electrolyte Imbalance. In rare cases, hyponatremia or hypernatremia, hypocalcemia, or hypomagnesemia may cause coma, and the correction of these electrolyte disturbances is central to treatment. More commonly, electrolyte abnormalities occur as secondary problems in children with CNS insults. Thus, a child with a head injury or increased ICP caused by, for example, Reye's syndrome may exhibit the syndrome of inappropriate antidiuretic hormone secretion. If free water is not restricted, hyponatremia with concomitant seizures and coma may result. Another potential iatrogenic electrolyte disturbance occurs when serum potassium level is allowed to drop, resulting in severe weakness that may confuse the clinical picture. In present-day intensive care facilities, frequent determination of serum electrolyte levels is often routine, and these problems are readily diagnosed.

Adjust Body Temperature. Hypothermia as a therapy is not generally used any longer in the management of coma. Studies with animals suggest that it may be effective in experimental head injury when it is implemented prior to the injury, an impractical approach in clinical situations. In rare instances, patients have survived prolonged periods of anoxia without apparent neurologic deficit because their body temperature had been reduced, for example, in near-drownings in ice water. In most cases, reduced body temperature may result in cardiac arrhythmias, and gradual warming is indicated.

Consider Specific Antidotes. Two specific antidotes are available: naloxone for the treatment of coma secondary to opiate overdose, and physostigmine for the treatment of anticholinergic poisoning. Of the two, naloxone is certainly safer and more specific. It may be given at a first dose of 0.01 mg/kg and if there is no response, 0.1 mg/kg.

Physostigmine is useful in treating the cardiac–central nervous system effects of anticholinergic agents. In contrast to the specificity of naloxone, physostigmine may cause nonspecific CNS stimulation and may, itself, cause seizures. It must be used cautiously, at doses of 0.5 to 2 mg. Once it is clear that the child is no longer in immediate danger from cardiac arrhythmias, the agent need not be continued. For more details, please see Chapter 5.

Control Agitation. It is particularly important to control agitation in children in coma due to increased ICP, but agitation may become a problem in coma secondary to toxic-metabolic disturbances, particularly when the child is beginning to recover. We generally recommend against the use of any other pharmacologic agent, and instruct our staff to try to restrain the children and prevent them from physically harming themselves during what is usually a very short-lived agitated period. Should the physician decide that some pharmacotherapy is needed, a benzodiazepine such as diazepam given intravenously or intramuscularly at a dosage of 0.25 mg/kg every 3 to 4 hours may be helpful. If diazepam proves ineffective, a neuroleptic such as haloperidol, 1 mg, or thioridazine, 25 mg, intramuscularly, 2 to 3 times each day may be necessary.

Laboratory Studies of Children in Coma

The studies listed in Table 8–5 represent those most relevant in the evaluation of the child in coma. Many of the tests follow directly from what has been discussed under "Management of Coma," and some may not be necessary at all, depending on the clinical situation.

The first group of investigations involve examination of the blood. Arterial blood gas (ABG) levels are necessary to monitor pulmonary status and to decide when intubation and controlled ventilation are indicated. Once the decision has been made to ventilate the child, ABG levels are needed to determine appropriate respiratory settings. A routine blood glucose determination will effectively exclude the uncommon occurrence of hypoglycemia as a cause of coma, whereas the routine determination of blood urea nitrogen (BUN) and electrolyte levels will help determine whether renal disease (uremic coma) or electrolyte abnormalities have occurred either as a primary cause (rare) or, more frequently, as an iatrogenic complication of a CNS disorder.

In general, both blood and urine samples should be sent to the laboratory for toxicologic analysis (see Chapter 5). The finding of drugs (barbiturates and other sedatives, neuroleptics, and anticonvulsants) may be diagnostic. Heavy-metal poisoning, such as lead intoxication, is diagnosed when blood lead concentrations exceed 40 μg/100 ml, though encephalopathy is not observed unless blood lead concentrations exceed 120 μg/100 ml. Erythrocyte protoporphyrin assay may also be helpful. However, a negative result does not necessarily exclude a toxic etiology for coma, and recent studies indicate that even in the best laboratories, specific toxic agents are identified in only 50 to 70 per cent of cases of poisoning.[15] Liver function tests are useful in the evaluation of hepatic coma or in the determination of hepatic damage secondary to ingestion of a toxin. Blood ammonia concentration is the single most valuable laboratory test in the diagnosis of Reye's syndrome and should be determined in any comatose child, particularly if there is a history of persistent vomiting. Blood should be obtained and cultured for bacteria in any child suspected of having a disseminated infection.

Table 8–5. LABORATORY STUDIES OF CHILDREN IN COMA

Arterial blood gas
Blood glucose
BUN, serum electrolytes
Computed tomography
CSF examination
Toxicology screen
Liver function tests, including blood ammonia
Blood cultures
EEG
Viral cultures (nasopharyngeal and rectal swabs)

The second group of studies incorporate investigations other than blood analysis. Of these, the single most important study is CAT scanning of the head, a radiologic procedure that has revolutionized the management of the child in coma. As noted previously, the principal differential diagnosis is between structural and toxic-metabolic disorders. By effectively diagnosing structural brain disease in a non-invasive and efficient manner, CAT scanning has become one of the most important tools in the physician's diagnostic armamentarium. In most large tertiary centers, CAT scanning may be obtained on an emergency basis and is often available within minutes. It should be employed in all cases of coma in which structural disorders are suspected or are included in the differential diagnosis.

CSF examination is another important and useful study. The principal purpose of this examination is the diagnosis or exclusion of infections of the CNS, and although beyond the scope of this chapter, the interpretation of CSF findings in meningo-encephalitis and meningitis are often diagnostic and lead to specific antibiotic therapy. Except in cases in which bacterial meningitis is strongly suspected, the CSF examination should not be performed until the CAT scan has been examined and structural brain disorders have been ruled out. Elevations of CSF pressure may be helpful in the diagnosis of increased ICP, and high CSF protein concentrations may indicate CNS tumor. With the advent of CAT scanning, the electroencephalogram (EEG) has little role in the diagnosis of structural brain disease. However, low-voltage, fast activity on the EEG may be indicative of drug ingestion. The EEG is also indispensable in the management of coma secondary to status epilepticus.

PROGNOSIS IN COMA

In many cases of coma of brief duration, recovery is immediate and complete. For example, in near-drowning, 90 per cent or more of children recover without residua.[44] When coma is of long duration, outcome is not nearly as favorable and depends to a considerable degree upon etiology. Thus, estimates based on several large series suggest a reasonable outcome after coma resulting from craniocerebral trauma.[41, 45–47] Most children, except for those in deepest coma, appear to recover with minor or perhaps no handicaps at all.

When coma is of non-traumatic origin the outcome is more problematic. Studies in adults who suffered cardiac arrest and were resuscitated provide the largest and, to date, the best estimates of outcome.[48–51] In general, such studies suggest neurologic recovery if consciousness is regained within 24 hours after the cardiac arrest. The absence of corneal or pupillary reflexes by the end of the first day was almost always associated with an unfavorable outcome. Structural brain disease such as cerebrovascular disease carried the worst prognosis, and metabolic problems the best, with hypoxia-ischemia intermediate.[48]

Prolonged coma (of at least 5 days duration) from non-traumatic causes in children is much less common than that from head injury, and in a recent review we were able to document only 41 cases of prolonged medical coma in children.[52] Except for the nearly uniformly poor prognosis in cases of herpes simplex encephalitis, more than half the children had either minor or no residua. In our series of 16 children with coma of 5 days or longer, 6 recovered without sequelae and another 6 had minor sequelae. Thus, 75 per cent of those in coma for five days or more made an excellent or reasonably good recovery. The results of such studies indicate that the physician's efforts in treating patients in coma will be rewarded when the children survive with normal neurologic functioning.

CRITERIA FOR DEATH

The pressing need to more rigorously provide a diagnosis of death has become increasingly apparent as state-of-the-art intensive care technology becomes widespread. In order to clarify a situation that all observers agree is chaotic, a recent presidential commission provided what appears to be a workable definition of death.[53] Their purpose was to eliminate any errors in classifying a living patient as dead, and to engender as few errors as possible in designating a dead body as alive. These criteria were designed to be used in a variety of clinical situations and to allow determination to be made quickly.

The criteria are embodied in a model law, termed the Uniform Determination of Death Act: "An individual who has sustained either (1) *irreversible cessation of circulatory and respiratory functions,* or (2) *irreversible cessation of all functions of the entire brain,* including the brain stem, is dead. A determination of death must be made in accordance with accepted medical standards."

Several points need to be emphasized about this definition. Note that no mention is made of "brain death," a concept that has remained ill-defined and controversial. Thus, in the United States, the concept of brain death was primarily a pathophysiologic one, whereas in England and other countries of Europe, the term referred to a pathologic process. Still another definition of brain death was prognostic, i.e., it was said to presage death of the rest of the body. The definition proposed by the task force eliminates these controversies by eliminating the term "brain death." Instead, death can be diagnosed by cessation and irreversibility either of respiratory and circulatory functions or of brain functions.

Irreversible cessation of circulatory and respiratory functions is evident by absence of heartbeat and respiratory effort that persists for an appropriate period of observation. Such criteria are generally easy to apply, though it is usual for ECG to be used as a confirmatory test.

Neurologic criteria of death are more difficult to apply. *Cessation of neurologic functions* is diagnosed when: (1) cerebral functions are absent, i.e., the patient is in coma (defined previously), and (2) brainstem functions are absent, though spinal cord reflexes may persist after death.[54, 55] The determination of cessation of neurologic functions mandates reliable testing of brainstem reflexes including pupillary light, corneal, oculocephalic, oculovestibular, oropharyngeal, and respiratory (apnea) reflexes. *Irreversibility* of cessation of neurologic functioning is recognized when: (1) The diagnosis is established and is sufficient to result in the clinical picture. It always presupposes a careful history, physical examination, and appropriate ancillary procedures, which may include CAT scanning, toxic and drug screening,

EEG, and more specific tests as required. (2) The possibility for recovery has been excluded. In practice, this determination necessitates excluding such important reversible conditions as sedation, hypothermia, neuromuscular blockade, and shock. (3) Cessation of all brain functions must persist for an appropriate period of observation.

Such diagnostic criteria mandate a great deal of physician responsibility in decision making. For example, the physician must decide what constitutes an "appropriate" period of observation. Clearly, the precise duration of an appropriate period may vary depending upon the circumstances, and the period sufficient to diagnose death in an adult may not be the same in children. Thus, in adults, observation for 6 hours may be sufficient in some cases, though a longer period, for example, 12 hours, may be desirable if the extent of damage is difficult to determine. The theoretically more plastic brain of the child would suggest that a longer time should be used, for example, 12 to 24 hours of observation.

The role of ancillary procedures in the diagnosis of death continues to evolve and it remains each physician's responsibility to decide on how these procedures are to be employed in satisfying criteria for death. However, such tests must be interpreted with a great deal of caution. In adults, an EEG that remains isoelectric for 30 minutes suggests absence of cerebral function, but an EEG is not mandatory for the diagnosis of death. It is well known that in rare instances drug (barbiturate) or metabolic intoxication may mimic death and must be excluded.[56, 57] In infants and young children the EEG may be misleading because it continues to demonstrate low-voltage cortical activity despite extensive brain liquefaction necrosis.[58] Brainstem-evoked responses may also be useful, but, here too, results may be misleading.[59] Four-vessel intracranial angiography is definitive for the diagnosis of cessation of circulation to the brain, but is not readily available except in large medical centers. Radioisotope bolus cerebral angiography and gamma-scintigraphy are easier to obtain. The assessment of blood flow to the brain using either test is sometimes a useful adjunct to the clinical examination in the diagnosis of death.

Despite these problems, the presidential commission has provided a practical framework that allows the application of the proposed criteria in most clinical situations. Furthermore, the new criteria permit investigators to verify their validity and utility in both children and adults.

SUMMARY

The medical approach to the child in coma was reviewed. Using a series of clinical case histories, the major categories of coma were explored. Differentiation of structural from toxic-metabolic disorders was emphasized, and management and prognosis reviewed. Status epilepticus as a cause of coma was examined, and, finally, the diagnosis of death discussed.

Coma is an important and common pediatric problem. Physicians dealing with the comatose child need to have at their command the principles elaborated here.

REFERENCES

1. Plum F, Posner, JB. The Diagnosis of Stupor and Coma. Philadelphia: FA Davis Co, 1980.
2. DeJong RN. The Neurologic Examination. Hagerstown: Harper and Row, 1979, 689–719.
3. Frowein, RA. Classification of coma. Acta Neurochir 1976; *34*:5–10.
4. Jennett B, Teasdale G. Management of Head Injuries. Philadelphia: FA Davis Co, 1981.
5. Jennett B, Plum, F. Persistent vegetive state after brain damage. Lancet 1972; *1*:734–737.
6. Sarwar M, Azar-Kia B, Batnitzky S. Basic Neuroradiology. St Louis: Warren H Green Inc, 1983.
7. Nyhan WL. Urea Cycle Disorders. *In*: Rudolph AM, Hoffman JIE. eds. Pediatrics. 17th ed. Norwalk: Appleton-Century-Crofts, 1982: 270–275.
8. Jennett B, Teasdale G. Aspects of coma after severe head injury. Lancet 1977; *1*:878–881.
9. Teasdale G, Jennett B. Assessment of coma and impaired consciousness. Lancet 1974; *2*:81–84.
10. Teasdale G, Jennett B. Assessment and prognosis of coma after head injury. Acta Neurochir 1976; *34*:45–55.
11. Teasdale G, Knill-Jones R, Van der Sande J. Observer variability in assessing impaired consciousness and coma. J Neurol Neurosurg Psychiatry 1978; *41*:603–610.
12. Jamieson KG, Yelland JDN. Extradural hematoma. Report of 167 cases. J. Neurosurg 1968; *29*:13–23.
13. Gascon G, Barlow C. Juvenile migraine presenting as an acute confusional state. Pediatrics 1970; 45:628–639.
14. Rumack BH. Anticholinergic poisoning: treatment with physostigmine. Pediatrics 1973; *52*:449–451.
15. Helliwell M, Hampel G, Sinclair E, et al. Value of emergency toxicological investigations in differential diagnosis of coma. Br Med J 1979; *2*:819–821.
16. Peden VH, Sammon TJ, Downey DA. Intravenously induced infantile intoxication with ethanol. J Pediatr 1973; *83*:490–493.
17. Dove DJ, Jones T. Delayed coma associated with salicylate intoxication. J Pediatr 1982; *100*:493–496.
18. Cutler EA, Barrett GA, Craven PW, Cramblett HG.

Delayed cardiopulmonary arrest after Lomotil ingestion. Pediatrics 1980; *65*:157–158.
19. Chisholm JJ Jr. Lead Poisoning. *In*: Rudolph AM, Hoffman JIE. eds. Pediatrics. 17th ed. Norwalk: Appleton-Century-Crofts, 1982: 739–746.
20. Reye RDK, Morgan G, Baral J. Encephalopathy and fatty degeneration of the viscera: a disease entity in childhood. Lancet 1963; *2*:749–752.
21. Johnson G, Scurletis T, Carroll N. Sixteen cases of encephalitis like disease in North Carolina school children. NC Med J 1963; *24*:464–468.
22. Shaywitz BA, Rothstein P, Venes JL. Monitoring and management of increased intracranial pressure in Reye syndrome: results in 29 children. Pediatrics 1980; *66*:198–204.
23. Goff WR, Shaywitz BA, Goff GD, et al. Somatic evoked potential evaluation of cerebral status in Reye syndrome. Electroencephalogr Clin Neurophysiol 1983; *55*:388–398.
24. Nugent SK, Bausher JA, Moxon ER, and Rogers MC. Raised intracranial pressure: its management in *Neisseria meningitidis* meningoencephalitis. Am J Dis Child 1979; *133*:260–262.
25. Bell WE. Treatment of bacterial infections of the central nervous system. Ann Neurol 1981; *9*:313–327.
26. Hirsch MS, Schooley RT. Treatment of herpes virus infections. N Engl J Med 1983; *309*:963–970.
27. Swaiman KF, Menkes JH, DeVivo DC, Prensky AL. Metabolic Disorders of the Central Nervous System. *In*: Swaiman KE, Wright FS. eds. The Practice of Pediatric Neurology. St. Louis: CV Mosby Co 1982: 472–600.
28. Menkes JH. Textbook of Child Neurology. Philadelphia: Lea & Febiger, 1974: 1–82.
29. Celesia GG. Modern concepts of status epilepticus. JAMA 1976; *235*:1571–1574.
30. Hauser WA. Status Epilepticus: Frequency, etiology, and neurological sequelae. *In*: Delgado–Escueta AV, Wasterlain CG, Treiman DM, Porter RJ. eds. Advances in Neurology, vol. 34. New York: Raven Press, 1983: 3–14.
31. Chevrie J, Aicardi J. Convulsive disorders in the first year of life: neurological and mental outcome and mortality. Epilepsia 1978; *19*:67–74.
32. Aicardi J, Chevrie JJ. Convulsive status epilepticus in infants and children: a study of 239 cases. Epilepsia 1970; *11*:187–197.
33. Rowan AJ, Scott DF. Major status epilepticus: a series of 42 patients. Acta Neurol Scand 1970; *46*:573–584.
34. Aminoff MJ, Simon RP. Status epilepticus: causes, clinical features and consequences in 98 patients. Am J Med 1980; *69*:657–666.
35. Hayakawa T, Sato J, Hara H, et al. Therapy and prognosis of status convulsivus in childhood. Folia Psychiatr Neurol. Jpn 1979; *33*:445–456.
36. Delgado–Escueta AV, Bajorek JG. Status epilepticus: mechanisms of brain damage and rational management. Epilepsia 1982; *23*:(suppl):s29–41.
37. Treiman DM. General Principles of Treatment: Responsive and Intractable Status Epilepticus in Adults. *In*: Delgado–Escueta AV, Wasterlain CG, Treiman DM, Porter RJ. eds. Advances in Neurology, vol. 34. Status Epilepticus. New York: Raven Press, 1983: 377–384.
38. Tasinari CA, Daniele O, Michelucci R, et al. Benzodiazepines: Efficacy in Status Epilepticus. *In*: Delgado–Escueta AV, Wasterlain CG, Treiman DM, Porter RJ. eds. Advances in Neurology, vol. 34. Status Epilepticus. New York: Raven Press, 1983, 465–475.
39. Delgado–Escueta AV, Enrile–Bascal F. Combination Therapy for Status Epilepticus: Intravenous Diazepam and Phenytoin. *In*: Delgado–Escueta AV, Wasterlain CG, Treiman DM, Porter RJ. eds. Advances in Neurology, vol. 34. Status Epilepticus. New York: Raven Press, 1983, 477–485.
40. Browne TR. Paraldehyde, Chlormethiazole, and Lidocaine for Treatment of Status Epilepticus. *In* Delgado–Escueta AV, Wasterlain CG, Treiman DM, Porter RJ. eds. Advances in Neurology, vol. 34. Status Epilepticus. New York: Raven Press, 1983, 509–517.
41. Bruce DA, Schut L, Bruno LA, et al. Outcome following severe head injury in children. J Neurosurg 1978; 48:679–688.
42. Dean JM, McComb JG. Intracranial pressure monitoring in severe pediatric near drowning. Neurosurgery 1981; *9*:627–638.
43. Todd, HH, Chadwick JS, Shapiro HN, et al. The neurological effect of thiopental following experimental cardiac arrest in cats. Anesthesiology 1982; *57*:76–86.
44. Fandel I, Bancalari E. Near drowning in children: clinical aspects. Pediatrics 1976; *58*:573–579.
45. Pagni CA, Signoroni G, Crotti F, et al. Severe traumatic coma in infancy and childhood. J Neurol Sci 1975; *19*:120–128.
46. Minami T, Ogawa M, Katsurada K. Clinical prediction of prognosis of coma. Neurol Med Chir 1975; *1*:67–72.
47. Carlsson CA, von Essen C, Lofgren J. Factors affecting the clinical course of patients with severe head injuries. J Neurosurg. 1968; *29*:242–251.
48. Levy DE, Bates D, Caronna JJ, et al. Prognosis in nontraumatic coma. Ann Intern Med 1981; *94*:293–301.
49. Caronna JJ, Levy DE, Finkelstein S, et al. Prognostic factors in hypoxic-ischemic coma. Ann Neurol 1981; *10*:79.
50. Longstreth WT Jr, Diehr P, Invi TS. Prediction of awakening after out of hospital cardiac arrest. N Engl J Med 1983; *308*:1378–1382.
51. Bedell SE, Delbanco TL, Cook EF, Epstein FH. Survival after cardiopulmonary resuscitation in the hospital. N Engl J Med 1983; *309*:569–576.
52. Margolis LH, Shaywitz BA. The outcome of prolonged coma in childhood. Dev Med Child Neurol 1980; *65*:477–483.
53. Guidelines for the Determination of Death: Report of the Medical Consultants on the Diagnosis of Death to the President's Commission for the study of Ethical Problems in Medicine and Behavioral Research. Neurology 1982; *32*:395–399.
54. Ivan LP. Spinal reflexes in cerebral death. Neurology 1973; *23*:650–652.
55. Mandel S, Arenas A, Scasta D. Spinal automatism in cerebral death. N Engl J Med 1982; *307*:501.
56. Bird TD, Plum F. Recovery from barbiturate overdose coma with a prolonged isoelectric electroencephalogram. Neurology 1968; *18*:456–460.
57. Kirshbaum, RJ, Carullo VJ. Reversible isoelectric EEG in barbiturate coma. JAMA 1970; *212*:1215.
58. Ashwal S, Schneider S. Failure of electroencephalography to diagnose brain death in comatose children. Ann Neurol 1979; *6*:512–517.
59. Taylor MJ, Houston BD, Lowry NJ. Recovery of auditory brainstem responses after severe hypoxic ischemic insult. N Engl J Med 1983; *309*:1169–1170.

CHAPTER

9

Reye's Syndrome

G. Robert DeLong, M.D.

Reye's syndrome (RS), an acute illness of children that follows a viral infection, is characterized by non-icteric hepatic dysfunction and encephalopathy. It was first described by Reye and colleagues in 1963,[1] under the name encephalopathy and fatty degeneration of the viscera. They described the major clinical and metabolic features, and the distinctive pathologic changes of microvesicular fat deposition without inflammatory change or necrosis in the liver that are associated with non-inflammatory swelling of the brain. These investigators also noted the biochemical features of elevated serum glutamic-oxaloacetic transaminase, abnormal prothrombin time, and decreased blood glucose. Johnson and coworkers[2] described an outbreak of 16 similar fatal cases in North Carolina at the same time; their cases were clustered within four months and occurred in association with an outbreak of influenza B. Other descriptions in earlier medical literature were recognized in retrospect.[3, 4]

RS is almost exclusively a pediatric disease that is rarely found in adults.[5] In the United States, 655 cases were reported in 1977 and 1978, of which 32 per cent were fatal. The incidence has been estimated as 3.6 cases per 100,000 persons less than 18 years of age with influenza B.[6, 8, 9] At other times, rates of 0.2 to 0.3 cases per year per 100,000 population less than 18 years of age have been described. RS primarily affects white children under the age of 18 years, with a mean age of 7.7 years; and bimodal incidence peaks in infancy and at age 6 to 7 years. The mean age of those affected has differed in different outbreaks. Although RS occurs infrequently in non-white children more than one year of age, there is a high incidence in black infants.[10, 11] These differences have been related to different patterns of exposure to the precipitating viruses. The case-fatality ratio in infants of all races is significantly higher than that in older children. The disease has been found worldwide, particularly in underdeveloped countries of Asia, the Middle East, and Latin America, but little accurate epidemiologic data is available. It seems to be uncommon in Europe.

The most common antecedent viral illnesses are influenza B, influenza A, and varicella.[6] Epidemics of influenza B or A tend to be associated with epidemics of RS. Flu-associated cases occur mainly between December and March. Sporadic cases are associated with varicella and usually involve younger children.[6]

The clinical pattern of development of RS is stereotyped and permits the physician or family of the child to suspect the diagnosis. Children typically have a viral illness from which they seem to be recovering. One to six days after the initial illness, they develop malaise and prolonged or intractable vomiting lasting up to 24 hours. Lethargy, confusion, ataxia, hyperventilation, disorientation, and combativeness follow. Hepatomegaly is noted initially in about 40 per cent of cases. The neurologic findings are non-localizing. The patient may progress to coma, rigidity, decerebration, and death, but the severity varies greatly, and the progression may halt at any point. A standardized scheme for staging the severity of neurologic involvement is given in Table 9–1. As suggested by the disparity in clinical severity, the presumed underlying toxic-metabolic disturbance may vary from mild to severe, as reflected by the abnormalities in laboratory values. Serum transaminase and ammonia levels are elevated. Prothrombin time is extended. Many other biochemical abnormalities are found, especially if the disease is severe (see later discussion). They include increased serum osmolality, a mixed metabolic acidosis and respiratory alkalosis, hyperlactatemia, elevated free fatty acids, a specific abnormal profile of elevated amino acids, and elevated creatine phosphokinase. Hypoglyce-

Table 9–1. DEFINITION OF STAGING—NEUROLOGIC CRITERIA FOR STAGING REYE'S SYNDROME

Stage	Criteria
Pre-coma: Stage 0	The patient is alert and oriented to place and time. There is an immediate normal appropriate response to painful, tactile, verbal, and visual stimuli.
Pre-coma: Stage 1	The patient is vomiting, lethargic and/or indifferent; the patient may be belligerent and uncooperative but can obey commands and does not lapse into sleep when left undisturbed. The younger child may have breathing abnormalities or be postictal.
Pre-coma: Stage 2	The patient is disoriented, delirious, combative when aroused; the patient lapses into sleep when not disturbed, may be hyperreflexive, may hyperventilate, and have abnormal breathing patterns (infants). The patient may be postictal, responds appropriately to noxious stimuli and has no abnormal posturing.
Coma: Stage 3	The patient is comatose and does not verbalize or respond to command; there is no appropriate motor response to pain, i.e., pinprick; instead, there may be a generalized nonspecific response including decorticate and/or decerebrate posturing or both. The patient has central hyperventilation, decorticate posturing and/or rigidity; there is preservation of pupillary light reflexes, although the pupils may be dilated. There is preservation of the oculovestibular reflex (response to iced-water calorics) and the oculocephalic (doll's-eye) reflexes. The infant and younger child may have Cheyne-Stokes or Biot's breathing pattern.
Coma: Stage 4	The patient has deteriorated. There is decerebrate posturing and rigidity, or loss of oculocephalic reflexes; the oculovestibular reflex is lost or dysconjugate; there are large "fixed pupils" with hippus on occasion; there may be other evidence of brainstem dysfunction, e.g., loss of corneal reflexes.
Coma: Stage 5	The patient is flaccid and has respiratory irregularities or agonal respirations, and fixed dilated pupils; there may be cardiovascular instability or signs of herniation, i.e., relatively small pupil on one side, a large unreactive pupil on the other side. Respiratory arrest ensues.

Adapted from Partin JC: Hepatic encephalopathy and Reye's syndrome. Pediatric Annals, *6*:346–354, 1977.

mia is seen only in young children (less than 5 years). Bilirubin is not elevated, and cerebrospinal fluid is normal.

Diagnostic definition depends on a typical clinical history. Criteria for diagnosis put forward by the Centers for Disease Control (CDC) include an acute non-inflammatory encephalopathy with microvesicular fatty metamorphosis of the liver confirmed by biopsy or at autopsy, or SGOT, SGPT, or serum ammonia greater than three times normal; if cerebrospinal fluid (CSF) is obtained, it should have less than eight leukocytes/mm^3, and in addition, there should be no other, more reasonable explanation for the neurologic or hepatic abnormalities.[12] For clinical purposes, reasonable diagnostic criteria include a typical history, elevated SGOT, prothrombin time, and serum ammonia level (preferably arterial), with normal CSF if examined, and normal bilirubin level and toxic screen results (except for salicylate). The diagnosis may be confirmed by liver biopsy showing typical fatty metamorphosis, although this is rarely necessary, and by amino acid analysis, showing the typical profile.[13] Hyperammonemia, lactic acidosis, and elevated serum osmolality tend to correlate with the severity of the clinical picture. Reye's-like syndromes clinically mimicking RS are discussed in detail later.

The metabolic storm runs its course in a matter of a few days. The child who survives usually recovers completely, but in up to 30 per cent of survivors who reached either stage 4 or 5 coma a residual neurologic deficit was reported.[7, 166] Survival rates have improved over the past decade, probably because of several factors. Milder cases are recognized and diagnosed. Supportive care, particularly management of increased intracranial pressure (ICP), has improved, which is probably chiefly responsible for the substantive improvement in survival. Programs to encourage earlier diagnosis, and thus earlier treatment, may have played a role in improved outcome. Mortality rates, previously in the range of 60 per cent in children with the most severe manifestations of the illness, are currently about 20–25 per cent; with optimal treatment they may be lower. In 1981 the reported death-to-case ratio was 28 per cent.[12] In order to be useful in evaluating treatment programs and comparing experience in different centers, mortality must be correlated with indices of severity. The most useful indices have been the clinical stage at admission,[7, 8] the peak blood ammonia level,[14] the total hyperammonemic burden (a function of hyperammonemia times duration),[15] and possibly the degree of lactic acidosis.[16, 17] Children who do not progress to stage 3 and beyond, or who have less than five-fold elevation of blood ammonia, usually recover fully.[14] The mortality rate of children with stage 4 disease on admission was 69 per cent, and with stage 5, 83 per cent.[7] With the recent advent of more vigorous measures to combat cerebral edema, more children with severe disease may be surviving with permanent neurologic and intellectual deficits. Crocker and Bagnell[29] have recently published a useful clinical review on Reye's syndrome.

As Reye's syndrome has become more widely recognized, it has become a bench mark for toxic-metabolic encephalopathies, and an increasing number of "Reye's-like" illnesses have been noted. These illnesses' clinical and metabolic features resemble those of Reye's syndrome, and they must be identified and differentiated from true RS. They will be discussed in more detail later.

RS, because of its dramatic clinical presentation, its devastating effects, and its unclear pathophysiology, has generated great interest for researchers, parents of victims, and the general public. This interest has resulted in the formation of national societies for the support and encouragement of studies of the disease.

PATHOPHYSIOLOGY

The pathophysiology of RS is complex. It is not clear how all the pieces of the puzzle fit together. The pathogenesis of RS has been reviewed in the medical literature.[18–21] The major pathophysiologic elements that have been identified are the following:

1. A preceding viral illness is reported, but the pathologic changes seen in organs of patients with RS do not suggest direct infection, and virus can be isolated from tissues only infrequently.

2. An acute and reversible insult affects the mitochondria particularly in the liver, and also in other organs, producing marked swelling and dissolution of cristae and a marked transient impairment of the activity of most liver mitochondrial enzymes. This results in impairment of urea cycle function[30, 31] and other hepatic metabolic functions.[33, 34]

3. A severe systemic metabolic disorder occurs, which is characterized by profound protein catabolism[15] and hyperammonemia, lipolysis and hyperfattyacidemia,[22–26] lactic acidosis,[17] and at times hypoglycemia.[1]

4. A toxic-metabolic encephalopathy produces coma and severe cerebral edema and increased ICP, without evidence of inflammation.

The causal relationships among these elements are complex and not unanimously agreed upon by all observers, but the following may be the most widely held hypothesis, and the one most in accord with the available data. It is given as a framework for the detailed discussion that follows.

The triggering virus may have a direct toxic effect on liver mitochondria, and to a lesser degree on those of other organs. Whether this effect may be mediated by a specific toxic protein is not known. The viral insult has two major effects: the first is on hepatic mitochondria, impairing enzyme activities and thus blocking major metabolic pathways of liver; and the second causes a severe catabolic disorder in muscle and lipid particularly, resulting in a massive increase in nitrogenous products and fatty acids presented to the liver for disposal. The combination of this increased mass of substrate and the impairment of liver metabolic capacity due to the mitochondriopathy, results in a tide of hyperammonemia and hyperfattyacidemia, lactic acidosis and at times hypoglycemia. The metabolic load presented to the liver may itself impair mitochondrial function: for example, organic acids such as propionate can impair ureagenesis.[35] In turn, hyperammonemia, perhaps in conjunction with the synergistic effect of elevated fatty acids, appears to be the primary cause of encephalopathy and brain swelling through its potent toxic effect on the brain's oxidative metabolism. The severity and mortality of the disease correlate strongly with the peak levels, and perhaps more importantly with the total burden, of hyperammonemia.

The Primary Insult

Many viruses have been associated with RS. The most common are influenza B and A, both of which occur in epidemics leading to epidemics of RS, and varicella, which is associated with sporadic outbreaks of RS. Other associated viruses that have been identified include the following: adenovirus type 3; Coxsackie A9, B1, and B4; Ebstein-Barr; ECHO 8 and

11; poliovirus type 1; parainfluenza; reovirus; rubella; herpes simplex; measles; and dengue.[6] How the viral illness produces RS is not known. Most investigators have not found viremia in RS patients.[55, 56, 81] Virus has been recovered only occasionally from liver, brain, or other organs.[57, 58, 59] Ultrastructural study of lymphocytes from a single RS patient showed marked nuclear changes, and also changes in mitochondria, which were interpreted as possibly the effects of virus infection.[60] It has been suggested that a virus protein may be toxic to mitochondria, but there is no direct evidence for it.[62] Davis et al.,[61] who recalled the work of Henle and Henle,[172, 173] presented evidence that influenza virus, inoculated intravenously in high doses, causes an illness in mice similar to RS. The mice develop coma and die in one to three days. Pathologic findings consist of fatty metamorphosis of the liver and no inflammatory change in the brain. Viral propagation does not occur in the liver or the brain. This model has many of the features of RS and raises interesting questions regarding a possible toxic—as opposed to infectious—role of influenza virus. The observation that only certain outbreaks of influenza A or influenza B are associated with epidemics of RS might suggest that a specific viral protein, present in only some strains of influenza, is pathogenic. Granular deposits of immunoglobulins G and M have been found in intramuscular vessels in RS, presumably representing antigen-antibody complexes; this suggests a possible mechanism of viral pathogenesis.[63] Circulating immune complexes were sought in the sera from 31 patients with the acute disease and found in six, and depression of complement components was found in 18. It was concluded that circulating immune complexes were not the cause of hypocomplementemia, and the study gives no strong support to a primary pathogenic role for antigen-antibody complexes in the disease.[64] An interaction between a virus and a second chemical toxin has also been proposed. Toxins proposed to have a possible adjunctive role include aflatoxins, pesticides, and aspirin.[6] The available data do not support convincingly a relationship between aflatoxin levels and RS, and aflatoxin levels were not different from controls in children with RS in the United States.[65] There is abundant evidence from animal and *in vitro* studies that viruses, insecticides, and insecticide carriers can be synergistic.[66, 67] Another possible interaction is suggested by the observation of a Reye's-like syndrome associated with the use of an insect repellent in a presumed heterozygote for ornithine carbamyl transferase deficiency.[69] Recent animal studies that attempted to model RS utilizing encephalomyocarditis virus and the toxins Atlox and hydroxylated hydroxytoluene produced some similar features, but not others.[68] Some chemical agents are capable of producing an illness similar to RS without the accompanying viral infection; these include tetracycline,[71] valproic acid,[72, 73] and margosa oil from Indonesia.[74] The common ground among these various agents seems to be that they interfere with metabolic functions performed by mitochondria. The data suggest that insults from viruses, toxins (whether exogenous or endogenous), or hereditary susceptibilities may be cumulative or synergistic in hepatic mitochondria. Different agents interfere with different functions; for example, aspirin and tetracycline interfere with oxidative phosphorylation.[71, 85] Valproic acid is reported to inhibit the mitochondrial contribution to ureagenesis by decreasing levels of *N*-acetyl glutamate, a necessary cofactor of carbamyl phosphate synthetase.[75] This drug is also reported to inhibit oxidative phosphorylation in rat liver mitochondria.[76]

It is not known why only a few children develop RS of the many who contract influenza or varicella. It was suggested earlier that affected children may have metabolic abnormalities rendering them susceptible to this syndrome when they are subjected to the stress of a viral illness.[77] However, children with RS routinely have had other viral illnesses without incident; they rarely have recurrence of RS, and affected mitochondrial enzymes (e.g., ornithine transcarbamylase) in kinetic study specimens[30] and in biopsy specimens taken after recovery[31] have shown no evidence of abnormality. The occasional patients who have recurrent RS are better considered to have partial genetic deficiencies, which become apparent during periods of metabolic stress, and are discussed later with the Reye's-like syndromes. Occasionally, two children in one family have RS, usually during the same epidemic; these children ordinarily cannot be shown to have genetic abnormalities and do not have recurrences. Thus the occurrence of RS in more than one child in a household is unexplained.[78]

The effects of toxic agents and genetic enzyme deficiencies illustrate the consequences of interfering with one or another metabolic function of liver mitochondria. In RS, however, there is a more global insult to hepatic mitochondria (and probably those of other organs), resulting in dysfunction of many, if not all, of the metabolic functions carried out by mitochondria. The activity of many mitochondrial enzymes is transiently decreased in liver from RS patients (see previous discussion). This decrease in activity implies that the effect of the causative virus somehow damages the entire mitochondrion as a unit, rather than specific metabolic enzymes. The mitochondriopathy is predominant in liver, is present in other visceral organs, and spares some organs and tissues. Mitochondria of many cells are normal morphologically, and mitochondrial enzyme activities have been found to be normal in brain and muscle, for example, in RS patients (see later discussion). This observation indicates a more or less specific attack on liver mitochondria in RS. The resulting disorders of hepatic metabolism must account in large part for the many biochemical abnormalities found in RS (discussed in more detail later).

Recent work has helped to clarify the relationship between varicella and RS. It has been suggested that hepatic dysfunction occurs in 77 per cent of children with varicella infection who have no other evidence of RS, and this condition has been called varicella hepatitis.[80–82] Recently, however, liver biopsies were performed on 14 children with varicella and repetitive vomiting alone, or vomiting and encephalopathy along with elevated transaminase.[80] All specimens demonstrated microvesicular fat deposition and mitochondrial swelling in hepatocytes, typical of RS, without evidence of inflammation. Only those children with elevated blood ammonia progressed beyond stage 1. The initial clinical course and histologic findings in the livers of the patients with a benign course were indistinguishable from those of patients who developed typical RS. Other workers have reported similar observations[81]; this extremely enlightening study suggests several points: (1) varicella virus commonly induces the liver lesion of RS, although it is usually mild; (2) only when the hepatic metabolic disorder is severe enough to cause hyperammonemia does progressive encephalopathy occur; (3) repetitive vomiting was found with microvesicular fat deposition in liver, but without hyperammonemia; thus the latter may not be the cause of vomiting in RS; and (4) the observation that the hepatic histological lesion commonly occurs without encephalopathy and that encephalopathy was observed only with hyperammonemia greatly strengthens the concept that the encephalopathy in RS is of hepatic metabolic origin, as opposed to a primary attack on brain mitochondria by a viral agent.

Similar observations have been made in the course of an influenza type A outbreak in Michigan in 1978–1979, in which SGPT values were elevated in 1.5 per cent of 860 school children tested.[48] Elevated SGPT was not associated with illness but was associated with recent influenza infection. The investigators estimated that at least 2.7 per cent of individuals infected by the particular strain of influenza A had associated elevated SGPT. This finding suggests that, as with varicella, subclinical effects on liver may be a relatively common feature of other viruses and may be related to the pathogenetic mechanism of RS. These observations afford a potentially important approach to clarifying the viral-mitochondrial interaction in RS.

Salicylate

Recently, it has been suggested that aspirin may play an important synergistic role in RS. Mortimer and Lepow[84] in 1962, prior to Reye's description, reported four patients with varicella who died. All had hypoglycemia and cerebral swelling, undoubtedly what would now be called RS. Three of the four had received excessive amounts of salicylate, which was considered to be the possible cause of the fatal illnesses. Aspirin uncouples oxidative phosphorylation[85] (thus it is a mitochondrial toxin), and salicylate intoxication is similar to RS in important aspects: vomiting, hyperventilation, metabolic acidosis with compensating respiratory alkalosis, and lethargy progressing to coma are prominent in both.[86] However, there are also important clinical and chemical differences: the mortality of patients with properly treated salicylism is quite low,[87] plasma amino acid profiles are different,[38] hyperammonemia is not a feature of salicylism,[19, 86] and the pathologic effects of salicylism in the liver are different from that of RS in experimental animals.[88] Thus, RS is not simply salicylism. However, the possibility remains that salicylates play some adjunctive role, along with the associated virus, in causing RS. Many investigators have found a high incidence of detectable salicylate levels at admission in patients with RS.[89] A high proportion of RS patients have received salicylates during their pre-RS illness.[91] This proportion was reported as 97 per cent in an Ohio group of 97 patients compared with 71 per cent in case controls; however, no relationship was found between dosage and stage of encephalopathy.[92] In one study, the mean serum salicylate level of 130 children with biopsy-confirmed RS was 12.3 mg/100 ml, and did not vary with neurological grade; however, the mean serum salicylate level at admission was significantly higher in those who died (15 mg/100 ml) than in survivors (10 mg/100 ml).[89]

Tonsgard and Huttenlocher[90] reviewed the use of salicylates in 43 consecutive patients with RS. No salicylates were found in the blood or urine in 15 of 43, and no significant difference was found between the salicylate levels in children with mild disease and those who died.

Fitzgerald found that 30 per cent of their 76 patients with RS had not received any salicylates during acute illness. Measured salicylate levels were less than 5 mg/100 ml in 26 of 51 patients.[93] In a study from Toronto, 13 of 18 patients with unequivocal cases of RS had undetectable salicylate levels.[94]

Andressen and colleagues[95] raise the important issue that the standard hospital laboratory assay method for salicylates does not necessarily reflect true blood concentrations of salicylate as obtained by a specific high pressure liquid chromatography (HPLC) technique; they suggest that interfering substances, elevated in the blood of RS patients, may cause artifactual elevations of salicylate values as measured by the standard method. Using HPLC, they found minimal or undetectable salicylate levels in CSF from seven RS patients when the standard assay showed elevated levels. HPLC assays likewise showed no correlation between salicylate levels and the grade of coma.

In summary, despite certain pathophysiological parallels, salicylism is different from RS, and RS occurs in the absence of salicylates. The evidence that salicylates may precipitate or exacerbate RS is inconclusive, indeed doubtful. No consistent correlation has been shown between dosage or serum levels of salicylates and stage or mortality of RS. In ferrets, salicylate intoxication showed no significant potentiating effect on the lesions or mortality induced by influenza infection.[88] The possibility remains that salicylate use may be an adjunctive risk factor statistically associated with occurrence of RS. The significance of this possibility for the current widespread use of aspirin in childhood illnesses is a topic of intense current discussion.[95–98] A careful methodologic review of the studies of salicylate use and RS has been done by Daniels and coworkers.[99]

The Lesion in the Liver

Reye recognized that the liver was involved in RS because he found a non-inflammatory, non-necrotic lesion characterized by a massive deposition of microdroplets of fat in hepatocytes. The weight of the liver was increased up to 20 per cent by this fat content, which imparted to the cut surface of the liver a bright yellow color. The original biochemical observations correlating with liver disease were the high SGOT and hypoglycemia; the latter occurred only in young children, and inconstantly. Bilirubin level was notably normal.[1]

Later, it was recognized that hyperammonemia was a consistent biochemical feature of RS.[36] Hyperammonemia tended to peak early, then decline over the next day or two regardless of the clinical course, so its importance in causing encephalopathy was uncertain. The pathogenesis of hyperammonemia in RS was clarified greatly by the finding of an abnormal profile of serum amino acids virtually identical to that seen in the heritable diseases of the urea cycle, carbamyl phosphate synthetase (CPS) and ornithine transcarbamylase (OTC) deficiencies.[37, 38] Subsequently, both CPS and OTC activities were found to be transiently and reversibly reduced in liver biopsies from RS patients.[30–32]

Electron microscopy of liver biopsy tissue in RS revealed, besides the accumulation of microvesicular fat droplets and depletion of glycogen, characteristic changes in the ultrastructural morphology of mitochondria in hepatocytes.[39] Mitochondria were uniformly swollen, with dissolution of cristae and loss of internal architecture. These changes were well-established in tissues from biopsies performed very early in the course of the illness, and returned to normal after several days, regardless of the fate of the patient. This finding focused attention on RS as a disease of mitochondria; CPS and OTC, mentioned previously, are located in mitochondria, whereas the other enzymes of urea cycle metabolism, levels of which are normal in RS, are cytoplasmic.[30]

Subsequently, activities of other enzymes of liver mitochondria have been found to be decreased in biopsy or autopsy material from

RS patients. These enzymes include succinate dehydrogenase, cytochrome oxidase,[40] pyruvate dehydrogenase and pyruvate carboxylase,[41] glutamic dehydrogenase, citrate synthase,[42] hydroxymethylglutaryl CoA lyase, and monamine oxidase.[11] All liver cytoplasmic enzyme levels measured have been normal including those of the urea cycle[30–32] and of gluconeogenesis.[41] Moreover, the serum level of the mitochondrial isozyme of SGOT is greatly increased in RS, leading to reversal of the normal ratio of cytoplasmic to mitochondrial SGOT ratio (normally 5:1 to 20:1). This reversal is seemingly specific to RS; it does not occur with hepatitis.[43]

The widespread alterations in mitochondrial enzyme activities in hepatocytes can presumably account for the impairment of major hepatic metabolic functions: (1) decreased CPS and OTC impair urea cycle function, and thus block detoxification of ammonia, (2) decreased pyruvate dehydrogenase and pyruvate carboxylase impair metabolism of pyruvate and gluconeogenesis, and (3) decreased glutamic dehydrogenase, succinate dehydrogenase, citrate synthase, and cytochrome oxidase impair oxidative metabolism. In this regard, liver ATP levels in biopsy samples from RS patients have been interpreted as normal[44] or low.[20] Decreased hydroxymethylglutaryl CoA lyase may impair ketogenesis, accounting for the low level of ketosis in RS,[45] and may also contribute to impaired fatty acid metabolism. In addition, hepatic protein synthesis may be impaired, including synthesis of the protein moiety of lipoprotein, thus resulting in a block of lipoprotein synthesis and release. Decreased monamine oxidase activity accounts for elevated levels of monamines such as tyramine and octopamine, which may affect central nervous system amine metabolism.[46, 47] In short, all major intermediary metabolic functions of liver—except bilirubin metabolism—are blocked by the mitochondrial lesion of RS.

The Lesion in Other Organs

A central question in the pathogenesis of RS has been whether the hepatic lesion is primary with secondary involvement of other organs, or whether the disease represents a generalized mitochondrial insult. Microvesicular fat deposition and mitochondrial swelling are found in other organs, especially the kidney, heart, and skeletal muscle,[48] but occur later and to a lesser degree than those in liver. Serial muscle biopsy specimens, in our experience, have shown normal features in light microscopic studies early in the disease (at a time when the hepatic lesion was well marked) and increased fat deposition at later stages.[48] Mitochondrial changes in skeletal muscle and brain are less extensive and less severe than those in liver.[49, 50] In brain, mitochondrial abnormalities have been limited to neurons[49]; these changes have involved only a portion of neuronal mitochondria and are different in appearance and milder in degree than those in hepatocytes. These brain changes are difficult to interpret because the available biopsy specimens have been from patients who have also suffered hypoxic-ischemic insults, which could account for the mitochondrial changes seen. In skeletal muscle,[50] changes are also milder and found only in about one-third of the mitochondria. As noted, the mitochondria in other locations have been morphologically normal, including astrocytes and capillary endothelial cells of brain. These findings, taken together, are best interpreted by assuming that the insult to liver mitochondria is predominant and that changes in other organs are milder than or secondary to hepatic disease.[42] This finding will be discussed in more detail later with reference to the brain, where the problem is most crucial. Whether the involvement of other organs, especially heart and kidney, causes functional impairment is unclear. Generally, such impairment does not occur; however, failure of both renal and cardiac function may occur late in severe cases of RS. It is not known to what extent this failure represents the effects of the basic disease process or secondary factors.

The Catabolic State

Excessive catabolism is characteristic of RS; there is evidence of massive net negative nitrogen balance,[15] indicating protein catabolism, and of prominent lipolysis.[24, 26, 27] These aspects have received relatively little attention, and several questions may be raised regarding them: Can the protein catabolism and lipolysis be explained simply as the result of a nonspecific illness and inanition, or do they reflect a more specific effect of the triggering virus, for instance an effect on muscle mitochondria resulting in muscle catabolism? Does this peripheral catabolism, flooding the liver with substrates, somehow induce the hepatic mitochondrial dysfunction, or indeed can it be a direct cause of the encephalopathy?

A tentative statement of current concepts might be as follows: Protein catabolism is probably greater than can be accounted for by nonspecific factors,[15] and may reflect an effect of the causative agent, presumably virus, on muscle and other peripheral tissues. The resulting flood of nitrogenous metabolites surely contributes to the hyperammonemia that is characteristic of the disease. Lipolysis may or may not represent a specific effect of the causative agent; it is comparable in magnitude to that found in fasting and can be reversed by supplying glucose.[26] Suggestions that elevations of fatty acids resulting from lipolysis may be the primary cause of the hepatic mitochondriopathy or the encephalopathy have little support, except for convincing experimental data showing that fatty acids are synergistic with hyperammonemia in producing encephalopathy and coma.[51, 52] It must be emphasized that the biochemical changes found in blood are the result not only of the hepatic enzyme changes but also of increased peripheral catabolism, i.e. of changes in the delivery of substrates to the liver. The relative contribution of the two factors can be assessed using turnover studies; these have been done for nitrogen metabolism, indicating both increased catabolism (increased delivery of substrate to liver) and impairment of hepatic detoxification of ammonia. DeLong and Glick[15] found net nitrogen excretion of 0.55 gm/kg/24 hours in 13 patients during the first hospital day; this value represents a greater protein catabolism than in most other acute catabolic illnesses, emphasizing the severity of the metabolic insult in RS. Urinary nitrogen excretion reached its highest levels about four to six hours after hyperammonemia peaked. The efficiency of urea cycle function may be estimated by the urinary ratios of urea to total nitrogen and ammonia to urea nitrogen. In a group of Reye's syndrome patients, urine urea to total nitrogen was 51 per cent (*versus* expected 90 per cent in normal individuals with a large protein load) and ammonia to urea nitrogen was 55 per cent (*versus* 2–5 per cent in normal individuals).[15] These data document both a severe catabolic state resulting in greatly increased delivery of nitrogenous products to liver, and a quantitative impairment of urea cycle function. Further evidence suggests that the total hyperammonemic burden, i.e., the integral of hyperammonemia over time, may be the most significant parameter of nitrogen metabolism in RS; this issue is discussed later.

Comparable studies have not been done with other substrates. Limited studies of lactic acid in Reye's patients found very high levels of lactate in jugular venous drainage, lower levels in femoral vein blood, and much lower levels in central venous blood.[53] These findings, showing that lactate is being produced by brain (as a consequence of impaired oxidative metabolism) and by muscle, and is being removed by liver, imply that hyperlactatemia in RS may be caused primarily by increased peripheral production, especially from brain, and not by impaired hepatic handling of lactate. More data of this kind would be of interest.

With regard to lipids, Chaves-Carballo and colleagues[54] recently reported that plasma levels of very low density lipoproteins (VLDL), the major form in which triglycerides are released by liver, were normal in RS patients. This finding indicates that release of triglycerides by the liver is probably normal, thus implicating excessive synthesis of fats by the liver as a major factor in the fatty liver production in this disease.[54] The elevated fatty acid levels in blood show significantly increased mobilization of lipids from adipose stores, as noted previously.

The Pathophysiology of the Encephalopathy

The encephalopathy of RS is the usual direct cause of death. There is general agreement that the cerebral lesion is non-inflammatory, that it is toxic or metabolic, and that the cerebral edema is cytotoxic. The several hypotheses put forward to explain the encephalopathy are examined in a recent review by DeLong and Glick.[18] They reduced the number of hypotheses to two: (1) a direct effect of the unknown viral-related toxin on mitochondria of brain, analogous to that on liver, or (2) a toxic or metabolic encephalopathy resulting from the hepatic lesion and the systemic metabolic disorder. The second appears to be favored in currently available data. Candidate toxic metabolites have included ammonia, fatty and organic acids, lactic acid, and monamines.

The evidence for a central role of hyperammonemia is strongest. In major series of RS patients, the mortality and severity of RS have correlated with peak levels of ammonia.[7, 14, 36, 100, 101] This correlation has been stronger than with any other putative toxic agent.[7] The inherited hyperammonemic disorders may have clinical courses indistinguishable from RS,[102, 103] as is true also of acute hepatic encephalopathy, in which hyperammonemia is considered to be a major toxic agent. Hyperammonemia has been shown to cause hyperventilation,[104] coma,[102] cerebral lactic acidosis,[104, 105] brain swelling,[106] and neuropathological changes,[107] both in experimental animal studies and in humans, similar to those found in RS.[18] A recent report documents severe intracranial hypertension similar to that seen in RS in a 4-month-old infant with hyperammonemia caused by argininosuccinic lyase deficiency.[103]

The effect of ammonia on the brain is complex. During hyperammonemia, nearly one-half of arterial ammonia is extracted during a single pass through the brain[108] and is rapidly converted to glutamine[109] in astrocytes, where glutamine synthetase is found. In this sense, astrocytes represent a "blood-brain barrier" for hyperammonemia, detoxifying ammonia and protecting neurons. Levels of glutamine in CSF and jugular effluent rise, representing the fate of detoxified ammonia. Arterial hyperammonemia can be detoxified safely in the brain as long as the levels do not exceed approximately 300 μg/100 ml. If this detoxification mechanism is overwhelmed, ammonia is capable of damaging neurons by impairing oxidative metabolism.

The mechanisms of the neurotoxicity of ammonia have been partially clarified.[19] Excess ammonia uptake by brain produces several changes, including increased glycolysis, which compensates for the utilization of α-ketoglutarate in forming glutamate and glutamine, increased cytoplasmic ratio of NADH to NAD^+, decreased phosphocreatine, and increased lactate production. ATP levels fall in severely intoxicated animals. Glutamate content and its release from neurons are decreased. This decrease may affect neutrotransmission. Excess ammonia and glutamine produce pathologic changes in astrocytes, primarily swelling and changes in nuclei.

In experimental animals, arterial hyperammonemia is associated with a linear increase in CSF and jugular venous lactate.[104] This finding may explain why hyperammonemic injury to brain tissue is essentially similar to that of hypoxia, i.e., both interfere with the brain's oxidative metabolism, which is necessary to cellular integrity.

There is recent evidence indicating that in RS the total burden of hyperammonemia presented to the brain correlates much more sensitively with severity and mortality than does peak ammonia level.[18] This observation is best explained by the concepts of ammonia uptake and detoxification previously outlined.

The role of other endogenous metabolic toxins in RS has been investigated. Organic acids (such as propionic and methylmalonic) are only modestly elevated (2–3-fold *versus* 1000-fold in genetic disorders of organic acid metabolism).[23] Fatty acid levels are elevated, and have been shown to affect cerebral function, but there is no evidence from either patients or experimental studies to indicate that these agents can cause the overwhelming encephalopathy and cytotoxic cerebral swelling that characterize RS.[110, 111] There are good data, however, indicating that excess fatty acids and hyperammonemia may have a synergistic effect, i.e., the effects of hyperammonemia are exacerbated by high levels of fatty acids.[51, 52] This synergism may well be important in RS. Blood lactate has been found to be elevated in RS, generally correlating with the severity of disease.[16, 17] Lactic acidosis in other circumstances may produce a severe metabolic encephalopathy resembling RS; it depends, however, on severe uncompensated acidosis,[112] which is not generally present in RS. Hyperlactatemia with a normal blood pH is not harmful: thus lactic acidosis cannot be the agent of encephalopathy in RS.

In summary, the weight of present data strongly indicates that the encephalopathy of RS is a type of hepatic encephalopathy, with hyperammonemia as the chief toxic agent producing, either alone or synergistically with fatty acids, the metabolic and pathologic changes found in the brain in this illness.

The neuropathologic examinations of RS patients show massive cerebral edema with brain weights up to 25 per cent greater than normal and with transtentorial and transforaminal herniation.[113] Diffuse or multifocal neuronal ischemia and laminar cortical necrosis are seen by light microscopy. Electron microscopic examination of brain biopsy tissue during the acute illness showed watery swelling of astrocytic somata and processes, injury of neuronal somata, and myelin bleb formation. The swollen astrocytes had normal mitochondria. Oligodendrocytes were normal. The neuronal somata showed changes consistent with ischemic injury, consisting of electron-dense cytoplasm, dilatation of endoplasmic reticulum, and swollen and rounded mitochondria. The appearance of these neuronal mitochondria was different from those in hepatocytes in RS[39]; in the former the changes are milder and involve only a portion of mitochondria. Mitochondria of the capillary endothelial cells were normal. The swelling in astrocytes with normal mitochondria is consistent with the effects of hyperammonemia.[107, 114] The neuronal abnormalities and myelin blebs are consistent with ischemic cell change and have been described as distinctive of cytotoxic edema.[111] Cerebral biopsy specimens, obtained 43 to 75 days after the acute illness, showed numerous reactive protoplasmic astrocytes typical of Alzheimer's type 2 astrocytes,[115] the neuropathologic hallmark of late hepatic and hyperammonemic encephalopathy.[114]

These neuropathological data are probably best interpreted not as evidence of a generalized mitochondrial lesion—for that is not found—but as the consequence of hyperammonemic encephalopathy with superimposed hypoxic-ischemic neuronal injury.

Pathophysiology of Osmolality, Blood Flow, and Renal Output

Many pathophysiologic events occur during the course of RS that must be recognized and dealt with by the clinician. Dehydration is usual; it tends to correlate with the severity of the illness. In one severely ill child with RS in whom an accurate weight had been recorded one week prior to her admission, a 7 per cent dehydration was estimated. The dehydration may be explained by vomiting and inanition; it is noteworthy that skin turgor does not reflect the dehydration and that urine output is maintained until a late stage of the illness. There may be a degree of osmotic diuresis, even without the use of mannitol, but good data are not available. Osmolality on admission is usually high, correlating well with the severity of illness; very severely ill children may have an osmolality of 320 or 330 mOsm/L (normal 285–295 mOsm/L) when admitted. Presumably this value reflects both dehydration and elevated levels of blood metabolites.

Anecdotal observations indicate that the cardiovascular system is hyperdynamic with markedly increased cardiac output, but systematic data are not available. In the late stages of the acute illness, cardiac failure, possibly related to direct myocardial injury, may result in pulmonary edema or a low-output state or both. This is a rare occurrence.

Renal output, initially well-maintained, commonly falls to oliguric levels in the late stages of the illness (typically two or three days after admission). The causes of oliguria include dehydration and hypovolemia resulting from repeated use of hyperosmolar agents, decreased cardiac output, and, possibly, direct renal involvement by the underlying toxic disease process.

Gastrointestinal involvement, not including the liver, includes gastric bleeding in later stages in perhaps one-fourth of severe cases and acute pancreatitis in a small number. Some observations have related the latter to severe increased intracranial pressure and the therapy instituted to combat it.[114] A coagulopathy, caused by failure of synthesis of hepatic coagulation factors, may be found. In severe cases, disseminated intravascular coagulation (DIC) may occur.

DIAGNOSIS AND STAGING

RS is quite stereotyped in its clinical progression and findings, varying only in severity and in the preceding viral illness. Diagnosis depends on the clinical history, physical examination, and biochemical evaluation. The clinical history is that of a common viral illness, usually influenza (in the setting of an epidemic of influenza A or B) or varicella (if sporadic); however, other viral illnesses may occasionally trigger the illness. The child seems nearly to recover from the initial illness, then after one to six days begins vomiting, which may continue up to 24 hours. This is followed by lethargy, ataxia, and confusion, progressing to hyperventilation, stuporous combativeness, and coma. The coma is metabolic with decortication or decerebration with initial preservation of doll's-eye movements. Doll's-eye movements are slow eye movements elicited by passively turning the patient's head; their absence in coma indicates loss of brainstem function. Absence of eye movements following iced-water caloric irrigation of the external ear canals has the same significance. In progressive coma, there is first hyper-reflexia, then increasing tone in the lower extremities in extension. In stage 3, withdrawal responses to stimulation, e.g., pinching, are replaced by decorticate then decerebrate responses, and in stage 4, rigidity and decerebration are maintained. With deepening coma, doll's-eye movements and pupillary responses are gradually lost, and respiratory arrest may supervene abruptly. This sequence of events may require from eight hours to three or four days, and it may stop progressing at any point. Seizures are usually not observed, except at the stage of deep coma. Seizures at an early stage of the illness may be seen in young children and in patients with hypoglycemia.[131] In the Far East, e.g., Singapore and Thailand, a seizure usually initiates the onset of coma.

The recognition of this sequence of events, and the corresponding clinical picture, leads one to suspect the diagnosis of RS. Any significant deviation from this clinical sequence should bring the diagnosis into question. The diagnosis is confirmed by the finding of typical biochemical abnormalities. Those readily available that are critical to the diagnosis include elevated SGOT and elevated blood ammonia (arterial ammonia level is more sensitive). Prothrombin time is nearly always moderately lengthened. The disease is differentiated from hepatitis by the absence of jaundice or hyperbilirubinemia and by the more fulminant course. Other corroborating biochemical parameters include a mixed metabolic acidosis and respiratory alkalosis with low bicarbonate, elevated osmolality, absence of marked ketosis, normal blood glucose or, in children less than 5 years, hypoglycemia,[10, 129] and absence of exogenous metabolic toxins on toxic screening. The specific blood amino acid profile is characteristic and strongly supports the diagnosis, though a similar pattern is found in CPS or OCT deficiency. Spinal fluid is normal, without pleocytosis. Other chemical abnormalities are found,[34] as noted in earlier sections, but are less useful for diagnosis; for instance, lactic acidemia and elevated creatine phosphokinase (CPK) are both commonly found, but they are inconstant and tend to occur relatively late.

It has been maintained by some investigators that liver biopsy is essential for definitive diagnosis of RS. This procedure probably does yield the most definitive confirmation, but it is not entirely clear that liver biopsy, during the acute illness, can rule out a partial genetic defect of CPS or OCT activity. These latter patients might be expected to have no fat deposition ("lean Reye's").[132, 133] Some information suggests that these genetic enzyme deficiencies may produce liver enlargement and microdroplet fat deposition during acute exacerbations; however, the mitochondrial appearance associated with these heritable urea cycle deficiencies is different from that associated with RS.[103, 134] Liver biopsy is not justified for diagnosis in the typical case of RS but should be employed when diagnosis is uncertain, in recurrent RS, or to meet research criteria for diagnosis. Similarly, lumbar puncture is probably not indicated in typical cases but should be done in the presence of atypical features, fever, nuchal rigidity, or possible encephalitis. It is advisable to save an admission serum specimen for later confirmation of diagnosis by amino acid analysis, if needed.[13]

Along with diagnosis, determining the severity of the illness is a crucial task when the patient is first encountered, for it will greatly influence not only prognosis but also management. The stages agreed upon by the NIH Consensus Conference,[135] following those proposed by Lovejoy,[136] reflect the stereotypic and predictable progression of illness outlined previously and are very useful for describing the patient's relative clinical state (see Table 9–1). The stages delineate a classic rostral-caudal deterioration of central nervous system function, essentially identical to that seen in severe hepatic encephalopathy. Taken alone, however, they are inadequate for accurate prognosis. Obviously, it is important to know whether the stage is determined at admission or at the nadir, and what the rate of progression is through the stages. One child admitted in stage 4 may stabilize and eventually begin to improve; another admitted in stage 2 may rapidly progress to coma and death. Nevertheless, there is a useful correlation between stage at admission and outcome.

A better index of prognosis may be the peak blood ammonia value. Blood ammonia usually peaks early, within a few hours of admission. Nearly all large series of RS patients studied showed a correlation between peak blood ammonia and mortality (see previous discussion).[14] Angelides and coworkers[14] have recently reported that if peak blood ammonia level was less than five times normal, all the children survived intact; if it were elevated greater than five-fold, mortality increased. These findings were independent of staging. DeLong and Glick[15] recently published calculations that indicate a very close correlation between the area under the hyperammonemic curve (a measure of the total ammonia burden presented to the brain) and mortality; they suggest that the total burden of hyperammonemia over time may be more critical than the peak level. The area under the curve, which is not available as a prognostic criterion early in the course, may be useful in predicting outcome as the course of RS progresses.

Many investigators have examined other chemical parameters as indices of prognosis in RS. Other useful indices include elevated serum osmolality, elevated blood lactate, low bicarbonate, and elevated CPK. No other early parameters have been found to correlate with severity and mortality as well as peak hyperammonemia. Levels of SGOT, invariably elevated early in the disease, do not predict outcome.

Electroencephalography is frequently employed to aid in prognosis; however, its usefulness is most equivocal in just that intermediate situation in which clinical and other prognostic indicators may be uncertain.[118] Nevertheless, it has a useful role especially in the paralyzed patient, and in monitoring barbiturate coma. It cannot be relied on alone for prognostication.

DIFFERENTIAL DIAGNOSIS

The Reye's-like syndromes discussed later are obviously pertinent to differential diagnosis. The major categories of differential diagnosis include primary central nervous system disease (especially encephalitis); other metabolic disorders that cause acute encephalopathy, particularly inherited metabolic disorders; and intoxication by exogenous substances. Acute abdominal illnesses, including pancreatitis and volvulus, have been mistaken for Reye's. Fulminant hepatitis is distinguished from RS by the presence of jaundice. Encephalitis must be excluded; seizures and fever usually are more prominent with encephalitis, CSF pleocytosis is usual but not invariable, and the characteristic biochemical abnormalities are not found.

Other metabolic encephalopathies must be excluded. Salicylism shares many features of RS. Two exceptions are the absence of prominent hyperammonemia and the presence of high blood salicylate levels. Diabetic ketoacidosis is readily distinguished by profound acidosis, ketosis, and hyperglycemia. Lactic acidosis is differentiated by the severe uncompensated metabolic acidosis and lack of prominent hyperammonemia. The genetic disorders of organic acid metabolism (propionic, methylmalonic, isovaleric) usually do not appear *de novo* in an otherwise previously healthy child but may indeed be intermittent. These disorders are characterized by acidosis, vomiting, and lethargy or coma, but the last is less severe and not accompanied by the overwhelming cerebral swelling found in RS. These syndromes are associated with moderate hyperammonemia caused by inhibition of urea cycle function by elevated organic acid.[135] As noted previously, children with intermittent episodic manifestations of genetic urea cycle disorders (especially CPS or OTC deficiency) may have a clinical picture indistinguishable from that of RS and are recognized only if liver biopsy tissue fails to show fat deposition or a recurrence prompts specialized study. Other family members may be affected. These genetic enzymatic disorders tend to arise as diagnostic issues in younger children. Other exogenous toxins besides salicylates must be excluded. Ethylene glycol and tetracycline both can produce coma with hyperventilation and mixed respiratory alkalosis and metabolic acidosis.[70] Tetracycline use can also produce microdroplet fat accumulation in liver, particularly during pregnancy as recorded in some reports.[71] Valproic acid may cause Reye's-like illness.[72] Usually, toxins can be readily excluded by lack of exposure. A toxic screen should be obtained on admission in all cases.

Lead poisoning should never be forgotten as a possible cause, in a young child, of vomiting, ataxia, confusion, and increased intracranial pressure.[137] Differentiation from RS is by history, serum lead and free erythrocyte protoporphyrin levels, and CSF abnormalities. Theophylline intoxication should be considered in the differential diagnosis. It is seen in children up to 6 years and is characterized by agitation, increased thirst, delirium, seizures, vomiting of brown bloody material, and hyperpyrexia. Diagnosis is obtained through history and the finding of elevated blood theophylline levels.[139] Rarely, acute abdominal disease, such as volvulus, may be confused with Reye's syndrome because of vomiting, dehydration, and lethargy.[140]

Reye's-like Syndromes

RS has become the paradigm of acute toxic-metabolic encephalopathies in childhood, with the result that a number of illnesses of similar pattern have been designated as "Reye's-like" and may require consideration in differential diagnosis. Some of these, when caused by genetic metabolic disorders, may cause recurrent illnesses and must be considered in cases of recurrent RS.[117] Disorders of urea cycle enzymes, especially partial deficiency of CPS or OCT,[119, 120] may produce recurrent episodes of disease clinically indistinguishable from

Reye's syndrome. This is one of the principal arguments for the central importance of the transient decrease in activity of CPS and OCT and hyperammonemia in the pathogenesis of Reye's. In the partial OCT cases, lack of fatty infiltration of the liver was a key finding alerting physicians to the possibility of another cause; however, in a partial CPS case (personal observation)—a four year old boy with a similarly affected sister—the liver showed typical microvesicular fat deposition during his third and fatal episode. LaBrecque and coworkers[121] have examined the liver histologically in 16 cases of heritable urea cycle deficiency; they found minor degrees of steatosis only in female heterozygotes for OCT deficiency. In none did the histologic picture resemble RS. However, a recent report describes a 4-month-old infant with argininosuccinic lyase deficiency who had hepatic steatosis indistinguishable from RS by light microscopy; electron microscopy did not show the marked mitochondrial swelling characteristic of RS.[103] Severe fatal intracranial hypertension was also a feature of the disease. This report re-emphasizes the very close parallelism between RS and genetic urea cycle disorders. The latter disorders may be diagnosable only after recovery from the acute illness, if ammonia intolerance and decreased enzyme activity are still demonstrable.

Genetic disorders of organic acid metabolism, such as propionyl CoA carboxylase deficiency, may produce episodic metabolic acidosis, lethargy or coma, and hyperammonemia that may mimic RS.[122] Robinson and colleagues[45] reported a case of hydroxymethylglutaryl CoA lyase deficiency mimicking RS; involvement of this enzyme in true RS may explain the minimal ketosis and reported increase in dicarboxylic acids. Systemic carnitine deficiency has also been reported to mimic RS.[123–125] In the cases described, the encephalopathy was relatively mild, and the cardiac involvement more prominent than is the rule in RS. The cases were marked by hypoglycemia without ketosis, progressive cardiomyopathy, and intermittent hepatic encephalopathy. Blood carnitine levels are normal in RS.[34, 126]

Several toxic agents have been reported to produce a Reye's-like syndrome. Jamaican vomiting sickness, caused by the toxic agent hypoglycin A found in the unripe akee fruit, was cited by Reye as similar to the disease he described. It is now known, however, that the biochemical changes caused by hypoglycin A are distinctly different from those found in RS.[127] Salicylate poisoning produces an encephalopathy and an acid-base disturbance similar to that of RS. However, hyperammonemia and the amino acid profile of RS do not occur in salicylate intoxication, and the prognosis of salicylism, properly treated, is much more favorable than that of RS. Recently, valproic acid has been reported to cause a Reye's-like syndrome with hyperammonemia and coma.[72, 73] This has been attributed to its similarity to other organic acids, and like propionate and isovalerate, valproic acid has been shown to inhibit oxidative phosphorylation.[76] Alternatively, elevated propionate levels resulting from metabolism of valproic acid may inhibit urea cycle enzymes by decreasing hepatic levels of *N*-acetyl glutamic acid.[75]

Aflatoxin has been implicated as a possible toxin producing Udorn encephalopathy, an illness that occurs in Thailand and is essentially similar to RS.[128, 129] Aflatoxin has not been found to have a role in RS in the United States.[127] Margosa oil has recently been reported to cause a Reye's-like illness in Indonesia.[74]

MANAGEMENT

The treatment of RS is not completely satisfactory, though definite gains have been made. All investigators agree that the encephalopathy, accompanied by cerebral swelling, is the chief life-threatening factor. The disease process in most organs is reversible as the acute illness subsides, but not always in the brain. However, because the insult to the brain is toxic-metabolic in origin and limited in time, it should theoretically be possible either to reduce the toxic-metabolic burden or to protect and sustain the brain through the limited critical period of the acute disease. The original treatment attempts aimed at supplying missing metabolites (Reye and coworkers[1] commented on the apparent benefits of glucose infusion) or removing unspecified toxins. Within a few years of Reye's description, it was recognized that hyperammonemia was frequently, if not uniformly, present in RS, and this finding focused therapeutic attempts on removing ammonia. Peritoneal dialysis[141, 142] and exchange transfusions[143, 144] both had extensive trials in the treatment of RS, but the results were disappointing, and therefore these modalities of therapy have been largely abandoned. Other therapy used to attempt to correct the metabolic disorder include the administration of metabolic precursors to maximize detoxification and removal of ammonia. These agents have included arginine,[147] α-keto acid analogs of amino acids,[146] sodium benzoate,[147] and citrulline.[15] It is beyond the scope of this chapter to discuss these therapies in detail. At present, the use of metabolic precursors is experimental, and they should not be employed except in research. The overall national data collected by the CDC[7] demonstrated no decrease in mortality rate resulting from the use of metabolic therapies such as exchange transfusion, peritoneal dialysis, and glucose and insulin. These negative results focused attention away from metabolic therapies and toward greater emphasis on supportive care,[150] including meticulous management of ICP.[151] This evolution has been aided by the use of hyperosmolar therapy, by the introduction of neurosurgical methods for precise monitoring of ICP, and by the advent of promising new modalities such as barbiturates for control of increased ICP. These methods form the mainstays of current therapy of severe RS and of the treatment approach described later. It should be noted, however, that these techniques have not been critically evaluated in RS, and they are not adequate to ensure control of increased ICP or full recovery in all severely ill RS patients. They are simply the best current therapies. More progress will probably require a return to metabolic approaches to treatment and better understanding of pathogenesis. It is increasingly recognized that cytotoxic damage to the brain and not simply increased ICP, may be the critical lesion that causes irreversible encephalopathy.

ICP monitoring was introduced in RS[152] and revealed clinically unrecognizable periods of severe intracranial hypertension, stimulating interest in aggressive anti–cerebral edema therapy.[153, 154] It was shown that exchange transfusion can rapidly reduce ICP as shown by monitoring.[155] Pentobarbital was introduced to control increased ICP[156]; its usefulness in RS has yet to be defined. A recent study found no decrease in mortality or morbidity when pentobarbital coma was instituted prophylactically for RS patients in coma, as when compared with its use only after other forms of treatment of ICP had failed.[157] A multicenter controlled study is currently under way to study the effectiveness of early pentobarbital therapy for RS.[158] The barbiturates are probably best regarded simply as additional adjunctive agents for control of increased ICP.

Detailed Management

There are several useful guides to management of acute RS.[21, 159–161] Not included here are several experimental treatments currently under evaluation in various centers; they include metabolic treatments to lower hyperammonemia,[15, 149] and early treatment with barbiturates to combat increased ICP.[156–158]

For patients in stage 1 and stage 2 with moderate elevation of blood ammonia (< 5 times the upper limit of normal), intervention is limited to non-invasive monitoring, maintaining fluid and electrolyte balance, providing adequate glucose, and using mannitol as necessary. Fluid management is best done by giving 10 to 20 per cent dextrose in one-third to one-half normal saline with 20 mEq/L of KPO_4 at maintenance rate (1500 ml/m^2/day). Potassium is given as phosphate because hypophosphatemia is usual in RS.[34] The rate of infusion will depend on osmolality, blood and urine electrolyte levels, and volume status. Children should be carefully monitored for body weight, fluid intake and output, and urine and blood osmolality. Blood glucose, electrolyte, and ammonia levels should be observed every 8 hours. Serial vital signs, mental status, and neurologic findings also should be recorded on a standard flow sheet hourly. Mannitol may be given to these patients (0.5 gm/kg initially, then 0.25–0.5 gm/kg q2h up to 3 ×) if necessary; if mannitol is used, osmolality should be checked 2 hours after administration. Hypovolemia or impending shock should be treated by administration of either normal saline (10–20 ml/kg) or colloid (5% albumin, 0.5–1.0 gm/kg) as a rapid infusion over 20–30 minutes. Repeated hypovolemia requires placement of a central venous pressure line. Patients in this favorable group rarely experience serious complications and may be expected to recover intact.

For patients in stage 3, 4, or 5, and those with arterial ammonia elevated more than fivefold, a more aggressive approach to treatment is needed, which requires invasive monitoring. In these stages the goals of controlling increased ICP and monitoring fluids and electrolytes require the ability to monitor and control cardiovascular, renal, and respiratory parameters as well as ICP. Several lines must be inserted. An arterial line is inserted for blood pressure monitoring and chemical studies. Two venous lines are placed, one of which is either a central venous pressure line or a pulmonary artery pressure (Swan-Ganz) catheter. The latter is preferable in the most unstable and severely ill patients. The bladder is catheterized with a Foley catheter, and all output measured hourly and recorded. A nasogastric tube is placed. Core temperature is continuously monitored. The use of an ICP monitor has become a standard part of management of the severely ill RS patient. Certain caveats must be made about its use: when muscle paralysis, morphine, and pentobarbital coma therapies are utilized, the pressure monitor supercedes direct neurologic observation of the patient. The clinicians must satisfy themselves that this trade-off is advantageous; and to do this, they must be certain that the monitor is functioning correctly and corresponds to the fluctuation in the patient's state as determined clinically. The pressure monitor must itself be closely scrutinized and its readings interpreted with care. There are at least three basic types of intracranial monitors: the subdural bolt, the intraventricular catheter, and the epidural monitor. The one selected depends on the experience and preference of the neurosurgeon. The subdural bolt, which is screwed into a burr hole in the skull table, records intracranial pressure via a catheter communicating with the subarachnoid space through a cruciate opening in the dura. The intraventricular catheter is inserted through a burr hole, then through the brain parenchyma into one lateral ventricle; whereas this has the advantage of permitting fluid removal, the ventricles are usually small and difficult to enter, and the risk of infection is considerable. The epidural monitor is a pressure-sensitive transducer slipped between the dura and the inner skull table via a burr hole. Probably the subdural bolt is the most widely used and most generally satisfactory.

The management of the comatose patient with RS may be discussed in two parts: general measures and those measures directed specifically at countering increased ICP.

General or supportive measures include the management of fluid administration, provision of adequate glucose, maintenance of oxygenation and adequate respiration, bowel cleansing to minimize ammonia production in the gut, prevention of bleeding, maintenance of normothermia, and simple general measures to prevent or treat increased ICP.

There are theoretical reasons to administer sufficient glucose to maintain blood glucose at two or three times normal levels: to minimize lipolysis and protein catabolism, and to increase substrate for brain energy metabolism.[34] The efficacy of producing elevated blood glucose levels by liberal glucose infusion has not been proved, however. Probably it is not necessary to administer insulin, because blood insulin levels are uniformly high in children with RS.[34]

Fluid management in conjunction with treatment of increased ICP is perhaps the most crucial issue in management of RS patients. Fluid management has as its goals the prevention and correction of increased intracranial pressure and cerebral swelling; maintenance of intravascular volume, cardiac output and blood pressure, and renal function; and prevention of excessive hyperosmolality. There are two contradictory issues in considering the problem of fluid replacement in RS: (1) the necessity to prevent cerebral edema by removing free water, which is done by maintaining an osmolar gradient across the blood-brain barrier, utilizing osmolar diuretics; and (2) removal of free water is countered by the need to maintain intravascular volume, blood pressure, and urine output and to prevent dangerous levels of hyperosmolality. The problem is made more difficult because severely ill RS patients are dehydrated (from inanition and vomiting) and hyperosmolar (osmolality occasionally up to 330 mOsm/L) at the time of admission. Blood pressure and urine output are usually well-maintained at the time of admission but may become problems after one or two days. These aforementioned problems are exacerbated by osmolar therapy. Mannitol, by withdrawing free water from the brain and ultimately from the body, decreases cerebral edema at a "cost" of a progressive increase in osmolality and decrease in intravascular volume. The use of mannitol incurs a "free water deficit," which is a reasonable trade-off to gain time. However, eventually this will lead to hypovolemia, oliguria, and circulatory collapse. Sufficiently high osmolality of itself may impair neurologic and possibly cardiac function. The answer to this dilemma requires judicious fluid replacement, including free water, crystalloid (normal saline), and colloid to maintain central venous pressure and intravascular volume, at the same time mannitol is being used. Specific goals of fluid therapy are to maintain cerebral perfusion pressure (CPP, equal to mean arterial pressure minus intracranial pressure: CPP = MAP − ICP) greater than 50 mmHg; to maintain serum osmolality at an appropriate level (305–315 mOsm/L); and to maintain adequate intravascular volume (CVP 5–8 mmHg or mean pulmonary artery

ALGORITHM FOR THE DIAGNOSIS AND MANAGEMENT OF REYE'S SYNDROME: PART A

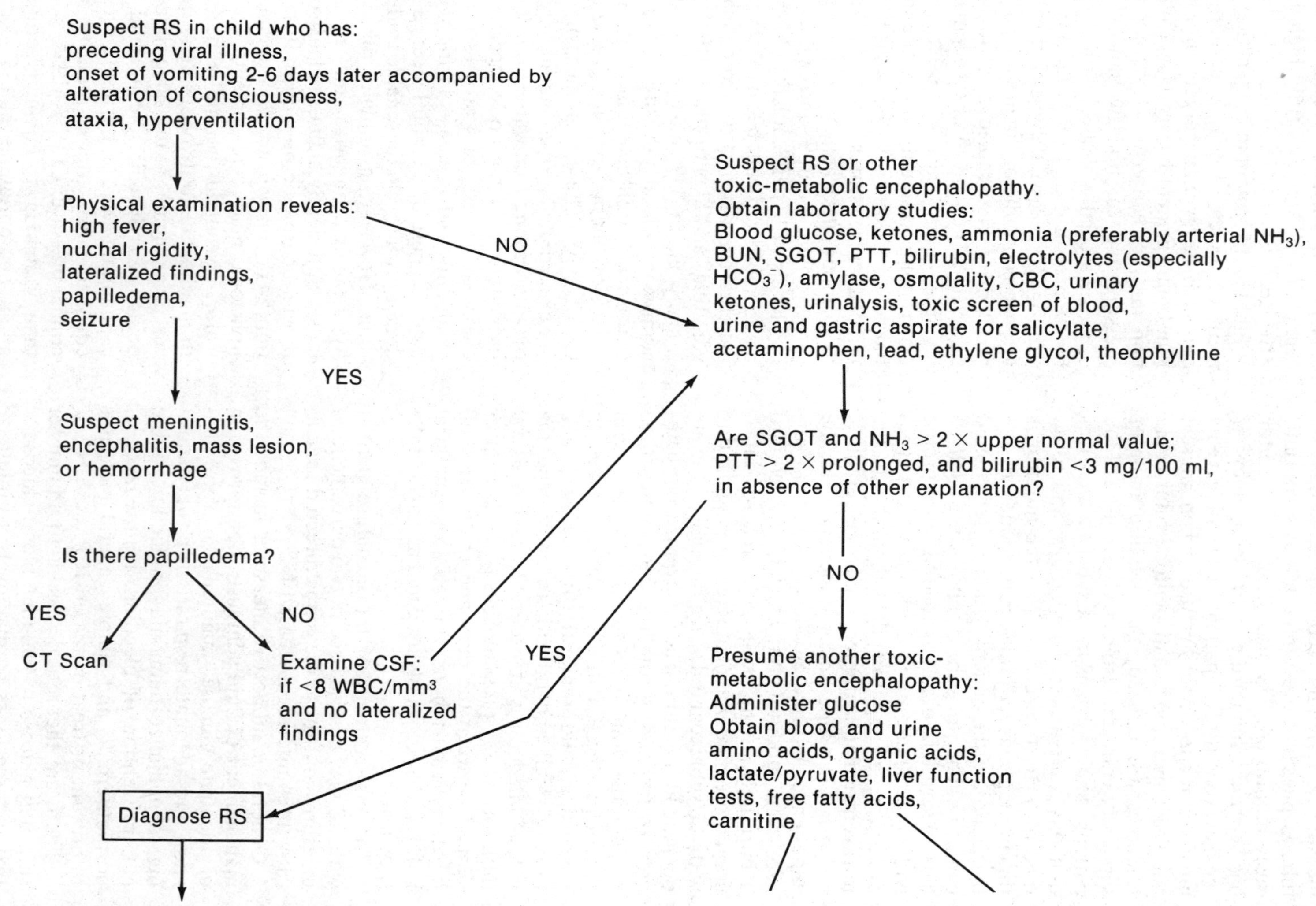

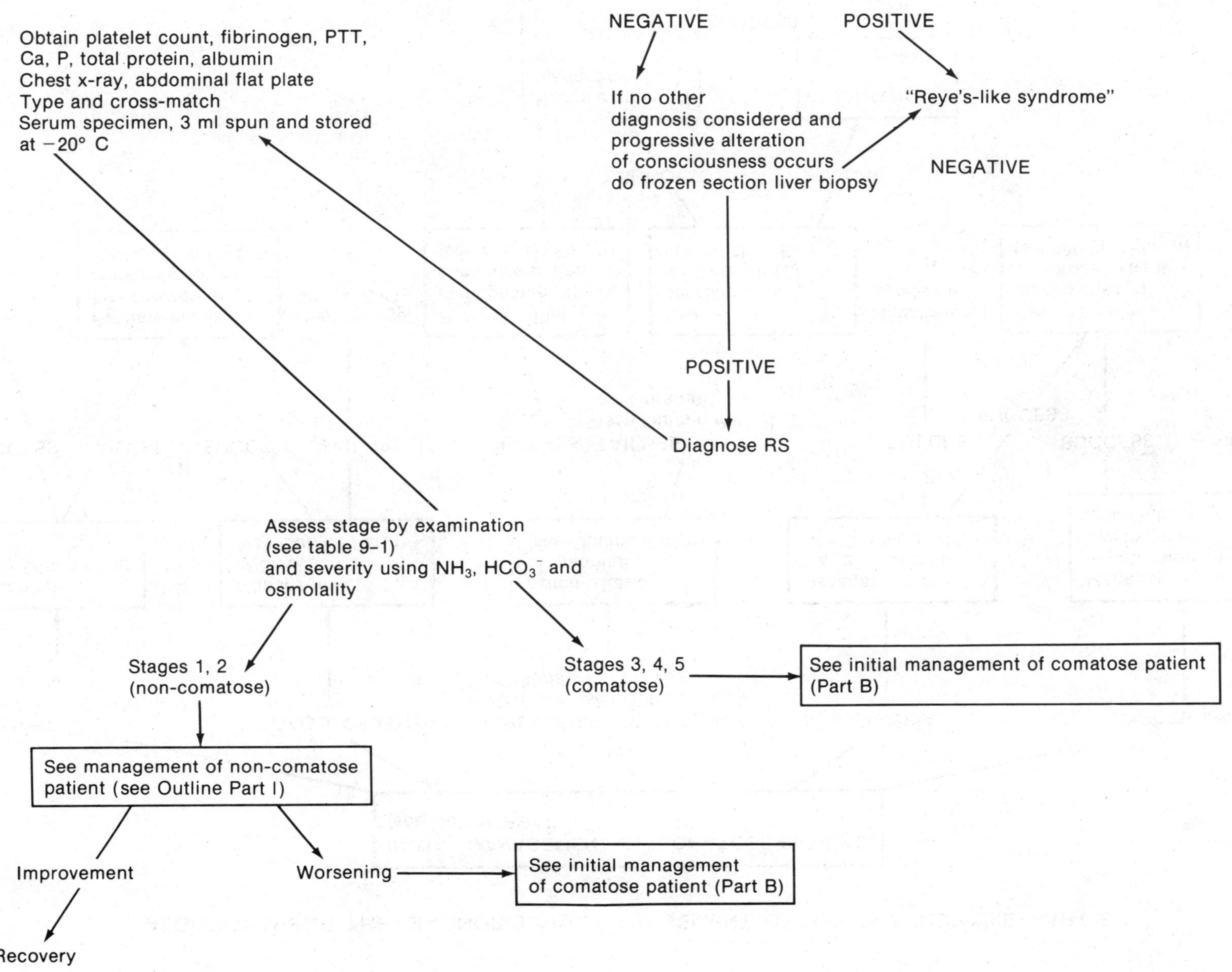
Obtain platelet count, fibrinogen, PTT, Ca, P, total protein, albumin
Chest x-ray, abdominal flat plate
Type and cross-match
Serum specimen, 3 ml spun and stored at −20° C
NEGATIVE
POSITIVE
If no other diagnosis considered and progressive alteration of consciousness occurs do frozen section liver biopsy
"Reye's-like syndrome"
NEGATIVE
POSITIVE
Diagnose RS
Assess stage by examination (see table 9–1) and severity using NH_3, HCO_3^- and osmolality
Stages 1, 2 (non-comatose)
Stages 3, 4, 5 (comatose)
See initial management of comatose patient (Part B)
See management of non-comatose patient (see Outline Part I)
Improvement
Worsening
See initial management of comatose patient (Part B)
Recovery

ALGORITHM FOR THE DIAGNOSIS AND MANAGEMENT OF REYE'S SYNDROME: PART B

INITIAL MANAGEMENT OF COMATOSE PATIENT (see Outline Part II)

- IMPROVEMENT (see Outline Part III for Criteria) → Weaning (see Outline Part III)
  - SUCCESS → Recovery
  - FAILURE → Resume initial management of comatose patient (see Outline Part II)
- COAGULOPATHY → Management of bleeding (see Outline Part IV)
  - SUCCESS → Resume initial management of comatose patient (see Outline Part II)
  - FAILURE → Hemorrhage, Shock, DIC
- INCREASED INTRACRANIAL PRESSURE (see Outline Part V for Criteria) → Administration of mannitol (see Outline Part V)
  - SUCCESS → Resume initial management of comatose patient (see Outline Part II)
  - FAILURE (see Outline Part VI for Criteria) → Use of pentobarbital to decrease ICP (see Outline Part VI)
    - SUCCESS → Resume initial management of comatose patient (see Outline Part II)
    - FAILURE → Craniectomy for decompression
      - SUCCESS → Resume initial management of comatose patient (see Outline Part II)
- OLIGURIA → Management of low urine output (see Outline Part VII)
  - FAILURE → Hepato-renal Syndrome
  - SUCCESS → Resume initial management of comatose patient (see Outline Part II)
- HYPOTENSION → Management of hypotension and hypovolemia (see Outline Part VIII)
  - SUCCESS → Resume initial management of comatose patient (see Outline Part II)
  - FAILURE → SHOCK

OUTLINE OF TREATMENT

I. Management of non-comatose patient.
  A. Manage in pediatric ICU.
  B. Institute non-invasive monitoring.
    1. Blood pressure, pulse, temperature, respiratory rate and pattern.
    2. Neurological monitoring, charted on a standard flow sheet.
    3. EEG and ECG.
  C. Obtain laboratory values every 8 hours.
    1. Blood glucose.
    2. Electrolytes, osmolality.
    3. Ammonia.
  D. Institute fluid management.
    1. One dependable venous line.
    2. Urinary collection for accurate I and O; catheterize if necessary.
    3. Give maintenance fluids; one-third to one-half normal saline, 1500 ml/m²/day, with KPO_4, 20 mEq/L, and 10–20% dextrose.
    4. Maintain blood glucose at 200 mg/100 ml.
    5. Adjust fluid volume and concentration as indicated by patient's volume and electrolyte status.
    6. Give mannitol, 0.5 gm/kg initially, then 0.25–0.5 gm/kg, as needed, q2h up to 3×.

II. Initial management of comatose patient.
  A. Place support and monitoring lines.
    1. Two dependable intravenous lines.
    2. Arterial line.
    3. Central venous catheter or Swan-Ganz pulmonary artery catheter.
    4. Foley catheter.
    5. Nasogastric tube.
      a. Give antacid, 10 ml q2h.
      b. Tube to gravity drainage.
      c. Neomycin, 100 mg/kg/day in 4 divided doses, nasogastrically.
    6. Monitor core temperature.
  B. Intubate with muscle relaxant and short-acting barbiturates; provide O_2.
  C. Treat coagulopathy with fresh frozen plasma, 5–10 ml/kg, and give vitamin K, 5 mg IM qd.
  D. Place intracranial monitor after rechecking coagulation parameters and correcting if necessary.
  E. Provide supportive therapy and fluid management.
    1. Maintain mean arterial pressure >60 mmHg.
    2. Control ventilation.
      a. Maintain Pa_{CO_2} at 22–27 mmHg.
      b. Maintain Pa_{O_2} at 100–150 mmHg.
    3. Give fluids at 1500 ml/m²/day initially. Replacement depends on matching urinary volume and electrolyte loss and gastric loss to maintain normovolemia, CVP of 5–8 mmHg, or pulmonary artery pressure of 12–20 mmHg, and normal BP and CPP.
    4. Give 10% dextrose; increase to 15% or 20% as needed to maintain blood glucose at 150–200 mg/100 ml.
    5. Give KPO_4, 2–3 mEq/kg, to maintain potassium level. If serum PO_4 is >5.5 mg/100 ml or if Ca is <8.0 mg/100 ml, do not give KPO_4 but KCL for potassium replacement.
  F. Control increased intracranial pressure (ICP).
    1. Maintain ICP at or below 15–18 mmHg and cerebral perfusion pressure >50 mmHg.
    2. Keep patient in head-up position (30°) while nursing.
    3. Maintain normothermia; use cooling blanket if necessary.
    4. Avoid unnecessary pain, procedures, and manipulations. Keep patient quiet and comfortable.
    5. Administer morphine, 0.1 mg/kg, q1–2h if necessary for sedation, and Pavulon, 0.1 mg/kg, q1–2h if necessary for muscle paralysis.
    6. Give mannitol, 1 gm/kg, initially, then 0.25–0.5 gm/kg, as needed if serum osmolarity is <340 mOsm/L. If no response within 10 minutes, increase dose to 1 gm/kg.

III. Criteria and procedures for weaning.
  A. Criteria.
    1. Stable ICP <13 mmHg for 24 hours (no mannitol for 24 hours).
    2. Cerebral perfusion pressure (CPP) >55 mmHg for 24 hours.
    3. Stable electrolytes.
  B. Procedures.
    1. Reduce pentobarbital to sedation levels.
    2. Stop paralysis.
    3. Allow P_{CO_2} to rise in 5 mmHg increments q1–2h.
    4. May use mannitol 1–2× for slight increase in ICP; if needed >2×, consider reinstituting therapy.
    5. Wean to spontaneous breathing, then extubate.

IV. Management of bleeding (major GI, pulmonary or mucous membrane).
  A. Recheck platelet count, PT, PTT, and fibrinogen.
  B. Administer fresh frozen plasma or cryoprecipitate.
  C. Administer platelets if indicated.

V. Criteria for increased ICP and administration of mannitol.
  A. Therapeutic guidelines for increased intracranial pressure.
    1. Hyperventilate to P_{CO_2} of 22–27 mmHg.

2. Induce paralysis and sedate; avoid stimuli. Chest physiotherapy and maintain tube clear.
3. Keep patient's head up.
4. Keep patient normothermic and normovolemic.

B. Administration of mannitol for ICP > 15 mmHg (in addition to previously listed therapy).
1. When ICP >15 and <20 mmHg, administer mannitol, 0.25–0.5 gm/kg.
2. If ICP remains >15 and <20 mmHg for 15 minutes administer mannitol again, 0.5 gm/kg.
3. If ICP increases to >25 mmHg for 1 minute, administer mannitol, 0.5–1.0 gm/kg, and increase hyperventilation.
4. If mean arterial pressure (MAP) drops so that CPP (MAP − ICP) is <50 mmHg, increase CVP up to 6 mmHg, or mean pulmonary artery pressure up to 12–20 mmHg, using albumin or plasma.

VI. Criteria for failure of mannitol therapy and use of pentobarbital to decrease ICP.
A. Criteria for failure of mannitol therapy.
1. Sustained elevation of ICP, i.e., ICP > 20 mmHg for 1 hour, or >30 mmHg for 10 minutes.
2. Refractory to two doses of mannitol, 1.0–1.5 gm/kg, given within 1 hour.
3. Serum osmolality >340 mOsm/L.
4. Progression to stage 5 coma.

B. Use of pentobarbital to decrease ICP.
1. Give pentobarbital, 10 mg/kg over 15–30 minutes, while observing BP; repeat with a second 10 mg/kg dose over 30 minutes.
2. Monitor and maintain BP, CVP, CPP, and pulse.
3. Monitor Pco_2.
4. Give pentobarbital, 2–5 mg/kg hourly, to maintain blood levels between 35–50 μg/ml.
5. Monitor pentobarbital blood level within 2 hours of starting infusion, then every 6 hours until stabilized.
6. If ICP persists, may given additional 5 mg/kg hourly × 2 hours.

VII. Management of low urine output.
A. Patient normotensive; output <1/ml/kg/hour.
1. If CVP >5 mmHg, give Lasix, 1 mg/kg IV.
a. Do not give if patient is hypotensive.
2. If CVP <5mmHg, double fluid administration rate until an adequate urine output is established or until CVP >5 mmHg.

VIII. Management of hypotension and hypovolemia.
A. Use fluid replacement liberally, including plasma and albumin colloid, to maintain CVP at 5–8 mmHg and to maintain mean pulmonary artery pressure at 12–20 mmHg.
B. Management of hypovolemia in normotensive or hypertensive patients.
1. If there is poor peripheral perfusion and evidence of renal failure give fluid challenge of saline, 10–20 ml/kg, and 5% albumin, 0.5–1.0 gm/kg.

C. Management of hypotension.
1. Evaluate fluid status.
a. If CVP <8 mmHg administer fresh frozen plasma, blood, or 5% albumin.
b. If CPP <50 mmHg administer albumin immediately to CVP of 10 mmHg, or mean pulmonary artery pressure of 15–22 mmHg (Swan-Ganz).
c. If CVP >8 mmHg administer dopamine at 2–5 μg/kg/min, continuous IV infusion to maintain CPP >50 mmHg.

---

pressure of 12–20 mmHg). Urine volume should be maintained at 1 ml/kg/hr or greater.

Initially fluids should be given at maintenance levels, 1500 ml/m²/day, as one-third to one-half normal saline with 20 mEq/L of KPO_4, as described previously, with further replacement depending on urine volume, gastric losses, and urine electrolyte losses as well as volume indices. Dextrose should be given as a 10 per cent solution, increased to 15 or 20 per cent as needed to maintain blood glucose at 150–200 mg/100 ml. Osmolality should be maintained at 305–315 mOsm/L. Central venous pressure should be maintained at 5–8 mmHg, or pulmonary artery pressure at 12–20 mmHg. In the event of hypotension, if CVP is less than 8 mmHg, fluid should be added, primarily as colloid (fresh frozen plasma, blood, or 5 per cent albumin) to raise CVP. If the cerebral perfusion pressure (CPP) is less than 50 mmHg, albumin should be administered immediately to bring the CVP to 10 mmHg, or mean pulmonary artery pressure to 15–22 mmHg (as measured by Swan-Ganz catheter). In the event of hypotension with CVP greater than 8 mmHg, dopamine should be administered by continuous intravenous infusion, 2–5 μg/kg/min, to maintain CPP greater than 50 mmHg. In the event of urine output falling to less than 1 ml/kg/hr despite normal blood pressure, if CVP is low (<5 mmHg) fluid administration should be doubled until urine output is adequate or CVP is greater than 5mmHg. If oliguria is present despite normotension and a CVP greater than 5 mmHg, Lasix, 1 mg/kg, should be given intravenously. Significant bleeding may require transfusion with whole blood. The requirements for fluid replacement may be substantially increased during treatment with pentobarbital, which expands the venous bed and thus intravascular volume requirements, but the principles remain the same. This approach has the rare but possible consequence of cardiogenic shock if the myocardium becomes critically affected, leading to vascular collapse or pulmonary edema. If these conditions supervene, the treatment is that used in similar circumstances generally, namely Lasix for high central venous pressure with pulmonary edema and dopamine for hypotension.[163]

Maintenance of adequate oxygenation requires a secure airway. Patients should be electively intubated when a decision is made for aggressive treatment as previously described. This procedure should be performed by a physician with experience in the intubation of patients with increased ICP and may require use of succinylcholine or thiopental (pentothal). Arterial oxygen should be maintained from 100–150 mmHg. Respiration should be controlled and the patient kept moderately hypocapnic (Pa_{CO_2} 22–27 mmHg; in general, Pa_{CO_2} should match the pre-intubation value) to combat increased ICP. Acute pressure rises should be controlled initially by prompt manual increase in hyperventilation, but this should not be prolonged for more than a few minutes without introducing other measures.

Management of the gut has as its purposes prevention of gastrointestinal (GI) bleeding and the consequent production and absorption of ammonia. To prevent gastric bleeding, a nasogastric tube is placed and Maalox, 10 ml, is given every two hours. Neomycin, 100 mg/kg/day, should be given by nasogastric tube in four divided doses. Cleansing saline enemas are given till gut is clear.

Clotting parameters (prothrombin time, partial thromboplastin time, platelets, and fibrinogen) should be determined initially, again before placement of an intracranial pressure monitor, and if significant bleeding occurs. Vitamin K, 5 mg/day intramuscularly, should be given. Significant bleeding (such as gastric bleeding, melena, or gross hematuria) should be treated with fresh frozen plasma or cryoprecipitate, and platelets given if indicated. Abnormal clotting values unaccompanied by significant bleeding should not be treated. Disseminated intravascular coagulation (DIC) may occur occasionally in severely ill RS patients and should be treated as it is in any other situation.

Most investigators advise maintaining a normothermic body temperature and preventing pyrexia by use of a cooling blanket if necessary while monitoring core temperature. Hyperthermia causes an increase in intracranial pressure and tends to increase body catabolism. Hypothermia may be employed in special circumstances to decrease ICP, but there is inadequate information to warrant its use as a routine procedure in management.

Certain simple and effective measures to reduce or prevent increased ICP should be employed at all stages in management; some have been mentioned. The patient should be nursed with the head elevated 30 degrees. The neck should not be turned or compressed. Procedures should be limited to the necessary minimum, and these performed with gentle care to prevent pain and agitation. Fever should be prevented. Excess hydration and elevated central venous pressure should be avoided. Hypercapnia, elevated mean airway pressure, and relative hypoxia should be avoided.

Beyond these simple measures, a range of procedures are available to lower the increased ICP. These measures include hyperventilation (hypocapia), osmotic dehydration, muscle paralysis and sedation, CSF drainage when a ventricular catheter is utilized, hypothermia, and barbiturate administration. The use of barbiturates will be discussed separately later. Rockoff and Ropper have recently published a complete description of therapy for increased ICP, to which the reader is referred.[163]

Muscle paralysis using Pavulon (pancuronium bromide), 0.1 mg/kg q1–2 h, and sedation with morphine, 0.1 mg/kg q1–2 h, or diazepam, 0.1 mg/kg q1–2 h, may be useful adjuncts for control of ventilation and agitation and thereby the lowering of the increased ICP. This therapy has the disadvantage of precluding clinical neurologic evaluation; for this reason, the patient's paralysis should be allowed to "lighten" periodically in order that his or her condition may be reassessed.

Perhaps more important than the agent chosen to reduce increased ICP is the timeliness of intervention. The treatment of increased

ICP must always be anticipatory; it is essential to be prepared for the possibility of rising pressure. Once herniation has occurred, with loss of brainstem function and respiration, the chance of recovery is greatly reduced if not virtually nil; it is necessary to anticipate increased ICP and treat the patient before this eventuality occurs, which may require constant vigilance for many hours or days.

Barbiturate Coma

The use of barbiturate, specifically pentobarbital, therapy to control increased ICP in severely ill children with Reye's syndrome is controversial.[156, 157, 163] Some investigators have found it useful and others have not. A multicenter controlled study currently underway may clarify the question. It is clear that pentobarbital is an effective agent to decrease increased ICP in some circumstances. It is also evident that pentobarbital can decrease cardiac output by weakening myocardial contractibility and increasing venous volume, and so may have dangers in treating Reye's syndrome. Pentobarbital-induced coma, along with pancuronium bromide and morphine, has the additional problem of obscuring the neurologic features, which are an index to the patient's progress. This is a significant, though perhaps not an insurmountable problem, even in deeply comatose patients. Frewen and colleagues[157] found no significant difference in outcome between early institution of pentobarbital and the use of hypothermia compared with the use of such therapy only in response to increases in ICP, and they found that the therapy was associated with significant morbidity, especially pulmonary complications. It was not known whether pentobarbital or hypothermia was more responsible for the pulmonary problems. Perhaps the best summary statement at present is that pentobarbital represents an adjunctive agent for control of increased ICP, which may be used in conjunction with other anti-ICP measures, but the clinician should be aware of its possible problems and complications.

Barbiturate therapy must be used before irreversible herniation has occurred. This prerequisite implies that its use must be anticipatory and raises the question of which patients should be selected for this treatment. There is no general agreement on the patient selection nor on the decision whether to use barbiturate coma at all. Fitzgerald[160] initiates pentobarbital coma in patients with more than five-fold elevation of serum ammonia level and disease at stage 3 or more severe. The multi-center Reye's syndrome study group proposes to use pentobarbital when therapy with mannitol and other measures to control increased ICP have failed. No generally agreed upon rule can be given. Our practice has been to use pentobarbital as an adjunctive agent to control increased ICP as needed and to consider pentobarbital coma in a child entering stage 4 whose condition deteriorates despite maximum treatment with other measures to counteract increased ICP.

The use of barbiturate necessitates maximal supportive care. Pentobarbital is the preferred agent, because it maintains cardiac output better than thiopental. Pentobarbital has the effect of increasing intravascular volume. Proper management requires the presence of a Swan-Ganz pulmonary artery catheter. Meticulous attention to fluid and volume management is essential. Large amounts of colloid and crystalloid may be needed to maintain central venous pressure at 5–8 mmHg, pulmonary artery pressure at 12–20 mmHg, and normal mean arterial blood pressure; in addition, continuous intravenous dopamine infusion up to 5 μg/kg/min may be necessary. Hypotension is the single greatest danger of barbiturate therapy in RS patients.

Pentobarbital may be given as a loading dose of 10 mg/kg, intravenously, over 15–30 minutes, which may be repeated up to a total of 20 mg/kg rapidly to lower ICP, then 2–5 mg/kg/h to maintain blood levels between 35–50 μg/ml. It is worth reiterating that the success of pentobarbital therapy may hinge on preventing hypotension, which requires careful monitoring, liberal fluid replacement, and liberal use of dopamine or another pressor.

Weaning from barbiturate coma is begun gradually after ICP has been normal for 24 hours. The dose is reduced to sedative levels. Muscle relaxants should be withdrawn intermittently, and stopped if ICP remains normal. Hyperventilation may then be eased, allowing P_{CO_2} to rise gradually. The child may then be allowed to breathe spontaneously and the tube may be removed.

Cranial decompression has been used in a few instances to control intractable increased ICP.[164] It must be performed before irreversible herniation occurs, and so the approach again must be anticipatory. In our experience, it is only in exceptional cases that an opportunity for decompression will present itself. A large proportion of children reported to survive after craniectomy have had residual neurological and intellectual damage.[143]

Outcome and Sequelae

In 1974 the death-to-case ratio of RS in the United States was 41 per cent.[6] In 1981 this ratio was 28 per cent.[12] Some of the decrease in death-to-case ratio may be due to increased recognition of mild cases. However, there also appeared to be a reduction between 1974 and 1978 in the death-to-case ratio in cases matched for neurologic status on admission; in 1974, mortality for cases admitted in stage 2 coma was 42 per cent, and in 1978 it was 26 per cent.[6, 165]

Indices predicting the severity of an individual case (mortality and morbidity) were discussed previously (see "Diagnosis and Staging"). Although mortality correlates with stage on admission, Angelides and coworkers[14] found a stronger correlation with peak ammonia levels. In their experience, all patients with peak ammonia levels less than five times normal survived intact. Of those with peak ammonia greater than five times normal, 41 per cent died.

Another group of workers have reported a mortality of 35 per cent and impaired survival in 17 per cent in a group of children with severe RS, despite an aggressive treatment program including barbiturate coma.[157]

Although most survivors of RS recover completely, some suffer significant morbidity. Severity of illness relates directly to severity of outcome. While many recover completely, 34 to 61 per cent of survivors have been found to have neuropsychological problems.[166–169] They may exhibit one or a combination of neurologic, behavioral, psychological, and intellectual sequelae. A recent study has noted relatively good intellectual and neurologic status of survivors, and emphasized the significant emotional problems of survivors and their families.[170] Younger children have higher morbidity and fatality rates than older children.

Reye's syndrome remains a dangerous and tragic illness. Current treatment methods are not adequate to effectively control the illness when it is severe. In planning therapy, and judging treatment results, it is essential to take account of the severity of the illness in each case. Staging has a role in assessing severity, but peak ammonia level or total hyperammonemic burden may be even more important as an index of severity.[175]

REFERENCES

1. Reye RDK, Morgan G, Baral J. Encephalopathy and fatty degeneration of the viscera. A disease entity in childhood. Lancet 1963; *2*:749–752.
2. Johnson GM, Scurletis TD, Carroll NB. A study of sixteen fatal cases of encephalitis-like disease in North Carolina children. NC Med J 1963; *24*:464–473.
3. Brain WR, Hunter D. Acute meningoencephalomyelitis of childhood: report of six cases. Lancet 1929; *1*:221–227.
4. Lyon G, Dodge PR, Adams RD. The acute encephalopathies of obscure origin in infants and children. Brain 1961; *84*:680–708.
5. Atkins JN, Haponik EF. Reye's syndrome in the adult patient. Am J Med 1979; *67*:572–578.
6. Sullivan-Bolyai JZ, Corey L. Epidemiology of Reye's syndrome. Epidemiol Rev 1981; *3*:1–26.
7. Corey L, Rubin RJ, Hattwick MAW. Reye's syndrome: clinical progression and evaluation of therapy. Pediatrics 1977; *60*:708–713.
8. Nelson DB, Hurwitz ES, Sullivan-Bolyai JZ, et al. Reye's syndrome in the United States in 1977–1978, a non–influenza B virus year. J Infect Dis 1979; *140*:436–439.
9. Corey L, Rubin RJ, Hattwick MAW, et al. A nationwide outbreak of Reye's syndrome: its epidemiologic relationship to influenza B. Am J Med 1976; *61*:615.
10. Huttenlocher PR, Trauner DA. Reye's syndrome in infancy. Pediatrics 1978; *62*:84–90.
11. Sullivan-Bolyai JZ, Nelson DB, Morens DM, et al. Reye syndrome in children less than one year old: some epidemiologic observations. Pediatrics 1980; *65*:627–629.
12. National surveillance for Reye syndrome, 1981: Update, Reye syndrome and salicylate usage. Morbidity Mortality Weekly Report 1982; *31*:53–61.
13. Romshe CA, Hilty MD, McClung HJ, et al. Amino acid pattern in Reye's syndrome: comparison with clinically similar entities. J Pediatr 1981; *98*:788–790.
14. Angelides AG, Wyllie R, Fitzgerald JF. The prognostic significance of peak ammonia levels in Reye's syndrome. Pediatrics 1982; *70*:997–1000.
15. DeLong GR, Glick TH. Ammonia metabolism in Reye's syndrome and the effect of citrulline. Ann Neurol 1982; *11*:53–58.
16. Isom JB. Lactic acidosis in Reye's syndrome: correlation with degree of encephalopathy, 24-hour urinary excretion of epinephrine and outcome. (Abstract) Ann Neurol 1982; *12*:200–201.
17. Tonsgard JH, Huttenlocher PR, Thisted RA. Lactic acidemia in Reye's syndrome. Pediatrics 1982; *69*:64–69.
18. DeLong GR, Glick TH. Encephalopathy of Reye's syndrome. A review of pathogenetic hypotheses. Pediatrics 1982; *69*:53–63.
19. Flannery DB, Hsia YE, Wolf B. Current states of hyperammonemic syndromes. Hepatology 1982; *2*:495–506.
20. DeVivo DC. Reye's syndrome: A metabolic response to an acute mitochondrial insult? Neurology 1978; *28*:105–108.
21. Trauner DA. Reye's syndrome. Curr Probl Pediatr 1982; *12*:1–31.
22. Mamunes P, DeVries GH, Miller CD, David RB. Fatty acid quantitation in Reye's Syndrome. *In*: Pollack JD ed. Reye's Syndrome. New York: Grune & Stratton, Inc. 1975:245–254.

23. Trauner D, Sweetman L, Holm J, et al. Biochemical correlates of illness and recovery in Reye's syndrome. Ann Neurol 1977; *28*:238–241.
24. Kang ES, Gates RE, Wrenn ELJ. Abnormal cellular regulation of lipolysis and phosphorylation in Reye's syndrome. Biochem Med 1982; *27*:180–194.
25. Pollack JD, Hilty MD, Haynes RE, et al. Serum lipid patterns in Reye's syndrome: elevated total free fatty acids. Pediatr Res 1973; *7*:164.
26. Pollack JD, Cramblett HG, Flynn D, Clark D. Serum and tissue lipids in Reye's syndrome. *In* Pollack JD ed. Reye's Syndrome. New York: Grune & Stratton, Inc. 1975:227–243.
27. Ogburn PL, Sharp H, Lloyd-Still JD, et al. Abnormal polyunsaturated fatty acid patterns of serum lipids in Reye's syndrome. Proc Natl Acad Sci 1982; *79*:908–911.
28. Simpson H. Encephalopathy and fatty degeneration of the viscera. Acid-base observations. Lancet 1966; *2*:1274–1277.
29. Crocker JF, Bagnell PC. Reye's syndrome: a clinical review. Can Med Assoc J 1981; *124*:375–382.
30. Snodgrass PJ, DeLong GR. Urea cycle enzyme deficiencies and an increased nitrogen load producing hyperammonemia in Reye's syndrome. N Engl J Med 1976; *294*:855–860.
31. Brown T, Hug G, Lansky L, et al. Transiently reduced activity of carbamylphosphate synthetase and ornithine transcarbamylase in liver of children with Reye's syndrome. N Engl J Med 1976; *294*:861–863.
32. Sinatra F, Yoshida T, Applebaum M, et al. Abnormalities of carbamyl phosphate synthetase and ornithine transcarbamylase in liver of patients with Reye's syndrome. Pediatr Res 1975; *9*:829–833.
33. Brown RE, Madge GE, Trauner DA, David RB. Lipid and lipoprotein studies in Reye's syndrome. Va Med Mon 1972; *99*:622.
34. Haymond MW, Karl IE, Keating JP, DeVivo DC. Metabolic response to hypertonic glucose administration in Reye's syndrome. Ann Neurol 1978; *3*:207–215.
35. Glasgow AM, Chase HP. Effect of propionic acid on fatty acid oxidation and ureagenesis. Pediatr Res 1976; *10*:683–686.
36. Huttenlocher PR, Schwartz AD, Klatskin G. Reye's syndrome: ammonia intoxication as a possible factor in the encephalopathy. Pediatrics 1969; *43*:443–454.
37. Kang ES, Gerald PS. Hyperammonemia and Reye's syndrome. N Engl J Med 1972; *286*:1216.
38. Hilty MD, Romshe CA, Delameter PV. Reye's syndrome and hyperaminoacidemia. J Pediatr 1974; *84*:363–365.
39. Partin JC, Schubert WK, Partin JS. Mitochondrial ultrastructure in Reye's syndrome (encephalopathy and fatty degeneration of the viscera). N Engl J Med 1971; *285*:1339–1343.
40. Bove KE, McAdam AJ, Partin JC, et al. The hepatic lesion in Reye's syndrome. Gastroenterology 1975; *69*:685–697.
41. Robinson BH, Gall DG, Cutz E. Deficient activity of hepatic pyruvate dehydrogenase and pyruvate carboxylase in Reye's syndrome. Pediatr Res 1977; *11*:279–281.
42. Robinson BH, Taylor J, Cutz E, Gall DG. Reye's syndrome: preservation of mitochondrial enzymes in brain and muscle compared with liver. Pediatr Res 1978; *12*:1045–1047.
43. Thaler MM. Clinical and enzymatic indices of hepatic dysfunction in Reye's syndrome. *In*: Crocker JFS, ed. Reye's Syndrome II. New York: Grune & Stratton, Inc. 1979:115–138.
44. Greene HL, Wilson FA, Gluck AD, et al. Hepatic ATP concentrations and glycolytic enzyme activities in Reye's syndrome. J Pediatr 1976; *89*:777.
45. Robinson BH, Oei J, Sherwood WG, et al. Hydroxymethylglutaryl CoA lyase deficiency: features resembling Reye's syndrome. Neurology 1980; *20*:714–718.
46. Lloyd KG, Davidson L, Price K, et al. Catecholamine and octopamine concentrations in brains of patients with Reye's syndrome. Neurology 1977; *27*:985–988.
47. Newman SL, Caplan DB, Camp VM, et al. Prolactin and the encephalopathy of Reye's syndrome. Lancet 1979; *2*:1097–1100.
48. Shapiro Y, Dechelbaum R, Statter M, et al. Reye's syndrome; diagnosis by muscle biopsy? Arch Dis Child 1981; *56*:287–291.
49. Partin JS. Brain ultrastructure in Reye's disease. II. Acute injury and recovery processes in three children. J Neuropathol Exp Neurol 1978; *37*(6):796–819.
50. Partin JC, Partin JS, Schubert WK. Muscle ultrastructure in Reye's syndrome (RS): evidence for a myopathy. Pediatr Res 1977; *11*:564A.
51. Zieve FJ, Zieve L, Doizaki W, Gilsdorf RB. Synergism between ammonia and fatty acids in the production of coma: implications for hepatic coma. J Pharmacol Exp Ther 1974; *191*:10–16.
52. Derr RF, Zieve L. Effect of fatty acids on the disposition of ammonia. J Pharmacol and Exp Ther 1976; *197*:675–680.
53. Shannon DC, DeLong GR, Bercu B, et al. Studies on the pathophysiology of encephalopathy in Reye's syndrome: hyperammonemia in Reye's syndrome. Pediatrics 1975; *56*:999–1004.
54. Chaves-Carballo E, Carter GA, Wiebe DA. Triglyceride and cholesterol concentrations in whole serum and in serum lipoproteins in Reye syndrome. Pediatrics 1979; *64*:592–597.
55. Moreus DM, Nobel GR. Reye's syndrome and influenza. Lancet 1977; *1*:807–808.
56. Noble GR, Corey L, Rubin RJ. Virologic components of Reye's syndrome. *In:* Pollack JD, ed. Reye's Syndrome. New York: Grune & Stratton, 1975: 189–197.
57. Partin JC, Schubert WK, Partin JS, et al. Isolation of influenza virus from liver and muscle biopsy specimens from a surviving case of Reye's syndrome. Lancet 1976; *2*:599–602.
58. Norman MG, Lowden JA, Hill DE, et al. Encephalopathy and fatty degeneration of the viscera in childhood: II. Report of a case with isolation of influenza B virus. Can Med Assoc J 1968; *99*:549.
59. Powell HC, Rosenberg RN, McKellar B. Reye's Syndrome: isolation of parainfluenza virus. Report of three cases. Arch Neurol 1973; *39*:135–139.
60. Lewinski UH, Djaldetti M. Ultrastructural alterations of the lymphocytes from a patient with Reye's syndrome. J Submicrosc Cytol 1981; *13*:697–701.
61. Davis LE, Cole LL. Comparison of Reye's syndrome and the experimental mouse model of influenza virus toxicity: a review. J Natl Reye's Synd Fndn 1980; *1*:99–103.
62. Johnson RT. Current concepts in neurology: the contribution of virologic research to clinical neurology. N Engl J Med 1982; *307*:660–662.
63. Hanson PA, Urizar RE. Ultrastructural lesions of

muscle and immunofluorescent deposits in vessels in Reye's syndrome: a preliminary report of serial muscle biopsies. Ann Neurol 1977; *1*:431–437.
64. Marder HK, Strife CF, Forristal J, et al. Hypocomplementemia in Reye's syndrome: relationship to disease stage, circulating immune complexes and C3b amplification loop protein synthesis. Pediatr Res 1981; *15*:362–365.
65. Nelson DB, Kimbrough R, Landrigan PS, et al. Aflatoxin and Reye's syndrome. A case control study. Pediatrics 1980; *66*:865–869.
66. Crocker JFS, Rozee KR, Ozere RL, et al. Insecticide and viral interaction as a cause of fatty visceral changes and encephalopathy in the mouse. Lancet 1974; *2*:22–24.
67. Pollack, JD. Models of chemical and virus interaction and their relation to a multiple etiology of Reye's syndrome. *In:* Crocker JFS, ed. Reye's Syndrome II. New York: Grune & Stratton, Inc. 1979: 341–360.
68. Hug G, Bosken J, Bove K, et al. Reye's syndrome simulacra in liver of mice after treatment with chemical agents and encephalomyocarditis virus. Lab Invest 1981; *45*:89–109.
69. Heick HMC, Shipman RT, Norman MG, et al. Reye-like syndrome associated with use of insect repellent in a presumed heterozygote for ornithine carbamyl transferase deficiency. J Pediatr 1980; *97*:471–473.
70. Parry MF, Wallach R. Ethylene glycol poisoning. Am J Med 1974; *57*:143.
71. Sherlock S. Patterns of hepatocyte injury in man. Lancet 1982; *1*:782–786.
72. Young RSK, Bergman I, Gang DL, Richardson EP Jr. Fatal Reye-like syndrome associated with valproic acid. Ann Neurol 1980; *7*:389–390.
73. Gerber N, Harland RC, Lynn RK, et al. Reye-like syndrome associated with valproic acid therapy. J Pediatr 1979; *95*:142–144.
74. Sinniah D, Baskaran G, Looi LM, et al. Reye-like syndrome due to margosa oil poisoning; report of a case with postmortem findings. Am J Gastroenterol 1982; *77*:158–161.
75. Coude FX, Rabier D, Cathelineau L, et al. A mechanism for valproate-induced hyperammonemia. Pediatr Res 1981; *15*:974–975.
76. Haas R, Stumpf DA, Parks JK, et al. Inhibitory effects of sodium valproate on oxidative phosphorylation. Neurology 1981; *31*:1473–1476.
77. Thaler MM, Hoogenrad NJ, Boswell M. Reye's syndrome due to a novel protein-tolerant variant of ornithine-transcarbamylase deficiency. Lancet 1974; *2*:438.
78. Engle D, Baublis JV, Duff TE, et al. Reye's syndrome in Michigan. *In:* Crocker JFS, ed. Reye's Syndrome II. New York: Grune & Stratton, 1979:195–213.
79. Pital PA, McCormick KL, Fitzgerald E, Orson JM. Subclinical hepatic changes in varicella infection. Pediatrics 1980; *65*:631–633.
80. Ludviggson P, Grover W, Brown LW. The fallacy of varicella hepatitis: evidence for Reye's syndrome. Ann Neurol 1981; *10*:300.
81. Partin JJ, Partin JC, Schubert WK: Varicella hepatitis or Reye's? Pediatrics 1981; *68*:610.
82. Ey JL, Smith SM, Fulginiti VA. Varicella hepatitis without neurologic symptoms or findings. Pediatrics 1981; *67*:285–287.
83. Monto AS, Ceglarek JP, Haynes NS. Liver function abnormalities in the course of a type A (HINI) influenza outbreak: relation to Reye's syndrome. Am J Epidemiol 1981; *114*:750–759.
84. Mortimer EA Jr, Lepow ML Varicella with hypoglycemia possibly due to salicylates. Am J Dis Child 1962; *103*:91.
85. Woodbury DM. Analgesic-Antipyretics, Anti-Inflammatory Agents, and Inhibitors of Uric Acid Synthesis. *In*: Gilman AG, Goodman LS, Gilman A, eds. The Pharmacological Basis of Therapeutics. New York: Macmillan Publishing Co, 1970:314–347.
86. Starko K, Ray CG, Dominguez LB, et al. Reye's syndrome and salicylate use. Pediatrics 1980; *66*:859–864.
87. Crichton JU, Elliot GB. Salicylate—a dangerous drug in infancy and childhood: a survey of 58 cases of salicylate poisoning. Can Med Assoc J 1960; *83*:1144.
88. Linneman CC Jr, Uede K, Hug G, et al. Salicylate intoxication and influenza in ferrets. Pediatr Res 1979; *13*:44–47.
89. Partin JJ, Partin JC, Schubert W, et al. Serum salicylate concentrations in Reye's disease. Lancet 1982; *1*:191.
90. Tonsgard JH, Huttenlocher PR. Salicylates and Reye's syndrome. Pediatrics 1981; *68*:747–748.
91. Linneman CC Jr, Shea L, Kauffman CA, et al. Association of Reye's syndrome with viral infection. Lancet 1974; *2*:179.
92. Halpin TJ, Holtzhauer FJ, Campbell RJ, et al. Reye's syndrome and medication use. JAMA 1982; *248*:687–691.
93. Clark JH, Fitzgerald JF. Doubts relationship of salicylate and Reye's syndrome. Pediatrics 1981; *68*:467.
94. Gall DG, Barker G, Cutz E. Doubts relationship of salicylate and Reye's syndrome. Pediatrics 1981; *68*:466.
95. Andressen B, Alexander M, Kwokei J, et al. Aspirin and Reye's syndrome: a reinterpretation. Lancet 1982; *1*:903.
96. Salicylate labeling may change because of Reye's syndrome. FDA Drug Bulletin 1982; *12*:1–2.
97. Brown AK, Fikrig S, Finberg L. Aspirin and Reye's syndrome. J Pediatr 1983; *102*:157–158.
98. RS Working Group. Reye's syndrome and salicylates: a spurious association. Pediatrics 1982; *70*:158–160.
99. Daniels SR, Greenberg RS, Ibrahim MA. Scientific uncertainties in the studies of salicylate use and Reye's syndrome. JAMA 1983; *249*:1311–1316.
100. Lovejoy FH, Smith AL, Bresnan MJ, et al. Clinical staging in Reye's syndrome. Am J Dis Child 1974; *128*:36–41.
101. Shaywitz BA, Rothstein P, Venes JL. Monitoring and management of increased intracranial pressure in Reye's syndrome: results in 29 children. Pediatrics 1980; *66*:198–204.
102. Shih VE. Congenital hyperammonemic syndromes. Clin Perinatol 1976; *3*:3–14.
103. Guertin SR, Levinsohn MW, Dahms BB. Small-droplet steatosis and intracranial hypertension in arginosuccinic lyase deficiency. J Pediatr 1983; *102*:736–740.
104. Hindfelt B, Siesjo BK. Cerebral effects of acute ammonia intoxication. I. The influence on intracellular and extracellular acid-base parameters. Scand J Clin Lab Invest 1971; *28*:353–364.
105. Hindfelt B, Seisjo BK. Cerebral effects of acute ammonia intoxication. II. The effect upon energy

metabolism. Scand J Clin Lab Invest 1971; *28*:365–374.

106. Kindt GW, et al. Blood/brain barrier and brain oedema in ammonia intoxication. Lancet 1977; *1*:201.
107. Norenberg MD, Lapham LW. The astrocyte response in experimental portal-systemic encephalopathy: an electron microscopic study. J Neuropathol Exp Neurol 1974; *33*:422–435.
108. Lockwood AH, McDonald JM, Reiman RE, et al. The dynamics of ammonia metabolism in man: effects of liver disease and hyperammonemia. J Clin Invest 1979; *63*:449.
109. Cooper AJL, McDonald JM, Gelbard AD, et al. The metabolic fate of 13-N labeled ammonia in rat brain. J Biol Chem 1979; *254*:4982.
110. Trauner DA, Huttenlocher PR. Short chain fatty acid–induced central hyperventilation in rabbits. Neurology 1978; *28*:940–944.
111. Hillman RE, DeVivo DC, Keating JP. Marked elevation of octanoic acid and other medium chain free fatty acids unassociated with cerebral symptoms. Pediatr Res 1978; *12*:507.
112. Kreisberg RA. Lactate homeostasis and lactic acidosis. Ann Intern Med 1980; *92*:227–237.
113. Manz HJ, Colon AR, McCullough DC. Temporal sequence in and pathogenesis of the neuropathology of Reye's syndrome. J Natl Reye's Syn Fdn 1981; *2*:3–19.
114. Cole M, Rutherford RB, Smith FO. Experimental ammonia encephalopathy in the primate. Arch Neurol 1972; *26*:130–136.
115. Partin JS, McAdams AJ, McLaurin RL, et al. Brain ultrastructure in Reye's syndrome; acute injury and repair. *In:* Crocker JFS, ed. Reye's Syndrome II. New York: Grune & Stratton, Inc. 1979:237–249.
116. Eichelberger MR, Chatten J, Bruce DA, et al. Acute pancreatitis and increased intracranial pressure. J Pediatr Surg 1981; *16*:562–570.
117. Pichichero ME, McCabe ERB. Recurrent Reye's syndrome. Am J Dis Child 1978; *132*:1097–1099.
118. Aoki Y, Lombroso CT. Prognostic value of electroencephalography in Reye's syndrome. Neurology 1973; *23*:333.
119. Yokoi T, Honke K, Funabashi T, et al. Partial ornithine transcarbamylase deficiency simulating Reye's syndrome. J Pediatr 1981; *99*:929–931.
120. Cox KL, Cannon RA. Recurrent Reye's syndrome without liver lipid deposition. Hosp Pract 1981; *16*:45–51.
121. LaBrecque DR, Latham PS, Riely CA, et al. Heritable urea cycle deficiency—liver disease in 16 patients. J Pediatr 1979; *94*:580–587.
122. Bergstrom T, Greter J, Levin AH, et al. Propionyl-CoA carboxylase deficiency: case report, effect of low protein diet and identification of 3-oxo-2-methylvaleric acid, 3-hydroxy-2-methylvaleric, and muleic acid in urine. Scand J Clin Lab Invest 1981; *41*:117–126.
123. Glasgow AM, Eng G, Engel AC. Systemic carnitine deficiency simulating recurrent Reye's syndrome. J Pediatr 1980; *96*:889–891.
124. Chapoy PR, Angelini C, Brown WJ, et al. Systemic carnitine deficiency—a treatable inherited lipid-storage disease presenting as Reye's syndrome. N Engl J Med 1980; *303*:1389–1394.
125. Ware AJ, Burton WC, McGarry JD, et al. Systemic carnitine deficiency. J Pediatr 1978; *93*:959–964.
126. Glasgow AM. Reye's syndrome mimickers. J Natl Reye's Syn Fdn 1980; *1*:104–114.
127. Tanaka K, Kean EA, Johnson B. Jamaican vomiting sickness. Biochemical investigation of two cases. N Engl J Med 1976; *295*:461–467.
128. Olson LC, Bourgeois CH, Keschamras N, et al. Encephalopathy and fatty degeneration of the viscera in three Thai children. Am J Dis Child 1970; *120*:1–2.
129. Nelson DB, Kimbrough R, Landrigan PS, et al. Aflatoxin and Reye's syndrome: a case control study. Pediatrics 1980; *66*:865–869.
130. Fox DW, Hart MC, Bergeson PS, et al. Pyrolizidine *(Senecio)* intoxication mimicking Reye's syndrome. J Pediatr 1978; *93*:980–982.
131. Hart ZH, Nelson KA, Kooi KA, et al. Reye's syndrome in children under two years of age: significance of electroencephalographic observations. Clin Electroencephalogr 1981; *12*:102–112.
132. Gosseye S, DeMeyer R, Maldagne P. Reye's syndrome without fatty liver. Helv Paediatr Acta 1975; *30*:509–513.
133. Glick TH: Lean Reye's syndrome. Am J Dis Child 1973; *125*:900–901.
134. Shapiro JM, Schaffer F, Tallan HH, et al. Mitochondrial abnormalities of liver in primary ornithine transcarbamylase deficiency. Pediatr Res 1980; *14*:775–789.
135. NIH Consensus Conference. The Diagnosis and Treatment of Reye's Syndrome. NIH Consensus Development Conference Summary, vol. 4, no. 1, 1981.
136. Lovejoy FH, Smith AL, Bresnan MJ, et al. Clinical staging in Reye's syndrome. Am J Dis Child 1974; *128*:36–45.
137. Conde FX, Ogier H, Grimber G, et al. Correlation between blood ammonia concentration and organic acid accumulation in isovaleric and propionic acidemia. Pediatrics 1982; *69*:115–117.
138. Magnus PD, Powers RJ, Leong A. Lead encephalopathy mimicking Reye's syndrome. J Pediatr 1979; *95*:495.
139. White BH, Doeschner CW. Aminophylline (theophylline ethylenediamine) poisoning in children. J Pediatr 1956; *49*:262–271.
140. Parke JT, Vargo TA, Fishman MA. Volvulus of the small intestine mimicking Reye's syndrome. (Abstract) Child Neurology Society, Salt Lake City, 1982.
141. Samaha FJ, Bleu E. The role of peritoneal dialysis in Reye's syndrome. *In:* Pollack JD, ed. Reye's Syndrome. New York: Grune & Stratton, 1975:295–299.
142. Editorial: Various regimens produce spotty results against Reye's syndrome. JAMA 1974; *228*:9.
143. Schubert WK, Partin JC, Partin JS, et al. Management of Reye's syndrome: Cincinnati experience. *In*: Crocker JF, ed. Reye's Syndrome II. New York: Grune & Stratton, Inc. 1979:155–171.
144. Bobo RC, Schubert WK, Partin JC, Partin JF. Reye's syndrome: treatment by exchange transfusion with special reference to the 1974 epidemic in Cincinnati, Ohio. J Pediatr 1975; *87*:881–886.
145. Donn SM, Swartz RD, Thoene JG. Comparison of exchange transfusion, peritoneal dialysis, and hemodialysis for the treatment of hyperammonemia in an anuric newborn infant. J Pediatr 1979; *95*:67–70.
146. Glasgow AM, Chase HP. Exchange transfusion to

remove ammonia. Am J Dis Child 1975; *129*:159–160.

147. Good TA, Tsai MY, Tang TT. Biochemical considerations in the serum amino acid patterns observed in Reye's syndrome. *In*: Pollock JD, ed. Reye's Syndrome. New York; Grune & Stratton, 1975:401–402.

148. McReynolds JW, Monteros S, Brusilow S, Rosenberg LE. Treatment of complete ornithine transcarbamylase deficiency with nitrogen-free analogues of essential amino acids. J Pediatr 1978; *93*:421–427.

149. Batshaw ML, Brusilow SW. Treatment of hyperammonemic coma caused by inborn errors of urea synthesis. J Pediatr 1980; *97*:893–900.

150. DeVivo DC, Keating JP, Haymond MW. Reye's syndrome: results of intensive supportive care. J Pediatr 1975; *87*:875–880.

151. Lovejoy FH Jr, Bresnan MJ, Lombroso CT, et al. Anticerebral oedema therapy in Reye's syndrome. Arch Dis Child 1975; *50*:933–937.

152. Mickell JJ, Reigel DH, Cook DR, et al. Intracranial pressure monitoring and normalization therapy in children. Pediatrics 1977; *58*:606–613.

153. Venes JL, Shaywitz BA, Spencer DD. Management of severe cerebral edema in the metabolic encephalopathy of Reye-Johnson syndrome. J Neurosurg 1978; *48*:903–915.

154. Shaywitz BA, Rothstein P, Venes JL. Monitoring and management of increased intracranial pressure in Reye's syndrome: results in 29 children. Pediatrics 1980; *66*:198–204.

155. Berman W, Pizzi F, Schut L, et al. The effects of exchange transfusion on intracranial pressure in patients with Reye's Syndrome. J Pediatr 1975; *87*:887–891.

156. Marshall LF, Shapiro HM, Rouscher A, et al. Pentobarbital in metabolic coma (Reye's syndrome). Crit Care Med 1978; *6*:1–5.

157. Frewen TC, Swedlow DB, Watcha M, et al. Outcome in severe Reye's syndrome with early pentobarbital coma and hypothermia. J Pediatr 1982; *100*:663–665.

158. Dobrin RS, Berman W: A prospective clinical comparison of osmotherapy (mannitol) *versus* pentobarbital augmented osmotherapy for the treatment of comatose patients with Reye's syndrome. (Abstract) *Presented at* Reye's Syndrome III Symposium, Detroit, November 1980.

159. Trauner DA. Treatment of Reye's syndrome. Ann Neurol 1980; 7:2–4.

160. Clark JH, Fitzgerald JF. Reye's syndrome in Indiana. J Indiana State Med Assoc 1981; *74*:785–789.

161. Consensus Conference. Diagnosis and treatment of Reye's syndrome. JAMA 246:2441–2444, 1981.

162. Perkin RM, Levin DL. Shock in the pediatric patient. Part II. Therapy. J Pediatr 1982; *101*:319–332.

163. Rockoff M, Ropper AH. Therapy of Increased Intracranial Pressure. *In:* Ropper AH, Kennedy S, Zervas NT, eds. Neurological-Neurosurgical Intensive Care. Baltimore, University Park Press, 1982.

164. Barker GA. The role of decompressive craniectomy in Reye's syndrome. J Natl Reye's Syn Fdn 1980; *1*:73–79.

165. Luscombe FA, Monto A, Baublis J. Mortality due to Reye's syndrome in Michigan: distribution and longitudinal trends. J Infect Dis 1980; *142*:363–371.

166. Shaywitz SE, Cohen PM, Cohen DJ, et al. Long-term consequences of Reye's syndrome: a sibling-matched, controlled study of neurologic, cognitive, academic, and psychiatric function. J Pediatr 1982; *100*:41–46.

167. Manz HJ, Colon AR. Neuropathology, pathogenesis, and neuropsychiatric sequelae of Reye's syndrome. J Neurol Sci 1982; *57*:377–395.

168. Brunner RL, O'Grady DJ, Partin JC, et al. Neuropsychologic consequences of Reye's syndrome. J Pediatr 1979; *95*:706–711.

169. Davidson PW, Willoughby RH, O'Tuoma LA, et al. Neurological and intellectual sequelae of Reye's syndrome. Am J Ment Defic 1978; *82*:535–541.

170. Benjamin PY, Levinsohn M, Drotur D, et al. Intellectual and emotional sequelae of Reye's syndrome. Crit Care Med 1982; *10*:583–587.

171. Wichser J, Kazemi H. Ammonia and ventilation: site and mechanism of action. Respir Physiol 1974; *20*:393.

172. Henle G, Henle W. Studies on the toxicity of influenza viruses. I. The effect of intracerebral injection of influenza viruses. J Exp Med 1946; *84*:623–637.

173. Henle W, Henle G. Studies on the toxicity of influenza viruses. II. The effect of intra-abdominal and intravenous injection of influenza viruses. J Exp Med 1946; *84*:639–660.

174. Myers MG. Hepatic cellular injury during varicella. Arch Dis Child 1982; *57*:317–319.

175. Lee SE, Painter MJ, Hirsch RP. Factors related to improved mortality in Reye syndrome: lack of effectiveness of intracranial pressure monitoring. Ann Neurol 1982; *12*:221.

CHAPTER

10

Head Injury

Darryl C. DeVivo, M.D.
Philip R. Dodge, M.D.

Head injury ranks high among the causes of death and disability in childhood.[1] The child who attains adulthood without ever having sustained a significant bump or blow to the head is rare. Although accurate statistics are not available, the majority of children who suffer such injury do not require hospitalization, and probably only a fraction of them are seen by the family doctor or pediatrician. Approximately 200,000 children are hospitalized each year for evaluation and treatment of head injuries and perhaps 5 to 10 per cent of them exhibit abnormal neurologic signs. From January 1974 to September 1975, 1522 children were evaluated for head injuries in our emergency room at St. Louis Children's Hospital, and of this group 200 (7.6%) were hospitalized for further observation and treatment. In addition, 224 children were admitted directly to our hospital usually as patient transfers from other hospitals. The total number admitted to St. Louis Children's Hospital for head injuries during this 21-month period was 424 children. Only 19 (4%) of them required neurosurgery.

Over the past 40 years many investigators have attempted to quantify the effects of closed head injury. Denny-Brown and Russell,[2] while developing an experimental model to study concussion, demonstrated that a much greater force is necessary to render an animal unconscious when the skull is held firmly in place than when the skull is free to move after impact. They named these two conditions compression concussion and acceleration concussion, respectively.

Acceleration-deceleration is more descriptive of the circumstances surrounding head injury in humans. Thus, the rate of change in head position after impact and the associated deformation of the skull at the time of impact are the major factors used in evaluating the effects of experimentally induced head injury. The force transmitted to the intracranial contents that produces acceleration and subsequent deformation of the skull gives rise to significant distortion and cavitation of the brain. There is little or no change in the volume of brain substance at the time of injury, but there is substantial change in its shape. This distortion causes bruising or laceration of the brain, which may occur at the site of the injury (coup) or at a distance from the site of injury (contrecoup).

A shearing force may tear small arteries and veins and produce parenchymatous bleeding or subdural hemorrhages in bridging vessels that course from the cerebral surface through the meninges to enter the dural sinuses. Less well recognized stretching or shearing effects can be transmitted to ascending and descending fiber tracts as they pass through the brainstem, separating these long processes from their cell bodies.[3] An appreciation of these several effects of a blow to the head leads to an understanding of the various clinical syndromes that follow an acute head injury (Fig. 10–1).

CLINICAL SYNDROMES AND PATHOLOGY

Concussion

The term concussion refers to the reversible neuronal dysfunction associated with loss of awareness and responsiveness (unconsciousness) that follows immediately upon a head injury and that persists for a brief time, usually measured in terms of minutes or hours. If the patient is observed carefully during this period, the duration of impaired consciousness can be

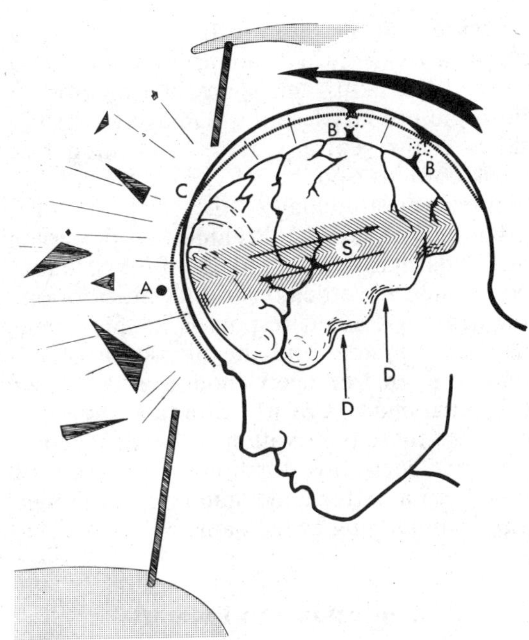

Figure 10–1. Diagrammatic representation of the mechanical distortions of the cranium following closed head injury. There is local deformation of the skull at the impact site with (*A*) representing the preinjury contour and (*C*) the immediate postinjury contour. Subdural veins (*B*) are torn as the brain rotates forward and the inferior temporal and frontal lobes (*D*) are traumatized by the restraining floors of the middle and anterior fossae. Shearing forces (*S*) are maximal at the brain surface and extend toward the center of rotation within the brain. (From Grubb, R. L., and Coxe, W. S.: Central nervous system trauma: Cranial. *In*: Eliasson, S. G., Prensky, A. L., and Hardin, W. B., Jr., eds. Neurological Pathophysiology. New York: Oxford University Press, 1974.)

noted precisely, but if one must rely on the history given by the patient at a later date, a false impression as to the duration of unconsciousness will be obtained, because the patient will be amnesic not only for the period of unconsciousness but also for events immediately before and after it. Loss of memory surrounding a concussion, termed post-traumatic amnesia (PTA), is considered by many investigators the single most important clinical phenomenon reflecting the extent and severity of injury to the brain following blunt trauma.[4, 5] The Glasgow Coma Scale has been developed to assess serially the degree and the duration of coma.[5] These observations are important in assessing the severity of diffuse brain damage. Three parameters are observed independently: eye opening, motor response, and verbal response (see Table 10–1).

Post-traumatic amnesia is composed of two parts: retrograde amnesia or the time before impact for which the patient has no memory; and anterograde amnesia or the period of memory loss after injury. Both periods tend to shrink with time, but the patient is always left with some permanent amnesia. Usually, no significant pathologic counterpart of concussion is found when the brain is examined by light microscopy. Concussion and PTA may not occur in injuries caused by sharp objects striking the head at high velocity and penetrating the skull (and even the brain) without producing significant deformities of the skull or acceleration-deceleration injury of the head. Under these circumstances severe focal damage to cerebral tissue and consequent neurologic defects can occur.[6]

Experimentally, concussion in animals is characterized by loss of consciousness, respiration, postural tone, and corneal and pinnal reflexes, is associated with a rapid rise in blood

Table 10–1. GLASGOW COMA SCALE

Parameter	Score
Eye Opening (E)	
Spontaneous	4
Responds to speech	3
Responds to pain	2
Nil	1
Best Motor Response (M)	
Obeys commands	6
Localizes pain	5
Withdraws	4
Abnormal flexion	3
Extensor response	2
Nil	1
Verbal Response (V)	
Oriented	5
Confused conversation	4
Inappropriate words	3
Incomprehensible sounds	2
Nil	1

The Glasgow Coma Scale is designed as a standardized assessment of the patient with disturbed consciousness. The tests can be performed serially to determine the patient's progress. The coma scale (E + M + V) = 3 to 15. All combinations equal to 7 or less define coma. Approximately 50 per cent of scores that equal 8 also define coma. Patients achieving a score of 9 or more are non-comatose.

pressure, and is followed by recovery. These findings relate to autonomic functions in the lower brainstem; and some investigators believe the primary lesion is damage to the large fibers in the ventral surface of the upper cervical cord caused by cervical extension and consequent stretching of the cord around the odontoid process.[7,8] Preliminary physiologic and pharmacologic studies of experimental concussion have demonstrated interruption in the sensory-evoked responses in the reticular activating system and the liberation of large quantities of free acetylcholine into the cerebrospinal fluid (CSF).[9] Although the significance of these observations at present remains unclear, such investigations may lead ultimately to a better understanding of the mechanism underlying concussion.

Contusion and Laceration

If visible injury to the brain exists, the terms contusion and laceration are used to describe the bruising and tearing of cerebral tissue, respectively, frequently accompanied by parenchymatous hemorrhage. The contusion or laceration is characteristically directly beneath the site of impact, but as noted earlier, the lesion may be remote from the site of direct trauma. Often in serious accidents there may be multiple sites of injury. The poles and undersurfaces of frontal and temporal lobes are injured most frequently.

Focal disturbances in strength, sensation, and visual awareness may result from such injury unless the damage involves so-called silent areas. The presence of these disturbances on examination need not, however, always imply this type of cerebral injury. Focal signs also may follow seizures (Todd's paresis) but are quite transient, usually resolving within two or three days after the cessation of seizure activity. Rapidly clearing focal findings in the absence of seizure activity may represent localized disturbances in neuronal function, referred to as "local concussion."[6] We have proposed that such a mechanism might underlie the transient loss of vision seen after mild head injury.[10] In some instances, development of such focal signs is delayed, suggesting that local edema and ischemia may be responsible.

Epidural and Subdural Hemorrhages

Hemorrhages developing between the calvarium and cerebral surfaces will compress the underlying brain. If the hemorrhage results from arterial bleeding, the temporal course of the resulting neurologic syndromes will be more rapid than if the bleeding is venous.

Epidural bleeding usually is accompanied by roentgenographic evidence of skull fracture; however, in children a fracture may be absent radiographically and at surgery in more than a fourth of the cases.[1] This fact presumably is attributable to the relative plasticity of the child's skull and the looseness with which the dura mater is attached to the overlying calvarium. For similar reasons, the hematoma may derive from diploic veins or dural sinuses rather than from an arterial source. Consequently, even in the absence of radiographic evidence of skull fracture, one must be alert to the possibility that an epidural hemorrhage can supervene.

Symptoms and signs of cerebral compression from acute subdural hemorrhage usually evolve within hours, or days of injury. When the hemorrhage develops more slowly, the patient may remain relatively asymptomatic; the clot will gradually undergo dissolution and a chronic subdural effusion will result. It is taught that symptoms and signs of epidural or subdural hemorrhage develop after a transient period of normality (lucid period) following concussion or other immediate effects of head injury. Clinically, however, this sequence of events is seldom recognized. More often in serious head injury, the effects of a developing mass lesion appear before recovery from the immediate effects of the trauma has occurred.

Skull Fracture

Breaks in the calvarium may be associated with any of the aforementioned clinical syndromes. The location and nature of the fracture may suggest additional complications. For example, if the fracture line extends through the squamous portion of the temporal bone, the possibility of an epidural hemorrhage from laceration of the middle meningeal artery is increased.

Fractures extending through the base of the skull may be associated with leakage of cerebrospinal fluid into either the auditory or nasal passages, resulting in otorrhea or rhinorrhea. The presence of these findings implies a break in the skull bone even if the fracture cannot be demonstrated radiographically.[1] The observation of intracranial air on x-ray films after trauma always means that there is anatomic continuity between nasal or ear cavities and the interior of the skull. This finding may exist even in the absence of obvious otorrhea or rhinorrhea. Rarely, such basal fractures also injure the pituitary stalk and cause transient or, less often, permanent diabetes insipidus. If the fracture line involves the rim of the foramen magnum, acute respiratory failure may occur secondary to direct injury of the lower brainstem or to subsequent compression of this region by a blood clot. Cranial nerve signs also may reflect direct injuries to these nerves, which have been captured in the line of fracture as they course through various bony canals.

The likelihood of a complicating intracranial infection is greater when there is a fracture, particularly when it extends through the base of the skull. Nuchal rigidity and peripheral leukocytosis frequently accompany head injury, particularly when there is bleeding into the subarachnoid space. Even though a low grade fever also may follow severe head injury as a direct consequence of the injury itself, its occurrence always should raise the possibility of a complicating meningitis or parameningeal infection, especially when there is evidence of disruption of the natural anatomic barriers to entrance of bacteria from the outside. In the presence of any of these findings, diagnostic lumbar puncture is indicated, *although this test should not be performed routinely following every head injury*. The potential risk of neurologic deteriorations developing in the patient with increased intracranial pressure after a lumbar puncture must be remembered; but this perhaps over-emphasized potential hazard should not countermand the use of such a test to evaluate the possible existence of an intracranial infection suggested by the clinical circumstances.

Cerebral Edema

Some degree of brain swelling is expected following significant craniocerebral trauma. Cerebral edema may coexist with any of the aforementioned clinical syndromes or it may be the only recognizable tissue alteration causing increased intracranial pressure.[11] Theoretically, cerebral edema may result from direct cellular injury (cytotoxic) or from vascular injury (vasogenic).[12] The fluid accumulation is intracellular in the cytotoxic form and interstitial in the vasogenic form, and plasma proteins leak into the brain when the vascular integrity is impaired. In fact, cerebral edema represents a mixture of both the cytotoxic and vasogenic forms in most clinical settings and certainly in relation to head injury.[13, 14]

HISTORY AND EXAMINATION

A detailed present and past history is essential even though the diagnosis of head injury seems obvious. Obviously, it is important in management to know that the unconscious child also may suffer from drug allergies, hemophilia, diabetes mellitus, or epilepsy, but it is surprising how frequently historical data germane to the problem are missed on the initial assessment of the patient.

Similarly, a precise knowledge of the details immediately surrounding the injury may help the examiner to interpret the significance of the injury. For example, if the child stumbles while running and strikes his head on the pavement, it is reasonable to assume that the resulting neurologic syndrome is the direct result of the injury. On the other hand if a child crumples to the ground and, in doing so strikes his head on the pavement, one would have to consider seriously why he fell and then search for predisposing factors, which could include a seizure or an intracranial hemorrhage. Similarly, if the injury is minor and the neurologic deficit profound, aggravation by the trauma of a pre-existing, clinically compensated intracranial disease process, such as a tumor, should be considered. Over the years, numerous examples of each of these several combinations have been witnessed.

Finally, a precise understanding of the circumstances surrounding the accident often will suggest to the physician sites of additional injury, which could prove to be important if shock or sepsis develops. It is axiomatic that multiple sites of trauma, as well as the presence of coexisting disease, demand consideration in every seriously injured child. The vigilant pediatrician can serve the vital function of coordinating the efforts of several other specialists, each focusing upon a particular facet of a complex problem. Unfortunately, this rarely obtains.

Following a minor head injury, such as might occur in a fall from bed, the child commonly will exhibit a transient period of lethargy usually associated with one or more episodes of vomiting. To the inexperienced parent or physician, this sequence of events may evoke great concern and immediately bring to mind the possibility of an evolving intracranial catastrophe. In the majority of such cases, however, this concern is unrealistic, particularly when consciousness has been preserved immediately after the injury. Preservation of consciousness is best assessed by determining whether the child cried immediately after injury. Nevertheless, careful evaluation of the infant or child is mandatory before one can justifiably return him to the care of his parents, who must continue to observe him until recovery is complete. The vast majority of children who sustain minor trauma with or without a brief period of unconsciousness can be managed with the expectation that they will recover uneventfully.

With severe head injury, as may occur following a fall from a significant height or as may be associated with a vehicular accident, prompt evaluation and recognition of developing complications and treatment are essential if the outcome is to be favorable. These situations constitute true emergencies demanding a thorough understanding of the nature of the problem requiring medical or surgical therapy.

Awareness of the rapidity with which complications of acute head injury can evolve may lead to fear and uncertainty and may impede the methodic evaluation of the patient by the pediatrician. All too frequently, recently injured patients will be sent for tests such as skull radiographs before an adequate clinical evaluation has been completed. Without accurate baseline clinical information, subsequent examinations of the patient are rendered more difficult and early recognition of developing complications may be delayed. Whenever possible, serial examinations by a single observer are strongly recommended. Only in this way can subtle worsening in the neurologic status over time be appreciated. Alterations in mental status, including increased difficulty in arousing the patient and mounting agitation, almost invariably imply an extension of the basic pathologic process. Developing focal or lateralizing neurologic findings or alarming changes in the vital signs, including those detailed later, should alert the examiner to the presence of a progressive lesion. Careful serial examinations of the child's level of alertness are fatiguing not only for the examiner but also for the patient. The patient's desire to fall asleep under these circumstances is not unreasonable and should not be confused with depression of consciousness due to progressing cerebral dysfunction.

The child's level of consciousness, heart rate, blood pressure, and breathing should be assessed rapidly, with primary attention to vital circulatory and ventilatory functions. Impaired circulation, hypoxia, and hypercapnia, if not life-threatening, will all compromise cerebral functions and will tend to elevate intracranial pressure further by increasing cerebral edema and vascular volume. Rising systemic blood pressure associated with slowing of the pulse rate and irregularity of breathing (Cushing's triad) usually implies increasing intracranial pressure. Rapid pulse with marked hypotension and irregular respiration must reflect disturbed brainstem function, as occurs with occipital fractures involving the foramen magnum; these alterations may lead to fulminant pulmonary edema. The same combination of findings in an injured child always should raise the possibility of occult hemorrhage, ruptured viscus, aspiration, sepsis, or massive fat embolization.

In the young infant, bleeding into the subdural space may be of such magnitude as to lower the hematocrit significantly; in such circumstances the associated rise in intracranial pressure should produce obvious evidence of the probable site of bleeding. The signs of acute subdural hemorrhage may include vomiting, enlarging head size, full fontanelle, squint, and retinal hemorrhage. In older children, the volume of blood lost into the cranial cavity is usually insignificant.

Although the relative fixation of the cranial bones at the suture lines precludes a significant increase in head size, other signs of increased intracranial pressure (ICP) should be evident. In the absence of significant intracranial hemorrhage, the prompt increase in ICP, which all too frequently follows head trauma in children, has been related to rapidly developing cerebral swelling ("flash edema").[11] Careful assessment of the patient's responsiveness to stimuli and of pupillary size can give important additional signs of such an increase in pressure. Surprisingly, perhaps, the significance of pupillary changes, always stressed in the evaluation of raised ICP, is incompletely understood by physicians. A dilated pupil, poorly reactive or unreactive to light, most often indicates compression of the third nerve on that side by the herniating mesial portion of the temporal lobe through the incisura of the tentorium, caused by increased pressure.[1, 14] Whereas this may be due to cerebral edema as well as to intracranial hematoma, the latter surgically remediable lesion should be kept foremost in mind, and appropriate contrast studies (computerized axial tomography [CAT scan]) should be performed to verify its presence.

This pupillary finding often is accompanied by paresis of the oculomotor nerve on the same side and contralateral, ipsilateral, or bilateral body weakness or intermittent decerebrate posturing.

It is important to be certain that no mydriatic preparation has been instilled into the conjunctival sac before concluding that the preceding circumstances apply. In general, mydriatic drugs should be avoided; but if it is administered, a sign should be placed on the patient's bed and on his or her chart to make this fact clear to all those involved in his or her care. The dilation of one pupil also may occur during a seizure.[15] Conjugate jerking of the eyes away from the side of the seizure discharge often accompanies the pupillary dilation, which may occur on either the contralateral or ipsilateral side. The intravenous administration of an anticonvulsant, such as diazepam (Valium), may result in prompt equalization of pupillary size, cessation of the ocular jerking, and return to consciousness of the patient. Direct injury to the eye or to the second or third cranial nerve also may result in a dilated and poorly reactive pupil.

Bleeding into the subarachnoid or subdural space may be suggested by retinal or preretinal hemorrhages. These hemorrhages usually develop in the presence of a marked rise in intracranial pressure and may be coupled with venous distention and early signs of papilledema. Well-developed papilledema usually is not seen during the first hours or days of injury. When it is, an associated but unrelated cerebral lesion, e.g., a brain tumor, must be considered. Spontaneous pulsations of the retinal veins usually reflect normal intracranial pressure, particularly if the systemic blood pressure is not elevated, and may be a reassuring finding in the child with head injury.

SPECIAL TESTS

After a thorough clinical evaluation, skull x-rays and other roentgenograms usually are indicated, especially if the patient lost consciousness following the injury. If hyperextension or flexion injury to the cervical spine is a consideration, appropriate x-ray films of this region should be obtained. Cervical cord injury is not uncommon following severe, blunt head injury and should be considered even in the absence of recognizable spinal fracture. CAT scanning of the cervical spine may reveal disease not visualized on plain cervical spine films. In fact, cranial and cervical spine CAT scanning often obviates the need for skull or cervical spine x-ray films in most instances.

In the infant or young child, paracentesis of the subdural spaces through the coronal suture may establish the presence of an extracerebral clot. Acute epidural or subdural hemorrhages are not associated with increased transillumination; rather, there is usually less of a glow about the rim of the light in such circumstances. Only when the subdural hematoma undergoes dissolution and the fluid becomes less turbid, and eventually xanthochromic, is excessive transillumination found.

Electroencephalography is not particularly helpful as an emergency procedure but may become so in the immediate period after head injury to define a focal destructive lesion or seizure activity, thus confirming or supplementing the clinical impression and assisting in the design of appropriate therapy. Echoencephalography (the recording of an ultrasonic echo from the interface of intracerebral structures normally midline), considered by some to be useful in the management of head injury, has been of limited value in our experience. Isotopic scan techniques similarly have contributed relatively little to diagnosis. Lumbar puncture is inadvisable as a routine procedure following craniocerebral injury but may be necessary when the diagnosis is obscure and should be performed if intracranial sepsis, especially meningitis, is a serious diagnostic consideration, as noted earlier. Cerebral angiography may contribute much to diagnosis and management. In particular, extracerebral and intracerebral hemorrhages may be outlined by this technique or, equally important, their presence rendered unlikely. Also, damage to the extracranial portions of the major blood vessels may be visualized during these studies. Special tests must be performed by physicians experienced in their use.

Computerized tomography has contributed enormously to the accuracy of neurologic diagnosis.[16] When it is available, the need for other diagnostic procedures frequently is obviated. CAT scanning is non-invasive and can be repeated serially to reassess intracranial relationships, particularly in the patient who remains comatose or who exhibits further neurologic deterioration. This technique permits identification of hemorrhage and cerebral edema and clearly outlines the ventricular cavities.

MANAGEMENT

The majority of infants and children who have not lost consciousness following head injury can be cared for by their parents, after a careful examination satisfies the physician that no serious intracranial disease exists. The decision regarding skull roentgenograms must be individualized. Most patients with minor head injuries do not require skull x-rays.[29] Palpation of the scalp may reveal an area of tenderness or crepitance overlying a fracture and skull films may confirm this clinical suspicion. Approximately one-third of young children with mild head injuries have linear skull fractures.[1, 29] However, this radiographic finding *per se* is not an indication for hospitalization. A second skull film should be obtained in three to six months to document healing of a demonstrated fracture of the cranial vault.

Patients who have focal or diffuse neurologic disturbances and all those who have been rendered unconscious, with or without an associated skull fracture, should be hospitalized until their condition is stable and the neurologic signs abate. Cranial CAT scanning should be performed to further define intracranial disease in all patients who are seriously injured or continue to demonstrate neurologic symptomatology for longer than 12 hours.

In the obtunded or comatose patient, intravenous fluids may be necessary, particularly if vomiting persists. Maintenance fluids of a balanced electrolyte solution such as 5 per cent dextrose and Isolyte-M should be restricted to 1000–1200 ml/m^2 body surface/day. This solution, although hypotonic after metabolism of the glucose, has proved to be safe if the volume administered is monitored carefully. The primary purpose of restricting fluids is to avoid hypotonicity, which will aggravate brain swelling so common after trauma. Accurate recording of fluid intake and output, daily weight, and serum osmolality (the serum sodium level in mEq/L $\times$ 2 plus 10 approximates the osmolality) should be monitored closely. When non-ionic solutes such as glucose and mannitol have been administered, the serum sodium level does not accurately reflect the osmolality, and the determination of serum osmolalities is essential. These data are absolutely necessary to avoid weight gain from water retention, excessive dehydration, and states of hypotonicity or hypertonicity. Hypertonicity also may occur when injury to the hypothalamus or pituitary stalk has produced diabetes insipidus. As stated earlier, this is usually a transient disorder. Sedatives and hypnotics should be avoided, although persistent vomiting may be treated with an appropriate antiemetic such as trimethobenzamide hydrochloride (Tigan).

Certain problems will require further consideration by a neurosurgeon. With skull fracture, rhinorrhea persists more commonly as a clinical problem than does otorrhea and may require surgical repair of the anatomic defect. Of course, the risk of intracranial infection remains as long as the defect exists. Depressed fractures should be referred to the neurosurgeon for possible elevation. Compound fractures require prompt surgical treatment, with debridement and removal of bone fragments, hair, and other foreign material that predisposes to intracranial infection.

When serial examinations suggest that the intracranial pressure is rising significantly, various measures to minimize this complication should be employed. Glucocorticoids, hyperosmolar agents, and assisted ventilation may help forestall herniation of cerebral tissue at either the tentorial opening or the foramen magnum.

Dexamethasone (Decadron) is the glucocorticoid most commonly used. It is administered usually in a dosage of 10 to 12 mg/m^2 of body surface area per day in four divided doses intramuscularly.[17, 18] Half of the first day's dose usually is given in the initial injection. Evidence suggests that glucocorticoids act primarily on the normal brain tissue to prevent cellular decompensation and increasing cerebral edema.[14, 19] Recently, some investigators have advocated "megadoses" of dexamethasone approximating 100 mg/m^2 body surface/day. There is little evidence to substantiate this recommendation, however.

Hyperosmolar agents are used to develop a transient osmotic gradient between the blood and the brain that will cause water to move from the brain tissues into the blood. Water moves from other cells as well, and the result is an expanded extracellular (including the vascular) space. Under usual circumstances, the solute and water are excreted by the kidneys. Mannitol, readily available for intravenous infusion as a 20 per cent solution (Osmitrol), contains 1.1 mOsm/ml. To increase the serum osmolality approximately 10 to 20 mOsm/L, it is given in a dose of 1 to 2 gm/kg. Smaller doses (0.25 gm/kg) may be given intravenously and may be preferable if the intracranial pressure is being monitored continuously (see later discussion). Intravenous infusion time should be 5 to 40 minutes with mannitol doses ranging from 0.25 to 2.0 gm/kg. Too rapid a rate of infusion of mannitol may produce a sudden increase in the intravascular volume with resulting cardiac decompensation. Following infusion of a hyperosmolar solution, a brisk diuresis develops, and catheterization of the bladder is necessary to prevent acute urinary retention in the unconscious patient.

Mannitol is most effective when the integrity of cerebral blood vessels has been maintained. This agent normally passes through these vessels into the cerebral tissue, but only to a small extent; after clearance by the kidneys, the resulting higher osmolality of the cerebral tissue draws water back into the brain, transiently increasing the intracranial pressure—the so-called rebound phenomenon. Risk of this phenomenon is increased in extensive injury to cerebral blood vessels, in which hyperosmolar solutions may pass more readily from the intravascular compartment into surrounding brain tissue.

The technique of assisted ventilation also can reduce the intracranial pressure transiently by producing cerebral vasoconstriction, thereby decreasing the size of the vascular compartment. Through this mechanism of action, brain perfusion is reduced, together with the intracranial pressure, which could accentuate the injury to brain tissue by enhancing the cerebral ischemia and resulting tissue anoxia.

Barbiturates are now used in the management of increased intracranial pressure, and their mechanism of action is partly understood. A reduction of the cerebral metabolic rate by 40 to 50 per cent has been demonstrated experimentally with serum concentrations of 30 to 50 μg/ml. Vasoconstriction also occurs, and like hyperventilation, it reduces the volume of the vascular compartment, thereby lowering the intracranial pressure. Barbiturates, however, have a negative inotropic effect on the myocardium. As a result, the decrease in intracranial pressure associated with the administration of pentobarbital (the most commonly used barbiturate under these circumstances) may be paralleled by a lessening of the cerebral perfusion pressure. The net benefit, therefore, may be diminished, and we have reservations regarding the utility of this treatment, especially since these drugs depress consciousness, making evaluation of the patient's progress more difficult.

However, when the clinical situation dictates emergency treatment—and action cannot be delayed while the precise nature or extent of the intracranial pathology is delineated—it is justified to utilize such temporizing maneuvers, despite the theoretical limitations of each method, until additional studies can be performed to define surgically remediable lesions. Extracerebral and intracerebral hematomas can be evacuated with very gratifying results. Unfortunately, there is no generally accepted surgical treatment for extensive contusion or laceration of brain substance or for cerebral edema.

Continuous monitoring of ICP has become a valuable technique in managing patients with cerebral edema resulting from head injury.[20, 21] It allows the physician to intercept elevations in intracranial pressure before further neurologic deterioration becomes manifest clinically. Uncontrolled elevation in ICP eventually compromises cerebral perfusion, in turn intensifying the edema and the probability of brain herniation. The outcome in any given case is the summation of the "primary" injury at the time of the accident and the delayed or "secondary" injury, which occurs in the immediate post-traumatic period. Vigorous control of brain edema to minimize ischemia and hypoxia appears crucial in attenuating the magnitude of the "secondary" injury. The ICP can be monitored by placing a sensing mechanism either in the lateral ventricle, subdural (subarachnoid) space, or extradural space. The ventricular catheter also permits the removal of CSF when the intracranial pressure is elevated. The choice of sites remains a local bias, each with its own virtues and disadvantages.

Other proposed adjuncts to treatment include the lowering of the body temperature to decrease the metabolic requirements of compromised cerebral tissue and the use of anticonvulsants. Hypothermia, to be truly effective in this regard, would require lowering of the body core temperature to 90 to 92°F, a level usually resulting in violent shivering and heightened metabolic activity that nullify the advantage sought in the treatment. Drugs such as promethazine hydrochloride (Phenergan) and chlorpromazine (Thorazine) will eliminate the shivering reflex but frequently will depress the level of consciousness and further accentuate any hypotensive tendency. Furthermore, at these low body temperatures, one can expect increasing cardiac irritability with the possibility of a serious arrhythmia. We therefore strive simply to keep the patient afebrile.

Although anticonvulsants probably do not lessen the liability to post-traumatic epilepsy, we advocate their use in severe head injury in which cerebral contusion or laceration is suspected, because of the impression that such therapy minimizes the occurrence of seizures during the immediate postinjury period. Either phenytoin (Dilantin) at a dosage of 5 mg/kg/day or phenobarbital at 4 mg/kg/day is an acceptable treatment, although the former is less likely to obtund the patient. Phenytoin should be administered intravenously for optimal effect. Phenobarbital may be administered either intravenously or intramuscularly.

PROGNOSIS

Children as a group demonstrate a remarkable capacity for recovery, even when substantial neurologic disturbances follow acute head injury. In general, the total duration of post-traumatic amnesia can be correlated directly with the degree of brain damage and, as Smith[22] has concluded, with the ultimate prognosis. The long-term effects of severe closed head injury and protracted coma have been summarized by Richardson.[23] He evaluated 10 children who were comatose for 7 to 47 days following severe head injury, with post-traumatic amnesia ranging from 25 to 65 days. All were rehabilitated and returned to school despite substantial residual neurologic and psychological deficits. Persisting specific defects in rote memory were demonstrated in most of these children on formal psychometric testing. Dencker[24] examined 117 head-injured children in a larger and less severely injured group, ten years following the acute injury, and as a control their uninjured twins; he failed to demonstrate any differences in the psychometric scores, range of symptoms, electroencephalograms, and personality integration. This study further substantiates the capacity of the young child to recover after significant closed craniocerebral injury.

This capacity for functional recovery must be remembered when evaluating any program of physical rehabilitation. Many sophisticated programs have been credited with the quality and quantity of recovery in the injured child and, as such, have unjustifiably increased the total financial expense incurred by parents. Yet there is no evidence that elaborate and time-consuming programs of physiotherapy offer any more than do simple passive and active range of motion exercises to minimize joint contractures and maintain muscle tone and strength.

The possibility of post-traumatic epilepsy is largely dependent on the site of injury. Certain areas of the brain, when damaged, give rise to epileptogenic foci more frequently than do others. The most vulnerable areas include the cortices of the medial temporal, posterior frontal, and anterior parietal lobes. In the given case the site of injury appears to be more important in the etiology of post-traumatic epilepsy than does an underlying genetic predisposition.[25] The incidence of post-traumatic epilepsy following closed head injury is probably 5 per cent or less. Patients with evidence of significant contusions or lacerations are especially prone to this complication. Those suffering from seizures at or shortly after injury may be more likely to develop post-traumatic epilepsy than those who have sustained comparable lesions without fits during the immediately post-traumatic period. Jennett and colleagues[26] have enumerated several determinants of post-traumatic epilepsy, which include seizures within the first week after injury, compound-depressed skull fractures, tearing of the dura mater, and post-traumatic amnesia exceeding 24 hours. Approximately 50 per cent of their patients destined to suffer post-traumatic epilepsy developed seizures within the first year after the accident.

Electroencephalography (EEG) is of little help in anticipating which children ultimately will develop a seizure disorder. Though many EEG recordings are focally or diffusely disordered and may show epileptiform activity during the immediate postinjury period, serial tracings usually show a gradual return toward a more normal pattern. Occasionally, an abnormal EEG with some epileptiform activity persists in a clinically asymptomatic patient; conversely, a large percentage of patients with post-traumatic epilepsy demonstrate a relatively normal EEG between seizures.

Chronic subdural effusions represent a major problem because of the lack of any uniformly effective treatment. Diagnostically, such a lesion may be suspected in a child whose head is increasing too rapidly in circumference, particularly if the contour is brachycephalic and transillumination shows a marked increase in the glow of light. The outcome in such cases appears to correlate primarily with the extent of damage sustained by the underlying cerebral substance during the acute head injury.[27] This realization, coupled with the knowledge that the efficacy of all forms of treatment remains unproven, encourages us to be conservative in

Table 10–2. TREATMENT #1—SEIZURE CONTROL

Drug	Dosage	Maintenance
Diazepam	0.2–0.3 mg/kg IV. Repeat ×2 q5–10 minutes prn.	None (immediately add phenytoin)
Phenytoin	10 mg/kg IV over 20 minutes. Repeat ×2 prn if seizures persist.	5–10 mg/kg/day IV in two divided doses. Maintain serum concentration of 15–20 μg/ml. Administer 3rd drug if seizures persist.
Phenobarbital	10 mg/kg IV. Repeat ×2 prn if seizures persist.	4–6 mg/kg/day IV in two divided doses. Maintain serum concentration of 30–50 μg/ml. Administer 4th drug if seizures persist.
Acetazolamide	10 mg/kg IV. Repeat ×2 prn if seizures persist.	30 mg/kg/day IV in three divided doses. Observe electrolytes for ↓ potassium and ↓ pH. Administer 5th drug if seizures persist.
Paraldehyde	4% solution IV at a rate sufficient to control seizures.	Taper rate prn to assess need—protect from light to avoid decomposition. Avoid plastic tubing.

our approach and to attempt only to lessen disproportionate increases in head size by periodic paracentesis.

Enlarging skull fractures associated with leptomeningeal cysts or erosion of the skull occur in a small minority of children who have suffered acute head injury. Taveras and Ransohoff[28] have suggested that rupture of the dura mater during the acute injury, with herniation of the arachnoid membrane into the fracture line, produces this condition. Aided by the normal pulsations of the brain, this entrapped arachnoidal hernia gradually erodes the edge of the bone and also may compress the underlying cerebral cortex.

Much of the management of the patient with acute head injury has been arrived at empirically, and many of the clinical regimens suggested, including the choice and dose of various therapeutic agents, are arbitrary (Tables 10–2, 10–3, and 10–4). Ritualistic adherence to any particular program will serve only to perpetuate our state of ignorance and preclude further clarification of the problems that attend head injury. Unfortunately, the cerebral insults that produce irreversible brain damage

Table 10–3. TREATMENT #2—INCREASED INTRACRANIAL PRESSURE (> 25 mm Hg)

Modality	Objective
Head in neutral position at 30 degrees of elevation	Facilitation of venous drainage from head.
Hyperventilation	Reduce Pa_{CO_2} to 20–25 mmHg.
Mannitol (20%)	0.2–2.0 mg/kg IV over 5–20 minutes. Repeat prn for ICP > 25 mmHg.
Dexamethasone	0.1–1.0 mg/kg IV every 6 hours.
Pentobarbital	1–3 mg/kg IV every 2–4 hours (maintain serum concentration of 30–50 μg/ml).
Surgical decompression	Usually advised only if there is a unilateral mass effect with impending herniation of uncus.

Table 10–4. GENERAL ASSESSMENT IN THE DIAGNOSIS AND MANAGEMENT OF HEAD INJURY (IF CONSCIOUSNESS IMPAIRED)

1. Secure airway
   a. Insure patency
   b. Intubate if necessary
   c. Ventilatory assistance as indicated
   d. Suction gently
2. Elevate head 20–30 degrees, stabilize head and neck in neutral position
3. Establish arterial and venous access routes for blood sampling, fluid, and drug administration
4. Ensure adequate circulation—isotonic volume expansion and vasoactive drugs if necessary to preserve cerebral perfusion
5. Nasogastric tube—intermittent suction to avoid aspiration
6. Urinary catheter
7. IV fluids—isotonic with 5% dextrose at 1000–1200 ml/m^2/day
8. Control seizures if necessary (see Table 10–2)
9. Evaluate for systemic injury
10. Monitor vital signs frequently

ALGORITHM FOR THE DIAGNOSIS AND MANAGEMENT OF HEAD INJURY

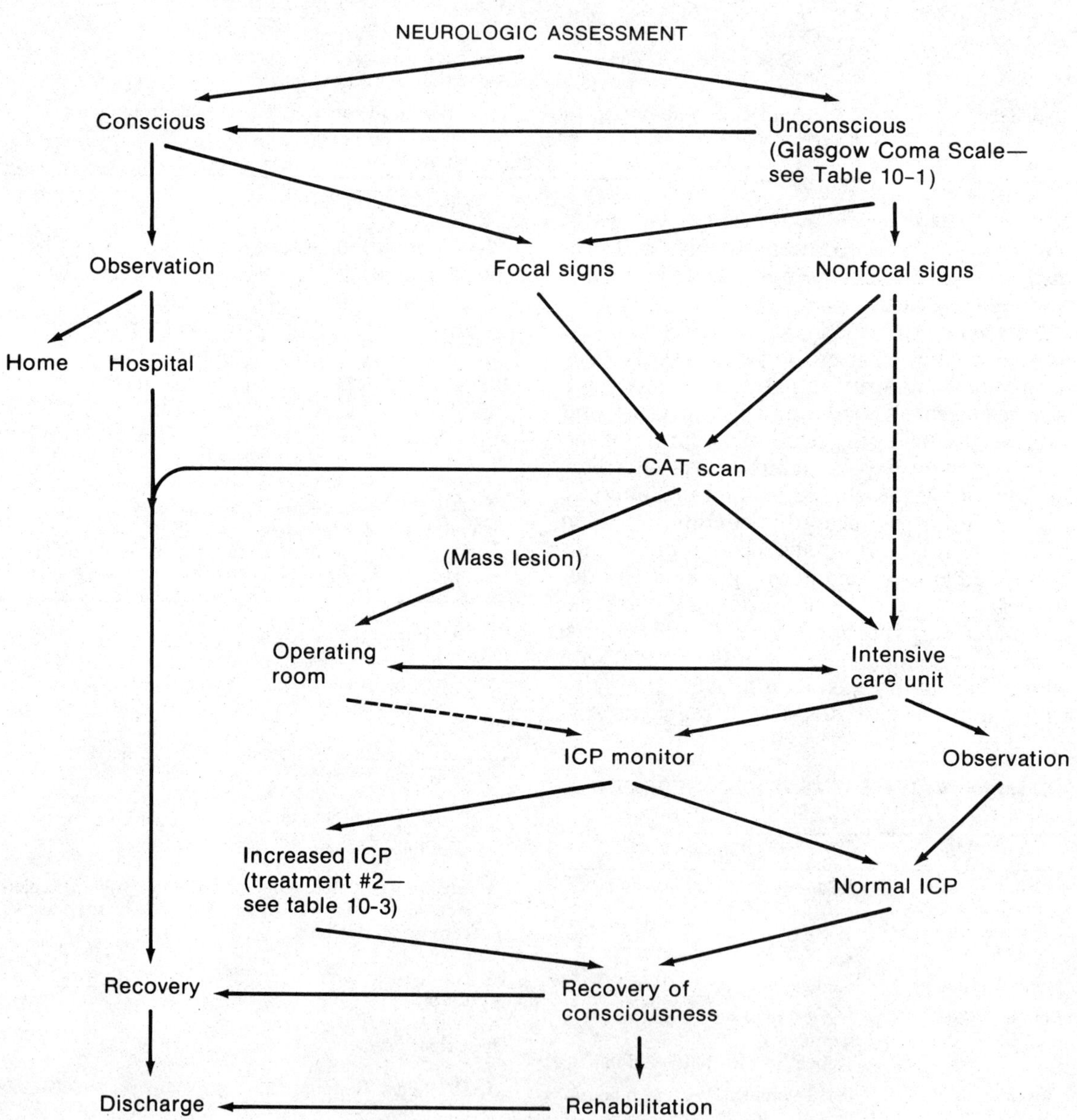

often have occurred before medical assistance is available. Much of the treatment we have outlined, therefore, is directed at the consequences of the primary brain insult rather than at the fundamental injury *per se*. As a result, the outcome in any given case may be determined in large part before effective medical care can be provided. Meticulous care and realistic goals are important elements in the management of infants and children with severe head injuries.

REFERENCES

1. Mealey J Jr. Pediatric Head Injuries. Springfield, Ill.: Charles C Thomas, 1968.
2. Denny–Brown D, Russell WR. Experimental cerebral concussion. Brain 1941; *64*:93.
3. Strich SJ. Shearing of nerve fibers as a cause of brain damage due to head injury. A pathological study of twenty cases. Lancet 1961; *2*:443.
4. Symonds CP. The differential diagnosis and treatment of cerebral states consequent upon head injuries. Br Med J 1928; *4*:829–832.
5. Teasdale G, Jennett B. Assessment and prognosis of coma after head injury. Acta Neurochir 1976; *34*:45–55.
6. Dodge PR. Tangential Wounds of Scalp and Skull. *In*: Heaton LD, Coates JB Jr, Meirowsky AM. eds. Neurological Surgery of Trauma. Washington DC, US Government Printing Office, 1965; 143–159.
7. Friede RL. Experimental acceleration concussion. Arch Neurol 1961; *4*:449.
8. Friede RL. Specific cord damage at the atlas level as a pathogenic mechanism in cerebral concussion. J Neuropathol Exp Neurol 1960; *29*:266.
9. Ward AA Jr. The Physiology of Concussion. *In*: Caveness WF, Walker AE. eds. Head Injury: Conference Proceedings. Philadelphia: JB Lippincott, 1966:203–208.
10. Griffith JF, Dodge PR. Transient blindness following head injury in children. N Engl J Med 1968; *278*:648.
11. Pickles W. Acute focal edema of the brain in children with head injuries. N Engl J Med 1949; *240*:92.
12. Klatzo I. Neuropathological aspect of brain edema. J Neuropathol Exp Neurol 1967; *26*:1.
13. Manz HJ. The pathology of cerebral edema. Hum Pathol 1974; *5*:291.
14. Fishman RA. Cerebrospinal Fluid in Diseases of the Nervous System. Philadelphia: WB Saunders Co, 1980.
15. Pant SS, Benton JW, Dodge PR. Unilateral pupillary dilatation during and immediately following seizures. Neurology 1966; *16*:837.
16. Hammock MK, Milhorat TH. Cranial Computed Tomography in Infancy and Childhood. Baltimore: Williams & Wilkins, 1981.
17. Sparacio RR, Lin TH, Cook AW. Methylprednisolone sodium succinate in acute craniocerebral trauma. Surg Gynecol Obstet 1965; *121*:513.
18. Long DM, Hartmann JF, French LA. The response of experimental cerebral edema to glucosteroid administration. J Neurosurg 1966; *24*:843.
19. McLaurin RL. Some Metabolic Aspects of Head Injury. *In*: Caveness WF, Walker AE, eds. Head Injury: Conference Proceedings, Philadelphia: JB Lippincott, 1966:142–157.
20. Lundberg N. Continuous recording and control of ventricular fluid pressure in neuro-surgical practice. Acta Psychiatr Neurol Scand (Suppl) 1960; *149*:1.
21. Miller JD, Becker DP, Ward JD, et al. Significance of intracranial hypertension in severe head injury. J Neurosurg 1977; *47*:501–516.
22. Smith A. Duration of impaired consciousness as an index of severity in closed head injuries. Dis Nerv Syst 1961; *22*:69.
23. Richardson F. Some effects of severe head injury. A follow-up study of children and adolescents after protracted coma. Dev Med Child Neurol 1963; *5*:471.
24. Dencker SJ. Closed head injury in twins. Arch Gen Psychiatry 1960; *2*:569.
25. Marshall C, Walker AE. The value of electroencephalography in the prognostification and prognosis of post-traumatic epilepsy. Epilepsia 1961; *2*:138.
26. Jennett R, Teather D, Bennie S. Epilepsy after head injury. Lancet 1961; *2*:138.
27. Rabe EF, Flynn RE, Dodge PR. Subdural collection of fluid in infants and children. Neurology 1968; *18*:559.
28. Taveras JM, Ransohoff J. Leptomeningeal cysts of the brain following trauma with erosion of the skull: a study of 7 cases treated by surgery. J Neurosurg 1953; *10*:233.
29. Burkinshaw J. Head injuries in children. Arch Dis Child 1960; *35*:205–214.

CHAPTER

11

The Bleeding Child

George R. Buchanan, M.D.

One of the most alarming experiences for parent and pediatrician alike is a child who is hemorrhaging. Coping with the acutely bleeding child is one of the most common hematologic emergencies in pediatric practice. A limited number of pathophysiologic mechanisms of excessive hemorrhage exist in infants and children, and differential diagnosis and management are quite straightforward in most cases. Usually, a brief history, physical examination (focusing on the presence or absence of underlying disease), and screening laboratory evaluation provide a specific diagnosis. Treatment, when necessary, then can be instituted rapidly. Many acute bleeding disorders in children are self-limiting, and others require only minimal intervention because the subsequent clinical course often depends upon the underlying disease (trauma, shock, sepsis, and malignancy) rather than the bleeding itself. The following discussion will focus on some of these issues in greater detail.

PATHOPHYSIOLOGY

Hemostasis, the process that prevents excessive hemorrhage following minor trauma, involves a complex interaction among three elements: blood vessels, platelets, and plasma proteins.[1–3] Failure or deficiency of one or more of these hemostatic bulwarks results in a tendency to bleed, a state that contrasts with overactivity of the hemostatic mechanism which results in thrombosis. The problems of thrombosis and thromboembolism are not discussed because they are far more relevant in adult patients.

Blood Vessels

The first line of defense against hemorrhaging is the blood vessel itself, particularly the endothelial layer of its wall, the subendothelial connective tissue, and the supporting structures. When large blood vessels are injured following major trauma or during or after a surgical procedure, excessive hemorrhage may result, and its cause is usually readily apparent. Compensatory mechanisms such as vasoconstriction and divergence of blood flow to more vital parts of the circulation usually intervene. Hemorrhage from smaller vessels—arterioles, venules, and capillaries—is often less obvious. Minor injuries to such vessels probably occur constantly in the normal individual. In children whose microvasculature has been damaged by antigen-antibody complexes, hypoxia, or toxins, vasculitis is a common result and purpuric lesions may become evident. However, gross external hemorrhage from diffuse small blood vessel injury is quite common.

Platelets

The next line of defense is the circulating blood platelet, the major function of which is to form hemostatic plugs in small blood vessels at sites of endothelial injury.[4] Under the light microscope, platelets are minute, nondescript granular fragments. However, electron microscopic examination reveals these cells to be highly complex packages of diverse secretory granules, microtubules, mitochondria, and irregular membrane-bound vesicles. The sequential series of reactions undertaken by platelets during the process of primary hemostasis is demonstrated in Figure 11–1.

Platelet adhesion, the sticking of platelets to a non-platelet surface, is the initial step following endothelial injury. Glycoprotein receptors in the platelet membrane recognize and bind to collagen, basement membrane, and other subendothelial connective tissue proteins. This interaction requires the presence of a plasma factor that has been named von Willebrand

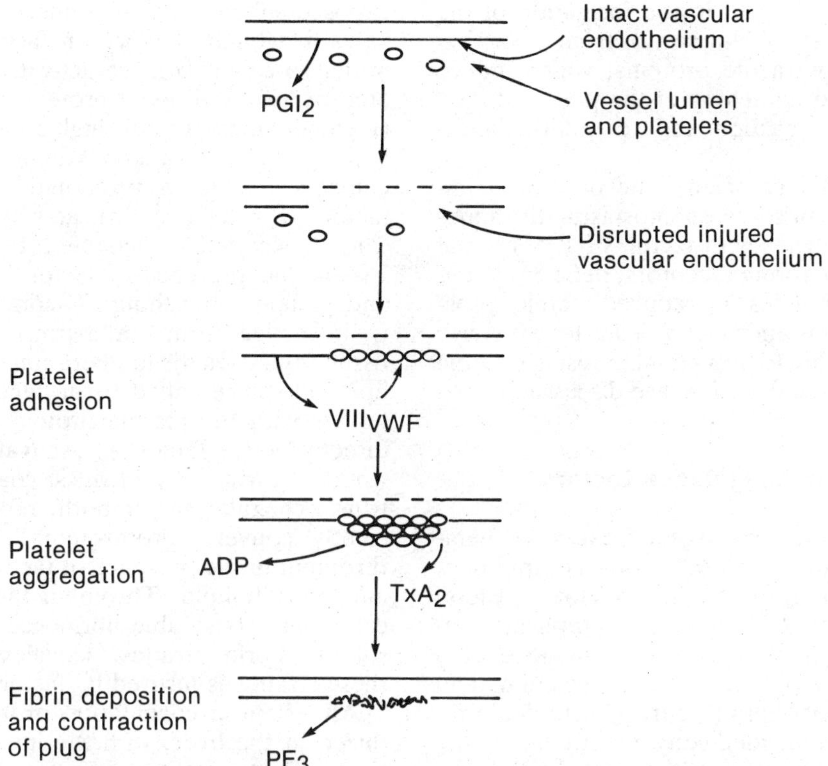

Figure 11–1. Platelet plug formation. This figure illustrates the sequential reactions taken by platelets when they are exposed to damaged vascular subendothelium. Endothelial cells normally secrete the antithrombotic substance prostacyclin (PGI_2), which prevents platelet activation. Following vascular injury, platelet adhesion, a process that requires the presence of factor VIII von Willebrand factor (VIII_{VWF}), occurs rapidly. Platelet adhesion is followed by primary and then secondary aggregation, accompanied by the platelet release reaction, in which the platelet secretes ADP from its dense granules and generates thromboxane A_2 (TxA_2), both of which recruit more platelets into the expanding hemostatic plug. Finally, platelet factor 3 (PF_3), a phospholipid intrinsic to platelet membranes, accelerates the blood coagulation mechanism, promoting the deposition of fibrin strands within the platelet plug. Contractile proteins then retract the plug and complete healing of the injury follows.

factor or ristocetin cofactor. This high-molecular-weight glycoprotein is part of the factor VIII complex and is synthesized in endothelial cells. It can be measured immunologically as well as assayed functionally using the antibiotic ristocetin.

Platelet adhesion is followed by *platelet aggregation,* which is defined as the sticking of platelets to one another (see Fig. 11–1). Aggregation occurs in two steps, primary and secondary. Primary aggregation is a rapidly reversible process in which platelets form small clumps. In secondary aggregation large numbers of platelets irreversibly bind to form an amorphous insoluble plug that usually stops the hemorrhage. Secondary aggregation is accompanied by internalization and then by rapid secretion of the platelets' granular contents, including adenosine diphosphate (ADP), calcium, and 5-hydroxytryptamine (serotonin). ADP induces still more platelet aggregation, so that a chain reaction of platelet aggregation, ADP release, and additional platelet aggregation is initiated. Granular secretion is accompanied by release of arachidonic acid from platelet membranes and its conversion by the enzyme cyclooxygenase to certain labile prostaglandin intermediates. These substances are the precursors of thromboxane A_2, the body's most potent vasoconstrictor and platelet aggregating substance. Thromboxane A_2 diffuses from the platelet and within seconds recruits still more platelets into the expanding hemostatic plug.[4]

Platelet adhesion and aggregation are accompanied by localized activation of blood coagulation, a process accelerated by platelet factor 3, a phospholipid complex in platelet membranes. Fibrin strands are thus deposited amid the mass of aggregating platelets. Some stimuli, thrombin in particular, induce simultaneous platelet aggregation and fibrin generation. The final event in the formation of the platelet hemostatic plug results from the action of platelet contractile proteins, which induce retraction and tightening of the plug and then a fibroblastic reaction and re-endothelialization.

An abnormality of any one of these components of primary hemostasis—thrombocytopenia, deficiency of factor VIII, abnormal platelet glycoprotein receptors, deficient platelet storage granules, or reduced platelet prostaglandin generation—can lead to excessive hemorrhage due to impaired hemostasis. Some of these specific disorders are discussed later.

Blood Coagulation Factors

The major defense against excessive hemorrhage from large blood vessels is rapid deposition of an insoluble fibrin clot.[1–3] Blood coagulation occurs following a complicated series of sequential reactions involving over a dozen soluble plasma proteins, calcium, and platelet phospholipid (Figure 11–2). These reactions can be divided conveniently but somewhat artificially into *intrinsic* and *extrinsic* coagulation systems. Intrinsic blood coagulation begins following endothelial cell injury, when

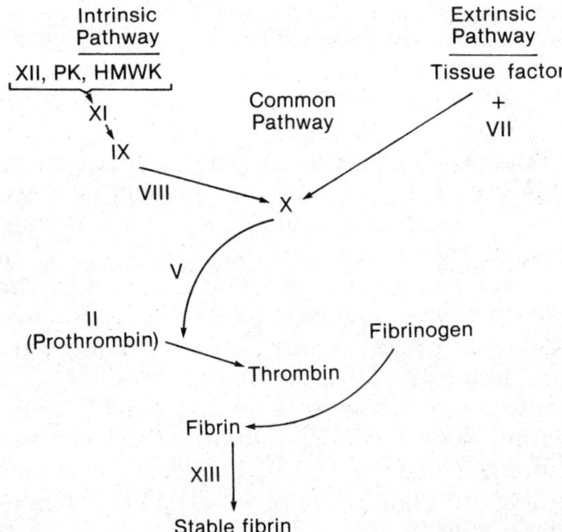

Figure 11–2. Blood coagulation mechanism. This figure illustrates a simplified version of the reactions of proteins involved in blood coagulation. Activated forms of the clotting factors, other than thrombin, and the necessary cofactors (calcium, phospholipid, etc.) are not shown. The partial thromboplastin time (PTT) is the screening test of the intrinsic system and prothrombin time (PT) screens the extrinsic system. PK = prekallikrein; HMWK = high-molecular-weight kininogen.

exposed subendothelial connective tissue activates Hageman factor, or factor XII. This initial so-called contact activation is accelerated by two additional proteins, prekallikrein (Fletcher factor) and high-molecular-weight kininogen (Fitzgerald or Williams factor). This complex results in proteolytic activation of factor XI, which in turn activates factor IX. The enzymatically activated form of factor IX—in the presence of factor VIII, calcium, and platelet phospholipid—converts factor X to its active form. In extrinsic coagulation, tissue injury results in liberation of a phospholipid substance called tissue factor, which interacts with the plasma protein factor VII to directly active factor X. Activated factor X, whether formed by intrinsic coagulation, extrinsic coagulation, or both, rapidly and efficiently converts prothrombin (factor II) to thrombin in the presence of factor V, calcium, and phospholipid. Thrombin then proteolytically converts soluble fibrinogen to friable insoluble fibrin strands. Covalent linkage of these strands is insured by factor XIII.

All of these coagulation proteins are produced in the liver, with the important exception of factor VIII.[2, 3, 5] Factors II (prothrombin), VII, IX, and X are synthesized as inactive precursors, which are then rendered functional within hepatic microsomes in a reaction requiring vitamin K. Work in several laboratories has recently shown that vitamin K promotes carboxylation of glutamic acid residues in these proteins, thus allowing for the calcium binding that is required for their participation in phospholipid-mediated reactions.[5]

Both intrinsic and extrinsic pathways are necessary *in vivo,* as evidenced by the presence of a hemorrhagic disorder unless both are intact. The relatively slow reactions in the contact activation pathway (involving factors XII, XI, prekallikrein, and high-molecular-weight kininogen) account for the greater duration of fibrin formation via the intrinsic pathway as compared with the extrinsic system. These slow reactions in part account for the fact that the partial thromboplastin time (PTT) is normally longer than the prothrombin time (PT) (to be discussed).

Deficiencies of contact factors usually result in no or only minimal hemorrhage, perhaps owing to the fact that their reactions can be bypassed *in vivo* by means of direct activation of factor IX by factor VII in the extrinsic pathway.[2, 3] However, deficiencies of most other coagulation factors to levels less than approximately 25 to 35 per cent of normal result in a tendency to bleed owing to impairment or delay in fibrin clot formation. These various congenital and acquired disorders, as they relate to acute bleeding emergencies, will be discussed.

Fibrinolysis and Other Protective Measures Against Excessive Thrombosis

Fibrin-clot formation must be counterbalanced by disolving or removing these clots in order to avoid tissue injury from vaso-occlusion.[2, 3] This task is carried out efficiently by the process of fibrinolysis, in which the enzyme plasmin, formed from the inactive precursor plasminogen, digests fibrin and fibrinogen into non-functional soluble fragments that are rapidly excreted in the urine or degraded by the reticuloendothelial system. Other key protective mechanisms against excessive blood coagulations are protein C and circulating antithrombin III, a protease inhibitor that inactivates thrombin, activated factor X, and other serine proteases. The acceleration of these reactions by heparin is discussed later.

Screening Laboratory Evaluation of Bleeding Disorders

Simple laboratory tests allow for evaluation of platelet numbers and function as well as the integrity of the blood coagulation cascade (Table 11–1). Laboratory procedures that evaluate blood vessel function are non-specific and imprecise.

Platelets can be enumerated by phase microscopy, by electronic cell counting, or by a glance at the peripheral blood smear. This last exercise can be extremely useful because the cause of a child's bleeding can often be ascertained at the same time as the platelet count estimation. Each platelet per oil-immersion field represents a count of approximately 20,000/mm.[3] Therefore, if the average number of platelets in a large number of randomly chosen fields is 4, the patient's platelet count will be approximately 80,000/mm.[3] Although the normal platelet count is between 175,000 and 450,000/mm^3, thrombocytopenia is rarely the sole cause of serious hemorrhage unless the platelet count is less than 20,000/mm.[3]

The best test of platelet function is the *bleeding time* as measured by the template

Table 11–1. SCREENING LABORATORY EVALUATION OF BLEEDING DISORDERS: NORMAL RANGES AND INDICATIONS FOR ORDERING

Test	Normal Range*	Indication
Platelet count	175,000–400,000/mm^3	Patients with serious or prolonged hemorrhage from any site
Prothrombin time (PT)	11–14 seconds	
Partial thromboplastin time (PTT)	25–35 seconds†	
Bleeding time	2–8 minutes	When platelet dysfunction is suspected
Fibrinogen	150–400 mg/100 ml	Patient with acute acquired bleeding that is serious or prolonged
Fibrin degradation products (FDP)	<10 μg/ml	
Thrombin time	15–20 seconds	When fibrinogen and FDP tests are unavailable
1:1 Mix of patient's plasma + normal plasma	Correction of abnormality indicates that inhibitor is not present	When coagulation inhibitor (e.g., heparin) is suspected as a cause of bleeding or abnormal laboratory test result
Platelet adhesion		Almost never indicated; tests are extremely non-specific and/or insensitive
Tourniquet test		
Clotting time		
Clot retraction		

*Normal values for all laboratory tests vary from one institution to another. Physicians should be familiar with the method and normal ranges for each test that is ordered from their hospital laboratory .

†Values are slightly longer in normal full-term infants (usually 30–40 sec) and markedly increased in premature infants (usually 40–65 sec).

technique, in which a small superficial incision is made on the volar surface of the forearm. The test is generally performed with a disposable device that standardizes the length and depth of the incision.[7, 8] The technique in children is similar to that in adults, although several modifications have been recommended for neonates.[8] The normal range deviates slightly from one laboratory to another but is usually between two and eight minutes. The bleeding time is prolonged whenever primary hemostatic plug formation is impaired, as in thrombocytopenia, von Willebrand disease, qualitative platelet defects, and microvasculature abnormalities. In patients with thrombocytopenia, the bleeding time is inversely proportional to the platelet count, making the bleeding time a useful test of platelet function even in the thrombocytopenic patient.[9] Other tests of primary hemostasis are sometimes necessary to arrive at a specific diagnosis in a patient with a prolonged bleeding time and clinical hemorrhage. These tests are discussed later.

The screening tests of the intrinsic and extrinsic blood coagulation systems are the *partial thromboplastin time* (PTT) and the *prothrombin time* (PT), respectively. Both tests can be performed easily in almost all hospital laboratories on a small specimen of venous blood mixed with citrate anticoagulant. The physician must be familiar with the normal ranges for these tests in the local diagnostic laboratory. Comparison of the patient's value with a "control" value can be misleading; the best interpretation of the results is made when the laboratory also reports normal ranges. Values for these tests are similar in children and adults, except newborns. As a general rule, if one or more factors in the intrinsic, extrinsic, or common pathway are reduced to less than 25 to 30 per cent of normal, the PTT or the PT or both are variably prolonged. Significant hemorrhage due to reduced coagulation factors in the critically ill patient is almost always accompanied by an elevated PT, PTT, or both, making them extremely useful screening procedures.

Other Screening Tests in the Acutely Bleeding Patient

In patients with apparent acquired bleeding disorders, two other tests are also extremely helpful, namely, measurement of *fibrinogen* level and quantitation of *fibrin degradation or fibrin split products* as a means of identifying compensatory fibrinolysis. Fibrinogen, present in a far greater quantity than any other blood coagulation factor, is easily measured by numerous techniques, usually on the same specimen of blood that is submitted for the PT and PTT. Whereas the non-specific PT and PTT are abnormal in many disorders, a diminished plasma fibrinogen level is found only in disseminated intravascular coagulation, severe liver disease, and congenital afibrinogenemia. Measurement of fibrin degradation products (FDP) is performed in most laboratories by one of a variety of simple techniques using a small sample of blood added to a tube containing thrombin and a fibrinolytic inhibitor. Markedly elevated FDP levels are quite specific for disseminated intravascular coagulation. Another test performed in many diagnostic laboratories is the thrombin time, in which dilute thrombin is added to a specimen of citrated plasma. A prolonged thrombin clotting time typically either results from a low fibrinogen level or is caused by an inhibitor of the fibrinogen-fibrin conversion reaction, such as heparin or increased FDP. The test is easy to perform but not specific. As mentioned earlier, an examination of the peripheral blood smear often serves as a useful screening test in the acutely hemorrhaging patient.

Several additional tests often ordered by the physician rarely provide useful information. These tests include the *whole blood clotting* time (an extremely insensitive test of intrinsic blood coagulation), the *clot retraction test* (abnormal only in the presence of thrombocytopenia and in the extremely rare qualitative platelet defect Glanzmann thrombasthenia), and the *in vivo* measurement of *platelet adhesion.* This last test is poorly reproducible and non-physiologic, and for the diagnosis of von Willebrand disease it has been supplanted by specific measurements of factor VIII components.

Definitive Laboratory Evaluation in Patients with Suspected Congenital Bleeding Disorders

It is rarely necessary to perform coagulation factor assays or sophisticated platelet function tests in children who are critically ill with acute hemorrhage. Most patients with congenital coagulation disorders will already have been specifically diagnosed, and children with acquired bleeding problems can usually be diagnosed and treated on the basis of screening tests alone. However, occasional patients with hemophilia or von Willebrand disease will have escaped detection prior to an acute life-threatening bleeding episode, and for these children specific blood coagulation factor assays are required. In the patient with a prolonged PTT and suspected hemophilia, an assay for factor VIII (and factor IX if the former measurement is normal) is necessary.

In a child with a platelet deficiency–type of bleeding (Table 11–2), normal platelet count, and prolonged bleeding time, the differential diagnosis includes *von Willebrand disease* and a *qualitative platelet defect.* These two disorders have similar clinical features but requires vastly different forms of therapy, so a specific diagnosis is mandatory. One or more components of factor VIII are defective or reduced in von Willebrand disease. Factor VIII can be measured functionally (in a blood coagulation assay), immunologically (as factor VIII–related antigen, determined usually by quantitative electroimmunossay), and by its von Willebrand factor or ristocetin cofactor activity.[7] This last test provides a measurement of the component of factor VIII that is responsible for platelet adhesion *in vivo,* and its reduction is a common abnormality in von Willebrand disease. Other new laboratory measurements of factor VIII components (crossed immunoelectrophoresis, factor VIII procoagulant antigen, etc.) are beyond the scope of this discussion.[10, 11, 73]

Patients with qualitative platelet defects usually have abnormal platelet aggregation *in vitro* when platelet-rich plasma is incubated in the presence of ADP, epinephrine, collagen, or thrombin. These studies are performed with a device called a platelet aggregometer. Their results, however, are subject to various artifacts, and important therapeutic decisions should never be made on the basis of aggregation tracings alone.

Artifacts in Blood Coagulation Testing

The results of blood coagulation tests are only as accurate as the methods used to obtain the necessary specimens. Ideally, samples should be drawn by an atraumatic venipuncture, immediately transferred to a tube containing the proper amount of anticoagulant, and rapidly transported to the laboratory for prompt analysis. A difficult venipuncture, an incorrect blood to anticoagulant ratio, a sample from indwelling catheters previously flushed with heparin, and a delay in plasma separation and sample analysis may all result in artifacts that cause confusion in diagnosis and delay in therapy.

DIAGNOSIS AND MANAGEMENT OF SPECIFIC BLEEDING DISORDERS

The cause of acute hemorrhage can usually be made with ease following a brief but careful history, physical examination, and screening laboratory tests.[2, 3] Excessive bleeding in the critically ill child is most commonly due to transection or disruption of blood vessels secondary to a distinct anatomic lesion such as trauma or ulceration. Patients with bleeding from multiple sites usually have a generalized impairment in one or more components of the hemostatic mechanism. However, even when bleeding occurs from only a single site (massive epistaxis, gastrointestinal hemorrhage, gross hematuria, etc.), a platelet or coagulation protein deficiency may contribute to an otherwise minor local vascular lesion. Therefore, screening laboratory tests should be performed for the patient with life-threatening hemorrhage of any type.

Unfortunately, in modern medical practice we increasingly expect the laboratory to provide us with the "answer" to our diagnostic

Table 11–2. DIFFERENTIATION OF PLATELET-VASCULAR ABNORMALITY FROM COAGULATION PROTEIN DEFICIENCY BY HISTORY AND PHYSICAL EXAMINATION

	Platelet or Vascular Abnormality	Coagulation Factor Deficiency
Ecchymoses	Small and superficial	Large and deep (often palpable)
Petechiae	Frequent	Never
Mucosal hemorrhage	Frequent	Uncommon in hemophilia; frequent in acquired disorders
Muscle, joint, or internal hemorrhage	Uncommon	Frequent
Prolonged bleeding from cuts and scratches	Frequent	Rare
Bleeding with trauma or surgery	Immediate; stops with pressure	Delayed (1–2 days later); does *not* stop with pressure

and therapeutic dilemmas. *Yet for bleeding disorders the patient's history provides far more information than any laboratory test* (see Table 11–2). For example, a laboratory test result can be strikingly abnormal (e.g., markedly prolonged PTT in factor XII deficiency) in the absence of a bleeding tendency. On the other hand, in vascular disorders and in mild forms of hemophilia and von Willebrand disease, the screening laboratory test results might be normal but clinically significant impairment of hemostasis might exist.[11, 12]

It is necessary to question the child's parents about the acute episode (onset and course of bleeding, antecedent drug history, measures taken to stop the bleeding, etc.) and it is equally important to ask about prior history of bleeding, focusing on type, extent, and duration of hemorrhage and previous surgical procedures. These details regarding bleeding history provide information about the chronicity (and thus probable inherited nature) of the disorder and also shed light on its pathophysiology, e.g., whether it is a platelet-vascular deficiency or clotting protein deficiency (see Table 11–2). Similar considerations apply to the family history. Thus, from the personal and family history alone, hemophilia usually can be differentiated easily from thrombocytopenia, von Willebrand disease, and a qualitative platelet defect, and acquired defects can be separated from congenital ones.

An important aspect of the past medical history is its focus on the presence or absence of an underlying condition (liver disease, cystic fibrosis, renal disease, immunodeficiency, etc.) that might predispose the child to an acquired basis for severe hemorrhage such as vitamin K deficiency, qualitative platelet defect, and disseminated intravascular coagulation. Attention to the psychosocial history is mandatory. Child abuse frequently enters into the differential diagnosis of a seriously ill infant or young child who is covered with bruises or has intracranial hemorrhage, or both. In contrast, many parents of newly diagnosed hemophiliacs previously have been wrongfully accused of child abuse.

The PT, PTT, and platelet count should be ordered on all children with excessive or unexpected bleeding (see Table 11–1). A bleeding time test should also be performed on children with suspected congenital hemorrhagic disorders, especially with mucosal bleeding or hematuria. For acute acquired bleeding problems, with or without an underlying non-hematologic disease (see later), a bleeding time test is usually unnecessary. Measurement of fibrinogen and FDP (or thrombin time if these more specific tests are unavailable) is recommended for these patients.

The most common bleeding disorders encountered in the critically ill child are discussed in the following sections. These conditions can be divided into those that are: (1) congenital and hereditary (most of which cause chronic intermittent bleeding), and (2) acute, acquired, and often associated with an underlying disorder.

Hereditary Disorders of Blood Coagulation

Congenital coagulation disorders, by far the most common of which are hemophilia A (factor VIII deficiency) and hemophilia B (factor IX deficiency or Christmas disease), are often responsible for acute bleeding, particularly in joints or muscles. These hemorrhagic episodes are indeed medical emergencies because severe pain and disability are acute symptoms and permanent joint or nerve injury may result if therapy is not administered promptly. A discussion of the management of acute hemarthrosis in hemophilia is beyond the scope of this chapter, because affected children are not critically ill.[13–15] Occasionally patients with hemophilia, whether previously diagnosed or not, develop life-threatening hemorrhage into the central nervous system or the iliopsoas muscle, or following a seemingly mild minor surgical procedure such as tonsillectomy or tooth extraction. An operation is a significant stress to the hemostatic mechanism and even in the patient with mild hemophilia is generally followed by delayed (1 to 2 days) hemorrhage that does not stop with pressure or other local measures and continues for days or even weeks. A history of male relatives with similar postoperative bleeding or musculoskeletal problems, a previous bleeding history in the patient, or a prolonged PTT suggests the diagnosis of hemophilia and dictates the performance of specific factor assays.[12, 15] Therapy with a concentrated preparation of the deficient factor is usually necessary, because fresh frozen plasma does not provide enough factor to achieve hemostasis following surgery or major internal hemorrhage. If the diagnosis of hemophilia is strongly suspected and the child is having serious bleeding, a specimen of blood should be collected and the plasma frozen at

−70°C for later assays. The patient should then receive 50 units/kg of factor VIII concentrate (or cryoprecipitate), immediately followed by a PTT to document its correction because 20 per cent of children with hemophilia have factor IX deficiency[15] and require prothrombin complex concentrates instead.

The most frequent cause of death in hemophiliacs is bleeding into the central nervous system.[16] These episodes may occur with minimal or no prior trauma and sometimes represent the first manifestation of the disease. Therefore all children with intracranial bleeding of uncertain etiology must have a PTT in order to exclude the diagnosis of hemophilia. Intracranial hemorrhage following open head trauma may cause both a prolonged PT and PTT, secondary to desseminated intravascular coagulation (DIC) (see later discussion).[17]

Other inherited bleeding disorders include von Willebrand disease,[11] hereditary thrombocytopenia,[18] and familial qualitative platelet defects.[19] Their diagnosis requires a detailed family and personal history and screening laboratory tests followed by definitive assays. Specific therapy in a critical setting is rarely necessary and it consists of providing the deficient component (platelet or plasma concentrates) as outlined in Table 11–3.

Acute Acquired Bleeding Disorders

Much more common than congenital bleeding disorders are the acute and acquired hemorrhagic syndromes that complicate the management of critically ill children with diverse metabolic, infectious, and cardiopulmonary problems. With regard to their differential diagnosis and management, these disorders fall into one of three categories: (1) isolated thrombocytopenia, with normal values for PT

Table 11–3. BLOOD PRODUCTS FOR TRANSFUSION REPLACEMENT THERAPY IN CHILDREN WITH SEVERE ACUTE HEMORRHAGE

Blood Product	Major Indications	Usual Dose	Comments
Whole blood	Hypovolemia Massive acute blood loss and exchange transfusion	As needed to treat hemorrhagic shock; 2 × patient's blood volume for exchange transfusion	There is no particular rationale for "fresh" (<24 hours old) whole blood
Packed red blood cells	Moderate and severe anemia, especially when secondary to subacute and acute blood loss	10–15 ml/kg over 4 hours; less (5–7 ml/kg) if patient is severely anemic (Hgb <5 gm/100 ml), hypertensive, or volume overloaded	
Cryoprecipitate	Hemophilia A von Willebrand disease	1 bag (approximately 100 units) per 5 kg for mild bleed and 1 bag per 2 kg for severe and/or life-threatening hemorrhage; repeat q12–24h as necessary	Occasionally useful for congenital afibrinogenemia or disseminated intravascular coagulation
Factor VIII or IX concentrate	Hemophilia A and B	Factor VIII, 50 units per kg for severe life-threatening hemorrhage Factor IX, 100 units per kg for severe life-threatening hemorrhage	Monitor factor VIII or IX level post-infusion and maintain levels over 50% of normal with q12–24h infusions
Platelet concentrate	Severe thrombocytopenia (especially due to decreased platelet production) Qualitative platelet defect	Approximately 1 unit per 5 kg body weight (newborns—1 unit; infant—2–3 units; young child 4–6 units; adolescent 8–10 units); repeat as often as necessary to maintain hemostasis	Each unit per m^2 body surface area usually raises platelet count by 10,000–15,000/mm^3
Fresh frozen plasma	Acquired coagulation disorders	10–15 ml/kg q12–24h	Avoid outdated, banked plasma
Plasma protein fraction	Volume expansion	As needed to replace intravascular volume	

and PTT; (2) a prolonged PT and PTT with or without concomitant thrombocytopenia; and (3) normal values for platelet count, PT, and PTT. Patients whose disorder is in the last category have either a qualitative platelet defect or a local vascular injury from an ulcer, hemangioma, or trauma.

Isolated Thrombocytopenia with a Normal PT and PTT. The three major disease entities in this differential diagnosis are *idiopathic thrombocytopenic purpura, consumptive thrombocytopenia due to mechanical factors or antigen-antibody complexes* (including hemolytic uremic syndrome, hyperviscosity, and infection), and *bone marrow failure syndromes.* Children whose diseases are in the first two of these categories usually have only mild bleeding and therefore require no specific therapy for their thrombocytopenia. However, severe hemorrhage, particularly in the gastrointestinal tract or in the brain, may occasionally intervene.

Idiopathic Thrombocytopenic Purpura (ITP). ITP results from immune-mediated platelet destruction within the reticuloendothelial system.[20–23] It usually occurs in a previously well child after a viral infection. Physical findings are normal except for petechiae, ecchymoses, and hemorrhage from the oral or nasal mucosa. The blood count is normal except for thrombocytopenia (platelet count usually <20,000/mm³). The bone marrow, which should be examined to exclude an infiltrative or aplastic process, contains abundant megakaryocytes. These children are not ill and usually recover spontaneously within several weeks. Since the frequency of intracranial hemorrhage is extremely low[20] and the rate of spontaneous recovery is high, no specific therapy is required except for avoidance of aspirin and aspirin-containing drugs and limitation of activities. "Overtreatment" is to be avoided; these children generally do not require hospitalization or daily platelet counts. There has been much controversy about the role of corticosteroids in the treatment of ITP.[24] There is no convincing evidence that they are of value,[20, 25] and certainly long-term high-dose corticosteroid therapy is absolutely contraindicated. Other forms of therapy include immunosuppressive agents,[26] intravenous gamma globulin,[27] and plasmapheresis,[28] but these treatment modalities are not of proven value in children with ITP. The occasional child with ITP who develops life-threatening hemorrhage is usually a teenager with acute intracerebral bleeding. Such a patient should be treated with high-dose corticosteroids (prednisone or methylprednisolone, 1–2 mg/kg every 4–6 hours) and platelet transfusions, and emergency splenectomy should be performed if the platelet count does not rise within several hours.[29, 30]

Other Conditions with Consumptive Thrombocytopenia. The most serious disorder in this disease category is the *hemolytic-uremic syndrome,* characterized by acute renal failure and hemolytic anemia.[31] Since affected patients usually have moderate thrombocytopenia and few bleeding symptoms, primary attention should be directed to the more important clinical problems of acute renal failure and hypertension. Microangiopathic hemolytic anemia, characterized by fragmented erythrocytes on the peripheral blood smear, is usually managed with slowly administered packed red blood cell transfusions. Affected children differ from those with ITP because of their ill appearance, volume overload, hypertension, and obvious anemia.

The most frequent cause of consumptive thrombocytopenia with a normal PT and PTT is *bacterial or viral infection,* particularly in neonates. Platelets may be injured directly by endotoxins, other bacterial products, or viral particles, or secondarily by vasculitis. Recent evidence also has suggested a role for immune complexes in mediating thrombocytopenia accompanying bacterial infection, both in newborn infants[32] and in older patients.[33] Despite profound degrees of thrombocytopenia, such children usually have little or no bleeding[34] and thus do not require platelet transfusions. As with DIC, treatment should be directed toward the underlying disease (see later discussion).

Other causes of consumptive thrombocytopenia include the hyperviscosity accompanying neonatal polycythemia and cyanotic congenital heart disease, mechanical destruction within a hemangioma (Kasabach-Merritt syndrome), and association with or following large vessel thrombosis, particularly in the renal vein.

Isolated Thrombocytopenia Secondary to Bone Marrow Failure. Children with leukemia, aplastic anemia, and post-chemotherapy myelosuppression may bleed secondary to thrombocytopenia. Their underlying disease is usually readily apparent on history and physical examination, and anemia and granulocytopenia are typically present. These children generally bleed more profusely than patients with similar platelet counts who have ITP or hemolytic-uremic syndrome, probably because their platelets are older and thus not particularly effective hemostatically. Platelet transfusions are unnecessary when the patient has a platelet count greater than 5000 to 10,000/mm^3 unless serious bleeding exists (gross hematuria, gastrointestinal hemorrhage, and evidence of intracranial hemorrhage). Platelet transfusions may be ineffective if the child has been alloimmunized by prior blood product transfusions.

Hemorrhage Associated with a Prolonged PT and PTT. The most common serious bleeding episodes in critically ill patients are in this category, in which multiple blood coagulation factors are diminished, resulting in abnormal values for both PT and PTT. The PT is the most valuable screening test in these children, particularly newborns.

Disseminated Intravascular Coagulation (DIC). DIC is a distinct clinical syndrome in which there is inappropriate activation of blood coagulation and consumption of circulating blood platelets secondary to one of several triggering events.[35, 36] This process may result in depletion of hemostatic elements, hemorrhage, thrombosis, microangiopathic hemolytic anemia, and multi-organ failure. Affected patients are always ill from one of a variety of underlying conditions (trauma, shock, hypoxia, acidosis, sepsis, massive hemolysis, and malignancy), which directly or indirectly activate the coagulation cascade. DIC exists in nearly all critically ill patients but is often low-grade and of minimal clinical significance because the liver and bone marrow are frequently able to generate clotting factors and platelets nearly as rapidly as they are being utilized.

DIC should be suspected in any critically ill patient who is bleeding from one or more locations, especially venipuncture and cutdown sites, ecchymoses, and the gastrointestinal tract. The PT and PTT are nearly always prolonged, sometimes strikingly (more than 50 and 100 seconds, respectively) owing to profound depletion of labile clotting factors. The platelet count is usually lowered, and about 50 per cent of patients have fragmented red blood cell on the peripheral smear, reflecting microangiopathic injury by fibrin strands that occlude the microcirculation. In contrast to other acute and acquired conditions in which the PT and PTT are prolonged, patients with DIC also have a reduced plasma fibrinogen level (usually $<$100 mg/100 ml) and elevated FDP, reflecting compensatory fibrinolysis. Thus, the thrombin clotting time is also usually quite prolonged. It is rarely necessary to perform specific clotting factor assays to confirm the diagnosis of DIC.[36]

Patients with DIC have an extremely high mortality, but their demise is usually secondary to the underlying disease rather than to hemorrhage or thrombosis.[35, 36] Therapy is directed at the primary disease by attempting to eliminate the factors inducing the consumption coagulopathy. No replacement transfusions are necessary in most patients with abnomal laboratory findings, since the most common type of bleeding—oozing from puncture sites—is controlled by application of pressure. Therapy should be considered only for those patients who require surgery, have internal bleeding, or exhibit superficial hemorrhage that does not cease with pressure. These patients will typically have grossly abnormal laboratory values such as PT and PTT two to three times normal, fibrinogen less than 50 mg/100 ml, and platelet count less than 50,000/mm^3. Therapy consists of fresh frozen plasma or platelets or both (see Table 11–3), depending upon which hemostatic abnormality is believed to be contributing most to the patient's bleeding. Fresh frozen plasma is administered at a dosage of 10–15 ml/kg every 8 to 24 hours, and platelet concentrates are given every 12 to 24 hours. It must be emphasized that these blood products will usually not correct the patient's abnormal laboratory values and may provide only temporary relief of the bleeding signs and symptoms. There are no convincing data that transfusions "add fuel to the fire" and thus worsen the thrombotic tendency.[37]

Ten years ago heparin was a fashionable therapeutic modality for DIC, but it now can be recommended only rarely.[35, 36] In theory, heparin should be of value because it neutralizes the proteolytic effects of thrombin and other activating clotting factors on their substrates.[38] However, heparin is effective only in the presence of heparin cofactor or antithrombin III, which is often depleted in DIC.[39] No information exists regarding the proper dose and duration of heparin therapy and no prospective studies attest to its efficacy.[38] Currently heparin should probably be used in two clinical situations in DIC: (1) when life-threatening hemorrhage is not controlled with vigorous replacement transfusions, and (2) when a thrombotic tendency is the primary manifestation of DIC. The recommended dose is 50–100 u/kg as an intravenous push followed by 15–25 u/kg/hour as a constant infusion. Heparin therapy is monitored by serial platelet counts, fibrinogen levels, FDP measurements, responses to subsequent transfusions, and clinical assessments of the hemorrhage tendency.

Bleeding Due to Impaired Liver Function. In severe liver disease, synthesis of nearly all clotting factors is diminished, particularly of fibrinogen, factor V, and the vitamin K–dependent factors II, VII, IX, and X.[1, 40] Vitamin K deficiency due to biliary obstruction, thrombocytopenia due to hypersplenism, and concomitant DIC may contribute to the bleeding tendency in children with liver disease, whether the damage is due to toxic, metabolic, or infectious agents.[1] Hemorrhage may be the first clinical manifestation of liver disease, and although the bleeding is often generalized, it may be restricted to the gastrointestinal tract, especially in the presence of esophageal varices, peptic ulcer, and gastritis.

Patients with liver disease and clinically significant hemorrhage have a prolonged PT and PTT but typically normal or only slightly abnormal values for platelet count and FDP. Fibrinogen level is variable but may be quite diminished when hepatic injury is severe.

Hemorrhage due to liver disease is usually accompanied by hepatomegaly, jaundice, and other obvious clinical and laboratory manifestations of liver failure.[40, 41] Treatment is not necessary for most children with altered laboratory values, but if serious bleeding occurs, even from a localized site, fresh frozen plasma should be administered along with vitamin K. Unfortunately, the risk of volume overload prevents the physician from administering enough plasma to entirely correct the defect. Thus, improvement in the hemorrhagic tendency is often transient, and bleeding remains a common cause of death. Prothrombin complex concentrates (Proplex and Konyne) should be avoided because of their high risk of hepatitis and of thrombosis due to contamination with activated procoagulants. Also these preparations do not contain fibrinogen or factor V.

Vitamin K Deficiency. Vitamin K is a fat-soluble vitamin obtained from dietary sources (particularly cow's milk and leafy green vegetables) and also absorbed from the colon where it is produced by certain microorganisms. Its ability to render factors II, VII, IX, and X functional was described earlier. Body stores of vitamin K are limited, so a deficiency may intervene rapidly in certain critically ill patients.[42] Vitamin K depletion is also observed in subacutely or chronically ill patients whose dietary intake has been reduced, particularly when malabsorption and broad-spectrum antibiotic therapy coexist.[43, 44] Vitamin K deficiency is a particular problem in children with biliary atresia and other disorders characterized by impaired fat absorption such as cystic fibrosis.[44] Coumarin anticoagulants are rarely used therapeutically in pediatrics. They are, however, contained in several types of rat poison, which may be ingested by young children. Other drugs inhibiting vitamin K coagulant action are phenytoin, vitamin E, and aspirin,[44, 45] but the only circumstance in which they have caused serious hemorrhage due to vitamin K deficiency is in the neonate whose mother is receiving phenytoin.[43]

Laboratory diagnosis of vitamin K deficiency is straightforward, with patients having both prolonged PT and PTT and normal values for fibrinogen and platelet count. Specific factor assays are unnecessary. The diagnosis is confirmed by administering vitamin K replacement therapy and documenting prompt cessation of hemorrhage and correction of the prolonged PT and PTT within several hours. For prophylaxis, vitamin K can be given orally (as a water-soluble analog) or intramuscularly, but patients with acute hemorrhage should receive vitamin K by slow intravenous push over several minutes. The dose is 2–3 mg for infants and 5–10 mg for older children.

Circulating Inhibitors. Another cause of prolonged PT or prolonged PTT or both in the bleeding child is an inhibitor of blood coagulation, most frequently heparin. The most common useful *in vitro* test results that demonstrate the anticoagulant action of heparin are a markedly prolonged PTT and thrombin time. The PT is less sensitive to heparin's inhibitory effects but can be prolonged when the plasma level is excessive. A heparin-induced prolonged PTT most frequently results from heparin contamination of a central catheter, needle, or syringe in a child who is not bleeding. Occasionally, unintentional systemic heparin anticoagulation can cause hemorrhage when a dose miscalculation has been made in a patient with a heparinized central arterial line.[47] Sometimes, excessive heparinization also occurs in children being therapeutically anticoagulated for thrombosis and during or immediately following cardiopulmonary bypass. In all of these cases the half-time of heparin in the circulation is extremely short,[48, 49] so specific therapy is not required.

Another type of coagulation inhibitor encountered in children is the lupus anticoagulant, in which an antibody exerts an *in vitro* inhibitory effect on the reaction leading to the generation of thrombin.[50] Paradoxically, affected children do not suffer from hemorrhage but may instead have venous thrombosis.[50] Circulating inhibitors against specific clotting factors may complicate the management of hemophilia[51, 52] and rarely may occur in otherwise normal children.[53] Serious hemorrhage is infrequently a problem in this latter case. The management of hemophiliacs with inhibitors must be individualized, because the specific transfusion regimen (factor VIII concentrate, prothrombin complex concentrate, activated prothrombin complex product, etc.) depends upon many variables, including inhibitor titer, nature of hemorrhage, and history of prior anamnestic antibody response.[51, 52]

If an inhibitor of blood coagulation is responsible for prolonging the PT or PTT or both, a 1:1 mixture of the patient's plasma with normal plasma will likewise show prolonged clotting times (see Table 11–1). In a coagulation-factor deficiency, on the other hand, normal plasma corrects the defect. A mixing study is therefore a useful diagnostic exercise when heparin, a lupus anticoagulant, or a specific inhibitor is suspected. The latter species of inhibitor sometimes requires incubation at 37° C for one to two hours to exert an effect. Specific laboratory tests are available to define each type of inhibitor, but their description is beyond the focus of this discussion.

Bleeding Associated with Normal Values for PT, PTT, and Platelet Count

Local Vascular Lesions. Screening coagulation tests should be performed for all children with massive hemorrhage from a single site. Yet the most common cause of massive epistaxis, hematemesis, lower gastrointestinal hemorrhage, and external hemorrhage from another site is a disruption or transection of blood vessel at which hemostasis does not occur despite normal concentration and function of platelets and coagulation proteins.[1] Attention must be directed to defining the presence or absence of a local vascular lesion, a task that may require ENT consultation for epistaxis, endoscopy for gastrointestinal bleeding, and surgical support for obvious arterial hemorrhage due to trauma. In addition, specific emergency measures may be necessary to treat shock resulting from acute blood loss and to manage anemia resulting from subacute or chronic hemorrhage.

Diffuse vascular inflammation or injury, such as in Henoch-Schönlein syndrome,[54] may result in extensive petechial and purpuric lesions and therefore may simulate a disorder of hemostasis. These children usually have multiorgan disease, including involvement of kidneys and gastrointestinal tract.[54]

Another important consideration in the differential diagnosis of the child with multiple bruises, with or without intracranial and intraabdominal hemorrhage, is *child abuse.*[55] This diagnosis should be suspected in any child with normal blood coagulation results, a suspicious or unbelievable history provided by the caretaker, and other physical findings consistent with neglect or abuse (malnutrition, lack of cleanliness, fractures, scars from old injuries or cigarette burns, etc.). Local child welfare and law enforcement authorities should be contacted immediately if child abuse is suspected.

Qualitative Platelet Defects. Platelet dysfunction is a common occurrence in clinical pediatrics and probably contributes to the bleeding tendency in many critically ill children. Yet, rarely is it the major cause for life-threatening hemorrhage. The bleeding time test should always be performed if platelet dysfunction is suspected. Platelet disorders can be classified as either inherited or acquired. The former constitute a rare and heterogenous group of conditions characterized by lifelong history of cutaneous and mucosal hemorrhage. Central nervous system or gastrointestinal tract bleeding may occasionally occur and is managed with platelet transfusions. Routine use of transfusions for minor bleeding is to be avoided because of the risk of alloimmunization. The most common inherited platelet defects include Glanzmann thrombasthenia, Bernard-Soulier syndrome, storage-pool disease, and aspirin-like release defects. These defects are discussed in detail in standard textbooks and recent review articles.[19, 56] In von Willebrand disease the platelets are intrinsically normal but lack the ability to adhere to subendothelial surfaces because of an abnormality or lack of factor VIII von Willebrand factor in plasma.[11] The clinical history is often similar to that in a patient with a qualitative platelet defect. It is important to differentiate intrinsic platelet disorders from von Willebrand disease because their therapies differ greatly. Platelet transfusions are administered to bleeding patients with platelet defects, whereas cryoprecipitates are given to children with von Willebrand disease. The vasopressin analog DDAVP raises plasma factor VIII components by uncertain mechanisms and recently has been shown to correct hemostasis in selected patients with von Willebrand disease and mild hemophilia.[57]

Acquired platelet disorders are most commonly due to extrinsic injury by a drug or mechanical lesion.[58] The drug that inhibits platelet function most frequently is aspirin, which irreversibly inactivates cyclo-oxygenase, the key enzyme in platelet prostaglandin synthesis. Since this inhibitory effect is permanent for the life span of the platelet, a single aspirin tablet may impair hemostasis for a number of days. In normal individuals this effect of aspirin is not usually clinically significant, but in patients with underlying conditions in which hemostasis is impaired (thrombocytopenia, hemophilia, intraoperative and postoperative states, etc.) aspirin may induce or accentuate a bleeding tendency.[59, 60] In addition, aspirin taken by women during the last week of pregnancy may promote hemorrhage in their newborns.[61] Accordingly, acetominophen, which does not impair platelet function, should be utilized for control of fever or mild pain in all of these circumstances. Other drugs that impair platelet function include non-steroidal anti-inflammatory agents, phenothiazines, sodium valproate, and high-dose parenteral penicillins.[58] The antiplatelet effects of these agents are rarely of clinical significance.

Bleeding in Uremia. Patients with acute renal failure usually have normal hemostasis unless they are thrombocytopenic owing to hemolytic-uremic syndrome. Patients with chronic renal failure, on the other hand, often experience severe cutaneous and mucosal hemorrhage secondary to platelet dysfunction. The bleeding time correlates well with the risk of hemorrhage and additional *in vitro* studies are rarely of value.[62] The exact cause of hemorrhage in uremia is uncertain but is likely due to one or another type of inhibitor, because the bleeding symptoms may improve following dialysis. Platelet transfusions are of no value, but two new therapeutic approaches for adults with bleeding associated with uremia are cryoprecipitate transfusion and DDAVP.[63, 64] The success with these two treatments suggests that the uremic inhibitor might in some way prevent the adhesion of platelets to subendothelium, which is mediated by high-molecular-weight multimers of factor VIII.[63] The bleeding defect in uremia can also be corrected with packed red blood cell transfusions,[65] suggesting that factors other than platelet inhibitors are of pathophysiologic importance.

Miscellaneous Causes of Acquired Hemorrhage

Cardiopulmonary Bypass. Profuse hemorrhage from chest tubes or other sites immediately follows cardiopulmonary bypass after some pediatric open-heart procedures. This bleeding may be due to excessive heparin, inadequate heparin neutralization, disseminated intravascular coagulation, enhanced fibrinolysis, or thrombocytopenia due to mechanical consumption in the pump oxygenator. Recently, it was demonstrated convincingly that the major hemostatic defect following open heart surgery was transient platelet dysfunction resulting in a long bleeding time.[66] Although excessive bleeding from the chest tubes is usually due to local factors and is not responsive to transfusion replacement therapy, platelet transfusions might be necessary when thrombocytopenia or unusually severe platelet dysfunction is documented. The other causes of hemorrhage mentioned previously should also be excluded by screening laboratory studies. Bleeding after open-heart surgery is most commonly observed in patients who were critically ill or who were cyanotic and polycythemic prior to surgery.[67] It should be emphasized that most children do not need platelet transfusion replacement therapy following open-heart surgery.

Massive Transfusion Therapy (Including Exchange Transfusion). The transfusion of more than one blood volume after traumatic blood loss or as an exchange transfusion results in depletion of clotting factors and platelets.[68] The synthetic capacity of the liver and the reservoir function of the spleen allow rapid restoration of clotting factors, but bone marrow reserve is limited. Therefore, dilutional thrombocytopenia is quite common following exchange transfusion or massive blood loss and should be monitored by serial daily platelet counts. Platelet transfusions are indicated if serious hemorrhage ensues.

GENERAL MANAGEMENT GUIDELINES

Management of bleeding in the critically ill child is nearly always dictated by the history and physical findings, not by the results of laboratory studies. Treatment should be directed at the underlying disease, whether it be induction chemotherapy for acute leukemia, management of acute renal failure for hemolytic-uremic syndrome, avoidance of drugs such as aspirin, or antibiotic therapy for the complicating infection. Many bleeding episodes are self-limiting and do not require therapy.

Often overlooked are local measures that

may successfully maintain hemostasis in children with platelet and vascular deficiencies. Prolonged application of firm pressure will usually stop nosebleeds, oral mucous-membrane bleeding, and superficial cutaneous hemorrhage following small vessel injury. Local pressure, however, is usually ineffective in hemophilia and acquired coagulation factor deficiencies. In addition to manual pressure and pressure dressings, other devices such as splints (around a tooth socket or to immobilize an extremity lesion) serve to reduce repetitive vessel injury from disruption of hemostatic plugs. Application of topical thrombin, Gelfoam, or microfibrillar collagen may also provide relief from hemorrhage of nasal mucosa and tooth sockets. For persistent epistaxis, nasal packing should be considered.

The child with extremely acute or massive blood loss must be monitored closely for hypovolemia or obvious clinical shock.[69] If the general appearance of the patient, magnitude of hemorrhage, or deteriorating vital signs (tachycardia, tachypnea, hypotension) suggests hypovolemia, rapid volume replacement is necessary. Whole blood need not be used, since saline, lactated Ringer's solution, and other colloid products provide acceptable volume expansion. If colloid replacement is given, plasma protein fraction (e.g., Plasmanate) is preferred over the more expensive purified albumin preparations or fresh frozen or outdated plasma with their attendant hepatitis risks. When red blood cell loss is excessive, packed red blood cell replacement transfusions may be required.[69]

Children with hemostatic failure due to any of the disorders discussed previously may require specific transfusion replacement therapy in addition to local measures (see Table 11–3).[70] When thrombocytopenia is contributing to major bleeding, particularly if the mechanism is decreased production, platelet transfusions are clearly indicated. The "dose" is somewhat empirical, since response (rise in platelet count and cessation of hemorrhage) is determined by innumerable factors, including the age and viability of the transfused platelets, underlying disease, presence of alloantibodies resulting from prior transfusions, and age of the patient. In general, one unit of transfused platelets per 30 kg body weight (1 m^2 of body surface area) will raise the platelet count by 10,000 to 15,000/mm^3. The dose that effectively stops hemorrhage is typically 2–3 units for an infant or toddler, 4–6 units for a young child, and 8–10 units for an older child or adolescent. Transfusions may need to be repeated once daily, depending upon clinical response. They are administered rapidly through a standard blood transfusion filter (microaggregate filters should be avoided). Platelets need not be ABO- and Rh-type specific, although ABO-type specificity is preferable in order to avoid coating of red blood cells by antibodies in the accompanying plasma. Response to platelet transfusions may be minimal in patients with rapid peripheral destruction (ITP, DIC, etc.).

Children whose bleeding is due to clotting factor depletion require replacement transfusions with plasma or the appropriate concentrated plasma products containing the missing factor. Hemophiliacs with serious bleeding should receive factor VIII concentrate or cryoprecipitate (hemophilia A) or the prothrombin complex concentrate Konyne or Proplex (hemophilia B). These products have numerous side effects, including hepatitis and possibly the acquired immunodeficiency syndrome[71, 72] and should be used with caution in patients whose prior transfusion history has not included extensive exposure to these products. Specific dosage guidelines are outlined in all standard reviews on hemophilia.[13, 15]

Children with acquired coagulation disorders who need plasma products should usually receive fresh frozen plasma, which contains all of the blood coagulation factors in hemostatically effective quantities, provided that an adequate amount can be given (see Table 11–3). Unfortunately, however, the maximally tolerated dose of fresh frozen plasma for a child is 10–15 ml/kg once or twice daily. Greater amounts may cause volume overload and pulmonary edema, even in the patient without pre-existing cardiopulmonary compromise. It is therefore impossible to achieve normal levels of blood coagulation factors in most children with massive hemorrhage due to DIC and liver failure.

Banked, outdated plasma contains reduced amounts of factor V and factor VIII and is not useful for patients with bleeding disorders. Use of cryoprecipitate is generally limited to hemophilia and von Willebrand disease, although an occasional patient with DIC and a profound fibrinogen deficiency may benefit from its administration. Recent work has shown that cryoprecipitate may also be of value in patients with septic shock whose plasma is depleted of fibrinectin, an adhesive glycoprotein that is cryoprecipitable and has a role in clearance of particulate matter from the circulation.[73]

ALGORITHM FOR THE DIAGNOSIS OF THE CAUSE OF ACUTE HEMORRHAGE

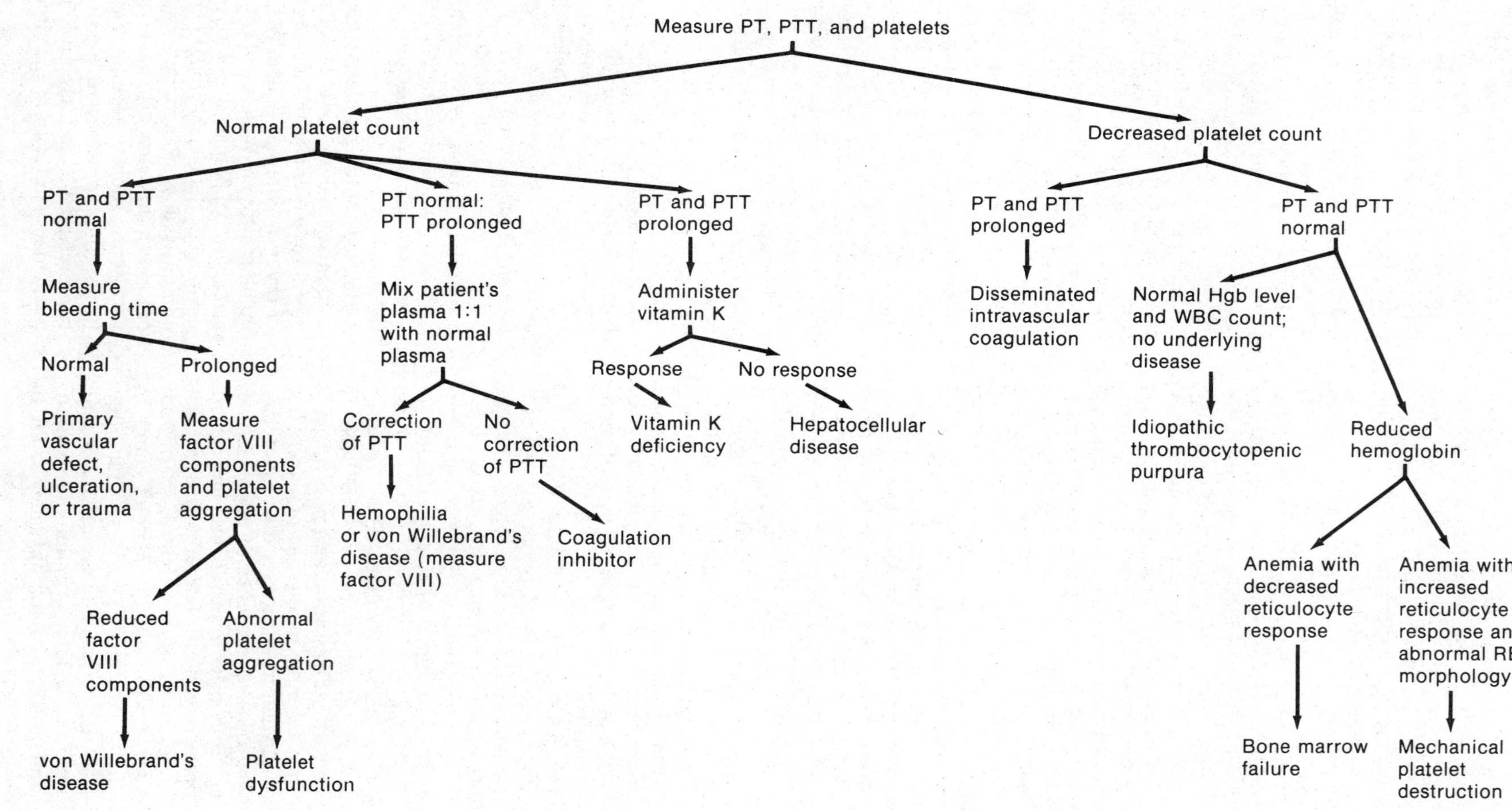

At all costs, it is crucial that the physician not administer treatments that add confusion to the diagnostic and therapeutic picture and possibly worsen the bleeding tendency. Invasive procedures (surgery, cutdowns, multiple arterial punctures, etc.) should not be performed on children with impaired hemostasis unless absolutely necessary. Aspirin and aspirin-containing drugs must be avoided. Side effects of blood products such as hepatitis and transfusion reactions must always be balanced against the risk of progressive and uncontrollable hemorrhage. Finally, the child should not be subject to excessive laboratory studies once a diagnosis has been made and therapy administered. A gratifying clinical response (i.e., cessation of hemorrhage) is more important than repetitive documentation of corrected PT and PTTs.

REFERENCES

1. Bowie EJW, Owen CA Jr. Hemostatic failure in clinical medicine. Semin Hematol 1977; *14*: 341–1364.
2. Bloom AL, Thomas DP, eds. Haemostasis and Thrombosis. New York: Churchill-Livingstone, 1981.
3. Thomson JM, ed. Blood Coagulation and Haemostasis: A Practical Guide. 2nd ed. New York: Churchill-Livingstone, 1980.
4. Harker LA, Zimmerman TS. eds. Platelet disorders. Clin Haematol 1983; *12*:1–360.
5. Rosenberg RD. Physiology of Coagulation: The Fluid Phase. *In*: Nathan DG, Oski FA, eds. Hematology of Infancy and Childhood, 2nd ed. Philadelphia: WB Saunders, 1981:1145–1167.
6. Bell A, Neely CL. Smear platelet counts. South Med J 1980; 73:899–901.
7. Babson SR, Babson AL. Development and evaluation of a disposable device for performing simultaneous duplicate bleeding time determinations. Am J Clin Pathol 1978; *70*:406–408.
8. Feusner HG. Normal and abnormal bleeding times in neonates and young children utilizing a fully standardized template technic. Am J Clin Pathol 1980; *74*:73–77.
9. Harker LA, Slichter SJ. The bleeding time as a screening test for evaluation of platelet function. N Engl J Med 1972; *287*:155–159.
10. Hoyer L. The factor VIII complex: structure and function. Blood 1971; *58*:1–13.
11. Zimmerman TS, Ruggeri ZM. von Willebrand's disease. Prog Hemost Thromb 1982; *6*:203–236.
12. Kitchens CS. Occult hemophilia. Johns Hopkins Med J 1980; *146*:255–259.
13. Buchanan GR. Hemophilia, Pediatr Clin North Am 1980; *27*:309–326.
14. Arnold WD, Hilgartner MW. Hemophilic arthropathy. Current concepts of pathogenesis and management. J Bone Joint Surg 1977; *59*-A:287–305.
15. Hilgartner MW, ed. Hemophilia in the Child and Adult. New York: Masson Publishing USA Inc, 1982.
16. Eyster ME, Gill FM, Blatt PM, et al and Hemophilia Study Group. Central nervous system bleeding in hemophiliacs. Blood 1978; *51*:1179–1188.
17. Miner ME, Kaufman HH, Graham SH, et al. Disseminated intravascular coagulation fibrinolytic syndrome following head injury in children: frequency and prognostic implications. J Pediatr 1982; *100*:687–691.
18. Murphy S. Hereditary thrombocytopenia. Clin Haematol 1972; *1*:359–367.
19. Weiss HJ. Congenital disorders of platelet function. Semin Hematol 1980; *17*:228–241.
20. Lusher JM, Iyer R. Idiopathic thrombocytopenic purpura in children. Semin Thromb Hemost 1977; *2*:175–199.
21. Cheung N-KV, Hilgartner MW, Schulman I, et al. Platelet-associated immunoglobulin G in childhood idiopathic thrombocytopenic purpura. J Pediatr 1983; *102*:366.
22. McMillan R. Chronic idiopathic thrombocytopenic purpura. N Engl J Med 1981; *203*:1135–1147.
23. McWilliams NB, Maurer HM. Acute idiopathic thrombocytopenia purpura in children. Am J Hematol 1979; 7:87–96.
24. Zuelzer WW, Lusher JM. Childhood idiopathic thrombocytopenic purpura. To treat or not to treat. Am J Dis Child 1977; *131*:360–362.
25. Buchanan GR, Holtkamp CA. Prednisone therapy for children with acute idiopathic thrombocytopenic purpura (ITP): results of a randomized clinical trial. Pediatr Res 1982; *16*:200A.
26. Joseph A, Evans DIK. Immunosuppressive treatment of idiopathic thrombocytopenic purpura in children. Acta Paediatr Scand 1982; *71*:467–469.
27. Ahn YS, Harrington WJ, Simon SR, et al. Danazol for the treatment of idiopathic thrombocytopenic purpura. N Engl J Med 1983; *308*:1396–1399.
28. Marder VJ, Nusbacher J, Anderson JW. One-year follow-up of plasma exchange therapy in 14 patients with idiopathic thrombocytopenic purpura. Transfusion 1981; *21*:291–298.
29. Woerner SJ, Abildgaard CF, French BS. Intracranial hemorrhage in children with idiopathic thrombocytopenic purpura. Pediatrics 1981; *67*:453–460.
30. Zerella JT, Martin LW, Lampkin BC. Emergency splenectomy for idiopathic thrombocytopenic purpura in children. J Pediatr Surg 1978; *13*:243–246.
31. Fong JS, de Chadarevian J-P, Kaplan BS. Hemolytic-uremic syndrome. Current concepts and management. Pediatr Clin North Amer 1982; *29*:835–856.
32. Zipursky A, Palko J, Milner R, Akenzua GI. The hematology of bacterial infections in premature infants. Pediatrics 1976; *57*:839–853.
33. Corrigan JJ Jr. Thrombocytopenia: a laboratory sign of septicemia in infants and children. J Pediatr. 1974; *85*:219–221.
34. Zipursky A, deSa D, Hsu E, et al. Clinical and laboratory diagnosis of hemostatic disorders in newborn infants. Am J Pediatr Hematol Oncol 1979; *1*:217–226.
35. Mant MJ, King EG. Severe, acute disseminated intravascular coagulation. A reappraisal of its pathophysiology, clinical significance and therapy based on 47 patients. Am J Med 1979; *67*:557–563.
36. Spero JA, Lewis JH, Hasiba U. Disseminated intravascular coagulation. Findings in 346 patients. Thromb Haemost 1980; *43*:28–33.
37. Corrigan JJ Jr. Heparin therapy in bacterial septicemia. J Pediatr 1977; *91*:695–700.

38. Feinstein DI. Diagnosis and management of disseminated intravascular coagulation: the role of heparin therapy. Blood 1982; *60*:284–287.
39. Bick RL, Bick MD, Fekete LF. Antithrombin III patterns in disseminated intravascular coagulation. Am J Clin Pathol 1980; *73*:577–583.
40. Roberts HR, Cederbaum AI. The liver and blood coagulation: physiology and pathology. Gastroenterology 1972; 297–320.
41. Gallus AS, Lucas CR, Hursh J. Coagulation studies in patients with acute infectious hepatitis. Br J Haematol 1972; *22*:761–771.
42. Ansell JE, Kumar R, Deykin D. The spectrum of vitamin K deficiency. JAMA 1977; *238*:40–42.
43. Clancy CM, Glew RH. Hypoprothrombinaemia and bleeding associated with cephamandole. Lancet 1981; *1*:250.
44. Corrigan JJ Jr. The vitamin K-dependent proteins. Adv Pediatr 1981; *28*:57–74.
45. Corrigan JJ Jr, Ulfers LL. Effect of vitamin E on prothrombin levels in warfarin-induced vitamin K deficiency. Am J Clin Nutr 1981; *34*:1701–1705.
46. Buchanan GR. Hemorrhagic Diseases. *In*: Nathan DG, Oski FA, eds. Hematology of Infancy and Childhood. 2nd ed. Philadelphia: WB Saunders, 1981; 119–143.
47. Schreiner RL, Wynn RJ, McNulty C. Accidental heparin toxicity in the newborn intensive care unit. J Pediatr 1978; *92*:115–116.
48. Wessley S, Gitel SN. Heparin: new concepts relevant to clinical use. Blood 1979; *53*:525–544.
49. Estes JW. Clinical pharmacokinetics of heparin. Clin Pharmacokinet 1980; *5*:204–220.
50. Shapiro S, Thiagarajan P. Lupus anticoagulants. Prog Hemost Thromb 1982; *6*:263–286.
51. Lusher JM, Shapiro SS, Palascak JE, et al. Efficacy of prothrombin-complex concentrates in hemophiliacs with antibodies to factor VIII. N Engl J Med 1980; *303*:421–425.
52. Roberts HR. Hemophiliacs with inhibitors: therapeutic options. N Engl J Med 1981; *305*:757–758.
53. Orris DJ, Lewis JH, Spero JA, Hasiba U. Blocking coagulation inhibitors in children taking penicillin. J. Pediatr 1980; *9*:426–429.
54. Silber DL. Henoch-Schoenlein syndrome. Pediatr Clin North Amer 1982; *19*:1061–1071.
55. Schmitt BD, Kempe CH. Abuse and neglect of children. *In*: Vaughn VC, McKay RJ, Behrman RE. Nelson eds. Textbook of Pediatrics. 11th ed. Philadelpha: WB Saunders, 1979:120–126.
56. White JG. Membrane defects in inherited disorders in platelet function. Am J Pediatr Hematol Oncol 1982; *4*:83–84.
57. Warrier AI, Lusher JM. DDAVP: a useful alternative to blood components in moderate hemophilia A and von Willebrand disease. J Pediatr 1983; *102*:228–233.
58. Malpass TW, Harker LA. Acquired disorders of platelet function. Semin Hematol 1980; *7*:242–258.
59. Kitchen L, Erichson RB, Sideropoulos H. Effect of drug-induced platelet dysfunction in surgical bleeding. Am J Surg 1982; *143*:215–217.
60. Kaneshiro MM, Mielke CH Jr, Kasper CK, Rapaport SI. Bleeding time after aspirin in disorders of intrinsic clotting. N Engl J Med 1969; *281*:1039–1042.
61. Stuart MJ, Gross SJ, Elrad H, Graeber JE. Effects of acetylsalicylic-acid ingestion on maternal and neonatal hemostasis. N Engl J Med 1982; *307*:909–912.
62. Steiner RW, Coggins C, Carvalho ACA. Bleeding time in uremia: a useful test to assess clinical bleeding. Am J Hematol 1979; *7*:107–117.
63. Mannucci PM, Remuzzi G, Pusineri F, et al. Deamino-8-D-arginine vasopressin shortens the bleeding time in uremia. N Engl J Med 1983; *308*:8–12.
64. Janson PA, Jubelirer SJ, Weinstein MJ, Deykin D. Treatment of the bleeding tendency in uremia with cryoprecipitate. N Engl J Med 1980; *303*:1318–1322.
65. Livio M, Marchesi D, Remuzzi G, et al. Uraemic bleeding: role of anaemia and beneficial effect of red cell transfusions. Lancet 1982; *2*:1013–1015.
66. Harker LA, Malpass TW, Branson HE, et al Mechanism of abnormal bleeding in patients undergoing cardiopulmonary bypass: acquired transient platelet dysfunction associated with selective α-granule release. Blood 1980; *56*:824–834.
67. Wedemeyer AL, Lewis JH. Improvement of hemostasis following phlebotomy in cyanotic patients with heart disease. J Pediatr 1973; *83*:46–50.
68. Miller RD, Robbins TO, Tong MJ, Barton SL. Coagulation defects associated with massive blood transfusions. Ann Surg 1971; *174*:794–801.
69. Levin DL, Patz J, Stein P. Shock. *In*: Levin DL, Morriss FC, Moore GC, eds. A Practical Guide to Pediatric Intensive Care. St. Louis: CV Mosby Co, 1979:58–63.
70. Buchanan GR. Coagulation Factors. *In*: Nathan DG, Oski FA, eds. Hematology of Infancy and Childhood. 2nd ed. Philadelphia: WB Saunders, 1981: 1536–1551.
71. White GC II, Zeitler KD, Hesesne HR, et al. Chronic hepatitis in patients with hemophilia A: histologic studies in patients with intermittently abnormal liver function tests. Blood 1982; *60*:1259–1262.
72. Desforges JF. AIDS and preventive treatment in hemophilia. N Engl J Med 1983; *308*:94–95.
73. Zimmerman TS, Ruggeri, ZM, Fulcher CA. Factor VIII: von Willebrand factor. Prog Hematol 1983; *13*:279.

CHAPTER

12

Sickle Cell Disease and Its Crises

Howard A. Pearson, M.D.

The population shifts that have characterized American demography during the past few generations have made it imperative that pediatricians throughout the country recognize the implications and consequences of the most common inherited hematologic abnormality of the black race—sickling of the red blood cells.

Approximately 8 per cent of American blacks carry a single abnormal gene for sickle hemoglobin (Hb S) and have the sickle cell trait. Although under most situations this fact has no meaningful clinical consequences, it has significant genetic implications. About 1 in 600 blacks has 2 genes for sickle hemoglobin that result in a hematologic disease of considerable severity. In these homozygous persons, life-threatening emergencies may endanger their health and even their survival. Successful management requires prompt recognition and diagnosis and application of rational therapy when possible.

GENETICS OF HEMOGLOBIN

The red blood cells of normal children and adults contain predominantly a type of hemoglobin designated Hb A (or Adult). Hb A is made up of two pairs of chemically different polypeptide chains designated alpha (α) and beta (β). Because there are two α- and two β-chains in each hemoglobin molecule, Hb A is designated as $\alpha_2\beta_2$.

Sickle hemoglobin is caused by a genetic mutation that results in a substitution of the amino acid valine for glutamic acid in the number six position of the β-chain.[1] Therefore, using chemical shorthand, Hb S is designated $\alpha_2\beta_2^S$.

The sickle gene may occur in either the heterozygous or the homozygous state. In the heterozygous state (sickle cell trait, Hb AS) both Hb A and Hb S are present in each red blood cell, and Hb S accounts for about 30 to 45 per cent of the total.

In contrast, when individuals are homozygous for the sickle gene, they have sickle cell anemia. The hemoglobin in the red blood cell is virtually all Hb S.

PATHOPHYSIOLOGY OF SICKLING

The biochemical characteristics of sickle hemoglobin have profound effects on its physical characteristics. Fully oxygenated Hb S does not differ from Hb A; however, upon deoxygenation, Hb S is insoluble and polymerizes into long filaments.[2] These filaments aggregate into large, linear crystals that distort the red blood cell into an elongated rigid sickle cell. In sickle cell anemia, *in vivo* sickling occurs spontaneously under normal conditions.

TESTS FOR SICKLING

Diagnosis of sickle cell conditions depends upon demonstration of the abnormal Hb S in the red blood cells. Several tests are available.

Sickle Cell Preparation. In the classic sickle cell "prep" of Daland and Castle, red blood cells are suspended in a fresh 2 per cent solution of the chemical-reducing agent sodium metabisulfite.[3] Red blood cells containing Hb S assume a sickled configuration that can be observed microscopically. Red blood cells from patients with sickle cell anemia sickle rapidly into elongated filamentous shapes. Red blood cells from individuals with sickle cell trait sickle more slowly and assume a "holly leaf" configuration. However, as ordinarily performed and interpreted, the sickle prep does not distinguish between sickle cell anemia, sickle cell trait, and other genetic variants. In addition, false-negative tests are not infrequent.

Solubility Tests. The fact that deoxygenated Hb S precipitates in aqueous solutions whereas all other hemoglobins remain soluble is the basis of the solubility tests for Hb S.[4] Blood is transferred by pipette into a solution containing saponin to lyse red blood cells and sodium dithionate to reduce the hemoglobin. When Hb S is present, the solution becomes turbid, whereas with all other hemoglobins the solution remains clear. Like the sickle prep, solubility tests are genetically non-definitive and do not differentiate between sickle cell anemia and other Hb S genetic variants. Another major problem with the solubility tests is that they give false-negative results if the patient's hemoglobin level is less than 5.0 gm/100 ml.[5]

Hemoglobin Electrophoresis. Hemoglobin electrophoresis is the definitive diagnostic test for hemoglobinopathies. Rapid and inexpensive techniques employ a cellulose acetate supporting medium and an alkaline buffer system (pH 8.2). These techniques definitively identify Hb A and S as well as many other variants, permitting a genotypic diagnosis in most cases.

In some instances it may be necessary to use other techniques such as acid–agar gel electrophoresis to differentiate hemoglobin variants such as Hb D, which resembles Hb S on alkaline electrophoresis. Since hemoglobin variants are inherited as co-dominant autosomal traits, family studies are frequently useful.

SICKLE CELL TRAIT

The heterozygous sickle cell trait (sickle cell trait, Hb AS) is clinically benign in almost every situation. It is important to stress the benign nature of heterozygous sickle cell trait because there have been many instances in which medical misinformation has been given individuals with the trait, resulting in inappropriate and unnecessary restrictions and concerns.

Other than the presence of 30 to 40 per cent Hb S in the red blood cells, there are no hematologic abnormalities present in individuals with sickle cell trait. Hemoglobin levels and reticulocyte counts are normal, indicating normal red blood cell life span. Longitudinal studies indicate no shortening of the individual's life expectancy.[6]

Perhaps the most important implication of sickle cell trait is a genetic one. Persons with sickle cell trait may pass the gene on to their offspring. If they mate with another person who has the trait, there is one chance in four that any child will have sickle cell anemia. The major aim of mass testing procedures should be to detect persons with sickle cell trait and to give them the information necessary for marital and family planning. Such information must be combined with meaningful educational and counseling programs to be effective.

SICKLE CELL ANEMIA

Sickle cell anemia (Hb SS disease) results from homozygosity for the Hb S gene. The red blood cells in sickle cell anemia contain large amounts of Hb S, variable amounts of Hb F (usually $<10\%$ in adults) and normal levels of Hb A_2 ($<3.5\%$). Because of the high concentration of Hb S, spontaneous sickling occurs *in vivo.* Sickled cells are also fragile and non-deformable and therefore rapidly destroyed. The clinical features of sickle cell anemia include symptoms such as pallor, weakness, and fatigability due to severe hemolytic anemia.

In addition to these features, which are found in any chronic and severe hemolytic state, unique clinical features of sickle cell anemia occur as a result of occlusion of small blood vessels by tangled masses of sickled cells. A consequence of this vaso-occlusion is tissue infarction. The clinical and hematologic manifestations of sickle cell anemia thus reflect two processes: (1) severe hemolysis and the compensatory mechanisms evoked by hemolytic anemia and (2) widespread vaso-occlusion and infarction involving many tissues and organs (Figure 12–1).

Laboratory Findings

Selected laboratory findings in sickle cell anemia are listed in Table 12–1. A moderately severe normochromic-normocytic hemolytic anemia with morphologic abnormalities (including Howell-Jolly bodies, target cells, polychromatophilia, and the presence of varying numbers of irreversibly sickled cells) is characteristic. The white blood cell (WBC) count is consistently elevated (10,000–15,000/mm^3) with polymorphonuclear leukocytosis. Platelet counts are increased. It is important to document and record "steady state" hematologic data (Hb, reticulocytes, WBC) for comparison when the patient later develops complications or "crises."

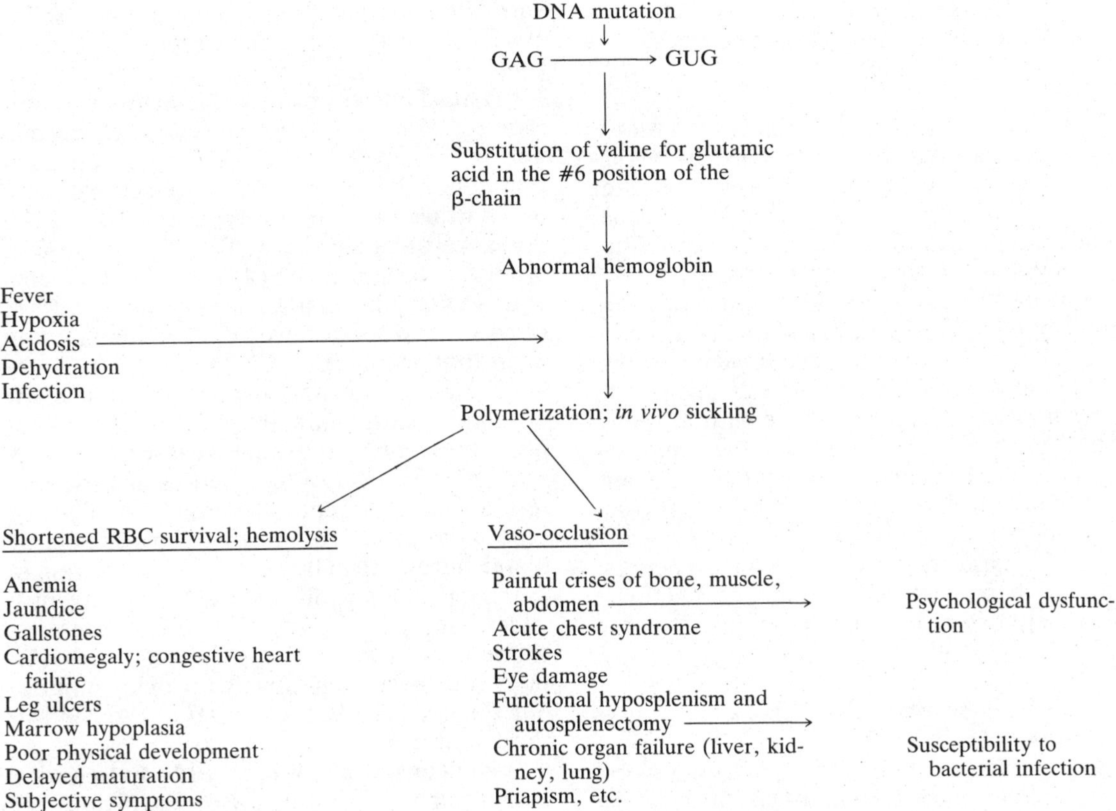

Figure 12–1. Pathophysiology of sickle cell anemia.

CONSEQUENCES OF HEMOLYTIC ANEMIA

Infants with Hb SS disease are not anemic at birth. The development of hemolytic anemia parallels the declining level of Hb F postnatally and is obvious by 4 months of age.

Sickle cell anemia has significant effects on growth. By about 4 years of age, the child's height and weight are usually below average, with weight being more affected. Delayed adolescence is a frequent occurrence.

Table 12–1. SELECTED LABORATORY VALUES IN SICKLE CELL ANEMIA AFTER EARLY CHILDHOOD

	Average	Range*
Hb (gm/100 ml)	7.5	5.5–9.5
Hct (%)	22	17–29
Reticulocytes (%)	12	5–30
Nucleated RBC (/100 WBC)	3	1–10
WBC ($\times 10^9$/L)	12	10–25

*The reasons for this variability are unknown. Steady state values should be determined for each patient.

Chronic, indolent ulceration about the ankles is a regular complication of sickle cell anemia. Ulcers are unusual in the first decade of life, but in some geographic areas as many as 75 per cent of adults develop them. These ulcers are thought in most instances to result from poor circulation and anemia, which impede healing of minor traumatic lesions. Conservative therapy, including clean dressings and immobilization, is indicated. In refractory or progressive cases, multiple transfusions with or without skin grafting and antibiotics may be necessary.[8]

Extreme hemolytic anemia results in a high frequency of pigmented gallstones, which are either radiolucent or radiopaque. About half are radiopaque and visualized on ordinary flat film of the abdomen. Oral cholecystography and gray scale ultrasonography are equally accurate in detection of gallstones. The prevalence of gallstones at 2 to 4 years of age is 12 per cent and increases to 42 per cent at 15 to 18 years of age.[9]

SICKLE CELL CRISES AND CONSEQUENCES OF INTRAVENOUS SICKLING

The clinical courses of patients with sickle cell anemia are punctuated by episodic events that threaten their comfort and lives. The onset of clinical symptoms attributable to intravascular sickling shows considerable variability. Symptoms may occur in children as early as 3 months of age, are noted in half the cases by 1 year of age, and appear in virtually all cases by 5 to 6 years of age. These acute events traditionally have been termed crises, but in fact a number of types of crises with different pathophysiologic mechanisms and symptoms occur and may require different types of therapy. These include the following: (1) vaso-occlusive or symptomatic crises, (2) acute splenic sequestration crises, (3) aplastic crises, (4) hyperhemolytic crises, and (5) functional hyposplenia and overwhelming infection.

Vaso-occlusive Crises

Vaso-occlusive or painful crises of several types are the most common seen in children with sickle cell anemia. Manifestations may vary markedly, depending on the tissues or organs involved and the extent of the ischemic damage. The basic cause of such a crisis is obstruction of blood flow by tangled masses of sickled cells and some degree of vasospasm. There are few or no changes in the hematologic parameters during these episodes. The events that trigger vaso-occlusion are largely undefined, although infections often are associated with or followed by painful crises, perhaps because of accompanying fever, acidosis, and dehydration. Exposure to cold is sometimes implicated, but there appears to be no seasonal variability in the United States. In most instances, there is no discernible antecedent cause.

"Hand-Foot Syndrome." Dactylitis is a common initial manifestation of sickle cell anemia during infancy.[10] This condition results from symmetric infarction of the metacarpals and metatarsals and causes painful swelling of the dorsa of the hands and feet. The hand-foot syndrome occurs in 10 to 45 per cent of patients and is often the first clinical symptom of the disease. Low-grade fever may accompany the hand-foot syndrome. Characteristic hematologic changes are not seen. X-ray films show no abnormalities initially, but areas of osteolysis, periostitis, and bone reabsorption may appear later. The diffuse and symmetric pattern of involvement of multiple bones and especially the lack of systemic signs and sterile blood cultures usually permit differentiation of the hand-foot syndrome from osteomyelitis, which may be suggested by roentgenograms. There is no specific therapy for dactylitis. Attacks may occur repetitively for many months, but do not usually recur after the second or third year of life.

Involvement of Joints and Extremities. Symptomatic, painful crises involving the joints and extremities usually begin after the age of 3 or 4 years. Pains in the extremities result from infarction of the small areas of the long bones or bone marrow or involvement of the periosteum and periarticular tissues of the larger joints. Swelling and moderate limitation of motion may occur, but redness and heat are not prominent. Episodes of joint pain may mimic acute episodes of rheumatic fever or rheumatoid arthritis. Vaso-occlusion and osteomyelitis may be very difficult to differentiate (Table 12–2). X-ray studies are usually unremarkable at the onset of crises. Scanning techniques employing radioisotopes are being

Table 12–2. DIFFERENTIATION OF BONE VASO-OCCLUSIVE CRISIS vs. OSTEOMYELITIS

Common Clinical Features	Features Favoring Osteomyelitis	Features Favoring Vaso-occlusion
Local pain, tenderness, swelling Fever Leukocytosis Abnormal x-ray (late) Abnormal ^{99m}Tc diphosphonate bone scan (late)	Single site Symptom complex unusual to patient Elevated bands (>1000/mm^3) Erythrocyte sedimentation rate >20 mm/hr Normal marrow uptake on ^{99m}Tc colloid scan (early) Positive results for blood and bone cultures	Multiple sites Symptom complex familiar and characteristic to patient Decreased marrow uptake on ^{99m}Tc colloid scan (early) Spontaneous recovery Negative results for blood and bone cultures

Adapted from Nathan DG, Oski FA. Hematology of Infancy and Childhood. 2nd ed. Philadelphia: WB Saunders, 1981.

used increasingly to assess the diagnosis of vaso-occlusive processes involving the marrow or the bones. Acute areas of decreased bone marrow perfusion are noted using ^{99m}Tc gelatin sulfur colloid; later, as healing takes place increased osteoblastic activity can be demonstrated with ^{99m}Tc diphosphonate.[11] In general, few hematologic changes occur during these painful crises, although the total white blood cell count may rise without a greater shift to the left. Significant elevations of temperature usually are not observed.

Osteomyelitis occurs with greater frequency in patients with major sickle cell diseases than in normal individuals. In the non–sickle cell population staphylococci account for more than 80 per cent of cases of hematogenous osteomyelitis, and salmonellae are decidedly uncommon pathogens. In contrast, in sickle cells states more than half the cases of osteomyelitis are caused by salmonellae of various types. Osteomyelitis is most common during the first 5 years of life.

The factors predisposing to salmonella osteomyelitis are no doubt many. Decreased and impaired reticuloendothelial activity facilitates bacteremia, but the propensity of salmonellae to grow in necrotic bone is probably the most important predisposition. Once salmonella infection is established, the immune mechanisms marshalled by the sickle cell patient are normal.

It may be difficult to differentiate bone infarction from osteomyelitis. The absence of fever, leukocytosis, and a markedly elevated erythrocyte sedimentation rate favor bone infarction. Diagnosis ultimately depends on the isolation of the organism from the blood or bone. Scanning techniques may also be useful.^{99m}Tc gelatin sulfur colloid uptake by the bone marrow usually is decreased in early vaso-occlusion, whereas ^{99m}Tc diphosphonate uptake by the bone characteristically is increased in osteomyelitis.

Abdominal Involvement. Episodes of abdominal involvement are thought to occur when infarction or hemorrhage within the liver, spleen, or abdominal lymph nodes results in capsular stretching. Occasionally, the pain may be incapacitating, severe, and episodic, and signs of peritoneal irritation may be present. However, peristalsis usually persists, and this finding helps to differentiate abdominal crises from inflammatory processes that require surgical intervention, such as appendicitis and peritonitis.[14] Clinical features that suggest painful crises as opposed to "surgical abdomen" are summarized in Table 12–3.

The duration of the painful crises averages three to four days. There may be early spontaneous termination, but protracted episodes lasting a week or more also can occur. Variability of individual crises and irregularity of their frequency, even in the same patient, make evaluation of any specific drug or other treatment difficult.

Central Nervous System (CNS) Crises. CNS involvement takes place in about 5 per cent of children with sickle cell anemia.[15] This involvement may be severe, resulting in hemiplegia and other neurologic findings suggestive of extensive CNS damage. The consequences of these "strokes" are variable. Some patients recover rapidly without residual disability, indicating that there had been significant vasospasm present. Others have permanent neurologic deficits, showing that infarction had occurred. Cerebral angiographic studies are not indicated until after the patient has been prepared with transfusions, because hypertonic contrast media produce immediate sickling of red blood cells exposed to them, which could well aggravate vaso-occlusion. However, when properly performed, these studies demonstrate abnormalities in the large cerebral blood vessels such as stenosis and obstruction that may reflect disease in the vasa vasorum with subsequent intimal hyperplasia.

The treatment of CNS crises includes prompt and vigorous hydration, administration

Table 12–3. FEATURES OF PAINFUL ABDOMINAL CRISIS vs. "SURGICAL ABDOMEN"

Painful Crisis	"Surgical Abdomen"
Clinical pattern familiar to patient	Clinical pattern unfamiliar to patient
No peritoneal irritation	Signs of peritoneal irritation
Normal peristalsis	Decreased peristalsis
No hematologic changes	Increased WBC and band count
Lack of significant pyrexia	Pyrexia
Response to symptomatic therapy	No response to symptomatic therapy

Adapted from Nathan DG, Oski FA. Hematology of Infancy and Childhood. 2nd ed. Philadelphia: WB Saunders, 1981.

of oxygen, and multiple transfusions of packed red blood cells. Several reports describe the effectiveness of a program of repeated transfusions for a year or more, resulting in marked improvement of vascular abnormalities in patients who have suffered strokes.[16] Such a program should be strongly considered because these strokes tend to be repetitive and progressive. In fact, some clinicians have advocated indefinite transfusions for these patients because of recurrences of stroke when transfusions were terminated. The relative risks and benefits of chronic transfusions *versus* recurrence of strokes remain to be determined.

Pulmonary Crises (Acute Chest Syndrome). Children with sickle cell anemia often have severe and protracted episodes of pulmonary disease. Although the precipitating event may be bacterial infection with either pneumococcal or even mycoplasmal organisms, infarction may also be a significant component. It may be impossible to differentiate infection from infarction, even with careful x-ray and scanning studies, unless they are done very early. In fact, both pneumonia and pulmonary infarction may be present (Table 12–4). After appropriate cultures have been taken, antibiotic therapy, including penicillin, should be administered. Multiple transfusions of packed red blood cells are also indicated if the pulmonary involvement is extensive or protracted and if it is causing significant pulmonary insufficiency or arterial desaturation. Such transfusions appear to hasten recovery.

Priapism. Priapism is an uncommon but distressing complication in adolescent boys and men with sickle cell anemia. There are two different types of priapism.[17] The first type is relatively brief with spontaneous detumescence usually occurring within three to four hours. The second type is prolonged, lasting more than 24 hours, and is associated with considerable pain. It is frequently followed by impotence.

Priapism appears to result from obstruction of communications between the corpora cavernosa and spongiosa. Sickling of the stagnant blood within the corpora cavernosa then occurs, aggravating obstruction.

Initially, a medical approach including analgesia, oxygenation, hydration, and replacement transfusions should be employed. Several types of surgical procedures have been suggested, including aspiration and irrigation of the corpora cavernosa and a variety of other shunting procedures. On many occasions, impotence has ensued.[18] A simpler surgical approach involving making temporary connections between the corpora cavernosa and spongiosa with a large bore needle has been suggested as being less likely to cause impotence.[19]

Management

At present, there is no specific effective pharmacologic therapy for vaso-occlusive crises.[20] Management of the vaso-occlusive crises is for the most part prophylactic, symptomatic, and supportive. It includes therapy directed at the following conditions that enhance the sickling process.

Hypertonicity, which enhances the sickling phenomenon *in vitro,* may occur *in vivo* by several mechanisms. The expanded plasma volume of these patients may become constricted during painful crises or infections. These patients have fixed hyposthenuria and polyuria and so may become dehydrated easily. Optimal hydration should be insured.

Oral fluids can be relied on in milder symptomatic episodes, but when the pain is severe and particularly when fever, vomiting, or diarrhea contributes to dehydration, parenteral

Table 12–4. DIFFERENTIATION OF PNEUMONIA vs. PULMONARY INFARCTION

Common Clinical Features	Features Favoring Pneumonia	Features Favoring Pulmonary Infarction
Chest pain	Age <5 years	Age >5 years
Infiltration	Chills	Associated painful crisis
Fever	Upper lobe involvement	Clear x-ray at onset
Leukocytosis	Elevated bands (>1000/mm³)	Positive V-Q scan
Rub or effusion	Erythrocyte sedimentation rate >20 mm/hr	Lower lobe disease
Hypoxia	Bacteriology: positive blood sputum cultures or cold agglutinins and mycoplasma titers	Negative cultures

Adapted from Nathan DG, Oski FA. Hematology of Infancy and Childhood. 2nd ed. Philadelphia: WB Saunders, 1981.

hydration is indicated. A mixture of equal amounts of normal saline and 5 per cent dextrose, infused at the rate of 2000–2500 ml/m²/day (1.5 times maintenance), should be given.

Because acidosis aggravates sickling, alkali therapy is often administered to rectify potential or actual acidosis. Although controlled studies showed little beneficial effect from such therapy, oral sodium bicarbonate or polycitrate solutions may be used in mild vaso-occlusive crises. When intravenous therapy is given, sodium bicarbonate is often added to the hydrating solution.

Reduced oxygenation and hypoxia increase sickling; therefore an atmosphere of well-humidified oxygen may be used when a child is experiencing pain. Although hyperbaric oxygen is probably effective, the modest increase in blood oxygenation accomplished with an oxygen tent or mask is of uncertain value.

Infection may be a precipitating cause of vaso-occlusive crises and in the tropics it may be the most important one. When evidence of bacterial infection is found, appropriate antibiotic therapy is indicated after cultures are taken.

Besides giving attention to the possible contributing factors, one should also consider the use of transfusions if the crisis is severe. Since the ordinary vaso-occlusive crisis is not associated with hematologic deterioration, blood is not usually given for anemia *per se*. In fact, the beneficial effects of a single blood transfusion in increasing oxygen transport may be counterbalanced by the greater blood viscosity resulting from an elevation in hematocrit. In severe or prolonged vaso-occlusive crises, vigorous multiple transfusion therapy designed to "dilute" the patient's sickle cells may be considered. If the number of sickle cells in the circulation can be reduced effectively, vaso-occlusive manifestations of the disease can usually be ameliorated. The most effective way to accomplish such a reduction is by transfusion of normal red blood cells from non–sickle cell donors. When at least 60 per cent of the patient's circulating red blood cells are replaced by normal cells, the progression of vaso-occlusive symptoms usually stops. Transfusions of fresh packed red blood cells, 10–15 ml/kg, can be given every 12–24 hours until the hemoglobin level has increased to 12–13 gm/100 ml. At this point simple dilution will have significantly reduced the proportion of the patient's circulating red blood cells. Because of their 10- to 20-day survival rate, the patient's own red blood cells, which predominantly contain Hb S, disappear rapidly. With small packed cell transfusions given to maintain the hemoglobin level greater than 12 gm/100 ml, the proportion of circulating cells containing Hb S will rapidly fall to low levels, thus producing the same effects as an exchange transfusion in a few days. Packed red blood cell transfusions every two to three weeks will usually insure that the circulating blood contains predominantly normal red blood cells. A quantitative sickle cell preparation, using sodium metabisulfite in which red blood cells of the patient and donor can be morphologically differentiated, is an accurate method for assessing the completeness of replacement transfusion and is more rapid than quantitative hemoglobin electrophoresis.

Although this "hypertransfusion regimen" is symptomatically effective, there are inherent risks of isoimmunization, hepatitis, and hemosiderosis. Patients with sickle cell anemia who receive transfusions on a regular basis develop hemosiderosis. A chronic transfusion program usually is advocated only for specific indications such as prolonged or severe vaso-occlusive crises, especially those involving the CNS; as preparation for anesthesia and surgery; as management of pregnancy; and as supportive therapy during complicating medical conditions. In critical situations, exchange transfusions with fresh blood may be the most effective way to rapidly reduce the proportion of cells containing Hb S.

Exchange transfusion with whole or reconstituted blood has been advocated when rapid reduction of the proportion of sickled cells is desirable. It can be done using a single peripheral intravenous line with successive withdrawal and infusion of 25–50 ml aliquots of blood. Alternatively, the patient's blood can be withdrawn from one vein while an equivolume of normal blood is infused in another blood vessel.

Sedation and Analgesia. Considerable relief of pain and discomfort may be obtained with the judicious use of sedatives and analgesics.

When pain is mild or moderate, painful events can often be managed at home using oral analgesics. Codeine sulfate (1 mg/kg) and aspirin or acetaminophen (10 mg/kg) should be given, every four hours.

When pain is more severe, hospitalization is often required. Parenteral morphine sulfate (0.1–0.2 mg/kg) or meperdine (1–2 mg/kg) should be given every 3 to 4 hours. In order to avoid periods of discomfort, these medications should be administered regularly rather than as needed or on request (prn). When the pain has been controlled for 12 hours, the dose of morphine sulfate or meperidine may be reduced 10 to 20 per cent. After the initial parenteral dose has been decreased about 50 per cent, it is often possible to resume oral analgesics. Compounds such as prochlorperazine and chlorpromazine are useful adjuncts for treatment of painful crises because of their sedating and tranquilizing action; their use may reduce the need for narcotics.

Pharmacologic Therapy. The history of sickle cell anemia is studded with enthusiastic preliminary reports of effective therapies. However, when these therapies have been subjected to tests in larger controlled studies, no significant benefit usually has been shown. The problem of evaluation is compounded by the extreme diversity and variability of the sickle cell crises. Ultimately any beneficial therapy of sickle cell anemia must be reflected in a reduction of *in vivo* sickling. Furthermore, careful, controlled crossover studies in which the patients serve as their own controls must demonstrate a decrease in the number and frequency of vaso-occlusive episodes. Unless unequivocal proof is demonstrated, a degree of healthy skepticism must be maintained, especially if the proposed therapy has some possibility of danger. The use of urea and cyanate merits special attention.

Considerable publicity extolled the possible benefit of intravenous urea in invert sugar for the painful crises of sickle cell disease.[21] The rationale for this therapy was that high concentrations of urea disrupt molecular bonds that participate in the sickling process. The therapeutic use of urea increases the patient's blood urea nitrogen level to 150–200 mg/100 ml and evokes a diuresis that must be treated vigorously if dehydration is to be avoided. Despite preliminary clinical reports of uncontrolled studies suggesting the efficacy of urea, the supposed therapeutic level of urea attained in patients was shown to have no effect on *in vitro* sickling, and controlled studies of both intravenous and oral urea administration did not demonstrate significant benefit. Therefore, the use of urea is not indicated in the management of sickle cell disease.

The possible value of cyanate has been investigated vigorously in patients with Hb SS disease.[22] This compound interacts with the sickle hemoglobin molecule by a process called carbamylation. Cyanate directly inhibits the sickling process, probably by changing the affinity between hemoglobin, oxygen, and 2,3-diphosphoglycerate or by altering molecular configuration.[22] Although oral cyanate treatment decreases the rate of hemolysis and leads to higher hemoglobin level, a controlled study did not demonstrate significant reduction in the number or severity of vaso-occlusive episodes. In addition, considerable drug toxicity was observed, including peripheral neuropathy, interference with nutrition, and in two patients the development of cataracts. The use of oral cyanate is not currently indicated in sickle cell disease.

A large number of compounds have the capacity to interfere with the sickling phenomenon in *in vitro* test systems. Some of these agents interact with the red blood cell membrane, whereas others interfere with hemoglobin polymerization. However, as of 1984, a safe and effective pharmacologic approach to sickle cell anemia remains elusive.

A novel investigative approach to the treatment of sickle cell anemia by genetic manipulation has recently been reported. Deactivation of the γ-gene is associated with methylation of DNA.[23] In the fetus with active γ-chain synthesis, the γ-gene is relatively hypomethylated, whereas in the older individual producing β-chains, it is heavily methylated. The cancer chemotherapeutic agent 5-azacytidine has been used to induce hypomethylation of the γ-gene and to reactivate Hb F synthesis in two adult patients with sickle cell anemia with apparent reduction in symptoms.[24] However, because the drug is toxic, with particular oncogenic potential, its use decidedly is experimental. A similar reactivation of Hb F synthesis has been described in an animal model study using the presumably non-carcinogenic agent hydroxyurea.[24a]

Splenic Sequestration Crises

Infants and young children with Hb SS disease whose spleens have not yet undergone multiple infarctions and subsequent fibrosis, and children with other major Hb S syndromes whose spleens remain enlarged into adult life, may suddenly have pooling of vast amounts of blood. In sickle cell anemia, these events may occur after 5 months of age but are unusual after 2 years of age.[25]

During these sequestration crises the spleen becomes enormous, fills the abdomen, and even reaches into the pelvis. The hemoglobin level may drop so precipitously that hypovolemic shock and death may occur. The exact pathogenesis of this syndrome is not known. It may result from temporary venous obstruction to blood flow and occurs in children who are functionally hyposplenic as indicated by ^{99m}Tc scans and percentage of "pocked" red blood cells (see "Diagnosis" of Functional Hyposplenism and Overwhelming Infection). Splenic sequestration is the most acutely dangerous crisis in the life of the young child with sickle cell anemia, and it must be recognized and treated promptly. Children between the ages of 8 months and 5 years are particularly susceptible and may die within hours of the first signs of this disturbance.

Diagnosis

The usual clinical indications of this complication are the sudden development of weakness, pallor of the lips and mucous membranes, breathlessness, rapid pulse, faintness, and abdominal fullness. Because large numbers of children with sickle cell disease have been diagnosed at birth and carefully followed sequentially, it has become apparent that minor episodes of splenic sequestration are common.[25] These minor episodes are characterized by moderate increases in spleen size associated with a reduction in hemoglobin levels of 2–3 gm/100 ml. Although these minor episodes usually resolve spontaneously, they may identify infants who are susceptible to the severe, life-threatening splenic sequestration episodes. Some centers have trained the parents to palpate the abdomen and assess the size of the spleen. If rapid enlargement occurs, they are instructed to seek immediate medical attention.

Management

Treatment of the sequestration crisis is directed toward the prompt correction of hypovolemia with plasma expanders and particularly with whole blood transfusions. If the shock can be reversed, much of the blood sequestered in the spleen is remobilized and dramatic regression of splenomegaly may occur in a short time. This phenomenon has been called the syndrome of the "yo-yo" spleen.[26] Because of the rapidity with which a sequestration crisis can occur and even recur and because of its potential fatality in a matter of hours, splenectomy should be considered strongly if a child has had one or more of these severe crises. Alternatively, a program of chronic transfusion can be employed in the infant less than 2 years of age, thus avoiding splenectomy in the very young child. However, if transfusions are discontinued, the child may then again be at risk.

Aplastic Crises

In patients with sickle cell anemia, red blood cell survival is only between 10 and 20 days, compared with 120 days in normal persons. Despite this extreme hemolysis the patient usually maintains a hemoglobin level of 5.5–9.5 gm/100 ml by increasing red blood cell production five- to eight-fold. If this maximal compensatory response is compromised, profound anemia develops rapidly. The patient quickly develops weakness, listlessness, rapid breathing, and tachycardia.

Pathogenesis

Diminished red blood cell production superimposed on the usual rapid destruction of red blood cells, rather than hyperhemolysis, is the basis of an aplastic crisis.

A number of infections, usually viral, may in some way damage the erythroid bone marrow and result in a cessation of red blood cell production that may persist for 10 to 14 days. Aplastic crises may occur in several members of a family (further evidence suggesting an infectious origin). It was recently noted that parvovirus-like infections were causally associated with asplastic crisis in children with sickle cell anemia in London and Jamaica.[27]

Diagnosis

During aplastic episodes, reticulocytes disappear from the blood and a markedly reduced number of erythroid precursors are present in the bone marrow.

The hematologic findings during aplastic crisis differ, depending on the stage at which the patient is studied. In the early stages, the degree of anemia is more extreme than usual, but jaundice may decrease. The numbers of reticulocytes in the blood and of nucleated red blood cells in the bone marrow are sharply reduced. Platelet and white blood cell counts are usually not affected. At the nadir of the aplastic crisis, the hemoglobin level may fall to 1 gm/100 ml and death may result from severe anemia and congestive heart failure.

Erythroid aplasia usually terminates spontaneously after about 10 days, and recovery is accompanied by a surge of reticulocytes and nucleated red blood cells in the blood. The reticulocyte count may then reach 50 to 60 per cent, and the hemoglobin quickly returns to its pre-crisis level. If the patient is studied early in the recovery stage from an aplastic crisis, a mistaken diagnosis of hyperhemolytic crisis may be reached because severe anemia and marked increase in reticulocytes are present.

Management

The treatment for an aplastic crisis is transfusion of fresh packed red blood cells, given slowly in a dosage of not more than 2–3 ml/kg every 6–8 hours until the hemoglobin level is increased by about 5 gm/100 ml. For the small child, a whole unit of packed cells (250–300 ml) can be divided and used sequentially, thereby reducing the risk of transfusion hepatitis and isoimmunization. Oxygen should be administered if the patient is dyspneic, but the use of digitalis is not indicated. Furosemide may also be administered. Parents of children with major Hb S diseases should be made aware of the manifestations of the aplastic crisis. They should seek medical attention promptly if the child becomes weak or pale, especially in the wake of infections.

Hyperhemolytic Crises

The frequency and even the existence of so-called hyperhemolytic crises are somewhat controversial because of the difficulty of proving a more rapid rate of hemolysis superimposed on an already severe process. Hyperhemolytic crises are probably very unusual.

Pathogenesis

Hyperhemolysis may ensue in association with certain drugs or acute infections. The concomitant presence of glucose-6-phosphate dehydrogenase deficiency has been suggested as a possible contributing cause of hyperhemolytic episodes, especially when combined with infections.

Diagnosis

During these episodes the patient begins to feel weak, look paler, and show more scleral icterus. There may be abdominal pain. The hematocrit falls from its usual 21 to 25 per cent to 15 per cent or less in a few days, and at the same time the reticulocyte count rises. The patient becomes more jaundiced. After several days the excessive hemolysis tends to gradually subside.

Management

If evidence of bacterial infection is found, appropriate antibiotic therapy is indicated. Oxidant drugs that may produce hemolysis should be discontinued. At the same time dehydration and acidosis should be corrected. Transfusions of packed red blood cells should be given to reverse or prevent incipient heart failure from anemic hypoxia.

Functional Hyposplenism and Overwhelming Infection

The spleen in sickle cell anemia undergoes characteristic changes during infancy and childhood. By six months of age, significant splenomegaly is apparent and persists during childhood. After 6 months of age, significant splenomegaly becomes less common. In the United States, persistence of splenomegaly after adolescence suggests a mixed sickle hemoglobin variant rather than homozygous Hb SS disease. The spleen, which is enlarged and congested in early years, undergoes progressive fibrosis, usually without clearly defined episodes of abdominal pain. Perivascular hemorrhage and infarction ultimately result in a minute siderofibrotic nubbin, a phenomenon designated as autosplenectomy.

Pathogenesis

A functional reduction of splenic activity regularly precedes autosplenectomy in early life. Functional hyposplenia is defined as defective splenic reticuloendothelial activity of the anatomically enlarged spleens of young children with sickle cell anemia.[28] This condition appears to be a consequence of altered intrasplenic circulation caused by intrasplenic sickling. It can be temporarily reversed by transfusions of normal red blood cells.[29] Functional hyposplenia is not a congenital but an acquired defect occurring between 5 and 36 months of age when the proportion of Hb F falls to less than 20 per cent.[30]

Diagnosis

Functional hyposplenism was first diagnosed using ^{99m}Tc gelatin sulfur colloid scans that showed no uptake of the radioactive colloid by the enlarged spleen. Study of developmental aspects of spleen dysfunction in sickle cell diseases has been made considerably easier by the use of a non-invasive technique involving examination of a patient's red blood cells, i.e., interference phase-contrast microscopy (Nomarsky optics). When red blood cells from asplenic patients are examined, using this optical system, approximately 20 per cent (range 12–40%) have one or more surface indentations resembling craters and can be designated as "pocked" or "pitted" red blood cells. In normal eusplenic persons, fewer than one per cent of the circulating red blood cells are pocked.[31] Values of pocked red blood cells greater than 3.5 per cent represent "hyposplenism." Interesting developmental changes of pocked RBCs have been documented in sickle cell anemia. At birth and for the first few months of life, the percentage of pocked RBCs is low, indicating normal splenic function. Thereafter, the pocked RBCs increase,[32] although there is considerable variability from patient to patient. A pocked RBC percentage of >3.5 per cent has been shown to have a predictive value of non-visualization of the spleen by ^{99m}Tc colloid spleen scan with >90 per cent accuracy.[33]

There are infectious consequences of functional hyposplenia. Children with functional hyposplenia are 300–600 times more likely to develop overwhelming pneumococcal and *Haemophilus influenzae* sepsis and meningitis than normal children.[34] This propensity to serious infection is similar to that following surgical splenectomy in young children.

Studies of sickle cell anemia in infancy indicate that the period of greatest risk for death from severe infection is during the first 5 years of life. To reduce this inordinately high rate in early life, populations at risk should be screened for sickle cell anemia, ideally at birth. Careful follow-up examinations and ready access to medical care can reduce mortality.

Management

It is important to recognize that fever in patients with sickle cell disease, like fever in children who are anatomically asplenic, may indicate potentially lethal sepsis.

The time of onset of functional hyposplenism may coincide with the onset of this susceptibility to infection. Functional hyposplenism is determined by interference phase contrast examination of a pocked red blood cell proportion of >3.5 per cent.[32]

Many physicians advocate the use of prophylactic penicillin (250 mg of Pen-V twice a day) or monthly depot penicillin injections. At the present time there are no controlled studies that validate the effectiveness of such a prophylactic regimen. Furthermore, compliance is a major problem with oral penicillin. In one study, despite frequent reinforcement and encouragement, only 64 per cent compliance could be documented.[35]

Immunization with pneumococcal polysaccharide vaccine at 2 years of age should be performed. Immunization before this age is not sanctioned by the FDA because it has unpredictable effects. However, cases of fatal pneumococcal infections have occurred in patients who have received the vaccine and others who were receiving prophylactic antibiotics.[36, 37] Therefore, in our institution, we have instructed the family to bring the child with sickle cell disease who develops a temperature of 102°F, or chills or toxicity at a lower temperature, to the hospital emergency room immediately. We have rather arbitrarily chosen this value of 102°F because of our experience that the child with sickle cell anemia and sepsis is almost always hyperpyretic (>103°F). The febrile child is evaluated, blood is drawn for culture, and 20 mg/kg of ampicillin is administered intravenously. Even if the child appears "well," he is observed for 4–6 hours and then is discharged to continue taking oral antibiotics. If clinical deterioration occurs, the child is admitted to the hosptial for intensive care. When access to the hospital is difficult, some physicians have provided oral antibiotics for immediate use at home if fever develops.

We recognize that our approach is a compromise because some children with sepsis may have temperatures lower than 102°F on presentation. However, we have seen that insisting upon intensive therapy, including hospitalization of the child for temperatures lower than 102°F, has led to non-compliance by the parents in reporting their child's episodes of fever to us. The use of the "arbitrary" temperature of 102°F has assured both continued compliance and recognition of potentially fatal infection.

The child with suspected sepsis should be hospitalized and monitored closely, preferably in an intensive care unit. Lumbar puncture should be performed. High dose intravenous antibiotics, such as penicillin and chloramphenicol, which are effective against pneumococci and *H. influenzae,* should be given. If the child appears critically ill, an exchange transfusion is indicated to reduce the risk of intravascular sickling, to provide opsonins, and to restore splenic function.

SUMMARY

An accurate definition of the prognosis of sickle cell anemia in the United States today is difficult. There is a paucity of careful, long-term prospective studies. Prognosis is markedly affected by the kind of available medical care and supervision. In a retrospective analysis of autopsy cases approximately 25 years ago, Diggs suggested that 20 to 30 per cent of patients die in the first 5 years of life.[38] The median age of death was less than 20 years, and survival past 40 years was unusual.

The causes of the inordinately high mortality rate during the first years of life are overwhelming sepsis and sequestration crises, complications that are preventable to a great extent by good medical supervision. Providing this supervision is the challenge of sickle cell disease to the pediatrician.

REFERENCES

1. Ingram VM. Abnormal human haemoglobins. I. The comparison of normal human and sickle-cell haemoglobins by fingerprinting. Biochim Biophys Acta 1957, *28*:539.
2. Noguchi CT, Schechter AM. The intracellular polymerization of sickle hemoglobin and its relation to sickle cell disease. Blood 1981, *58*:1057.
3. Daland GA, Castle WB. A simple and rapid method for demonstration of sickling of the red cells: the use of reducing agents. J Lab Clin Med 1948, *33*:1082.
4. Nelbandian RM, Nichols BM, Camp FR, et al. Dithionate tube test—a rapid inexpensive technique for detection of hemoglobin S and non-S sickling hemoglobin. Clin Chem 1971, *17*:1028.
5. Schmidt, RM, Wilson S. Standardizations in detection of abnormal hemoglobin solubility tests for hemoglobins. JAMA 1973, *225*:1225.
6. Boyle E Jr, Thompson C, Tryoler HA. Prevalence of sickle cell trait in adults of Charleston County. Arch Environ Health 1968, *17*:891.
7. Kramer MS, Rooks Y, Washington L, Pearson HA. Pre- and postpubertal growth and development in sickle cell anemia. J Pediatr 1980, *96*:857.
8. Serjeant GR. Leg ulceration in sickle cell anemia. Arch Intern Med 1974, 133:690.
9. Samiak S, Soorya D, Jim J, et al. Incidence of cholelithiasis in sickle cell anemia using ultrasonic gray scale techniques. J Pediatr 1980, *96*:1005.
10. Watson RJ, Burko H, Megas H, Robinson H. The hand-foot syndrome in sickle cell disease in young children. Pediatrics 1963, *31*:975.
11. Hammel CB, DeNardo GL, Lewis JP. Bone marrow and bone mineral scintigraphic studies in sickle cell disease. Br J Haematol 1973, *25*:593.
12. Diggs LW. Bone and joint lesions in sickle cell diseases. Clin Orthop 1967, *52*:119.
13. Powars DR. Natural history of sickle cell disease—the first ten years. Semin Hematol 1975, *12*:267.
14. Kudsk KA, Tranbaugh RF, Sheldon GF. Acute surgical illnesses in patients with sickle cell anemia. Am J Surg 1981, *142*:113.
15. Portnoy RA, Herron JC. Neurological manifestations in sickle cell disease. Ann Intern Med 1972, *76*:643.
16. Russell MO, Goldberg HL, Reis L, et al. Transfusion therapy for cerebrovascular abnormalities in sickle cell disease. J Pediatr 1976, *88*:382.
17. Edmond EM, Holman R, Hayes RJ, Serjeant GR. Priapism and impotence in homozygous sickle cell disease. Ann Intern Med 1980, *140*:1434.
18. Snyder GB, Wilson CA. Surgical management of priapism and its complications in sickle cell disease. South Med J 1966, *59*:1393.
19. Winter CC. Priapism cured by creation of fistulas between glans penis and corpora cavernosa. J Urol 1978, *119*:227.
20. Dean J, Schechter AN. Sickle cell anemia: molecular and cellular basis of therapeutic approaches. N Engl J Med 1978, *299*:804 and 863.
21. Nalbandian RM. Urea for sickle cell crisis. N Engl J Med 1971, *284*:1381.
22. Gillette PM, Lu YS, Peterson CM. The pharmacology of cyanate with summary of its initial usage in sickle cell disease. Prog Hematol 1973, *5*:181.
23. Ley TJ, DiSimone J, Aganow NP, et al. 5-Azacytidine selectively increases γ globin synthesis in a patient with β-thalassemia. N Engl J Med 1982, *307*:1469.
24. Charache S, Dover G, Smith K, et al. Treatment of sickle cell anemia with 5-azacytidine. Proc Nat Acad Sci 1983, *80*:4842.

24a. Letvin NL, Linch DC, Beardsley GP, et al. Augmentation of fetal-hemoglobin production in anemic monkeys by hydroxyurea. New Engl J Med 1984, *310*:869.

25. Topley JM, Rogers DW, Stevens CG, Serjeant GR. Acute splenic sequestration and hypersplenism in the first five years in homozygous sickle cell disease. Arch Dis Child 1981, *56*:765.
26. Pearson HA. Sickle Cell Disease Crises and Their Management. *In:* Smith CA, ed. The Critically Ill Child. 2nd ed. Philadelphia: WB Saunders, 1977.
27. Patterson JR, Jones SE, Hodgson J, et al. Parvovirus infections and hypoplastic crisis in sickle cell anemia. Lancet 1981, *1*:664.
28. Pearson HA. Functional asplenia in sickle cell anemia. N Engl J Med 1969, *281*:923.
29. Pearson HA, Cornelius EA, Schwartz EA. Transfusion reversible functional asplenia in sickle cell anemia. N Engl J Med 1970, *281*:334.
30. O'Brien RT, McIntosh LS, Apnes GT, Pearson HA. Prospective study of sickle cell anemia in infancy. J Pediatr 1976, *89*:205.
31. Pearson HA, Johnston D, Smith KA, Touloukian RT. The born-again spleen. N Engl J Med 1978, *298*:1389.

32 Pearson HA, McIntosh LS, Ritchey AK. Developmental aspects of splenic function in sickle cell disease. Blood 1978, *53*:358.

33. Pearson HA. Splenic function in sickle cell anemia. Pediatr Res 1983, *17*:204A.
34. Barrett-Connor E. Bacterial infection and sickle cell anemia. Medicine 1971, *50*:97.

35. Buchanan GR, Siegel JD, Smith SJ, DePasse BM. Oral penicillin prophylaxis in children with impaired splenic function: a study of compliance. Pediatrics 1982, *70*:926.
36. Ertel IJ, Babes ET. Infections after splenectomy. N Engl J Med 1977, *296*:1174.
37. Overturf GD, Field R. Death from type II pneumococcal septicemia in a vaccinated child with sickle cell disease. N Engl J Med 1979, *300*:143.
38. Diggs LW. Anatomic Lesions in Sickle Cell Diseases. *In:* Abramson H, Butler JF, Wethers DL, eds. Sickle Cell Disease: Diagnosis, Management, Education, and Research. St. Louis: CV Mosby, 1973:189.
39. Nathan DG, Oski FA. Hematology of Infancy and Childhood. 2nd ed. Philadelphia: WB Saunders, 1981.

CHAPTER

13

Cardiac Arrhythmias

Welton M. Gersony, M.D.
Allan J. Hordof, M.D.

Childhood cardiac arrhythmias have been encountered more commonly in recent years. Spontaneous arrhythmias now are identified more accurately in pediatric patients, and there are a significant number of survivors of surgical repair of congenital heart disease who are prone to rhythm disturbances. Early diagnosis is required in order to anticipate untoward cardiac events. As a result of the current technology revolution, improved diagnostic techniques have evolved, which are being used with greater frequency in pediatric units at most major medical centers. These techniques include 24-hour ambulatory electrocardiographic monitoring and exercise studies for the clinical evaluation of rhythm disturbances, and sophisticated intracardiac electrophysiologic procedures for the delineation of complex rhythm abnormalities.[1–3]

Essentially, the risk of a severe cardiac rhythm disorder is that of severe tachycardia or bradycardia leading to decreased cardiac output, further deterioration of cardiac rhythm, syncope, and even death. The threat of ectopic cardiac activity, even without frank tachyarrhythmia or bradyarrhythmia, is that certain types of aberrant activity, while relatively benign in their early phases, may deteriorate to severe arrhythmia. On the other hand, some rhythm abnormalities, notably single premature atrial or ventricular beats, are common in the general population and under most circumstances do not pose a threat, especially among individuals with normal cardiac dynamics. Accurate differential diagnosis of cardiac arrhythmias is critical.

Table 13–1 indicates the possible diagnoses for pediatric patients in whom cardiac arrhythmias are a special risk. A great majority of such patients have congenital heart disease and many have had surgery. In some patients, arrhythmias may be the first manifestations of an unusual congenital abnormality or acquired condition (e.g., cardiac tumor, myocarditis, right ventricular dysplasia syndrome). However, even in children with "normal" hearts, severe arrhythmias may occur. Some patients have predisposing conduction abnormalities such as prolonged QT intervals, pre-excitation syndromes, and other forms of familial conduction disturbances.

An improved understanding of the electrophysiologic basis of rhythm abnormalities as well as the advent of new diagnostic tools have led to advances in pharmacologic and surgical management. An increasing number of pharmacologic agents are now available for the treatment of significant rhythm disturbances.

Problems with frequency of administration, compliance, and side effects remain, and selection of an antiarrhythmic agent still involves a great deal of empiricism. Nevertheless, various treatment regimens, including single and multiple agents, have been successful in controlling a number of cardiac arrhythmias. Surgical intervention to eliminate bypass tracts associated with pre-excitation syndromes or unusual electrically active areas in the heart is now available in extreme situations. Furthermore, in recent years, implanted pacemakers have become more sophisticated and much less prone to technical failure than early models.[2, 3]

PATHOPHYSIOLOGY

Before we review the mechanisms for abnormal electrical activity responsible for ar-

The authors wish to acknowledge the invaluable assistance of Linda D. O'Neill, R.N., M.A., and Eugene W. Greene in the preparation of the manuscript.

Table 13–1. DIAGNOSES FOR PEDIATRIC PATIENTS IN WHOM CARDIAC ARRHYTHMIAS ARE A SPECIAL RISK

Acquired
Cardiomyopathy
Acute and chronic inflammatory heart disease
Thalassemia
Sickle cell disease
Diphtheria
Congenital
Postoperative transposition of great vessels
Postoperative tetralogy of Fallot
"Corrected" transposition of great vessels
Idiopathic hypertrophic subaortic stenosis
Mitral valve prolapse
Ebstein anomaly*
Right ventricular dysplasia*
Cardiac tumor*
Pulmonary vascular disease
Mitral and tricuspid valve disease†
Primary Conduction System Disease
Prolonged QT
Pre-excitation syndrome
Congenital heart block

*Also may be categorized as Primary Conduction System Disease.
†Also may be categorized as acquired.

rhythmia induction, it is important to understand the electrical and ionic events which form the basis of normal cardiac electrical activity. In the normal heart, electrical activity is initiated in the sinus node and spreads radially to the adjacent atrial myocardium. Propagation occurs along presumed specialized atrial fibers to the atrioventricular node and to the left atrium. Electrical activation of the atrial myocardium is recorded from the body surface as the P wave. Conduction through the AV node, His bundle, and Purkinje fibers (left and right bundle branches) occurs during the PR interval. Because the electrical activity is of such low magnitude at this time, only an isoelectric segment is evident during this portion of the electrocardiogram (ECG). The QRS complex is the result of ventricular myocardial activation, and the T wave is the result of ventricular myocardial repolarization. It is apparent therefore that the electrical function of the heart depends on repetitive impulse initiation at a single site in the heart, usually the sinus node, and an orderly sequence of propagation and repolarization.

Much of what is known about the pathophysiology of arrhythmias has come from studies of the transmembrane action potentials recorded from isolated cardiac tissue.[4] In this section we will briefly review some of the important information related to normal electrical activity in single cardiac cells.

The high level of resting membrane potential in Purkinje fibers is primarily due to the potassium concentration gradient maintained across the cell membrane by active transport, resulting in a high intracellular potassium concentration compared with the external potassium concentration.[5, 6] The resting cell is highly permeable to potassium and relatively impermeable to sodium and behaves like a potassium electrode.[5, 6] This results in a linear relationship between the resting membrane potential and the log of the external potassium concentration.[4] When a stimulus of appropriate strength and duration depolarizes the cell to a critical level of membrane potential (the threshold potential), there is an increase in sodium permeability. The electrical and concentration gradients to sodium result in a rapid entry of sodium into the cell (Fig. 13–1A).[7] A rapid depolarization to a positive level of membrane potential occurs. This phase of the action potential is referred to as phase 0.[8] It is followed by a phase 1 depolarization associated with a reduction of sodium entry and a passive chloride entry into the cell.[9] Phase 2, the plateau phase, is due in part to a slow inward calcium current as well as a slow sodium entry.[10] Phase 3, a repolarization phase, is associated with an outward potassium current, causing an outward flow of positive ions that results in a return to the resting membrane potential.[11] In non-pacemaker cells, phase 4 is a period of electrical quiescence between action potentials. The ion fluxes that occur during the action potential are passive processes. However, an active transport process is necessary for restoration and maintenance of the appropriate concentrations of ions across the cell membrane at the end of full repolarization via the sodium-potassium ATPase pump.[4]

Cardiac cells have important properties that differentiate them from other types of muscle and nerve cells. These properties include *automaticity, excitability, conductivity,* and *refractoriness. Automaticity* is defined as the ability to initiate action potentials spontaneously in the absence of an extrinsic stimulus.[4] The dominant specialized area of the heart that has the property of automaticity is the sinus node. However, automaticity is also present in specialized atrial conducting fibers, fibers in the atrial surface of the mitral and tricuspid valves, fibers in the lower or junctional region of the AV node, and fibers in the His-Purkinje system.[4, 12, 13] Automaticity is responsible for the function of the escape pacemakers at times of sinus node depression or atrioventricular

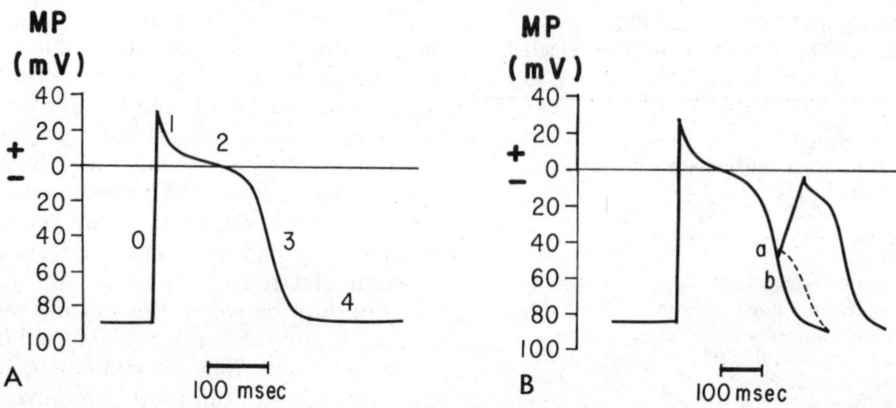

Figure 13–1. *A*, The transmembrane action potential. Cardiac cell has a resting membrane potential of approximately −90 millivolts. When a stimulus of appropriate strength and duration is applied, the cell is depolarized to a critical level of membrane potential (threshold potential), resulting in a transmembrane action potential. Phase 0 is during rapid depolarization; phases 1, 2, and 3 are during repolarization; and phase 4 is the period of electrical diastole. *B*, Refractory periods. The premature depolarization (a) occurs too early during repolarization, resulting in a non-propagated local response (dotted line). The premature stimulus (b), occurs later during repolarization, resulting in a propagated premature action potential (solid line).

block. Enhanced automaticity in cardiac fibers can also result in pacemakers competing with the sinus node in initiating arrhythmias.

Excitability refers to the electrical responsiveness of the heart to external stimuli.[4, 7] All cardiac cells are excitable; given a stimulus of adequate strength and duration, they will respond by initiating an action potential.

The velocity at which the cardiac impulse is propagated is dependent on the passive properties of the cardiac fibers, or *conductivity*.[4, 8] These passive properties of the cardiac fibers allow them to function as a cable that is capable of conducting an electrical current. Following excitation of a fiber segment, its membrane potential changes rapidly as it is depolarized. Current then flows from the depolarized, excited segment to adjacent unexcited portions of the fiber, resulting in depolarization of these areas and propagation of the impulse.[4, 14]

The fourth property that is important to the understanding of the physiology of cardiac fibers is that of *refractoriness*. Once a cell has responded to a stimulus by initiating an action potential, it will fail to respond to a second depolarizing stimulus until it has repolarized to approximately −50 to −60 millivolts. The period during which the cell is repolarizing and is unable to respond to a premature stimulus by initiating a propagating or second action potential is referred to as the effective refractory period.[4] The effective refractory period is important because it determines whether or not a premature depolarization will propagate further in the specialized conduction system (Fig. 13–1B).

Mechanisms of Arrhythmias

There have been many classifications of the mechanisms of arrhythmias. A common approach to the pathophysiology of cardiac arrhythmias has been outlined by Hoffman and Cranefield.[15] They defined the mechanisms of arrhythmias as (1) abnormal impulse generation, (2) abnormal impulse conduction, and (3) simultaneous abnormalities of both impulse generation and conduction (Table 13–2). We will briefly describe the characteristics of each type of mechanism in the next section.

Table 13–2. MECHANISMS OF ARRHYTHMIAS

I. Abnormal impulse generation
  A. Automaticity
    1. Normal mechanism
    2. Abnormal mechamism
  B. Triggered Activity
    1. Early after-depolarizations
    2. Delayed after-depolarizations
II. Abnormal impulse conduction
  A. Block
    1. Partial
    2. Complete
  B. Reentry
    1. Unidirectional block and slow conduction
    2. Reflection
    3. Summation
III. Simultaneous abnormalities of impulse generation and conduction
  A. Parasystole

Abnormal Impulse Generation

Abnormal impulse generation occurs when either the function of the normal sinus node pacemaker is depressed or the pacemakers elsewhere in the heart are accelerated and compete with the sinus node. The sinus node is generally the dominant pacemaker because it has a more rapid rate of phase 4 depolarization. Because of its property of automaticity and its more rapid rate, the sinus node pacemaker overdrive suppresses potential subsidiary pacemakers. Under normal conditions, all other pacemaker tissues are discharged by conducted impulses from the sinus node before they are manifested. These pacemakers are subsidiary and are manifested only when the sinus node fails to function. In other words, potential pacemakers are suppressed because of dominance of the primary pacemaker's faster rate. In addition, a sudden suppression of the dominant pacemaker is followed by a period of quiescence before the subsidiary pacemaker begins to discharge ("overdrive suppression").[16] This period of quiescence is longer than the interval between the beats of the newly established subsidiary rhythm. If the sinus node is excessively slow or is arrested completely, subsidiary pacemakers become the actual pacemakers of the heart.

Different degrees of automaticity of subsidiary pacemaker tissues in the atrium and ventricle provide a regulation for overdirve suppression.[16] If the sinus node fails to function, the subsidiary pacemaker tissue is released from its block and becomes the dominant pacemaker, usually in the atrium. This would be expected because the atrial pacemaker is faster intrinsically than the subsidiary idioventricular pacemakers and is therefore less suppressed by the sinus node. When the sinus node function is depressed, the initiation of the cardiac rhythm and the survival of the patient are dependent upon the function of these subsidiary pacemakers elsewhere in the specialized conduction system.

It is important to understand that the phenomenon of overdrive suppression is dependent upon multiple factors, including the rate and the duration of stimulation and also the location of the subsidiary pacemaker. For example, idioventricular pacemakers are more likely to be overdrive suppressed and are less reliable as the dominant pacemaker when compared with pacemakers originating in the atrial and junctional regions.

A second type of abnormal impulse generation is due to enhanced phase 4 depolarization in latent pacemakers that is not associated with depression of sinus node function. In these instances impulse initiation in the subsidiary pacemakers competes with the normally functioning sinus node. Depending upon the location of an accelerated subsidiary pacemaker, competition can result in either suppression of the sinus node activity or interference AV dissociation or both. This type of automaticity occurs in diseased cardiac tissue with a low resting membrane potential, an excessive catecholamine concentration, a toxic concentration of digitalis, or a low extracellular potassium concentration.[17]

Another form of abnormal impulse generation is *triggered activity*. This has been defined by Cranefield as repetitive activity arising from after-depolarizations.[18] These after-depolarizations never occur spontaneously, an action potential always is required to initiate them. There are two kinds of after-depolarizations, early and delayed. Early after-depolarizations occur during repolarization of a normal action potential. They appear as a change in membrane potential in a positive direction instead of the expected negative direction during normal repolarization. Repetitive activity can be initiated by early after-depolarizations from a low level of membrane potential. Delayed after-depolarizations are transient depolarizations that occur after completion of repolarization of an action potential. Delayed after-depolarizations are enhanced as the heart rate increases. When a rapid enough rate is achieved, they can attain threshold potential resulting in a tachyarrhythmia. This type of activity displays the unusual electrophysiologic characteristic of overdrive enhancement. The likelihood of arrhythmia induction is greater with increased spontaneous and paced cardiac rates.[18] The mechanisms responsible for early and delayed after-depolarizations and resultant tachyarrhythmias have not been well defined.

Abnormal Impulse Conduction

Abnormalities in conduction result when conduction proceeds with normal or abnormal velocity along abnormal pathways such as in pre-excitation, or when conduction velocity in any site of the normal conducting system is altered or propagation is blocked.[4, 18] The conduction velocity of the cardiac impulse is determined in part by the level of membrane potential at any site in the conduction system as well as the amplitude and the upstroke

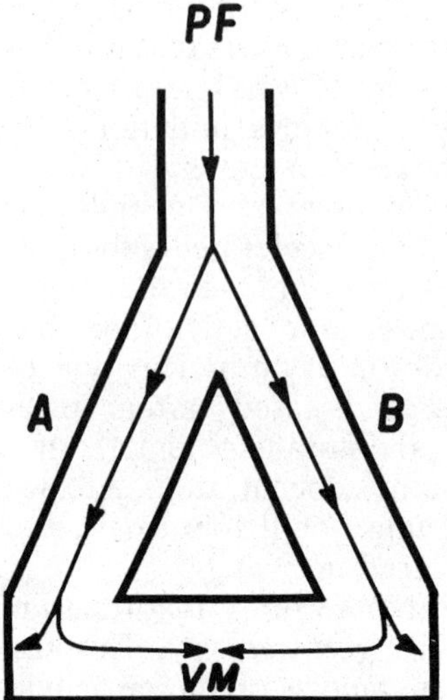

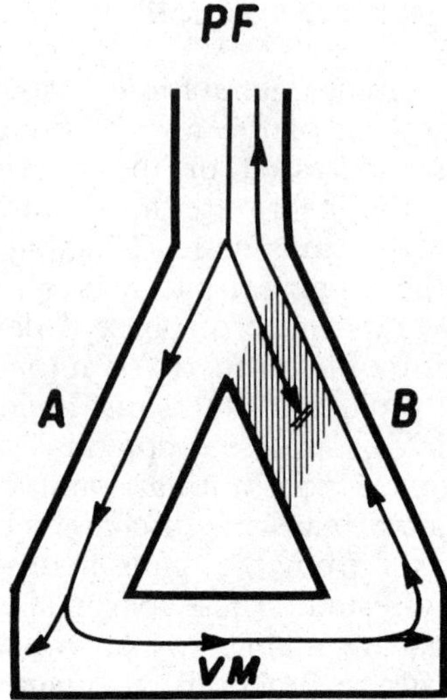

Figure 13–2. *A,* This diagram shows the pathway of excitation under normal conditions in the distal ventricular conduction system. Purkinje fibers (PF) divide into two branches (A and B) before entering the ventricular muscle (VM). The normal impulse, after leaving the main Purkinje fiber bundle, conducts through both branches simultaneously and enters the ventricular muscle. *B,* This diagram shows the conditions for initiation of re-entry. The impulse can conduct through branch *A* after leaving the main Purkinje fiber bundle, but is blocked in the antegrade direction in branch *B (shaded area).* The impulse that enters branch *A* conducts into the ventricular muscle and continues to conduct into branch *B* in a retrograde direction. If the impulse then re-enters the main Purkinje fiber bundle after it has fully recovered excitability, re-entrant excitation can occur.

velocity of the action potential.[4, 14] Any conditions that lower resting membrane potential within the area surrounding the SA or AV node (e.g., surgical injury, ischemia, hyperkalemia, and dilatation) can result in conduction block either from the SA node or through the AV node. This type of block can also occur in the His-Purkinje system. The probability of an arrhythmia being produced is dependent upon the degree of block. A significant degree of block in the specialized conduction system will most often result in bradyarrhythmias.

The mechanism believed to be responsible for most tachyarrhythmias is abnormal conduction, i.e., re-entry.[19] Under physiologic conditions, the conducting impulse ceases after sequential activation of the atrium and ventricles. For re-entry to occur, the cardiac impulse, after exciting a region of the heart, must persist somewhere in the heart until the cardiac fibers it has just excited regain excitability. The impulse may then re-enter and re-excite the region, resulting in a premature beat.[20] The refractory period of cardiac fibers is quite long. Therefore, the impulse that is destined to re-enter or re-excite the heart muscle must survive for a relatively long time if it is to outlast the refractory period and initiate cardiac arrhythmia. The cardiac impulse is conducted at a velocity between 0.5 and 4 meters per second in cardiac fibers other than the sinus and atrioventricular nodes.[4] At these speeds there is no way that it could travel along a pathway of sufficient length and survive. Therefore, anatomic restraints must exist that permit the impulse to conduct very slowly so that it may persist long enough to re-enter and re-excite the myocardium.[20] The most common form of re-entry is due to circus movement and is often associated with slow conduction and unidirectional conduction block.[19] Under normal circumstances propagation proceeds at an equal velocity through both branches of a conducting system, entering the myocardium and uniformly activating the cardiac muscle (Fig. 13–2A). Under conditions necessary for re-entry, one of the two branches of the fiber bundle must be depressed or partially depolarized. At this site antegrade conduction is blocked. The action potentials in these situations lose their efficiency as stimuli for impulse propagation, leading to slowing of conduction and block.[20–22] Activation proceeds normally to the other fiber bundle, enters the myocardium, and returns toward the depressed region. On reaching the depressed segment the impulse may be blocked from further conduction by the mechanisms just described or may be propagated through this segment. For the propagation to occur, the conditions for depression of conduction must be less operative in the retrograde than in the antegrade direction. If the impulse is propagated through the depressed segment and reaches a site of normal tissue, a premature beat occurs (Fig. 13–2B). This particular mechanism is referred to as unidirectional block and re-entry.[20–22] Additional mechanisms have also been described for the occurrence of re-entry in cardiac tissue.[19, 23, 24]

Abnormalities of Impulse Generation and Conduction

The classic example of this mechanism is the parasystolic focus. Parasystole occurs when an ectopic pacemaker has a fixed rate of firing independent of the normal pacemaker.[25] Manifest premature beats appear when the ectopic focus discharges at a time when the exit pathway and the surrounding cardiac tissue are excitable. The association between the abnormalities of automaticity and conduction is important when one is considering parasystole.[26] If there is no entrance block into the region of the ectopic pacemaker, the automatic focus could not exist since each sinus impulse would depolarize the potentially automatic site. Whether or not parasystolic foci can initiate tachyarrhythmia is controversial. They do not generally fire at a very rapid rate. However, they could alter local conduction and, acting like any other premature impulse, set up conditions for re-entry.[27] In addition, a properly timed premature impulse from a parasystolic focus could initiate an arrhythmia due to the R on T phenomenon (premature QRS occurring in the vulnerable period of the T wave).

DIAGNOSIS

In determining the diagnosis of a patient with suspected cardiac arrhythmia, one has to consider the following: First, does the patient have an arrhythmia, and if he does, what is its origin and mechanism? Second, in patients with severe syncopal or cardiorespiratory arrest, are these episodes of potential cardiac origin and possibly caused by an arrhythmia? Third, what, if any, drug or pacing therapy is appropriate in the management of this arrhythmia? When one is assessing a cardiac arrhythmia from an ECG, it is extremely important to maintain a systematic approach. *First,* the cardiac rate is determined and *second,* the P waves in each of the standard leads (I, II, III, AVR, AVL, and AVF) are identified. Normal atrial depolarization should occur downward and to the left. This depolarization should result in positive P waves in leads I and AVF. Each ventricular depolarization, as manifested by the QRS inscription, should be preceded by a P wave of similar configuration in each lead. Thus, the presence of a normal leftward and downward P wave axis (0–90°) and consistent P-QRS relationship defines a sinus rhythm. A sinus mechanism that results in a fast rhythm is referred to as sinus tachycardia, and a slow rhythm is referred to as sinus bradycardia. Minor variations in cardiac rate with respiration are referred to as sinus arrhythmia, which is always a normal phenomenon.

Bradycardia

Sinus bradycardia in older children and adolescents is defined as a heart rate less than 60 beats per minute. Among infants and young children, bradycardia has been classified on an age-dependent basis.[1–3] Sinus bradycardia occurs because of abnormalities in sinus node automaticity and sinoatrial conduction. It may, however, be a normal phenomenon, particularly in a well-conditioned individual. Bradycardia may also occur as an abnormality secondary to central nervous system disease, hypoxia, metabolic disease, drug effects, or trauma to the sinus node region. In patients in whom the sinus node has been injured, e.g., following an intra-atrial baffle procedure for transposition of the great arteries (Mustard operation), an aberrant atrial or junctional escape rhythm may ensue, which is characterized by a relatively slow heart rate with absent or "abnormal" P waves. This aberrant rhythm may be associated with alternate bradycardia and tachycardia (see "Sick Sinus Syndrome").

Another cause of abnormally slow cardiac rhythm is the slowing of AV conduction through the AV node or the His-Purkinje system or both. In this situation, the sinus impulse is initiated normally and depolarizes the atrium in the usual fashion. However, the impulse is not propagated normally through the junctional area to the ventricles. The nature and degree of the block of conduction through this region define the severity of the problem in the individual patient. When conduction is slowed through the AV node, a prolonged AH interval (septal atrial electrogram to His bundle electrogram) can be meas-

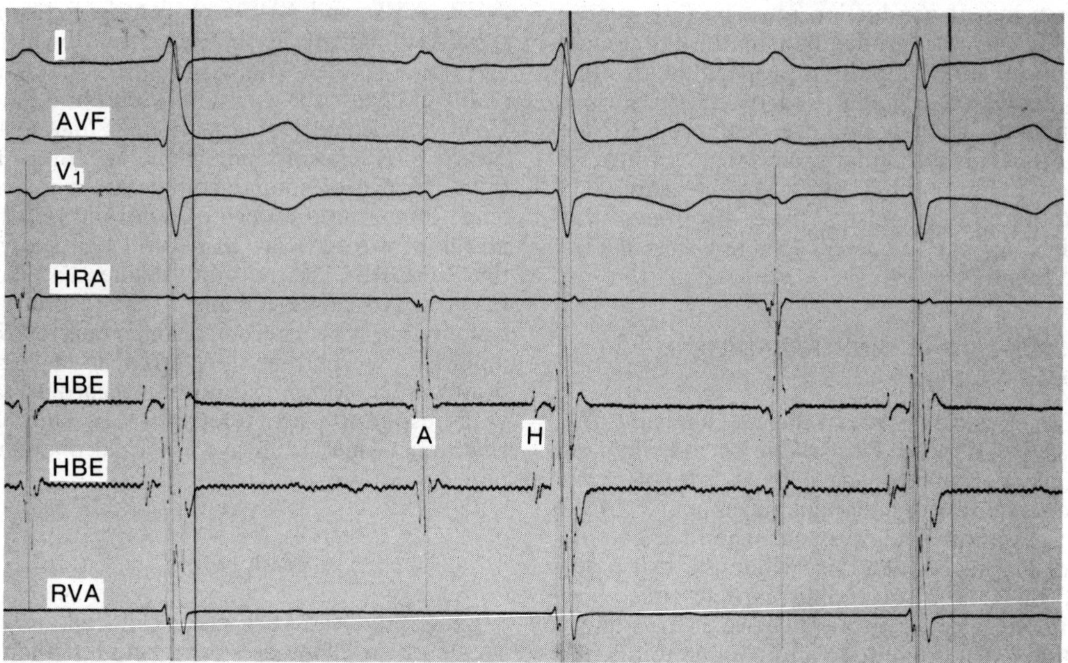

Figure 13–3. His bundle electrogram in a patient with first degree AV block secondary to slow conduction through the AV node. The three top tracings are surface electrocardiographic leads I, AVF, and V_1. The four bottom tracings represent intracardiac electrocardiographic recordings, high right atrium (HRA), His bundle electrogram (HBE), and right ventricular apex (RVA). There is markedly prolonged conduction from the septal atrial electrogram recorded on the His bundle electrogram (A) to the His bundle electrogram (H) of 320 msec (normal range 60–120 msec).

ured during intracardiac electrophysiologic recordings (Fig. 13–3). Slowing in the His-Purkinje system results in His to ventricle (HV) prolongation (Fig. 13–4).

The observation of a prolonged PR interval or first-degree AV block on a standard ECG does not assist in the differentiation of the areas of conduction abnormality, because a His potential is not recorded on the standard ECG. *First-degree AV block* may occur as a result of slowing of conduction within the AV node because of surgical injury, congenital structural abnormality, or inflammatory disease. The latter effects AV conduction either directly or, in the case of acute rheumatic fever, by enhanced vagal activity. In first-degree AV block, impulses initiated by the sinus node eventually propagate to the ventricle despite delay in the AV node.

Second-degree AV block occurs when some impulses are completely blocked within the AV node or His-Purkinje system. When prolongation of the PR interval is incremental with each beat until a sinus beat is completely blocked and the cycle begins again, Mobitz type I or Wenckebach phenomenon is present (Fig. 13–5). This condition almost invariably is the result of slowing of conduction within the AV node producing an increasing prolongation of the AH interval with each beat. It is usually a benign manifestation and is rarely a precursor of greater degrees of AV block.[1–3] Wenckebach phenomenon is often a result of increased vagal tone and, along with sinus bradycardia, may be observed among highly trained athletes, especially when they are sleeping. However, when second-degree AV block occurs as a result of HV prolongation, the prognosis is more guarded. In most cases, Mobitz type II AV block is the result of disease in the His-Purkinje system rather than the AV node.[1–3] Less reliable distal subsidiary pacemakers of the idioventricular type are all that remain if a greater degree of block evolves. A Mobitz type II rhythm is manifested on the surface ECG by failure of AV conduction without changes in the preceding PR intervals. There is no increment in AV conduction (PR interval) prior to the non-conducted impulses. The conducted PR interval may be normal or prolonged (Fig. 13–6). In cases of 2:1 AV block (2 P waves for each QRS complex) the differentiation between Mobitz type I (Wenckebach) and Mobitz type II is not possible by

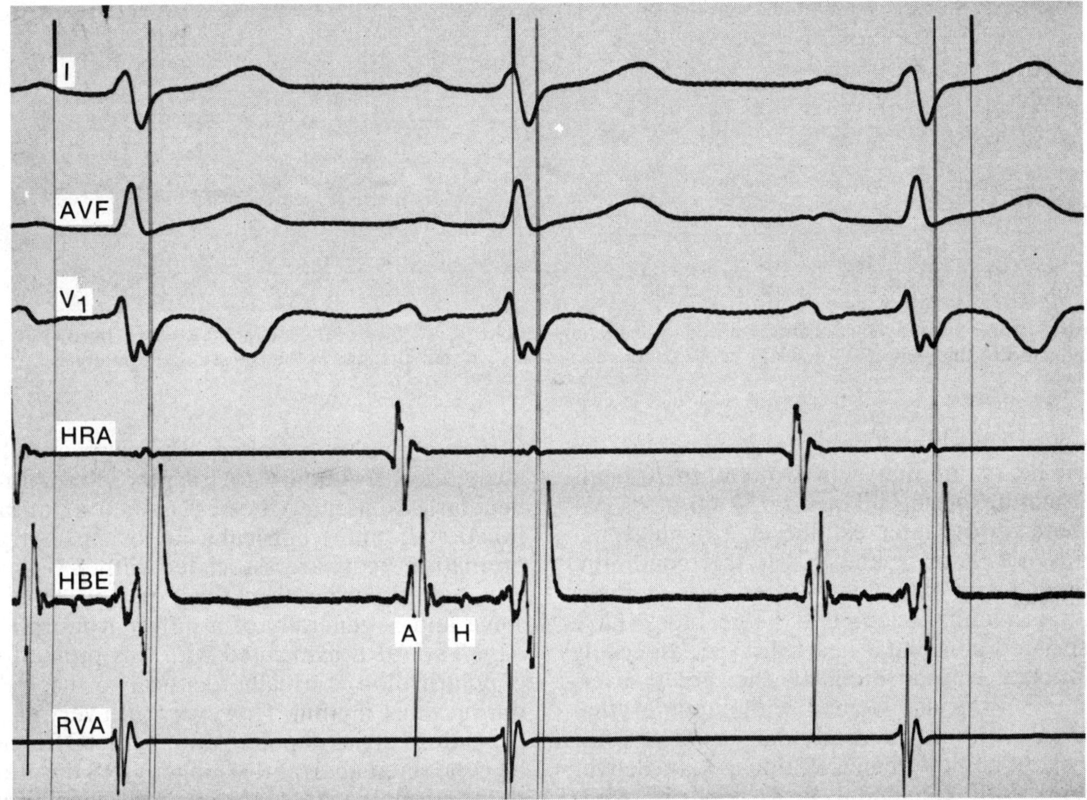

Figure 13–4. His bundle electrogram in a patient with slow conduction through the His-Purkinje system. The top three tracings are surface electrocardiographic recordings of leads I, AVF, and V_1. The bottom three tracings are intracardiac electrocardiographic recordings of the high right atrium (HRA), the His bundle electrogram (HBE), and the right ventricular apex (RVA). The AH interval on the His bundle electrogram is at the upper limit of normal (120 msec). However, there is markedly prolonged conduction in the His-Purkinje system as evidenced by the prolonged HV interval of 75 msec (normal range 30–55 msec).

standard ECG. In most instances, however, children with 2:1 block have AH rather than HV disease.

When complete interruption occurs between the atrium and ventricles and a His-Purkinje or idioventricular rhythm ensues at a slow rate, the condition is defined as *third-degree or complete heart block*. In this situation, the atrial rate is always faster than the ventricular rate. The ECG shows no consistent relationship between the P wave and the QRS, and the P wave can be seen classically to "march through" the QRS (Fig. 13–7). Complete heart block is either acquired or congenital. Congen-

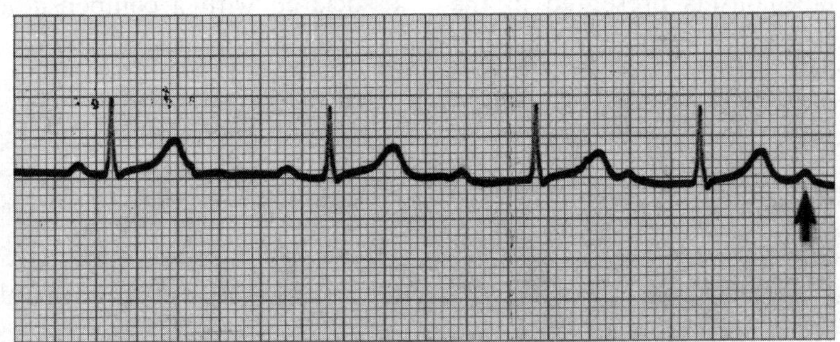

Figure 13–5. Surface electrocardiogram demonstrating AV Wenckebach. There is a gradual prolongation of the PR interval from 200 msec in the first beat to 380 msec in the fourth beat. The fifth P wave (*arrow*) is not conducted to the ventricle.

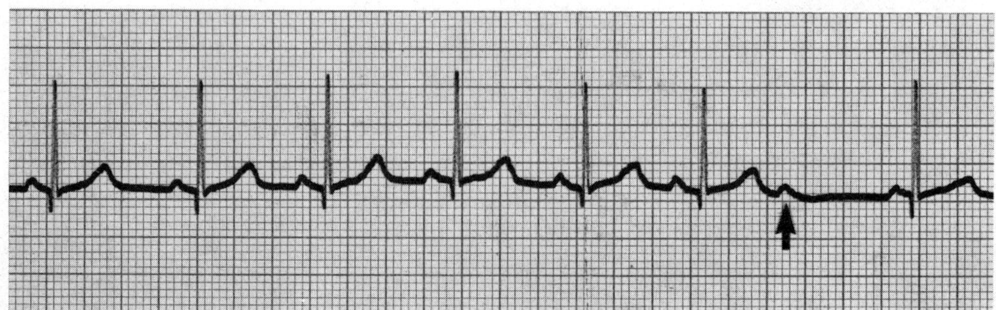

Figure 13–6. Surface electrocardiogram demonstrating Mobitz II AV block. The seventh P wave (*arrow*) is not conducted to the ventricle. The failure of AV conduction occurs without changes in the preceding PR intervals.

ital heart block may be noted *in utero* and the basic heart rate may slow from 60 to 70 beats per minute during infancy to 30–40 beats per minute during later childhood.[28] In most patients no cause is known for this condition, although approximately 30 per cent of those with congenital, complete heart block have associated congenital heart disease, especially corrected transposition of the great arteries.[1, 2, 28] Pregnant women with lupus erythematosus, either previously diagnosed or prior to overt clinical manifestations, may deliver babies with congenital heart block.[29] As a general rule, newborns with congenital heart block do not require treatment such as cardiac pacing unless the heart block is associated with a significant anatomic cardiac defect. However, complete heart block due to surgical intervention for congenital heart disease is more often associated with an unreliable idioventricular pacemaker, recurrent syncopal episodes, or sudden death and requires treatment with an artificial pacemaker.[1, 2, 30]

Premature Depolarizations

Premature depolarizations can be the result of any of the mechanisms presented in the section on pathophysiology. They appear to be most often secondary to re-entry. Premature depolarizations have been classified as atrial, junctional, and ventricular in origin. Atrial premature beats are associated with a P wave that occurs earlier than the expected sinus P wave and is generally of a different morphology. The QRS associated with this premature depolarization is usually identical to the QRS during sinus rhythm. However, with very early premature atrial depolarizations, the QRS can be conducted aberrantly (longer QRS duration than normal). Atrial premature depolarizations generally are not associated with a compensatory pause. The premature depolarization occurs close enough to the sinus node so that it is conducted retrogradely into the sinus node and resets the sinus pacemaker. If one measures from the last normal QRS prior to the atrial premature depolarization to the first normal QRS following the premature depolarization, the interval is less than the interval of two normal R-R intervals (Fig. 13–8).

Junctional premature depolarizations are generally identical to atrial premature depolarizations except that the P wave preceding the premature beats is not observed. Junctional premature depolarizations may or may not be associated with a compensatory pause. They

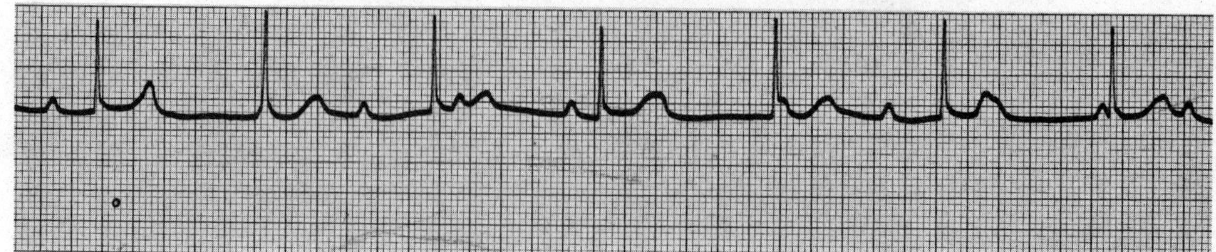

Figure 13–7. Surface electrocardiogram of a patient with third degree or complete AV block. There is a sinus arrhythmia with the atrial rate varying from 75 to 100 beats per minute. The ventricular rate is 55 beats per minute. There is no constant relationship between the P waves and the QRS, and the P waves can be seen to "march through" the QRS complexes.

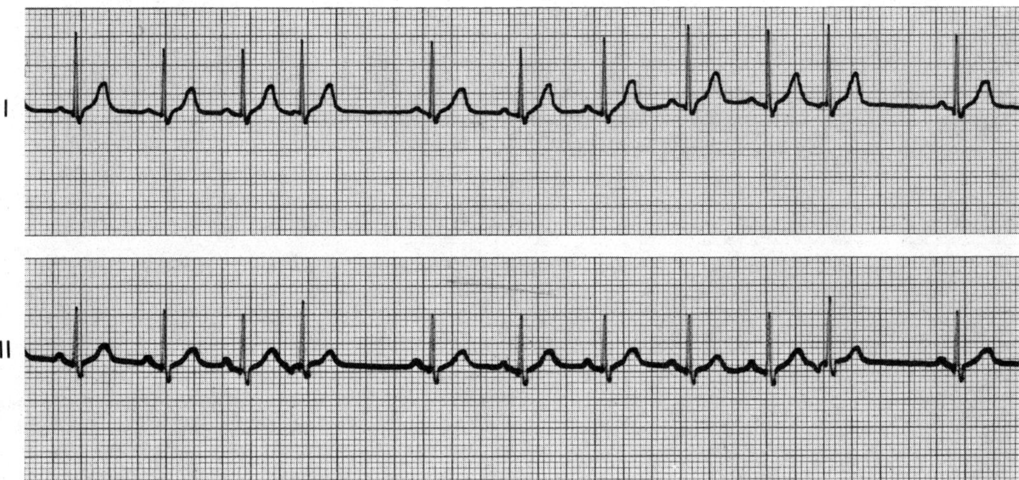

Figure 13–8. Simultaneous surface electrocardiographic leads I and II in a patient with atrial premature depolarizations. The fourth and tenth beats in the sequence are atrial premature depolarizations. Each beat is associated with a P wave of different configuration, which occurs earlier than the expected sinus P wave. The QRS morphology is identical to that during sinus rhythm. In this patient, the atrial premature depolarization is associated with a full compensatory pause.

can originate anywhere from the low atrial region to the region of the His bundle prior to its bifurcation.

Ventricular premature depolarizations (VPDs) do not have a preceding P wave and generally are of a different configuration from that of the normal QRS. This occurs because the sequence of activation of the ventricle is abnormal. In addition to occurring prematurely, VPDs are generally aberrant in configuration and are associated with a discordant T wave (the T wave direction is opposite to the QRS). VPDs are usually associated with a full compensatory pause. Since a VPD originates distally in the specialized conduction system, it usually does not depolarize or reset the sinus node; the sinus node "fires on time." It is not manifested because it is concealed within the wide QRS of the premature depolarization. The next sinus beat comes "on time" as one expects when sinus rhythm is not interrupted. If one measures from the last normal QRS preceding the premature depolarization to the first normal QRS following the premature depolarization, the interval is equal to two normal R-R intervals (Fig. 13–9).

In evaluating the significance of premature depolarizations one has to consider their origin. Both atrial and junctional premature depolarizations are of no clinical significance unless they are precursors or inducers of supraventricular tachycardia. Episodes of supraventricular tachycardia are generally initiated by premature depolarizations.[31] Therefore suppression of premature beats can prevent initiation of tachycardia. Atrial and junctional premature depolarizations do not require further evaluation or therapy in patients with no history of either underlying structural heart disease or tachyarrhythmia.

Uniform, fixed-coupled VPDs are a frequent finding in children.[32] By *"fixed coupling"* we mean that the interval from the last normal QRS to the premature QRS is constant (see Fig. 13–9). VPDs secondary to a parasystolic focus have no fixed relationship between the normal QRS and the abnormal QRS, but the interectopic interval can be determined to be a multiple of a fixed denominator. Uniform, fixed-coupled VPDs are often seen in children. They appear to be rare in infants and more common in adolescents. Generally, the concern is not about the premature depolarizations themselves, but rather about whether they represent a potential initiator of episodes of sustained ventricular tachycardia or fibrillation.

In an attempt to assess whether or not venticular premature depolarizations may be precursors of a more serious arrhythmia, the following findings must be considered.

1. *Association with structural heart disease.* It has been demonstrated that an abnormal myocardium is more likely to respond to premature depolarizations with the initiation of a sustained arrhythmia. This response probably relates to the presence of areas of potential slow conduction and unidirectional block that can sustain a tachyarrhythmia.[15, 18, 19]

2. Patients who have VPDs with *variable*

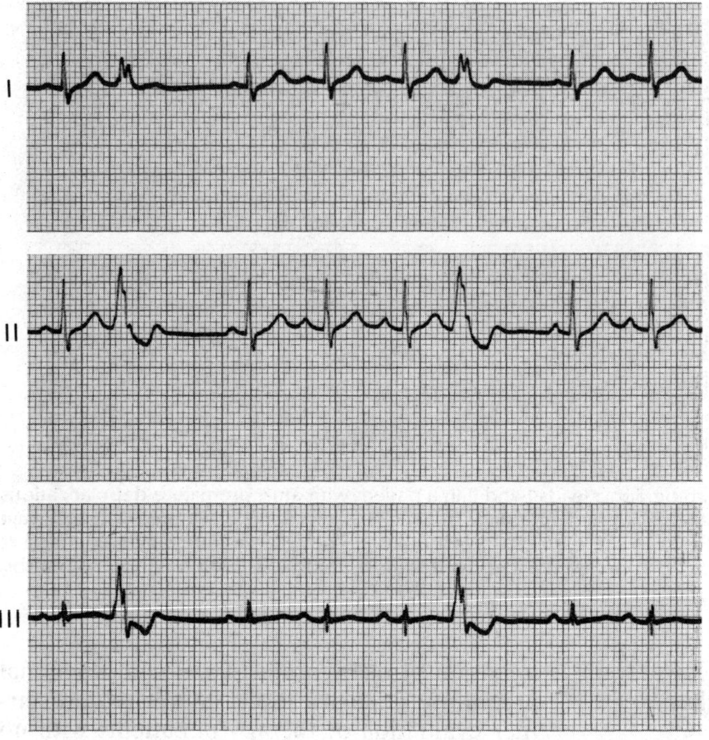

Figure 13–9. Simultaneous surface electrocardiographic leads I, II, and III in a patient with uniform fixed coupled ventricular premature depolarizations. The second and sixth beats in the series are ventricular premature depolarizations. There is no preceding P wave, and the QRS is of a different morphology from the QRS during sinus rhythm. As expected, there is a full compensatory pause. Premature depolarizations are uniform in configuration and also demonstrate fixed coupling, i.e., the interval from the last normal QRS to the premature QRS is constant.

coupling intervals appear to have a worse prognosis especially if there is associated underlying heart disease. At present, there is no evidence showing that parasystole in pediatric patients with normal hearts increases the risk for ventricular tachycardia or fibrillation. Even closely coupled premature depolarizations or those occurring with the R on T phenomenon are unlikely to induce tachyarrhythmias in patients with normal hearts. In patients with structural heart disease, variable coupling intervals with the potential for R on T phenomenon are a more ominous finding.[1–3]

3. *Multiform ventricular premature depolarizations* are VPDs that have different morphologies in the same ECG lead. Multiform configurations are associated with a more ominous prognosis in patients with underlying heart disease.[1–3]

4. The presence of a *prolonged QT interval* on a resting ECG associated with VPDs has a potentially ominous prognosis. Patients with prolonged QT intervals are at risk for paroxysmal episodes of ventricular tachycardia, ventricular fibrillation, and sudden death.[33–35]

5. *A family history* of lethal ventricular arrhythmia is a concern in any child with ventricular ectopic activity.

6. *The response to exercise has been used as an important predictor of VPD significance.*[38–40] In patients with benign VPDs, an exercise stress test will show suppression of the ventricular depolarizations. Patients in whom exercise causes an increased frequency in VPDs require further evaluation. Increased frequency of VPDs during physical activity can be secondary to either catecholamine-induced automatic beats or exercise-induced subendocardial ischemia in a diseased myocardium. In either case, these patients are at greater risk to develop significant ventricular arrhythmias.

7. Patients who have VPDs with extremely short coupling intervals (*R on T phenomenon*) can be at a greater risk for development of ventricular tachycardia. This phenomenon appears to be more important in the induction of ventricular tachycardia in patients with significant structural heart disease. As is the case with other risk factors, the abnormal myocardium has a lower threshold for the induction of ventricular tachycardia or fibrillation caused by a VPD that occurs in the vulnerable period of repolarization.

8. Patients with VPDs *associated with symptoms possibly secondary to cardiac arrhythmias* such as syncope and undocumented tachycardia require further evaluation of the ventricular arrhythmia. In the majority of these pa-

tients, except for those with structural heart disease, the VPDs are not related to the associated symptoms.

Supraventricular Tachycardia

Supraventricular tachycardia originates from an abnormal non-sinus mechanism in which the rate exceeds the maximum sinus rate based on age. In children, the rapid atrial rate is almost always associated with one-to-one conduction to the ventricles. Aberrant conduction and various degrees of AV block may be seen occasionally but are uncommon in children. The non-sinus supraventricular tachycardias include all rapid rhythms originating above the His bundle. The atria or the ventricles or most often both are rapidly activated. Both antegrade and retrograde block can be seen in association with supraventricular tachycardia. When one-to-one AV conduction is present, the ventricular rate often exceeds 220 beats per minute and some times may even exceed 300 beats per minute. In most pediatric patients with supraventricular tachycardia and one-to-one AV conduction, the heart rate ranges between 150 and 250 beats per minute.[1–3] P waves on the surface ECG may or may not be present during tachycardia. When P waves are present, the P wave axis in the frontal plane usually is abnormal. In children, because of the rapid rate of the tachycardia, the P wave is often located on the preceding T wave, resulting in a peaked, pointed T wave. A relatively long PR interval can often be appreciated, particularly when it is compared with the PR interval of a tracing during normal sinus rhythm. The QRS duration is often normal but may be prolonged in patients with bypass tracts, associated congenital heart diseases, and surgically induced right bundle branch blocks. Rate related bundle branch aberrancy also occurs and is usually of right bundle branch block as in the adult population.[1–3] Supraventricular tachycardia is the most common tachyarrhythmia in children and can occur at any time, including fetal life.[1–3] In most instances supaventricular tachycardia is not associated with structural heart disease.

The mode of initiation and termination of a tachycardia episode is important in providing a clue to diagnosis. The abrupt initiation or termination of a tachycardia episode by a premature atrial depolarization is a strong indication of the presence of supraventricular tachycardia, just as gradual changes in heart rate are suggestive of sinus tachycardia. Classic paroxysmal supraventricular or atrial tachycardia is initiated by a premature atrial depolarization that is conducted slowly through the AV node during the relatively refractory period. If a critical delay occurs, AV nodal reentry is established, resulting in tachyarrhythmia (Fig. 13–10).[31, 41, 42]

The cardiac rate during supraventricular tachycardia can vary from 150 to 300 beats per minute, depending upon the age of the patient. The clinical manifestations of supraventricular tachycardia are related to heart rate, duration of abnormal rhythm, and the patient's age.[42] Paroxysmal supraventricular tachycardia develops abruptly and terminates dramatically. Attacks may last for a few seconds to several days. Prolonged tachycardia is more common in the small infant. In a baby with prolonged tachycardia the first sign may be congestive heart failure. The parents sometimes realize in retrospect that the baby was not feeding well or was pale or irritable prior to the first definite symptoms of cardiac decompensation. Fetuses with supraventricular tachycardia are frequently born with evidence of congestive heart failure. In its extreme form, hydrops fetalis may develop that requires *in utero* conversion.[43] Symptoms in older children are similar to those in adults i.e., palpitations, chest pain, and feeling "sick." Occasionally, the present-

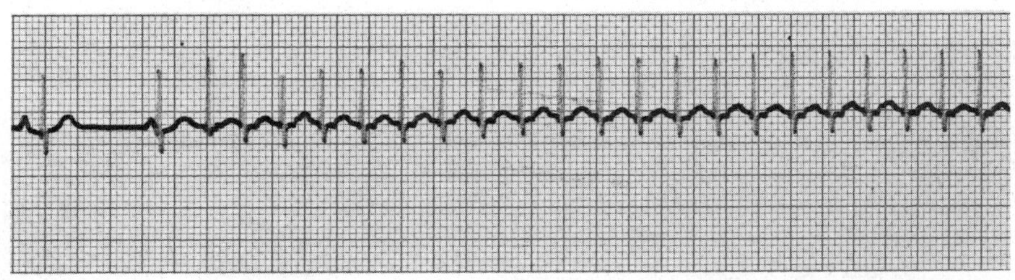

Figure 13–10. Surface electrocardiogram in a patient with supraventricular tachycardia initiated by a premature atrial depolarization. The third beat in this sequence is a premature atrial beat, resulting in a supraventricular tachycardia with a rate of 250 beats per minute.

ing symptom may be abdominal pain or vomiting. Anxiety tends to compound the symptoms. In the absence of additional organic heart disease, supraventricular tachycardia in older children is usually tolerated well and rarely leads to the clinical manifestations of frank congestive heart failure. Syncope is a rare presenting symptom of supraventricular tachycardia in older children. Associated cardiac malformations reduce the hemodynamic tolerance to tachycardia episodes and may enhance the appearance of congestive heart failure and cardiac decompensation.

Ectopic Atrial Tachycardia

Ectopic atrial tachycardia is a form of supraventricular tachycardia due to a rapid nonsinus rhythm attributed to increased automaticity of ectopic atrial pacemakers.[44] If P waves are identified, the axis is abnormal, suggesting that the origin of the rhythm is outside of the sinus node. Similar to sinus tachycardias, these rhythms often start and subside gradually rather than abruptly and may be interspersed with short episodes of sinus rhythm during which a normal P wave morphology can be identified (Fig. 13–11). At times it may be difficult to differentiate this arrhythmia from other forms of supraventricular tachycardia or even sinus tachycardia. The gradual initiation and termination of this rhythm differentiate it from the former, while the abnormal P wave morphology and at times extremely rapid rates differentiate it from the latter.

Junctional Tachycardia

Junctional tachycardia is an arrhythmia in which the tachycardia is initiated in the junctional region. Junctional tissue can be defined as anywhere from the low atrial region through the AV node to the His bundle. Junctional tachycardia is an uncommon form of supraventricular tachycardia in the absence of underlying structural heart disease. This rhythm disturbance is seen most often in children immediately following open heart surgery.[45] The mechanism of junctional tachycardia appears most likely to be abnormal automaticity, although in some instances it may be secondary to re-entry. Triggered automaticity and afterdepolarization were recently suggested as leading to the development of this arrhythmia in the postoperative patient.[46] The rate of a junctional tachycardia is from 120 to 280 beats per minute and is related to the patient's age and hemodynamic status. The ECG usually shows a narrow QRS complex with no obvious P waves because of simultaneous activation of the atria and ventricles or, at times, AV dissociation with a ventricular rate faster than the atrial rate (Fig. 13–12). This mechanism is called interference dissociation, in which the atria and ventricles are dissociated from one another because of "collision" of the impulses in the AV node that prevents the atria and the ventricles from activating one another. Occasionally, the QRS complexes are followed by a negative P wave when the atria have been activated by the ventricles in a retrograde fashion. In patients who have had a right ventriculotomy and have postoperative right bundle branch block, a junctional tachycardia may simulate ventricular tachycardia on the surface ECG, since both may be seen with AV dissociation. However, the QRS morphology during junctional tachycardia should always be a right bundle branch block pattern and should be identical to that seen during sinus rhythm. In comparison, in patients with ventricular tachycardia, the QRS morphology often will be a left bundle branch block pattern and also will be different from that seen during sinus rhythm.

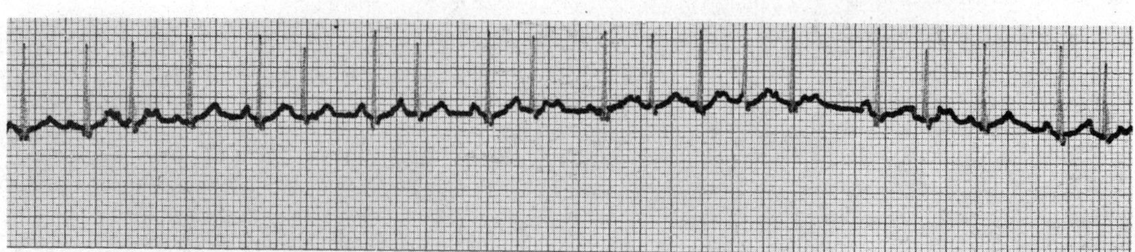

Figure 13–11. Surface electrocardiogram in a patient with a chaotic atrial tachycardia. There is a very rapid irregular atrial rate with changing P wave configuration. At times the ectopic tachycardia appears to be interspersed with episodes of sinus rhythm.

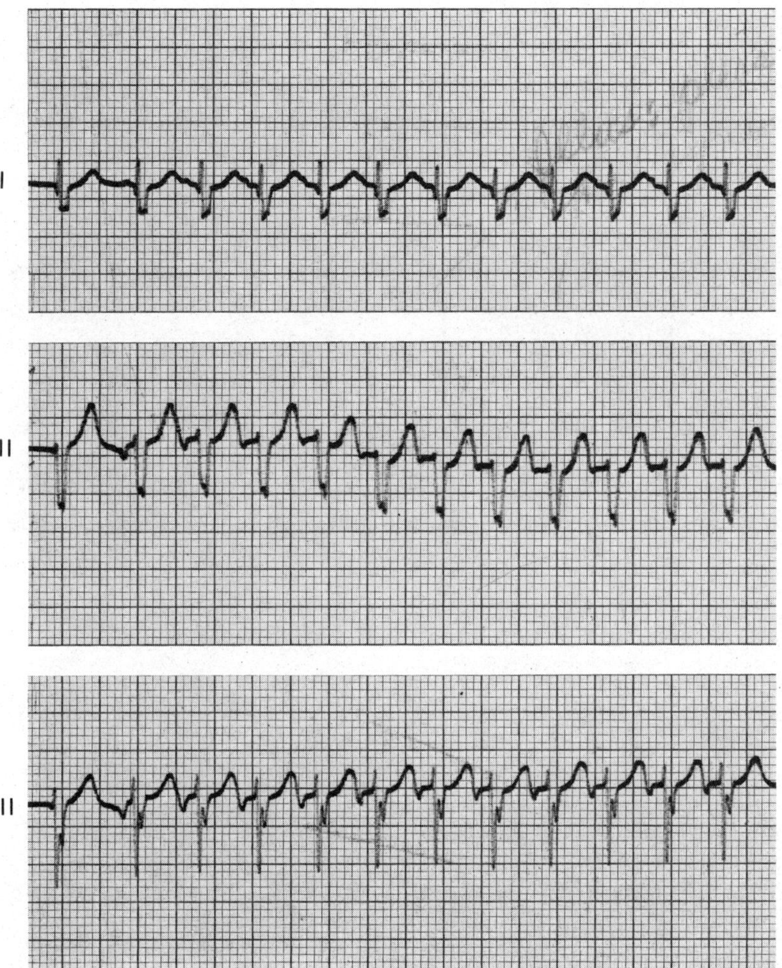

Figure 13–12. Simultaneous surface electrocardiographic leads I, II, and III in a patient with a rapid junctional tachycardia. The P waves, which can be seen in the second and third beats in lead II, are no longer visible as the rate increases. The junctional rate exceeds the sinus rate, resulting in either retrograde activation of the atrium or AV dissociation.

Atrial Flutter and Atrial Fibrillation

Idiopathic atrial flutter and atrial fibrillation not associated with congenital or acquired heart disease are rare in children.[1–3] Atrial flutter is a regular or regularly irregular rhythm. The atrial rate is usually between 250 and 400 beats per minute, and distinct P waves are commonly observed on the surface ECG, often with a typical "saw-toothed" pattern. Atrial fibrillation is an irregularly irregular rhythm. There are no distinct P waves on the surface ECG, only low amplitude fibrillatory waves are noted (Figs. 13–13 and 13–14).

Atrial Flutter

The atrial rate in children with atrial flutter varies from 250 to 400 beats per minute.[1–3] Because the AV node may not conduct 1:1 at these rates, there is virtually always some degree of AV block associated with this arrhythmia. The ventricular response is related to the capability of the AV conduction system to transmit the rapid atrial impulses and often is regularly irregular. This is dependent upon the patient's age and the electrophysiologic characteristics of the AV node. The ventricular rate may vary as a result of 2:1, 3:1, or 4:1 AV block. The characteristic atrial flutter waves or F waves are best seen in the right precordial chest leads (see Fig. 13–13). In older children, the atrial rate and ventricular responses are slower than in neonates and infants.

Atrial Fibrillation

Atrial fibrillation in children is rare.[47] Low-amplitude fibrillatory waves are seen on the

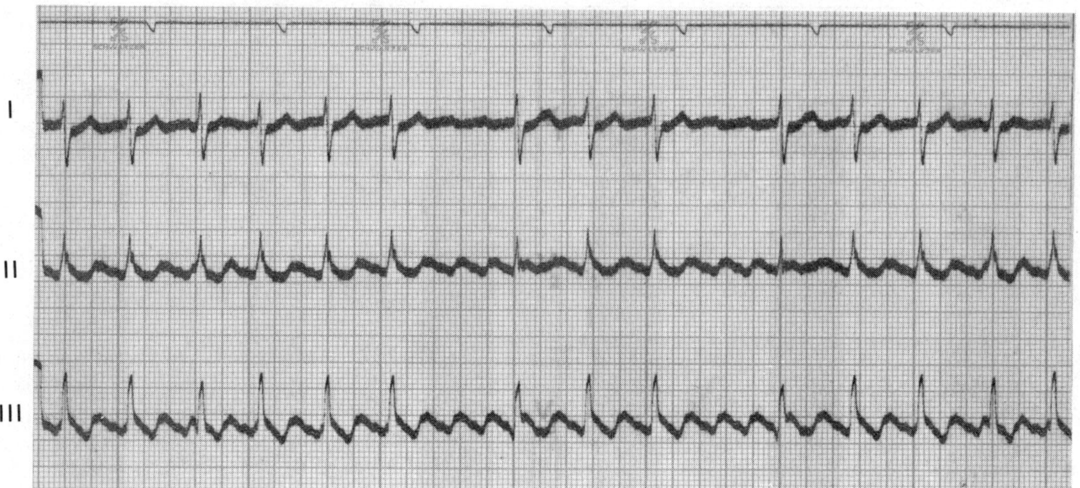

Figure 13–13. Simultaneous surface electrocardiographic leads I, II, and III in a patient with atrial flutter. A regularly irregular rhythm with typical flutter waves is seen particularly in leads II and III. The irregular rhythm is secondary to a variable degree of AV block.

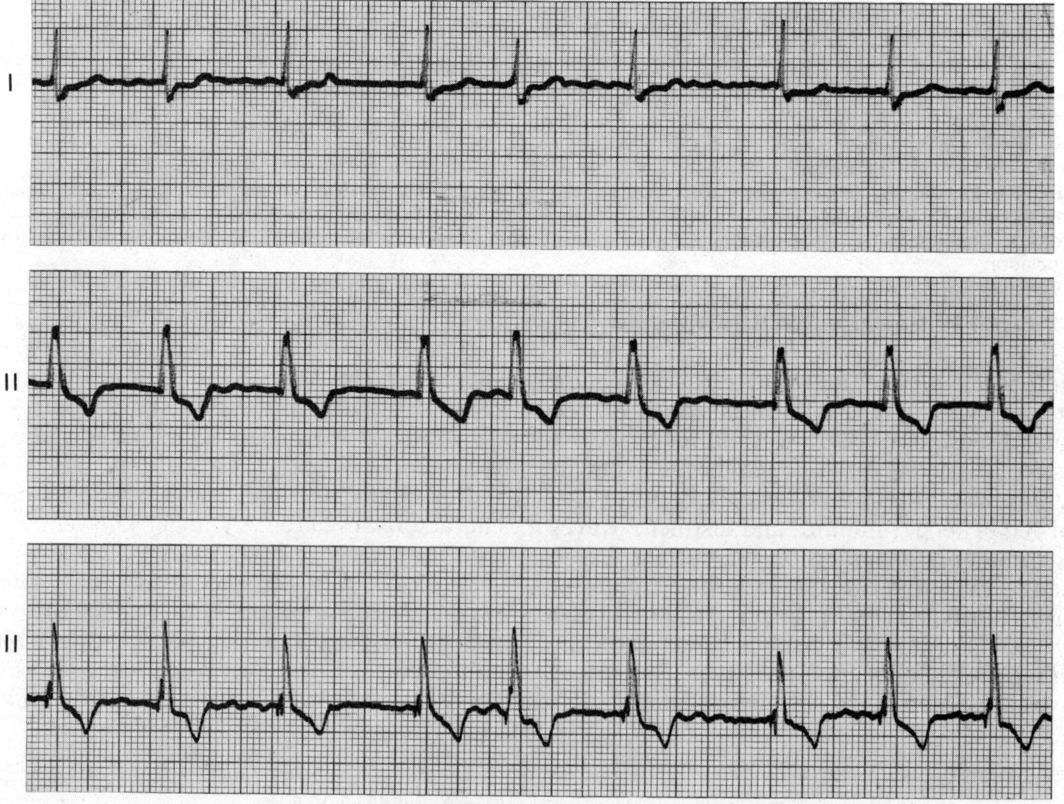

Figure 13–14. Simultaneous surface electrocardiographic leads I, II, and III in a patient with atrial fibrillation. An irregularly irregular rhythm with typical low-amplitude fibrillatory waves is seen on the surface electrocardiogram.

surface ECG. The ventricular rhythm is typically irregularly irregular. The rate will vary with the capability of the atrioventricular conduction system to transmit impulses to the ventricle (see Fig. 13–14). Atrial fibrillation is most often seen in association with acquired or congenital malformations of the heart that lead to atrial dilatation, e.g., cardiomyopathies, AV valve stenosis, and insufficiency.[1–3] The hemodynamic consequences of both atrial flutter and fibrillation are similar to those of supraventricular tachycardia and depend primarily on the age of the patient, the rate of the ventricular response, the duration of the arrhythmia, and the associated cardiac malformations.

Sick Sinus Syndrome

Sinus node dysfunction is being recognized in a greater number of infants and children. It is more often caused by surgical injury to the sinus node than to intrinsic disease of the node.[48–50] Clinical and electrocardiographic manifestations may include sinus bradycardia, sinoatrial block, sinus arrest with or without AV junctional escape, tachycardia-bradycardia syndrome, and paroxysmal atrial flutter or fibrillation. In pediatric patients, sick sinus syndrome may follow open heart repair of transposition of the great vessels using the Mustard or Senning procedure. Chronic damage may occur due to incision of the sinus node or extensive suturing of atria in its vicinity.[48] Interruption of the sinus node blood supply may also lead to degeneration and fibrosis of the approaches to the sinus node or of the sinus node itself.[49] This may lead to clinical manifestations of sick sinus syndrome months or even years following open heart repair.[51, 52] In children, sick sinus syndrome more often results in excessive sinus bradycardia and junctional escape rhythms rather than tachycardia-bradycardia syndrome (Fig. 13–15). Sick sinus syndrome seldom causes symptoms in children because of the bradycardia alone.[51, 52] The junctional escape rhythms usually are reasonably well tolerated. In some patients, however, the rhythm will often vary between a low atrial or junctional rhythm and atrial flutter or supraventricular tachycardia, simulating the common form of paroxysmal supraventricular tachycardia. The symptoms of sick sinus syndrome tend to develop more rapidly in patients in whom residual anatomic lesions are present. Syncopal attacks secondary to bradycardia or tachycardia require vigorous therapy including insertion of permanent pacemakers.[51–53]

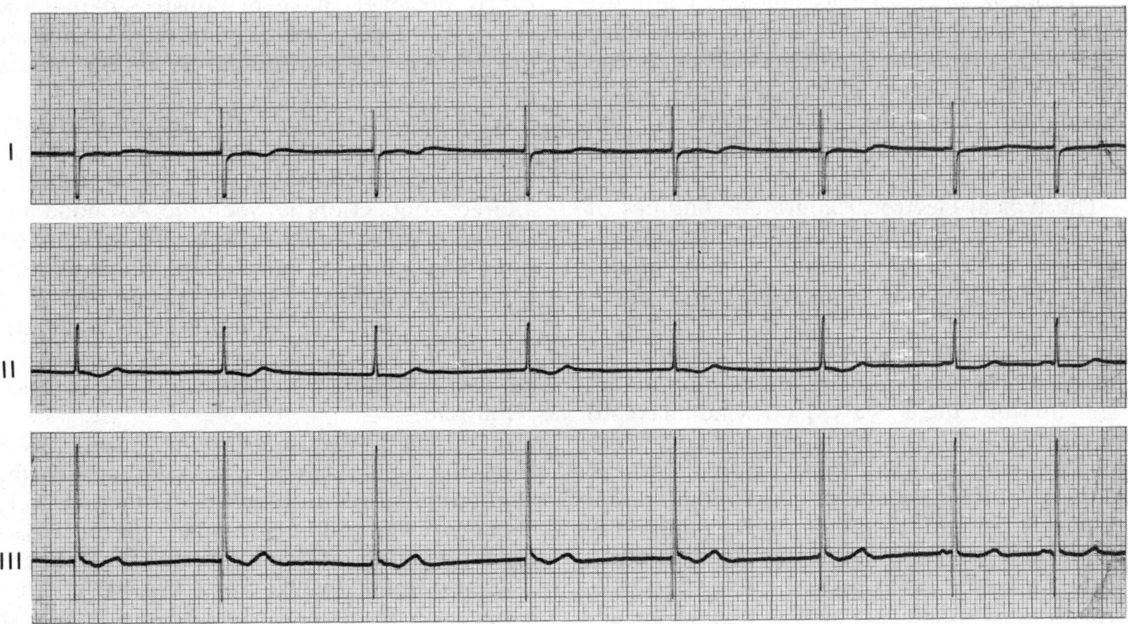

Figure 13–15. Simultaneous surface electrocardiographic leads I, II, and III in a patient with sick sinus syndrome and a slow junctional rhythm. The junctional rate is approximately 50 beats per minute.

Pre-excitation Syndromes

Pre-excitation syndromes have generally been known as the Wolff-Parkinson–White syndrome. In actuality, Wolff-Parkinson–White syndrome is one form of the pre-excitation syndromes that involve the presence of accessory or bypass tracts that bypass the AV node and activate the ventricles in an abnormal fashion. Among children with supraventricular tachycardia, pre-excitation syndrome is common.[42, 54–56] It is estimated that up to 50 per cent of pediatric patients with bypass tracts may have episodes of supraventricular tachycardia.[2, 3] In the pediatric population, the incidence of bypass tracts is estimated to be approximately 0.1 per cent.[57, 58] However, in patients with congenital heart disease the incidence is somewhat higher and is estimated to be approximately 0.5 per cent.[57, 58] Up to 58 per cent of infants with supraventricular tachycardia may have associated pre-excitation syndrome. However, the episodes of supraventricular tachycardia associated with bypass tracts in the first year of life seem to decrease or disappear by the second year. It has been suggested that this decrease is secondary to a change in the electrophysiologic properties of the bypass tract with growth and development.[42, 54]

Pre-excitation syndrome associated with supraventricular tachycardia may occur throughout childhood, and can be a particularly difficult problem in the adolescent.[42, 54] The most common congenital heart lesions that have been associated with pre-excitation syndrome are Ebstein anomaly of the tricuspid valve, congenitally corrected transposition of the great arteries, and familial cardiomyopathies.[2, 3, 59]

The typical electrocardiographic findings of pre-excitation syndrome can be best understood if they are related to the normal impulse propagation from the sinus node to the ventricles. The short PR interval is the result of the impulse bypassing the AV node. Because the sinus impulse (after it depolarizes the atrium and inscribes the P waves) does not have to conduct through the AV node but can reach the ventricles via the "bypass tract," the PR segment (primarily secondary to AV nodal delay) is absent, resulting in the short PR interval. The abnormal QRS configuration seen, i.e., the "delta wave," the wide QRS, and the discordant T wave, is due to an abnormal sequence of activation of the ventricle. The delta wave represents early abnormal ventricular activation by the bypass tract. Thus, the pre-excitation syndrome is present when all or part of the ventricular muscle is activated by the atrial impulse sooner than would be expected if the impulse were to reach the ventricles only by way of the normal AV conduction system (Fig. 13–16). The major clinical significance of this syndrome is the high frequency of associated supraventricular tachycardias in these patients, who are often very difficult to treat with standard pharmacologic therapy.[56, 60]

The pre-excitation syndromes have also been classified using anatomic connections or eponyms, e.g., Kent, James, and Mahaim fibers. However, detailed electrophysiologic studies have demonstrated a more precise classification of this anomaly:

1. *Atrial-ventricular bypass tracts* originate in the atrial myocardium and insert in the ventricular myocardium, forming direct connections between the atria and ventricles.[60] These previously have been known as the Kent bundles and are the most common form of pre-excitation syndrome. Atrial-ventricular bypass tracts produce the classic short PR interval and delta wave pattern on the surface ECG. They are located in the free wall and septal regions of both the right and left sides of the heart. A previous classification of these tracts into type A and type B is no longer applicable, because there are many potential sites for the AV bypass tracts.[60, 61] Analysis of surface ECGs however, have demonstrated that the vector of the delta wave can be used to indicate the site of the ventricular insertion of the bypass tract.[60, 62]

2. *Nodo-ventricular tracts* are bypass tracts that originate in the AV node and insert into the ventricular myocardium.[60, 61] This results in a direct connection between the AV node and the ventricular myocardium. These connections were previously labeled as Mahaim fibers. The surface ECG will often show a normal PR interval with the delta wave and abnormal QRS configuration. Nodo-ventricular tract is an uncommon form of pre-excitation syndrome.

3. *Fasciculoventricular connections* occur from the His-Purkinje system directly to the ventricular myocardium.[60, 61] They are very similar to the nodo-ventricular type of bypass tracts and also have been called Mahaim fibers.

4. *AV nodal bypass tracts* involve a direct connection from the atrium to the bundle of His or to the lower portions of the AV node via specialized perinodal or intranodal

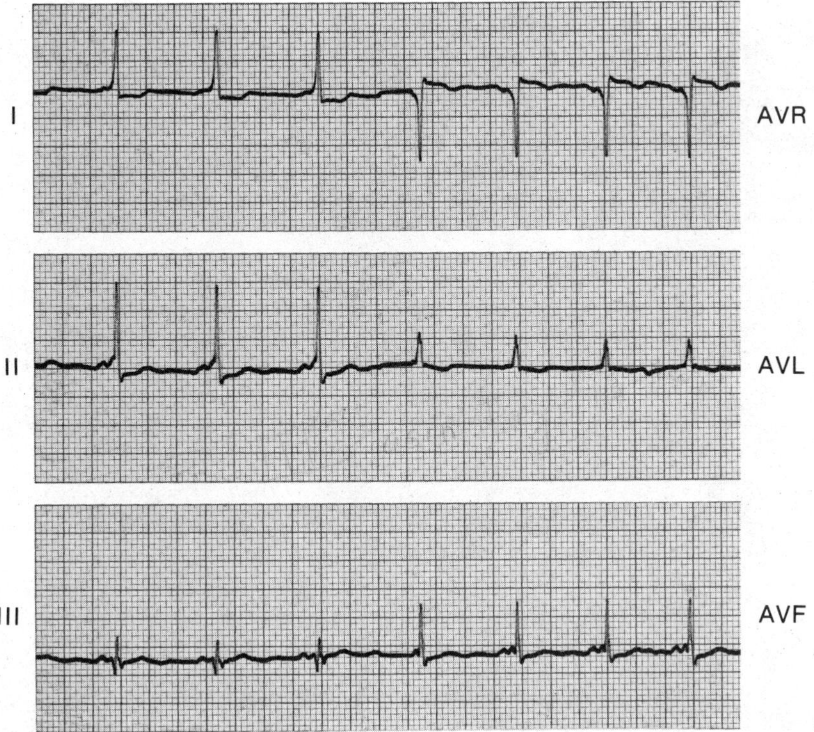

Figure 13–16. Six standard electrocardiographic leads in a patient with the pre-excitation syndrome. The typical findings of a short PR interval, delta wave, and abnormal QRS configuration are seen.

tracts.[60, 61] The resultant surface ECG shows a short PR interval and a normal QRS complex. This finding has been previously considered to be secondary to James fibers and has been known as the Lown-Ganong-Levine syndrome.

During episodes of supraventricular tachycardia in most patients with the pre-excitation syndrome, the QRS morphology is normal (Fig. 13–17). This is because the antegrade limb of the re-entrant loop is through the AV node, and the retrograde limb is through the bypass tract (see "Pathophysiology"). Thus, the ventricles during tachycardia are activated in the normal fashion, resulting in normal QRS morphology. It is therefore difficult, if not impossible, to determine from a surface ECG taken during episodes of supraventricular tachycardia whether a patient has a bypass tract.[60] Following conversion of the arrhythmia to sinus rhythm, the typical electrocardiographic pattern seen in the pre-excitation syndrome becomes manifest (Fig. 13–17B).

Some patients with bypass tracts have conduction only in a retrograde fashion. Evidence of pre-excitation syndrome, therefore, is never seen in sinus rhythm. However, these patients can still have episodes of supraventricular tachycardia because the bypass tract can be the retrograde limb of the re-entrant pathway. Such a bypass tract is "concealed" and is demonstrable only during intracardiac electrophysiologic studies.[63–65]

Ventricular Tachycardia

Ventricular arrhythmias are less common clinical problems in the pediatric population than supraventricular arrhythmias. In the past, they were considered clinical curiosities,[66, 67, 68] but in recent years ventricular arrhythmias have become an increasingly important problem in children for two reasons: the first is the heightened awareness of and improved methods for diagnosis of arrhythmias in children.[2, 3] The second is the improved survival of patients with congenital heart disease who have undergone palliative and/or open heart repair. Some of these patients are more prone to develop ventricular arrhythmias.[69–71] Furthermore, right ventriculotomy for repair of septal defects produces a scar in the ventricle that may be a potential arrhythmogenic focus.[40, 72–74] In this group of patients, particularly those with sig-

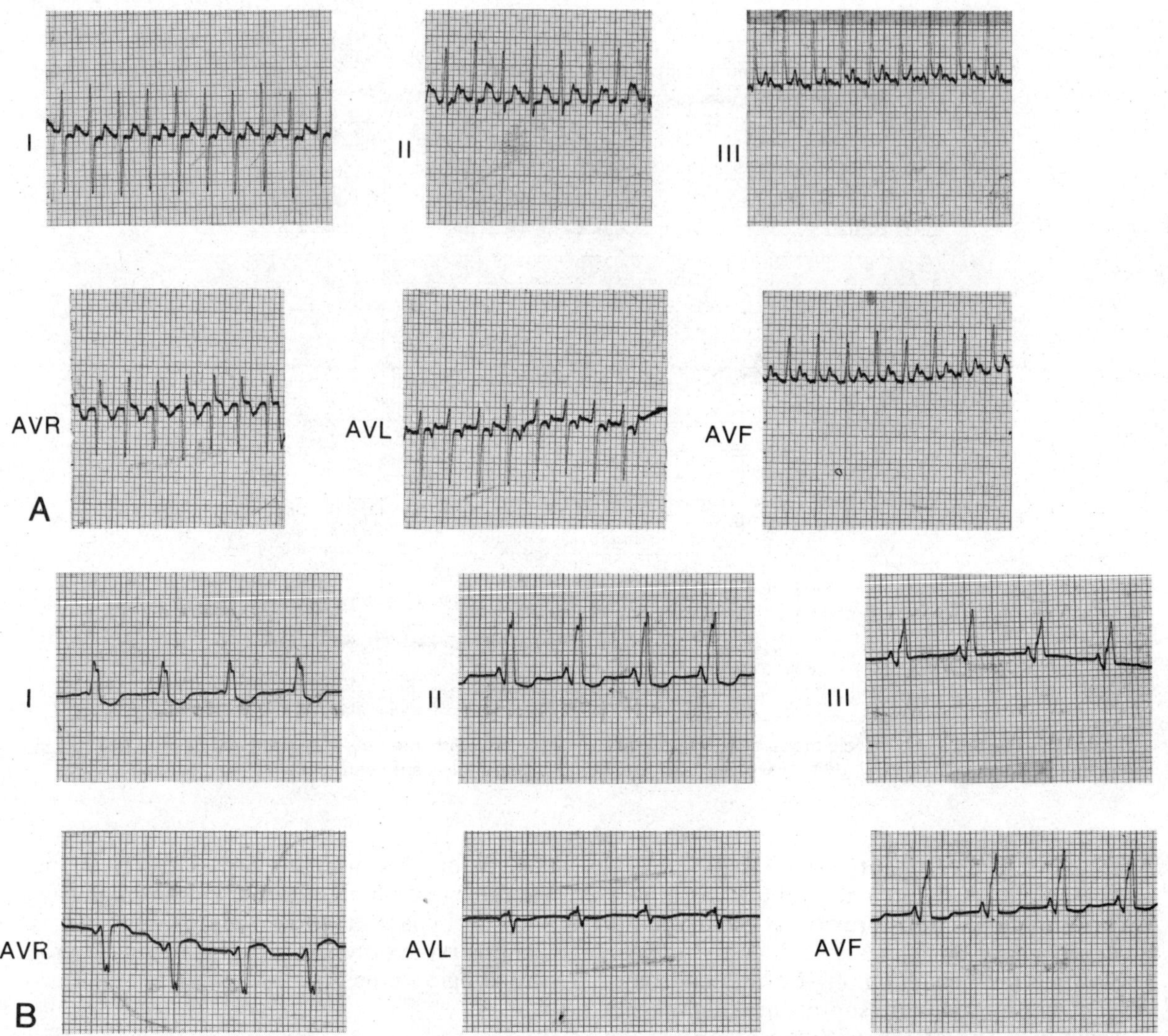

Figure 13–17. *A,* Six standard electrocardiographic leads from a patient with pre-excitation syndrome during an episode of supraventricular tachycardia. The tachycardial rate is between 275 and 300 beats per minute. A narrow QRS exists with what appears to be normal QRS morphology. The diagnosis of pre-excitation syndrome cannot be made during the episode of supraventricular tachycardia. *B,* Following conversion to sinus rhythm, the typical features of the pre-excitation syndrome are seen.

nificant residual hemodynamic defects, ventricular arrhythmias significantly increase morbidity and mortality.[40, 69–74]

Ventricular tachycardia has been defined as a rhythm disturbance originating distal to the bifurcation of the bundle of His and including three or more ventricular beats in succession.[75] The diagnosis of ventricular tachycardia on the surface ECG and the differential diagnosis from other tachycardias may be difficult, particularly in the infant or in the postoperative child. In children, most tachyarrhythmias with rates greater than 250 beats per minute are supraventricular in origin. However, many instances are known, particularly in infants, in which the rates of ventricular tachycardias exceed 250 beats per minute and are as fast as 300 beats per minute.[2, 3] More important than the rate is the relationship of the P wave to the QRS during the tachycardia. The presence of AV dissociation is an important finding in the diagnosis of ventricular tachycardia. However, in infants and children with very rapid heart rates, it may be difficult to evaluate the presence of a P wave. In addition, many patients with ventricular tachycardia, particularly infants, may have one-to-one retrograde VA conduction, and some patients with certain forms of supraventricular tachycardia may have AV dissociation.[2,3]

The presence of fusion beats, i.e., the intermittent capture of the ventricles by a supraventricular beat, is an excellent electrocardiographic observation in favor of ventricular tachycardia (Fig. 13–18). If the patient was having ectopic beats prior to the onset of the tachycardia, evaluation of these beats is also helpful in differentiating supraventricular from ventricular tachycardia. However, in patients with the pre-excitation syndrome, ventricular premature depolarizations may initiate episodes of supraventricular tachycardia.

The presence of a wide QRS may be helpful in diagnosing ventricular tachycardia in children. Rate related aberrancy is less common in the pediatric population, and therefore the presence of a wide QRS complex favors the diagnosis of ventricular tachycardia.[1-3] However, as discussed later under differential diagnosis, wide QRS supraventricular tachycardia may be present in patients with certain forms of pre-excitation[76] as well as in patients who have had a right ventriculotomy during open heart surgery and have residual complete right bundle branch block. Thus, it may be impossible to identify the origin of a wide QRS tachycardia with a right-bundle branch block pattern from the ECG alone in patients who have had cardiac surgery.

DIFFERENTIAL DIAGNOSIS OF TACHYARRHYTHMIAS

From the standpoint of prognosis and treatment, it is important to accurately diagnose the type of tachyarrhythmia that is present. Often the differential diagnosis is clear-cut on a clinical and electrocardiographic basis, but in some instances it may be difficult. It is also important to develop a systematic approach to diagnosis based on heart rate, presence and configuration of the P wave, duration of the QRS deflection, and rhythmicity (Table 13–3). First, it should be determined whether the patient actually has a *sinus tachycardia*. Time is lost from proper treatment of an infection, acute anemia, or other illness that results in sinus tachycardia while tachyarrhythmia is considered, wrongly diagnosed, or even treated. Heart rates much faster than 220 beats per minute are generally too rapid for sinus tachy-

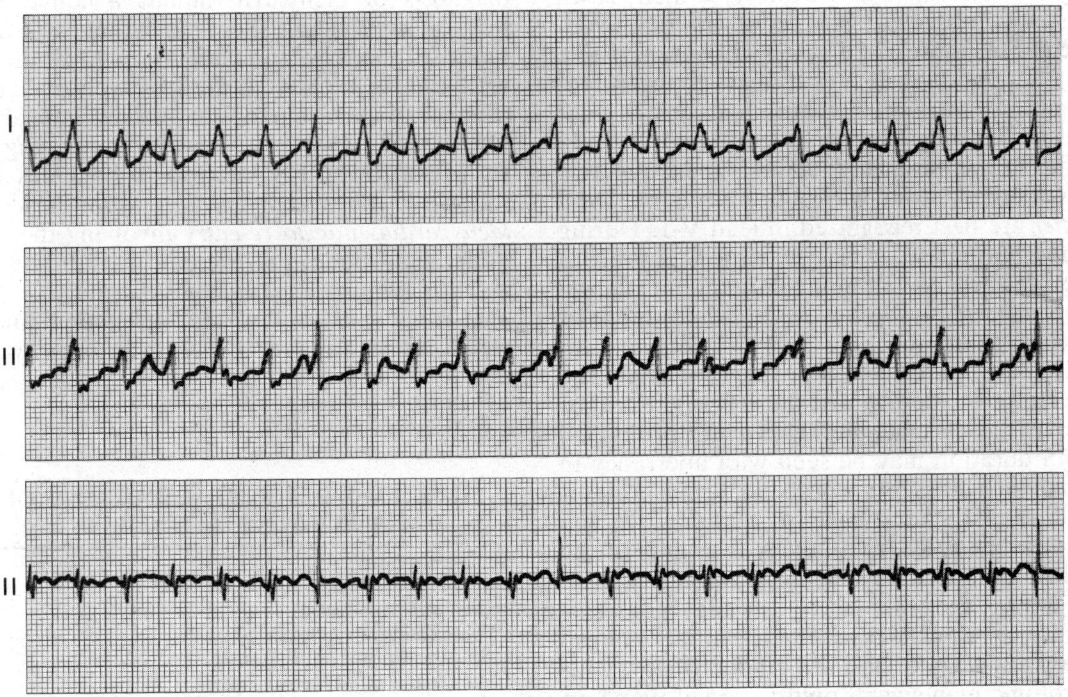

Figure 13–18. Simultaneous electrocardiographic surface leads I, II, and III in a patient with ventricular tachycardia. The tracing shows a wide QRS tachycardia with a ventricular rate of 165 beats per minute. There is evidence of AV dissociation with the P waves "marching through" the QRS complexes. The ventricular rate is faster than the atrial rate. In addition, fusion beats (seventh, twelfth, and last beat in the series) are seen.

Table 13–3. DIFFERENTIAL DIAGNOSIS OF TACHYARRHYTHMIAS

	Electrocardiographic Findings			
Tachyarrhythmia	*Heart Rate (beats/minute)*	*P Wave*	*QRS Duration*	*Regularity*
Sinus tachycardia	<225	Always present (normal axis)	Normal	Rate varies with respiration
Atrial tachycardia	150–320	Present—50% (superior axis common)	Normal or prolonged (RBBB pattern)	Regular
Atrial fibrillation	100–200	Fibrillatory waves	Normal or prolonged (RBBB pattern)	Irregularly irregular
Atrial flutter	Atrial rate: 250–400 Ventricular response: variable (100–320)	"Saw-toothed" flutter waves	Normal or prolonged (RBBB pattern)	Regular ventricular response (e.g., 2:1, 3:1, 3:2)
Ventricular tachycardia	120–240	Absent	Usually prolonged	Slightly irregular

cardia, but rates between 140 and 220 beats per minute could be an arrhythmia or of sinus origin. Ventricular tachycardia is generally slower than supraventricular tachycardia.

Although it is possible to have *supraventricular tachycardia* with P waves that display a normal configuration (upright in leads 1, 2, and AVF), in most instances P wave morphology is abnormal. Unfortunately, in many cases of supraventricular tachycardia with rapid ventricular response, the P wave will not be visible on the standard ECG. It may be useful to obtain Lewis-Golub leads (exploring right chest electrodes) or an esophageal lead in order to demonstrate P waves. The distinctive saw-toothed atrial waves produced by *atrial flutter* are best recognized in lead V-1. During *atrial fibrillation,* atrial activity is simply a chaotic baseline variation. Throughout *ventricular tachycardia* the P wave is either absent or out of phase with the QRS deflection. An extremely narrow QRS suggests that the rhythm is of supraventricular origin, i.e., at or above the His bundle. However, prolonged QRS duration may be seen with aberrancy in a patient with supraventricular tachycardia as well as with ventricular arrhythmia. In the former, the QRS morphology is usually of the right-bundle branch block morphology.

Finally, the rhythmicity should be determined. In sinus tachycardia the rate will vary every few seconds and will gradually slow with vagotonic maneuvers, only to speed up again when they are discontinued. Ventricular tachycardias will display beat-to-beat variations, and most atrial tachycardias will be extremely regular except at the onset or prior to termination. Atrial flutter will either be regular, or with block, the ventricular response consistently will be some multiple of the interval between the flutter waves (see Fig. 13–13). In atrial fibrillation, ventricular response will be irregularly irregular (see Fig. 13–14).

For further consideration of the differential diagnosis of tachyarrhythmias, a convenient way of subdividing these arrhythmias is into those with narrow and wide QRS. Most tachyarrhythmias in children are supraventricular in origin and have narrow or normal appearing QRS (Table 13–4).[2, 3] The differential diagnosis of narrow QRS tachycardia includes the following: *sinus tachycardia; supraventricular tachycardias due to re-entry* involving the AV node, sinus node, pre-excitation syndrome, or atrium; *automatic atrial tachycardia; accelerated junctional tachycardia; atrial fibrillation; atrial flutter;* and, rarely, *ventricular tachycardia.*

Table 13–4. DIFFERENTIAL DIAGNOSIS OF NARROW QRS TACHYCARDIA

- Sinus tachycardia
- Supraventricular tachycardia
  - AV node re-entry
  - Pre-excitation syndromes
  - Sinus or intra-atrial re-entry
  - Automatic atrial tachycardia
- Accelerated junctional tachycardia
- Atrial flutter
- Atrial fibrillation
- Ventricular tachycardia (extremely rare)

Table 13–5. DIFFERENTIAL DIAGNOSIS OF WIDE QRS TACHYCARDIA

Ventricular tachycardia
Supraventricular tachycardia without pre-excitation
Associated with rate-related aberration
Associated with post–open heart surgery right bundle branch injury
Supraventricular tachycardia with pre-excitation
Orthodromic tachycardia associated with rate-related aberration
Antidromic tachycardia
Atrial flutter or fibrillation with antegrade conduction via bypass tract
Nodo-ventricular tachycardia (Mahaim)

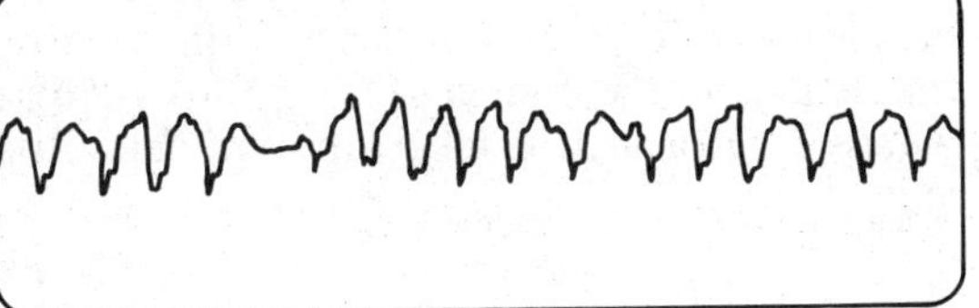

Figure 13–19. An irregularly irregular, rapid, wide QRS tachycardia in a patient with pre-excitation syndrome. This tracing is an example of atrial fibrillation in a patient with pre-excitation syndrome with antegrade conduction via the bypass tract. This syndrome results in a very rapid ventricular response, indicating that the bypass tract has a very short antegrade effective refractory period.

Recent information has demonstrated that the mechanism of wide QRS tachycardias in infants and children can be quite varied (Table 13–5).[2, 3, 76] Although ventricular tachycardias remain the most common causes of wide QRS tachycardias in children,[2, 3] a number of supraventricular tachyarrhythmias have a wide QRS morphology. The majority are associated with pre-excitation syndrome.[2, 3, 76] However, on rare occasion, a child will have a *supraventricular tachycardia with bundle branch aberration.* The differential diagnosis of wide QRS tachycardias in children also includes bypass tracts. When a patient has a wide QRS tachycardia in association with a possible *pre-excitation syndrome*, the differential diagnosis includes the following entities:

1. The presence of a *bundle branch aberration* associated with a supraventricular tachycardia of the "orthodromic type," i.e., conduction antegrade via the AV node and retrograde in the bypass tract with bundle branch block that develops during the tachycardia because of delayed conduction in one of the limbs of the bundle branches.[3, 76]

2. *Antidromic tachycardia* in which conduction during the tachycardia is antegrade via the bypass tract and retrograde via the AV node. Since antegrade conduction occurs via the bypass tract, there is an abnormal sequence of activation of the ventricles. The morphology of the QRS is therefore abnormal.[3, 76, 77]

3. *Atrial flutter or fibrillation* with ventricular pre-excitation with conduction during the flutter and fibrillation over the bypass tract. Atrial flutter may result in a very rapid regular rhythm. In fibrillation it would be an irregular rapid tachycardia (Fig. 13–19).[3, 76]

4. Antegrade tachycardia using a *Mahaim or nodo-ventricular bypass tract.* In this tachycardia the nodo-ventricular connection is the antegrade limb, with the His-Purkinje system or a portion of the AV node the retrograde limb. Patients with this tachycardia have been described with only a left bundle branch pattern (Fig. 13–20).[3, 76, 78]

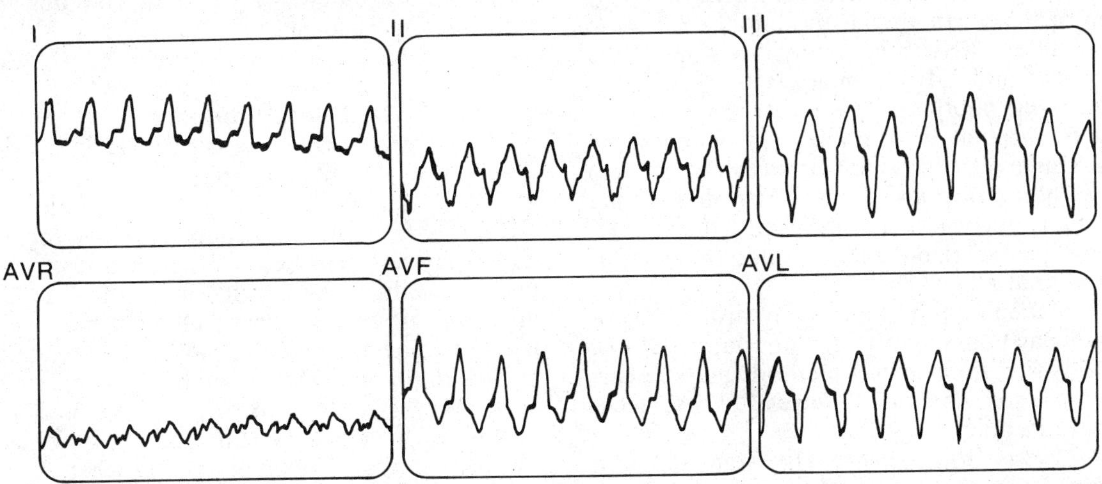

Figure 13–20. Six standard electrocardiographic leads showing a regular rapid wide QRS tachycardia with a ventricular rate of approximately 200 beats per minute. This patient was initially diagnosed as having ventricular tachycardia. An intracardiac electrophysiologic study demonstrated that this patient had supraventricular tachycardia with a variant of pre-excitation syndrome (Mahaim or nodo-ventricular bypass tract).

The differential diagnosis of the more complex wide QRS tachycardias is difficult from the surface ECG alone and frequently requires invasive intracardiac electrophysiologic studies.

TESTS FOR DIAGNOSIS

Evaluation of Arrhythmias

The signs and symptoms associated with cardiac arrhythmias range along a wide spectrum. Many patients will be asymptomatic whereas others will complain of being aware of "skipped beats," "tickling," and "pounding." Infants with marked tachyarrhythmias appear to be listless and pale, and often seem to be suffering from mild infections. When heart rates are in the range of 250 beats per minute or more for an extended period, infants may show signs of overt congestive heart failure. Patients with tachyarrhythmias, which under certain circumstances may progress to ventricular flutter or fibrillation, may die suddenly, or may be revived by cardiopulmonary resuscitation. Children with heart block may exhibit dizzy spells or fainting episodes of the Stokes-Adams variety.

A physical examination carried out at the time the rhythm disturbance is occurring will assist in differentiating an arrhythmia from normal sinus rhythm. The rate and regularity of the heart beat may suggest a specific diagnosis, but essentially, initial evaluation of any cardiac arrhythmia is carried out via the surface ECG.

Whether one is dealing with bradyarrhythmia or tachyarrhythmia, the initial evaluation should be to determine the relationships of the P waves and QRS complexes to themselves and to one another: (1) whether the P-P interval is constant or variable, (2) whether the QRS interval is constant or variable, and (3) how the P wave and QRS are related to one another and whether they have a fixed relationship, a variable relationship, or no relationship at all.

In patients with rapid tachycardias, the P wave may not be easily seen on routine ECGs. In this situation various methods may be carried out to "find the P waves." These techniques include:

1. Lewis-Golub lead: The standard arm (limb) leads are converted to precordial leads and the right precordium is "searched" for the location of atrial depolarization (P wave).
2. Esophageal lead: An electrode catheter is inserted into the esophagus so that the lead lies in the esophagus behind the left atrium. This technique puts the lead in close proximity to the atrium and is another way of recording atrial activity in patients in whom one cannot record P waves on a routine surface ECG. The esophageal lead can also be used for pacing, either for diagnostic or therapeutic purposes. This use is discussed in more detail in the section on treatment.
3. Vagal maneuvers utilize the autonomic nervous system in attempting to diagnose cardiac rhythm disturbances, particularly tachyarrhythmias. In patients with tachyarrhythmias, vagal maneuvers can be carried out while the surface ECG is recorded. These maneuvers include immersion (using the diving reflex), carotid or orbital massage, and gagging. They may convert a rhythm such as supraventricular tachycardia to sinus rhythm or slow an atrial flutter so that flutter waves may be better identified.[42, 79, 80, 82, 83]
4. Exercise testing at the bedside can be carried out to determine the response of either premature beats or arrhythmia to increased sympathetic tone. It is particularly useful in determining the significance of ventricular premature depolarizations.[1–3, 38–40]

All of the foregoing techniques can be carried out rapidly at the bedside of a patient who presents with an arrhythmia that requires immediate evaluation and therapy.

However, once the patient is stabilized, more sophisticated testing is carried out. Subsequent evaluation of the patient should include a careful physical examination, a chest x-ray, a 12-lead ECG, and often a 2-dimensional echocardiogram in order to rule out an associated cardiac defect.

24-Hour Ambulatory Electrocardiography (Holter Monitoring)

Twenty-four hour ambulatory electrocardiography has now become a standard procedure in evaluation of arrhythmias in all pediatric age groups.[81–83] This technique has been useful in diagnosing both bradyarrhythmia and tachyarrhythmia. Holter monitoring can record every heart beat over a 24-hour period, or longer if necessary. Information obtained by this technique helps determine whether or not a patient is having a cardiac arrhythmia that was not recognized during recording of the surface ECG. In addition, the recordings carried out on the ambulatory ECG can be related to a patient's symptoms. Twenty-four hour ECGs carried out in healthy newborns and older children have demonstrated that "cardiac arrhythmias" occur in the normal population.[84–87] These include episodes of sinus bradycardia, sinus pauses with junctional escape rhythms, first-degree AV block, second-degree AV block of the Wenckebach type, and premature atrial and ventricular beats. In healthy newborns and older children, uniform ventricular premature beats were not a rare finding. However, complex ventricular ectopy was extremely uncommon.[84–87] Ambulatory electrocardiography has also been used to detect significant arrhythmias in patients with various forms of heart disease and in patients after open heart surgery.[51, 73, 74, 88] Similarly, significant ventricular arrhythmias have been detected with ambulatory electrocardiography in patients with mitral valve prolapses, congenital complete AV blocks, and in patients with various other forms of heart disease.[81–83] In addition to diagnosing cardiac arrhythmias, ambulatory electrocardiography can be utilized to evaluate drug efficacy in their treatment.[89, 90]

Exercise Stress Testing

Exercise stress testing has become a very useful tool for evaluation of cardiac arrhythmias in children, particularly ventricular arrhythmias. Exercise can be carried out using a treadmill for children as young as 4 to 5 years of age and a bicycle ergometer for children as young as 2 to 3 years of age. Many reports have demonstrated the value of exercise stress testing for the evaluation of ventricular arrhythmias in children.[38, 40, 74, 82, 91, 92] Studies in large normal pediatric populations have indicated the absence of exercise-induced ventricular arrhythmias.[38, 91, 93–95] Exercise stress testing is extremely useful in the evaluation of ventricular arrhythmias in children who have had open heart surgery.[40, 74, 91, 96] In studies of patients after open heart repair of tetralogy of Fallot, as many as 30 per cent had ventricular arrhythmias induced during exercise stress testing that were not present at rest.[40, 74, 91] Exercise-induced ventricular arrhythmias have also been detected in patients with mitral valve prolapses and in patients with chronic complete AV blocks; these patients had a poorer prognosis than patients with no evidence of ventricular arrhythmias.[81, 82] In a child with a cardiac arrhythmia, a small risk is entailed in carrying out an exercise stress test, i.e., induction of a hemodynamically significant arrhythmia. However, induction of the arrhythmia under controlled conditions with trained personnel and resuscitation equipment available is preferred to the occurrence of the arrhythmia during spontaneous activity. Exercise-induced or exercise-enhanced cardiac arrhythmias, particularly those of ventricular orgin, often require long-term anti-arrhythmic drug therapy.

Intracardiac Electrophysiologic Studies

Intracardiac electrophysiologic studies of children have enhanced the understanding of normal impulse initiation and conduction and have improved the diagnosis and treatment of cardiac arrhythmias.[1–3] Intracardiac electrophysiologic studies can be carried out on children of any age. These studies often require the insertion of from two to four special electrode catheters into the heart. Intracardiac electrophysiologic studies can assist in answering many questions that cannot be answered from non-invasive electrophysiologic studies alone. Rapid atrial pacing studies and programmed extra-stimulus techniques aid in the evaluation of both sinoatrial and atrioventricular node functions.[1–3] These techniques are used to induce and terminate tachyarrhythmias in order to determine the mechanisms of these arrhythmias and the responses to pharmacologic agents.[1–3]

Intracardiac electrophysiologic studies are invasive and entail some minimal risk to the patient. Therefore, there must be specific indications for this type of study in an individual patient. These include: (1) evaluation of the cause of symptoms of severe syncope or cardiorespiratory arrest suspected to be of cardiac origin and possibly an arrhythmia; (2) determination of the mechanism of a tachycardia so as to improve drug therapy; (3) evaluation of the efficacy of anti-arrhythmic drugs in treating specific arrhythmias; (4) mapping of a tachycardia in a candidate for surgical ablation of a bypass tract or ectopic focus; and (5) evaluation of the integrity of the specialized conduction system following open heart surgery.

TREATMENT OF CARDIAC ARRHYTHMIAS

Prior to the institution of therapy, a correct diagnosis of a cardiac arrhythmia must be made. Therapy may have to be instituted to treat the arrhythmia, or treatment may have to be directed towards a secondary underlying cause of a cardiac rhythm disturbance, e.g., hyperkalemia. Four major forms of therapy are available for the management of cardiac arrhythmia:

1. Antiarrhythmic drugs.
2. Maneuvers involving the autonomic nervous system, including the use of pharmacologic agents and vagal stimulation.
3. Electrical cardioversion and cardiac pacing.
4. Surgical ablation of bypass tracts in patients with the pre-excitation syndrome or surgical removal of foci within the atrium or ventricle that initiate life-threatening cardiac arrhythmias resistant to standard therapy.[60, 97, 98]

Bradyarrhythmias

Brief episodes of sinus bradycardia or sinus pause with a junctional escape rhythm do not generally require therapy. Acute episodes of bradycardia or sinus arrest with slow junctional rhythms are seen in children secondary to noncardiac causes such as hypoxia and acidosis. The underlying causes must be diagnosed and managed. However, patients with sick sinus syndrome who develop severe sinus bradycardia, sinus pauses, and a very slow junctional escape rhythm may require antiarrhythmic therapy.[48–53]

For patients with intrinsic abnormalities in sinus node automaticity or conduction and slow cardiac rates that result in inadequate cardiac output, treatment must be directed towards increasing heart rate (e.g., intravenous atropine or an intravenous infusion of a β-adrenergic catecholamine such as isoproterenol). Some patients with sick sinus syndrome and symptomatic sinus node dysfunction may have syncopal episodes due to the slow cardiac rate and may require insertion of a permanent cardiac pacemaker.[2, 3, 53] It is unusual for these symptomatic patients to have bradycardia alone; most have an alternating bradycardia-tachycardia syndrome.[48–53] Treatment of this syndrome is discussed in the tachyarrhythmias section.

Bradyarrhythmias can also result from abnormalities in AV conduction. They can be secondary to diseases in the AV node or His-Purkinje system that are congenital, secondary to surgical injury or, secondary to an acute or chronic inflammatory process. Similar to patients with sinus bradycardia, those with bradycardia secondary to abnormalities in AV conduction can benefit from atropine therapy if there is transmission of some impulses through the AV conduction system and if the disease is in the AV node or above the AV node.

In patients with His-Purkinje disease, a slow idioventricular pacemaker, or other forms of complete heart block in which there is no transmission of impulses from the atrium to the ventricle, atropine will generally not increase the rate of the subsidiary idioventricular pacemaker. In these situations, β-adrenergic catecholamines such as isoproterenol are used to increase the cardiac rate. Should this therapy be ineffective, ventricular pacing remains as the only alternate mode of therapy.

Atropine is a true competitive inhibitor of acetylcholine and blocks the so-called muscarinic responses to acetylcholine in the heart. Atropine (0.01–0.02 mg/kg IV; maximum 1.0 mg) is particularly effective in treating supraventricular bradycardias. The same dose is used to enhance atrioventricular conduction in transient heart block. However, in unusual circumstances, the acceleration of sinus rate may exceed the improvement of AV conduction caused by the atropine and may result in a rate-related increase in the degree of block with a reduction in the ventricular rate. Occasionally, atropine-induced parasympathetic block may be preceded by brief mild cholinergic stimulation with transient bradycardia secondary to stimulation of the vagus. The transient vagal hyperactivity produced by atropine generally occurs at low doses and is not a contraindication for continued administration.[1–3]

Isoproterenol is used for the treatment of supraventricular bradycardia and atrioventricular block. It is the agent of choice for symptomatic complete heart block until a cardiac pacemaker can be introduced. Isoproterenol is titrated to desired effect or until toxic effects are observed. The usual dosage range is 0.05–0.5 μg/kg/min. This agent enhances atrioventricular and His-Purkinje conduction and increases the automaticity of both atrial and ventricular pacemakers. However, isoproterenol can also produce excessive sinus tachycardia and precipitate episodes of supraventricular tachycardia, ventricular premature beats, ventricular tachycardia, and even ventricular fibrillation in patients with intrinsic heart disease and susceptibility to catecholamines.[1–3] Beta adrenergic stimulating agents should be used with caution in patients with hypoxia, acidosis, or who are taking digitalis preparations.

Tachyarrhythmias

Supraventricular Tachycardias

Immediate Management

In most infants and children who have supraventricular tachycardias without associated cardiac diseases, adequate hemodynamic status is maintained for extended periods. Therefore, in a hemodynamically stable patient a gradual approach for termination of the tachycardias can be carried out. The length of time that these arrhythmias will be tolerated is a function of (1) the underlying state of the myocardium, (2) the rate of the tachycardia, and (3) the duration of the abnormal rhythm. It should be emphasized that electrical cardioversion is the treatment of choice in any patient in whom the cardiac output is significantly compromised.

The first measure is that of vagal stimulation. Initiation of a strong vagal discharge by inducing the diving reflex is the most effective maneuver to enhance vagal tone in children.[42, 79, 80] In a neonate or infant, induction of the diving reflex is carried out by suddenly placing an ice-cold wet towel or washcloth on the patient's face and holding it there for several seconds. In older children, facial immersion in ice-cold water is similarly effective. Other vagal maneuvers such as carotid sinus massage, stimulating the gag reflex, inducing vomiting, or occular pressure have not been as effective in infants as in older children and adults. Often, a "vagal maneuver of choice" may exist for each patient, even a bizarre method such as a headstand.

A second measure to induce an increase in vagal tone is the intravenous administration of an α-adrenergic agent such as phenylephrine in order to increase systolic blood pressure and initiate a responding baroreceptor reflex.[1–3] Phenylephrine (0.05–0.5 μg/kg/min; titrated to desired effect or until toxicity occurs) should be infused slowly until the systolic blood pressure is 150 to 200 per cent of the baseline measurement. An effective venous route is essential in order to avoid local infiltration, which can result in significant injury to the surrounding tissue.

A third method of increasing vagal tone is the use of edrophonium (Tensilon). Edrophonium is an acetylcholinesterase inhibitor that enhances vagal tone by inhibiting the breakdown of acetylcholine by the enzyme acetylcholinesterase.[1–3] A test dose of approximately a tenth of the recommended dose should be given prior to the administration of the entire dose (0.1–0.2 mg/kg intravenously). Occasionally, a patient may have a significant "overreaction" to the drug. The effect of edrophonium may be profound, with the induction of extreme sinus bradycardia, junctional rhythm, or AV block. Atropine (0.01–0.02 mg/kg IV: maximum 1.0 mg) should be available when edrophonium is to be used. The maximum dose of edrophonium should not exceed 5 mg per dose. If the initial dose does not convert the arrhythmia, a second dose can be administered.

Digitalis preparations have been the drugs of choice for patients in whom anti-arrhythmic drug therapy is to be used to convert supraventricular tachycardias. Digoxin can be administered intravenously, intramuscularly, or orally. The mode of administration is dependent upon how rapid an effect is required. A number of different digitalis glycoside preparations are available. One should become familiar with one type of digitalis glycoside and use that preparation only. We have found digoxin to be the most versatile form of digitalis. It has a relatively rapid onset of action when used intravenously and has a long enough half-life so that it does not have to be given very frequently when administration is long-term. Digoxin is administered intravenously as a total digitalizing dose of 25–50 μg/kg in divided doses, with a maximum total digitalizing dose of 1 mg. The oral dose is 40–70 μg/kg in divided doses with a maximum dose of 1.5 mg. The lower dose is recommended for neonates. Premature infants and patients with renal failure must be evaluated on an individual basis, and even lower doses are required because of decreased rates of excretion.

Digoxin is generally administered in divided doses with a quarter to a half of the "digitalizing" dose given initially, followed in 2 to 8 hours by subsequent doses. The timing of the doses depends upon how rapidly it is necessary to convert the supraventricular tachycardia to sinus rhythm. The onset of action of intravenous digoxin is approximately 30 minutes, and the peak action occurs within 2 hours. Therefore, if the arrhythmia remains unchanged 2 hours after the initial dose, one can give a second dose of digoxin intravenously at that time.

Once conversion of the tachyarrhythmia occurs, digitalization of the patient can be completed at a more leisurely rate, orally rather than intravenously. For an oral dose, a third greater than the intravenous dose should be calculated. Maintenance digoxin dosage is a quarter to a third of the digitalizing dosage and usually is between 10 and 20 μg/kg/day orally, with a maximum maintenance dosage of between 0.25 and 0.5 mg/day. Digoxin has a relatively long half-life of 36 hours and therefore the maintenance dose is either administered once daily or in divided doses twice daily.

Digoxin is extremely effective in converting most supraventricular tachycardias to sinus rhythm.[1–3] It has a marked vagotonic effect and is especially effective for the common supraventricular tachycardias that involve the AV node as part of the "re-entrant pathway." In addition, there are direct effects on conduction and refractoriness of the AV node.[99, 100, 101] Atrial flutter or fibrillation is also treated with digoxin, which slows the ventricular rate on the basis of the mechanisms previously described. Rarely, digoxin will convert atrial flutter to sinus rhythm. However, digoxin often will convert atrial flutter to atrial fibrillation, resulting in a slower ventricular rate.

Digoxin must be used with care in patients with the pre-excitation syndrome, especially in those with short antegrade effective refractory periods of the bypass tract. Digoxin may shorten the antegrade effective refractory period of the bypass tract, resulting in enhanced conduction to the ventricle, particularly in patients with atrial fibrillation. This effect can result in very rapid ventricular rates that can lead to ventricular tachycardia or fibrillation.[102] This mechanism is very uncommon in infants and children. However, it is a significant potential risk in older children and adults. Another concern about the use of digoxin is the potential for post-digitalis cardioversion–induced ventricular arrhythmias.[103, 104] This possibility is only theoretical and in practice is very uncommon in children. It would be of major concern primarily in patients with severe underlying structural heart disease and would be unlikely to occur in patients with no structural heart disease unless digoxin has been given in near toxic doses.

Verapamil is extremely effective for use in terminating supraventricular tachycardias, particularly those involving the AV node.[105, 106] Verapamil is a blocker of the slow inward current carried primarily by calcium. Since the action potentials of the AV node are "slow response type" calcium action potentials, verapamil is very effective in treating rhythm disturbances that originate in this region.[4, 18] Its advantage over digoxin is that it has a very rapid onset of action (3–5 minutes) and the effects are seen immediately. However, the immediate effects also can dissipate fairly rapidly and another dose may be required. The usual initial dose of verapamil is 0.075–0.15 mg/kg intravenously with a maximum dose of 5 mg. It can be repeated between 10 and 30 minutes following the initial dose. Verapamil is also useful in slowing the ventricular response in patients with atrial flutter and fibrillation, particularly as an adjunct to digitalis therapy. However, as with digoxin, verapamil has been shown to shorten the effective refractory period of the bypass tract in patients with pre-excitation syndrome, and therefore the same potential risks are present for these patients that exist with digitalis.[107] Although verapamil has been proven to be more efficacious in the immediate pharmacologic conversions of supraventricular tachycardias than digitalis, it also has a higher incidence of side effects, including a high degree of AV block, extreme bradycardia, asystole, hypotension, and congestive heart failure.[108] The adverse cardiovascular effects can generally be overcome by treatment with β-adrenergic agents such as isoproterenol and parenteral administration of calcium. Verapamil is also available as a long-term oral preparation. The starting oral dosage in children is approximately 4 mg/kg/day in 3 divided doses. This dosage can be increased until either therapeutic or early "toxic" effects are seen. The upper limits of the dosage for long-term oral preparation (approximately 10 mg/kg/day) in infants and young children has not been clearly determined.[105, 106]

A third antiarrhythmic drug that can be used immediately for the treatment of supraventricular arrhythmias is the β-adrenergic blocking agent propranolol. As with the other agents, the major effects are on the AV node. The blocking of sympathetic input to the AV node results in an unbalanced parasympathetic (vagal) effect. The intravenous dose of propranolol is 0.1–0.15 mg/kg. The maximum immediate dose should not exceed 5 mg and the maximum rate of administration should not be greater than 1 mg/minute. This dose can be repeated in approximately 20–30 minutes if no effect is seen. As with verapamil, side effects can include a high degree of AV block, extreme bradycardia, asystole, hypotension, and congestive heart failure. The adverse cardiovascular effects can be effectively treated with a β-adrenergic agent such as isoproterenol.

On occasion, supraventricular tachycardia may be detected *in utero*. If the arrhythmia persists, the fetus may develop congestive heart failure that is manifested by evidence of hydrops fetalis. The administration of an antiarrhythmic drug such as digoxin to the mother at usual therapeutic doses will often convert the arrhythmia to sinus rhythm *in utero*. Thus, early delivery by cesarean section is avoided.[79]

Electrical cardioversion using defibrillation and DC cardioversion is the emergency treatment of choice for any patient with a supraventricular tachycardia in an unstable hemodynamic state or severe congestive failure. This includes most forms of supraventricular tachycardia, atrial fibrillation, and atrial flutter with rapid ventricular response. Cardioversion is also used for elective conversion of these arrhythmias in stable patients who are refractory to routine long-term anti-arrhythmic therapy. Such patients should be "anesthetized" by an agent such as Valium or Pentothal (thiopental) prior to the attempted cardioversion. Electrical cardioversion of an awake, fully alert patient is "unkind." The usual dose for cardioversion is 1–2 watt-seconds/kg.[109, 110]

Electrical conversion of supraventricular arrhythmias can also be carried out by electrical pacing. Supraventricular tachycardia can be converted either by inducing properly timed premature atrial beats or by rapid atrial pacing.[111, 112] Atrial flutter can be converted using rapid atrial pacing of the atrium at rates significantly faster than the flutter rate (entrainment).[113]

Long-term Management

Long-term therapy of supraventricular tachycardias can be carried out with a variety of anti-arrhythmic drugs either alone or in combination. These include digoxin, beta-blocking agents (propranolol, nadolol, atenolol), verapamil, quinidine, procainamide, and disopyramide. In addition, new "experimental drugs" such as amiodarone are being tested and will be available for anti-arrhythmic therapy.[114, 115] The decision as to which anti-arrhythmic drug to use is often made on an empiric basis. However, if the exact mechanism of the tachycardia is known, a more rational choice of drug can be made. For example, in patients with AV nodal re-entrant supraventricular tachycardias, agents that effect the AV node, such as digoxin, verapamil, and beta-blocking agents, are the drugs of choice.[42] However, in patients with ectopic automatic tachycardias, an agent such as propranolol that affects atrial automaticity is a more rational choice.[44, 45] In treating patients with pre-excitation syndrome one can choose drugs that primarily affect the AV node or drugs that primarily affect the bypass tract, such as quinidine, procainamide, and disopyramide (Table 13–6).[56, 60] Long-term treatment of atrial flutter or fibrillation is commonly carried out with either digoxin to control the ventricular rate or a combination of digoxin and quinidine to prevent recurrence of the flutter or fibrillation. When treating atrial flutter, one should "protect the AV node" by digitalizing the patient prior to instituting quinidine therapy. This treatment prevents the occurrence of a more rapid ventricular response that may follow quinidine administration because of the anticholinergic effects of quinidine on the AV node. In addition, because of the interaction between digoxin and quinidine, the dose of digoxin must be decreased 25 to 33 per cent when quinidine therapy is prescribed for a "digitalized" patient.[116–118] Other than digoxin, most of the pharmacologic agents just discussed have to be taken three to four times a day and therefore patient compliance is often not optimal. These agents also have significant side effects that limit their usefulness. The dosages and side effects of the commonly used antiarrhythmic drugs are outlined in Table 13–6.

A form of therapy that may be useful in selected cases is surgery. Patients with the pre-excitation syndrome who display life-threatening or refractory arrhythmias require careful endocardial and epicardial mapping to determine the location of the bypass tract, which is followed by surgical division.[60, 97] This procedure has been successful not only in patients with drug-resistant cardiac arryhythmias due to pre-excitation, but recently has also been utilized in patients with refractory atrial tachycardias secondary to ectopic atrial foci. The focus is removed surgically after careful mapping, which locates the area of disease from where the arrhythmia originates.[98]

Ventricular Arrhythmias

The management of the child with a ventricular arrhythmia is dependent upon the severity of arrhythmia, the associated hemodynamic

Table 13–6. COMMONLY USED ANTI-ARRHYTHMIC DRUG SCHEDULES IN PEDIATRIC PATIENTS

Drug	Oral Administration		Intravenous Administration*			Comments and Side Effects
	Maximal Dose	*Maintenance Dose*†	*Loading Dose*	*Maximal Dose*	*Comments*	*Side Effects*
Digoxin	0.5 mg	0.01–0.02 mg/kg/day DD‡ q12h	0.025–0.05 mg/kg in 3 DD q4–8h	0.5 mg	Oral loading dose 0.04–0.07 mg/kg/day DD q8. See text for age-related differences.	APDs, VPDs, conduction defects, bradycardia, nausea, vomiting, anorexia.
Quinidine sulfate	2.4 g	20–60 mg/kg/day DD q6h	—	—	Oral test dose 2 mg/kg.	Nausea, vomiting, diarrhea, cinchonism, QRS and QT prolongation, AV block, asystole, syncope, thrombocytopenia, hemolytic anemia, blurred vision, convulsions, allergic reactions, exacerbation of periodic paralysis, enhancement of digoxin effects.
Quinidine gluconate	2.0 g	20–60 mg/kg/day DD q8–12h	10–15 mg/kg as 250 μg/kg/min	20 mg/min to 1.0 g		
Procainamide	6.0 g	50–100 mg/kg/day DD q4–6h DD q6h†	10–20 mg/kg as 300 μg/kg/min	20 mg/min to 1.0 g	Intravenous maintenance 20–40 μg/kg/min	PR, QRS, QT prolongation, anorexia, nausea, vomiting, rash, fever, agranulocytosis, thrombocytopenia, Coombs-positive hemolytic anemia, lupus erythematosus–like syndrome, hypotension, exacerbation of periodic paralysis.
Disopyramide	1.2 g	8–12 mg/kg/day DD q6h DD q12h†	—	—	—	Anticholinergic effects, urinary retention, blurred vision, dry mouth, QT and QRS prolongation, exacerbation of periodic paralysis, negative

Phenytoin	600 mg	3–6 mg/kg/day DD q12h	10–15 mg/kg as 250 μg/kg/min	20 mg/min to 1.0 g	—	Rash, gingival hyperplasia, CNS manifestations, ataxia, lethargy, vertigo, tremor, macrocytic anemia.
Lidocaine	—	—	1 mg/kg repeat q5/min × 3	50–75 mg	Intravenous maintenance 30–50 μg/kg/min.	CNS effects, confusion, convulsions, high degree AV block, asystole, coma, parasthesias, respiratory failure.
Verapamil	480 mg	4–10 mg/kg/day DD q8h	0.075–0.15 mg/kg q 20 min ×2	5 mg	—	Bradycardia, asystole, high degree AV block, hypotension, congestive heart failure, enhancement of digoxin effects.
Propranolol	Not established	1–4 mg/kg/day DD q6h	0.1–0.15 mg/kg	1 mg/min to 10 mg	Long-acting beta-blocking agents (nadolol, atenolol) are preferred for long-term therapy (less frequent administration and CNS side effects)	Bradycardia, loss of concentration or memory, bronchospasm, hypoglycemia, hypotension.

*Intravenous administration of anti-arrhythmic drugs should always be given slowly with constant monitoring of blood pressure and electrocardiogram, particularly in patients with compromised cardiac function or compromised renal or hepatic function. Dose must be modified in patients with abnormal renal or hepatic function.

†Sustained-release preparations available for clinical use.

‡Divided doses.

effect of the arrhythmia, and the presence of associated cardiac and extra-cardiac disease. Premature ventricular depolarizations in a child with a normal heart, whether they are uniform with fixed coupling, uniform without fixed coupling, multiform or even couplets, do not require emergency therapy. This applies even if the premature ventricular depolarizations are in a bigeminal pattern unless they are interfering with cardiac hemodynamics or are a precursor to the development of ventricular tachycardia or fibrillation. In patients with abnormal cardiac function or conditions such as the prolonged QT syndrome, one attempts to suppress the ventricular ectopy. Ventricular tachycardia should be treated in most patients regardless of their hemodynamic state. Occasionally, if a child does not have associated heart disease and the tachycardia is "non-sustained" or well tolerated, long-term anti-arrhythmic drug therapy may not be required. If the patient with ventricular tachycardia has severely compromised hemodynamics, electrical cardioversion with 1–2 watt-seconds/kg is the treatment of choice.[109, 110] For ventricular fibrillation, it is the only treatment available.

If the patient is stable enough so that emergency electrical cardioversion is not immediately necessary, an intravenous access route can be established and treatment with intravenous lidocaine can be carried out. The initial dose should be 1 mg/kg as a rapid bolus. The maximum amount administered in one dose should never exceed 75 mg. In our experience, lidocaine is effective in suppressing ventricular arrhythmias in approximately 85 per cent of pediatric patients. When recommended doses are used, lidocaine has no significant electrophysiologic effects on the AV conduction system, and other than suppression of the ventricular arrhythmia, changes in the PR interval, QRS duration, or QT interval are not seen.[119, 120] If the initial dose does not result in conversion of the arrhythmia, a bolus can be repeated every 5 to 10 minutes to a maximum dose of 3 to 5 mg/kg. Generally, if three doses do not convert the arrhythmia, then lidocaine is not going to be useful. Once lidocaine has been demonstrated to be effective, the intravenous bolus should be followed by an intravenous infusion at a rate of 30 to 50 μg/kg/minute. It takes approximately three to five half-lives to reach the steady state of the intravenous infusion (lidocaine half-life of approximately 90 minutes). If after one or two hours following the start of the intravenous infusion ventricular ectopy returns, rather than increasing the infusion rate, one should give another bolus of lidocaine at half the initial dose or 0.5 mg/kg. Since the infusion may not have reached steady state at this time, the lidocaine level may have decreased below the therapeutic range.

To properly evaluate the efficacy of any of the anti-arrhythmic drugs, one should obtain plasma drug levels to ensure that the dose being administered will result in therapeutic blood levels for that particular agent. Dosing schedules for children have not been well standardized and so have been adapted from adult dosing schedules. Since there are significant differences in both the pharmacokinetics and responsiveness of the developing heart, one has to be very careful in extrapolating the adult's dosage to the child's dosage.

One should use caution in administering lidocaine to patients with significant AV block. In children with complete heart block, lidocaine may acutely suppress the automaticity of the idioventricular pacemaker.[120] Therefore, in any patient with complete heart block who has significant ectopy and requires lidocaine administration, a ventricular pacemaker should be inserted prior to initiation of lidocaine therapy. Since lidocaine is almost totally metabolized in the liver, it has to be used with caution in patients with significant hepatic dysfunction. Dosage modification and careful monitoring of the drug's blood levels is especially important under these circumstances and must be carried out to prevent toxicity.

In patients with ventricular tachycardia that does not respond to intravenous lidocaine, the drug of choice is intravenous procainamide. The intravenous administration of procainamide must be done slowly and carefully. Procainamide has a direct effect on the peripheral vascular bed and can cause profound systemic hypotension with rapid administration.[121, 122] Procainamide has negative inotropic effects that may be exaggerated by rapid intravenous administration, particularly in patients with abnormal hemodynamic function. In addition, procainamide has a marked effect on AV conduction and can enhance or induce AV block.[121, 122] Despite these potential side effects, when used properly procainamide is an effective anti-arrhythmic agent for the immediate management of ventricular arrhythmias.

In adults, procainamide is administered as 100-mg boluses every 5 minutes to a maximum of 1 g or to a therapeutic or toxic effect.[123] We have modified an intravenous protocol for procainamide for use in children, in which a dose of 300 μg/kg/minute mixed as 1 g of procainamide in 100 ml of normal saline is infused slowly at an appropriate rate for weight. A maximum rate of 20 mg/minute and a maximum dose of 20 mg/kg is recommended.[124] Once a therapeutic effect is achieved, blood should be obtained to determine the plasma level necessary to control the arrhythmia. Following conversion of the arrhythmia to normal sinus rhythm the rate of the infusion is decreased to 20–40 μg/kg/minute.

One advantage of procainamide over lidocaine is that once a therapeutic effect has been established, intravenous therapy can be converted to long-term oral therapy using the same drug (see Table 13–6). No long-term oral lidocaine preparation is available for routine use in children.

During rapid administration of procainamide careful monitoring of the surface ECG should be carried out. Specifically, measurements of PR interval, QRS duration, and QT interval should be made. None of the intervals should increase more than 25 per cent of the pre-treatment value. A greater prolongation may indicate that toxic effects are imminent, including high degree of atrioventricular block, ventricular arrhythmia, and asystole.[121, 122] As with lidocaine, procainamide should be used with caution in the presence of AV or intraventricular conduction defects, and ventricular pacing should be available for any patient with complete heart block.

Another intravenous drug that is available for refractory ventricular tachycardia or fibrillation is bretylium tosylate. This drug is presently used in patients whose arrhythmia is refractory to recurrent electrical cardioversion, intravenous lidocaine, or procainamide.[125] Because there is little experience with this drug in pediatric practice, it is rarely administered to children except under extreme circumstances. The initial dose is 5 mg/kg as an intravenous bolus. It can be repeated in 15 to 30 minutes with a second dose of 5 or 10 mg/kg (maximum 500 mg). Should this drug prove to be efficacious, a long-term infusion can be carried out as either an intermittent or as a constant infusion (1–2 mg/minute in adults). The maximum immediate dose should never exceed 30 mg/kg and the maximum dose per day should not exceed 30 mg/kg with a long-term infusion.[125]

Occasionally, intravenous propranolol will be effective in the immediate treatment of ventricular tachycardia. The dosages and precautions are similar to those discussed for the treatment of supraventricular arrhythmias. Phenytoin is available as an intravenous preparation, but is rarely used for the rapid conversion of ventricular tachycardia.[126]

In addition to administration of anti-arrhythmic drug therapy, at the same time one should correct any acid-base or other metabolic abnormalities that exist. All of the agents discussed are much more effective in the presence of normal pH and PaO_2. Therefore, adequate ventilation should be established, and correction of acidosis should be carried out using sodium bicarbonate. Improvement in spontaneous cardiac activity and hemodynamic status with a β-adrenergic agent may frequently aid in the conversion of arrhythmias. However, these agents must be used with caution in a patient with ventricular ectopy because they can also be arrhythmogenic.

The choice of anti-arrhythmic agent for the long-term suppression of ventricular arrhythmias in children often must be made on an empiric basis. There are no detailed studies of drug efficacy available to help determine the best choice of anti-arrhythmic agents and the proper dosages for pediatric patients of different age groups. The age-related differences in the effects of therapeutic agents are well recognized. Recent studies of quinidine, procainamide, amiodarone, and disopyramide have indicated important differences between children and adults.[115, 119, 127–136] Careful monitoring of plasma blood levels of all drugs administered (Table 13–7) and the subsequent modification of dosages is required in patients who are not responsive to the recommended drug schedules.

The long-term suppression of ventricular ectopy can be accomplished by one of the drug schedules outlined in Table 13–6. At our institution, most patients are treated with quinidine or procainamide. Disopyramide has also been an effective agent. Newer anti-arrhythmic

Table 13–7. PLASMA LEVELS FOR COMMONLY USED THERAPEUTIC ANTI-ARRHYTHYMIC DRUGS IN PEDIATRIC PATIENTS

Digoxin	1–2 ng/ml*
Quinidine	2–5 μg/ml
Procainamide	4–10 μg/ml
Disopyramide	2–4 μg/ml
Propranolol	50–150 ng/ml†
Phenytoin	15–20 μg/ml
Lidocaine	2–5 μg/ml

*Many infants tolerate higher levels with no clinical evidence of toxicity.

†Therapeutic levels not clearly demonstrated.

drugs such as amiodarone and mexiletine await further evaluation to determine their place as effective and safe alternative therapy in children. The development of sustained-release preparations has been helpful in encouraging compliance in patients taking the antiarrhythmic agents discussed.

In selected groups of patients, specific antiarrhythmic drug therapies have been recommended. For example, in patients with prolonged QT syndrome, mitral valve prolapse, or obstructive cardiomyopathy, propranolol is usually the initial drug of choice.[33–35, 82, 92, 137] Phenytoin has been suggested in some centers as the agent of choice in postoperative pediatric patients with ventricular arrhythmias and residual hemodynamic abnormalities.[71, 92, 126, 138]

Surgical treatment of ventricular tachycardia in children is rarely required.[98] However, surgical excision of an arrhythmogenic focus located at the right ventricular outflow tract in patients with postoperative tetralogy of Fallot has been carried out successfully.[72] In addition, surgery has been carried out in children with arrhythmogenic right ventricular dysplasia[139] and cardiac tumors.[140–142]

Antitachycardia pacemakers used in selected adult patients for control of ventricular tachycardia[143–145] are of limited value in pediatric patients. Pior to using this type of pacemaker, a detailed intracardiac electrophysiologic study must be carried out to determine the mode of pacing that will terminate the tachycardia.

Our experience, as well as that of others, has indicated that it is difficult to completely suppress chronic ventricular arrhythmias in children.[92, 137] It is estimated that long-term drug treatment is effective in approximately 60 per cent of children with no underlying heart disease. The lack of data concerning the reproducibility of the 24-hour ambulatory electrocardiogram and exercise stress test in assessing drug efficacy in children with chronic ventricular arrhythmias limits the usefulness of these noninvasive studies. At present, the role of intracardiac electrophysiologic studies for the identification of patients at risk for sudden death from ventricular arrhythmia and the evaluation of drug efficacy has not been determined and awaits further study. However, with the thoughtful use of available noninvasive and invasive electrophysiologic testing and with the careful monitoring of anti-arrhythmic drug plasma levels, most pediatric patients who require long-term suppression of ventricular arrhythmias can be managed appropriately.

Cardiac Pacing

Cardiac pacemakers are used for treating patients with bradyarrhythmias to control the cardiac rate and recently have also been used to convert cardiac arrhythmias.[1–3] Many of the modern pacemaker's functions can be controlled by external means after its insertion. In children, the most common indications for cardiac pacing are complete heart block, either post-surgical or congenital, and sick sinus syndrome. The latter is common after open heart surgery for transposition of the great vessels (Mustard procedure), but most patients do not require a pacemaker.[1–3]

Pacing is most commonly carried out from the right ventricle; however, recently, atrial pacemakers have been used more frequently, with pacing wires inserted in the right atrium.[1–3] The pacing wires can be inserted either transvenously or via a thoracotomy on the epicardial surface of the heart. Generally, in infants and children for long-term pacing, epicardial wires are employed. In older children and adults, transvenous pacemaker insertion is the preferred method of electrode implacement.

The pulse generators of the pacemakers have been symbolized by a three-letter code. The first letter indicates the chamber paced; the second letter the chamber sensed; and the third letter the mode of response to the sensed event; so that *A = atrium, V = ventricle, D = double, O = none, I = inhibited* and *T = triggered*.

There are various kinds of pacemakers that can potentially be used in children. The initial pacemakers developed 25 years ago were *asynchronous or fixed-rate pacemakers, (AOO, VOO)*. These pacemakers can be placed in the atrium, ventricles, or both atrium and ventricles simultaneously. They stimulate the cardiac chamber into which they are inserted at a constant fixed rate regardless of the spontaneous rhythm or patient's intrinsic heart rate. In a patient in whom there is no or very low potential for spontaneous activity, these pacemakers will assume total pacemaker control of the heart. However, in many patients, chronic use of asynchronous or fixed-rate pacemakers commonly will create competing rhythms. Although in theory these circumstances could initiate life-threatening arrhythmias, in fact this has rarely occurred.

With the development of more reliable noncompetitive stimulation pacemakers (AAI, VVI; Fig. 13–21), the asynchronous or fixed-rate pacemaker is no longer utilized.

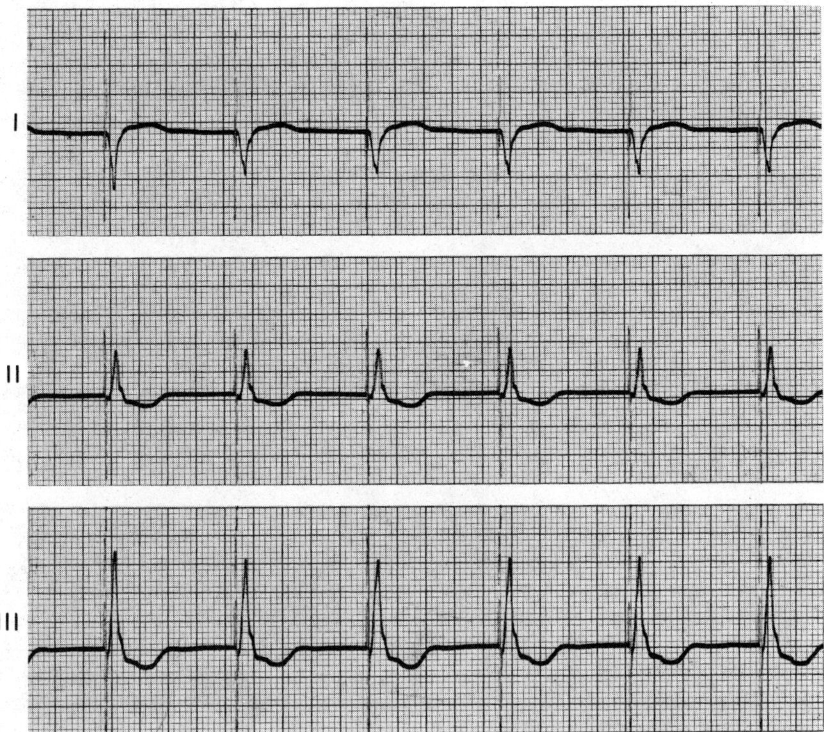

Figure 13–21. Simultaneous surface electrocardiographic leads I, II, and III in a patient with a ventricular pacemaker. The ventricular pacing artifact precedes each QRS complex. This tracing could represent either VOO or VVI pacing mode.

In addition to having the ability to pace the heart, these pacemakers have a sensing system that allows them to sense the patients' spontaneous rhythms. The most commonly used ventricular pacemakers are the R-wave inhibited pacemakers. If the pacemaker senses the spontaneous R-wave of the patient's inherent rhythm, the output of the pacing mechanism is inhibited. The rate at which the pacemaker will discharge and will inhibit is preset. The pacing mode of the non-competitive stimulation pacemaker will be inhibited at all spontaneous rates that are more rapid than the set pacemaker rate. This inhibition theoretically prevents the occurrence of competitive arrhythmias. Non-competitive atrial P wave–inhibited pacemakers are also available.

In certain patients with complete heart block and associated structural heart disease, ventricular pacing alone may not allow adequate cardiac output. These patients may be dependent upon synchronous atrioventricular contraction. An "atrial kick" is required in order to maintain adequate cardiac output. To accomplish this, one can use the *atrial synchronous pacemaker*. (There are two variants of this kind of pacemaker, *VAT* and *VDD*.) They require two leads, one in the atrium and one in the ventricle. The atrial lead is used for sensing the P wave. After sensing of the P wave, there is a preset AV delay, following which the ventricular lead is triggered to stimulate the ventricle *(VAT)*. An additional sensing device can be added in the ventricular electrode to prevent premature atrial beats from causing ventricular activation and to prevent potential competition between spontaneous ventricular activity and ventricular pacing *(VDD)*. Should the patient have severe sinus bradycardia or sinus arrest, these pacemakers switch to a function identical to non-competitive ventricular pacemakers *(VVI)* at a preset low rate. When the patient's spontaneous atrial rate exceeds a preset upper limit rate, an artificial Wenckebach AV block is established.

Another type of pacemaker is the *atrioventricular sequential and synchronous pacemaker (DVI)* (Fig. 13–22). This type is best suited for patients who require pacing and in whom constant augmentation of cardiac output by sequential atrioventricular contraction is desired. These pacemakers also require pacing electrodes to be inserted in both the atrium and ventricle. In this type of pacemaker both the atrium and the ventricle are paced in a se-

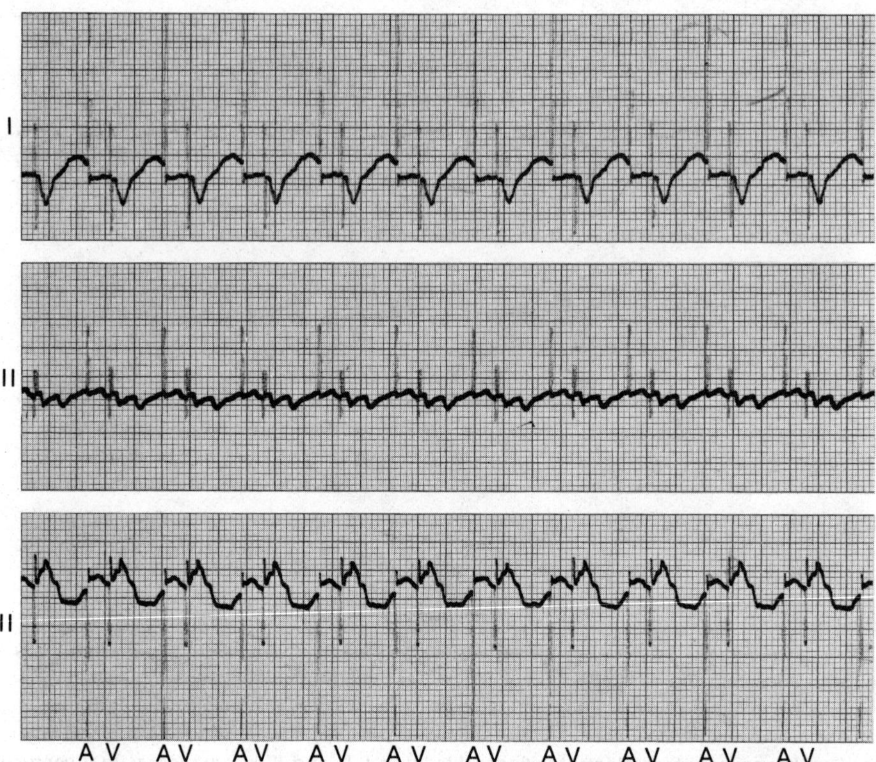

Figure 13–22. Simultaneous surface electrocardiographic leads I, II, and III in a patient with an atrioventricular sequential and synchronous pacemaker (DVI). A pacing artifact can be seen preceding each P wave (A) and QRS (V). There is a preset AV delay.

quential fashion. There is a preset AV delay. These pacemakers are generally ventricularly inhibited. However, at times they can be atrially triggered and ventricularly inhibited. Their major advantage is that they allow consistent atrioventricular sequential pacing. However, unlike the atrial synchronous pacemakers, they do not allow for changes in heart rate that might occur with spontaneous activity.

The most sophisticated type of pacemaker produces *atrioventricular sequential pacing at all pacing rates (DDD)* (Fig. 13–23). As with the previous mode of pacing, these pacemakers also require two leads, one in the atrium and one in the ventricle. The atrial and ventricular leads are both used for pacing and sensing. In a patient with normal sinus rhythm these pacemakers function identically to the atrial synchronous pacemakers *(VDD)*. However, should the patient have severe bradycardia or sinus arrest, these pacemakers function as atrioventricular sequential and synchronous pacemakers *(DVI)* at a preset low rate. When the patient's spontaneous atrial rate exceeds the

Text continued on page 283.

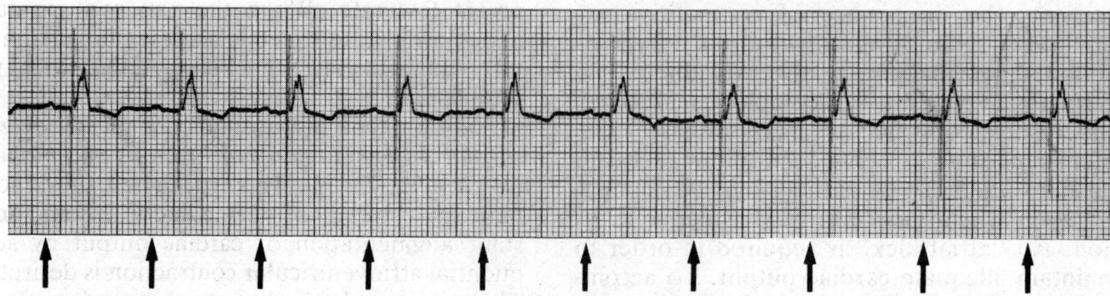

Figure 13–23. Surface electrocardiograms demonstrating atrial synchronous pacing in a patient with a dual-chambered universal type pacemaker (DDD). After each P wave *(arrows)* there is a preset delay, followed by ventricular pacing. A pacing artifact precedes each QRS.

DIFFERENTIAL DIAGNOSIS OF TACHYARRYTHMIAS BASED ON WIDE OR NARROW QRS MORPHOLOGY (IA)

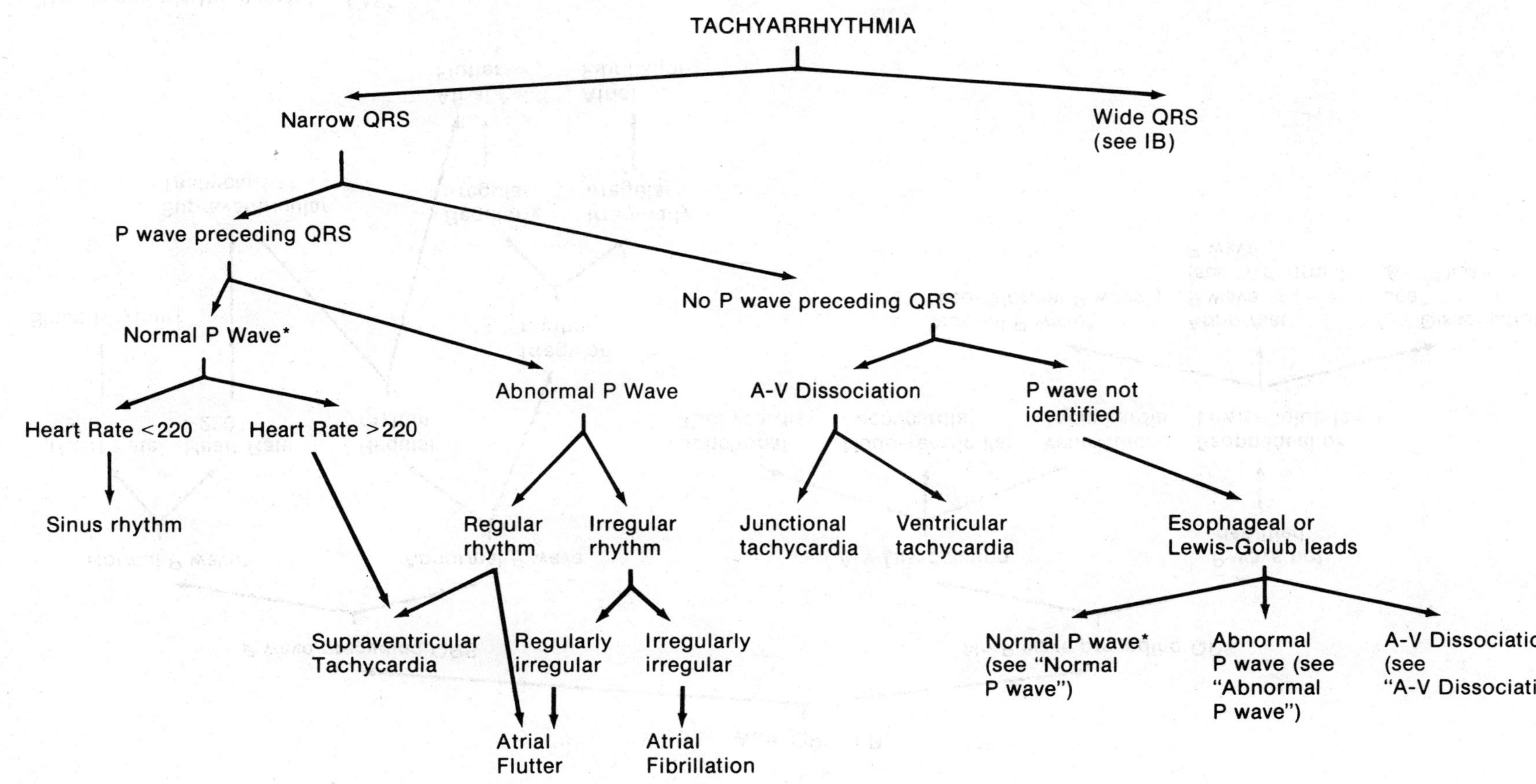

*Upright or isoelectric in leads I and AVF.

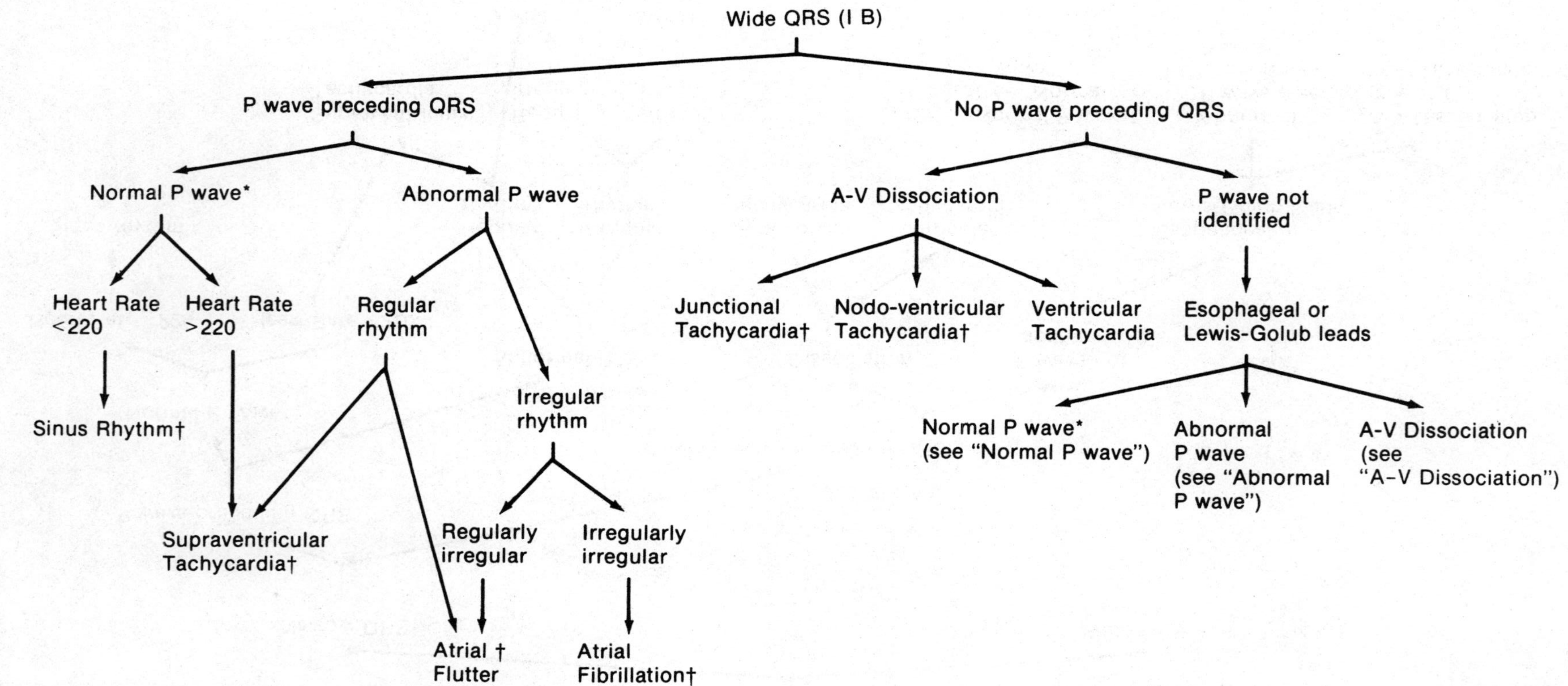

*Upright or isoelectric in leads I and AVF.
†Wide QRS secondary to postoperative right bundle branch block pattern, pre-excitation syndrome with antegrade conduction via bypass tract or rate related aberrancy.

MANAGEMENT OF CRITICALLY ILL PATIENTS WITH ASYSTOLE, BRADYCARDIA, VENTRICULAR TACHYCARDIA, OR FIBRILLATION; AND OF PATIENTS RECENTLY CONVERTED TO SINUS RHYTHM (II A)

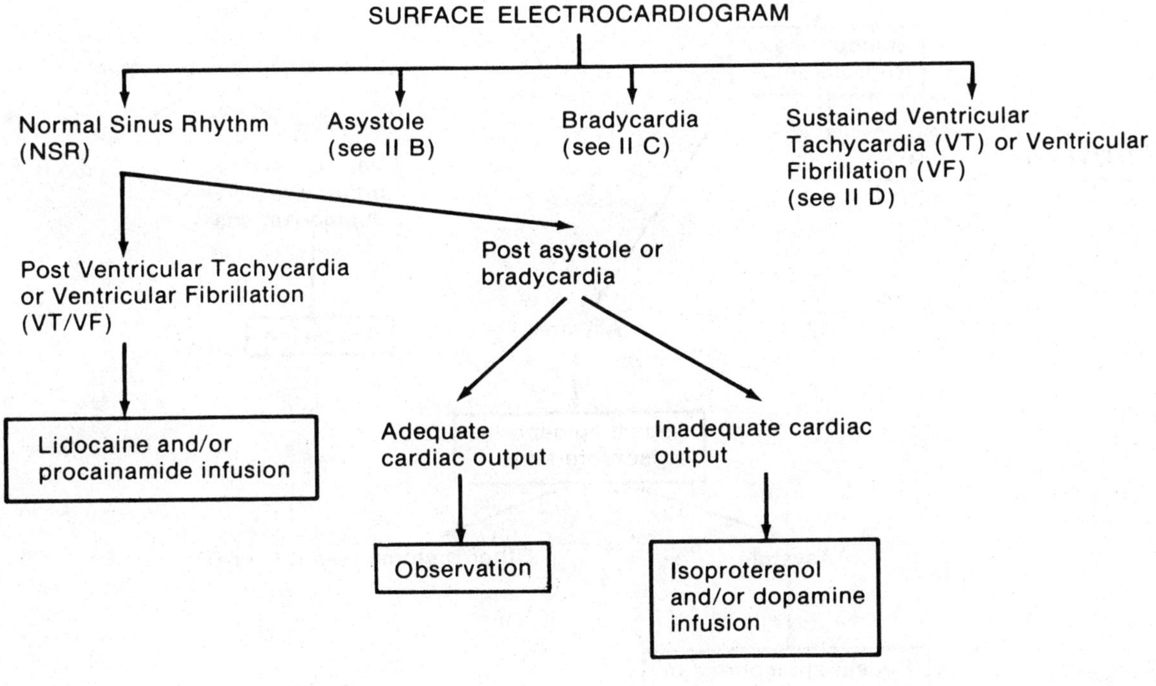

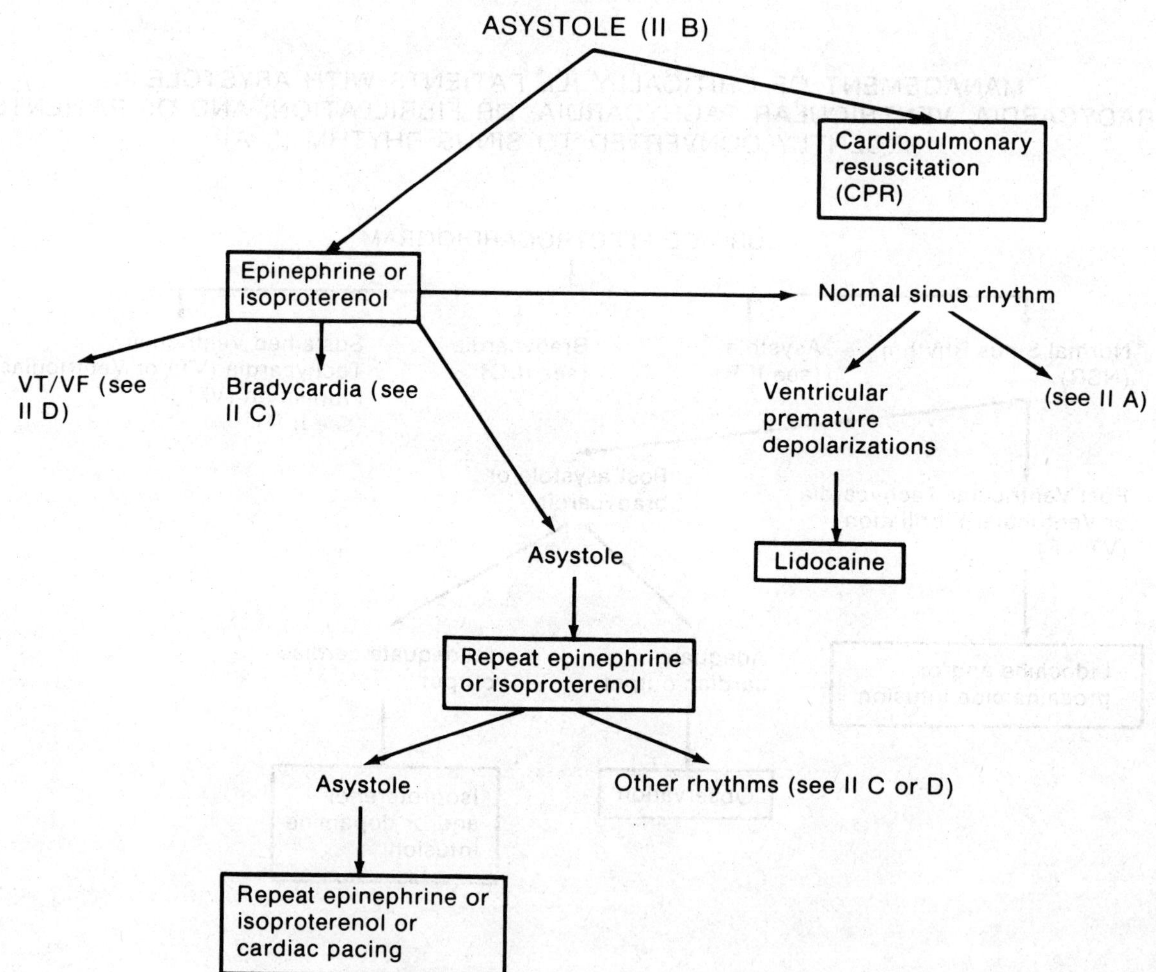
ASYSTOLE (II B)
Cardiopulmonary resuscitation (CPR)
Epinephrine or isoproterenol
Normal sinus rhythm
VT/VF (see II D)
Bradycardia (see II C)
Ventricular premature depolarizations
(see II A)
Lidocaine
Asystole
Repeat epinephrine or isoproterenol
Asystole
Other rhythms (see II C or D)
Repeat epinephrine or isoproterenol or cardiac pacing

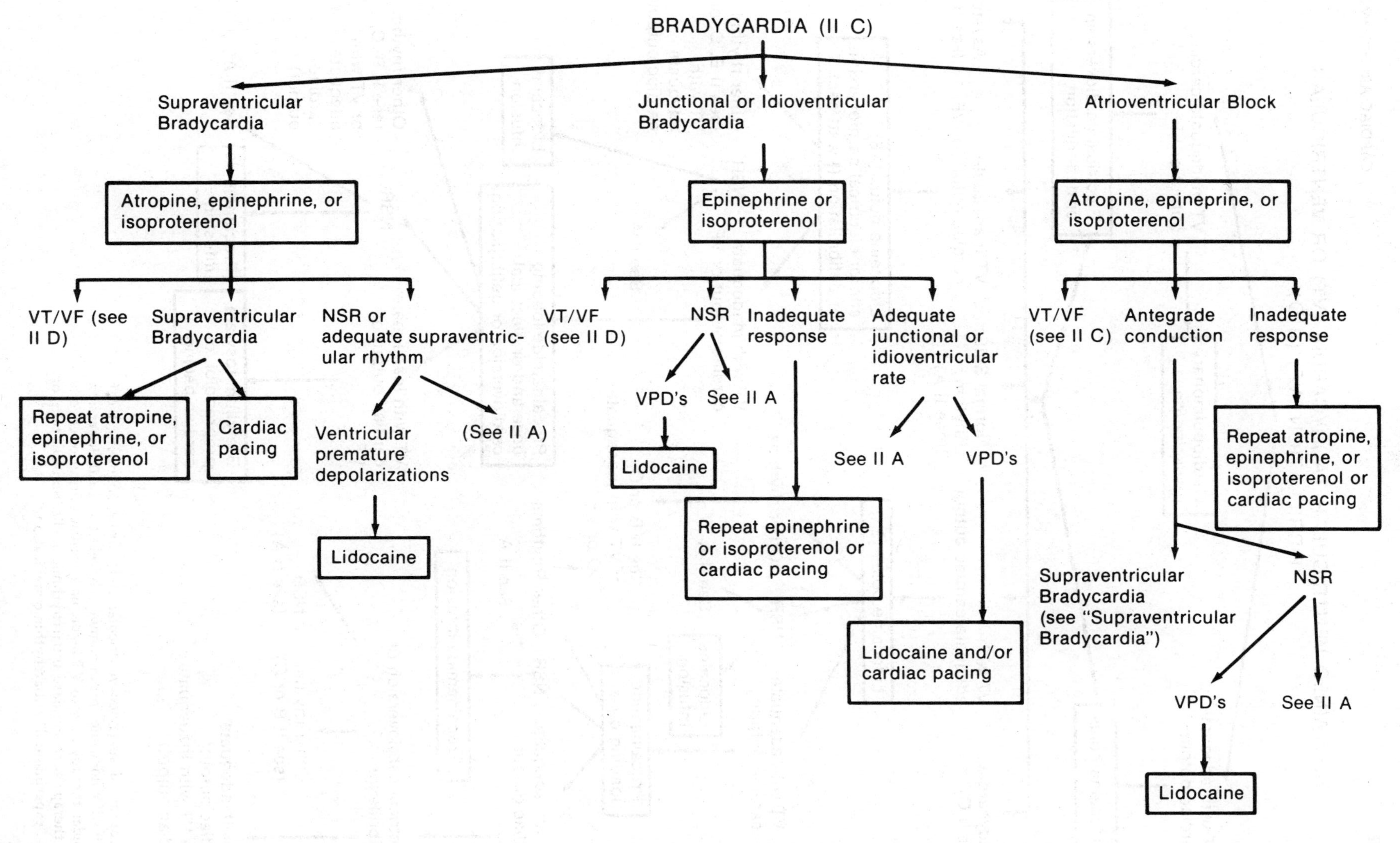
BRADYCARDIA (II C)
Supraventricular Bradycardia
Junctional or Idioventricular Bradycardia
Atrioventricular Block
Atropine, epinephrine, or isoproterenol
Epinephrine or isoproterenol
Atropine, epineprine, or isoproterenol
VT/VF (see II D)
Supraventricular Bradycardia
NSR or adequate supraventricular rhythm
VT/VF (see II D)
NSR
Inadequate response
Adequate junctional or idioventricular rate
VT/VF (see II C)
Antegrade conduction
Inadequate response
Repeat atropine, epinephrine, or isoproterenol
Cardiac pacing
Ventricular premature depolarizations
(See II A)
VPD's
See II A
Repeat atropine, epinephrine, or isoproterenol or cardiac pacing
Lidocaine
Lidocaine
See II A
VPD's
Repeat epinephrine or isoproterenol or cardiac pacing
Supraventricular Bradycardia (see "Supraventricular Bradycardia")
NSR
Lidocaine and/or cardiac pacing
VPD's
See II A
Lidocaine

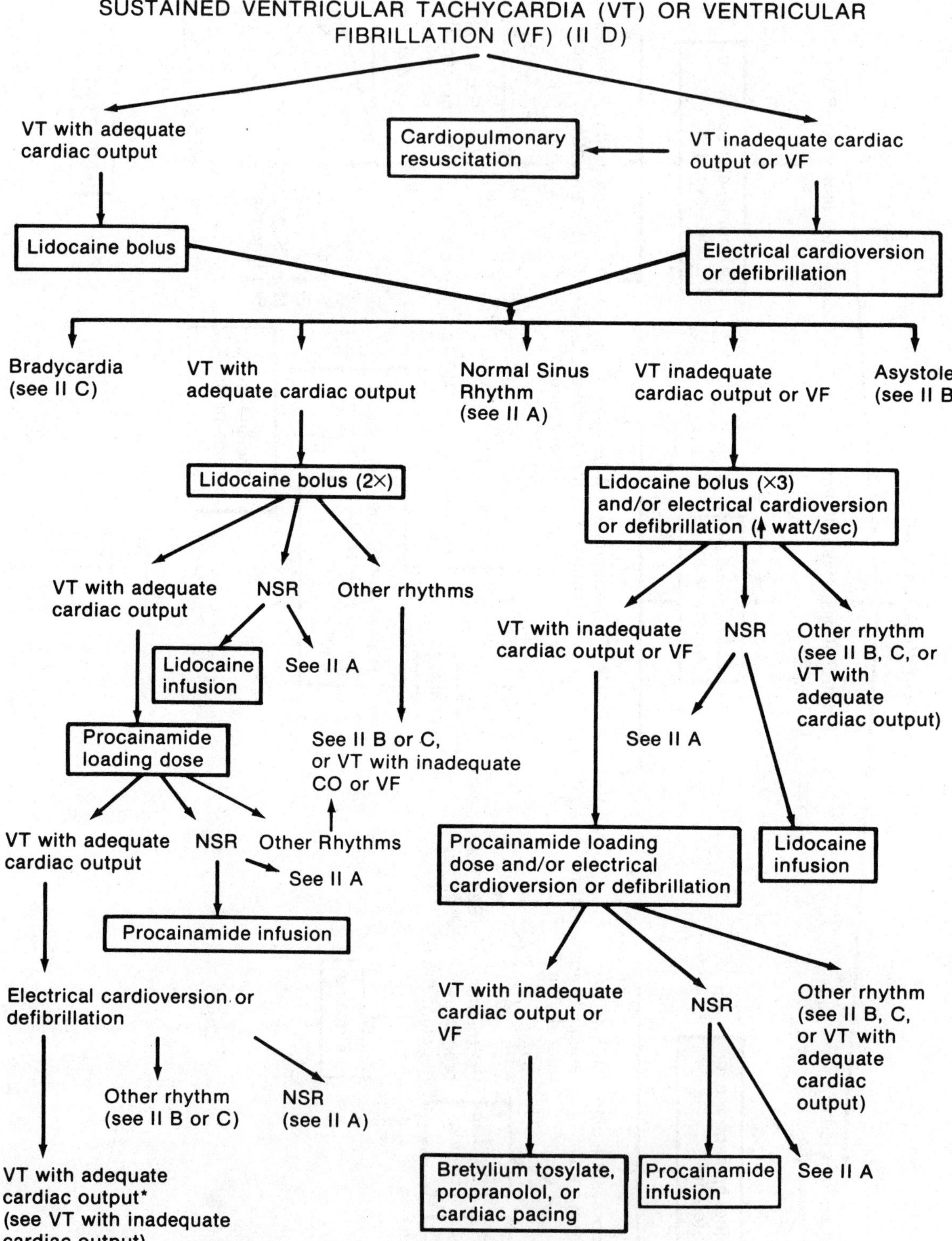

*Continued sustained ventricular tachycardia, following treatment with lidocaine, procainamide, and electrical cardioversion: consider therapy as with VT inadequate cardiac output or chronic oral therapy with standard antiarrhythmic medication (see text) or with "experimental" antiarrhythmic medication.

pacemaker's upper preset rate, an artificial Wenckebach AV block is established. The DDD pacemaker provides for every contingency of cardiac pacing under all physiologic conditions, and is replacing the other types of atrioventricular sequential pacemakers.

Automatic antitachycardia pacemakers are used in extreme circumstances for patients with tachyarrhythmias that are refractory to standard medical or surgical intervention. These pacemakers can be activated by the patient in response to symptomatic tachycardia, or they have automatic devices that sense the tachycardia and deliver a train of impulses or a single defibrillatory shock to terminate the arrhythmia. These devices can be used for intractable atrial arrhythmias, for ventricular arrhythmias, and for the conversion of ventricular fibrillation.[143–145] Prior to using this type of pacemaker, detailed intracardiac electrophysiologic testing must be carried out to ascertain whether a particular type of pacing will terminate the tachyarrhythmia.

REFERENCES

1. Roberts NK, Gelband H, eds. Cardiac Arrhythmias in the Neonate, Infant and Child. New York: Appleton-Century-Crofts, 1977.
2. Gillette PC, Garson AJ, eds. Pediatric Cardiac Dysrhythmias. New York: Grune & Stratton Inc, 1981.
3. Roberts NK, Gelband H. eds. Cardiac Arrhythmias in the Neonate, Infant and Child. New York: Appleton-Century-Crofts, 1982.
4. Hoffman BF, Cranefield PF. Electrophysiology of the Heart. New York: McGraw-Hill, 1960.
5. Hodgkin AL, Keynes RD. Movement of cations during recovery in nerve. Symp Soc Exp Biol *8*:423, 1954.
6. Hodgkin AL, Keynes RD. The potassium permeability of a giant nerve fiber. J Physiol *128*:61, 1955.
7. Weidmann S. Effect of current flow on the membrane potential of cardiac muscle. J Physiol *115*:227, 1951.
8. Draper MH, Weidmann S. Cardiac resting and action potentials recorded with an intracellular electrode. J Physiol *115*:74, 1951.
9. Trautwein W. Generation of the Cardiac Action Potential. *In*: Manning GW, Ahuja SP. eds. Electrical Activity of the Heart. Springfield, Ill: Charles C Thomas Publisher, 1969; 9–22.
10. Reuter H. Divalent cations as charge carriers in excitable membranes. Prog Biophys Mol Biol *26*:3, 1973.
11. McAllister RE, Noble D. The time and voltage dependence of the slow outward current in cardiac Purkinje fibers. J Physiol *186*:632, 1966.
12. Wit AL, Fenoglio JJ Jr, Wagner BM, Bassett AL. Electrophysiological properties of cardiac muscle in the anterior mitral valve leaflet and the adjacent atrium in the dog: possible implications for the genesis of atrial dysrhythmias. Circ Res *32*:731, 1973.
13. Wit AL, Fenoglio JJ Jr, Hordof AJ, Reemtsma K. Ultrastructure and transmembrane potentials of cardiac muscle in the human anterior mitral valve leaflet. Circulation *59*:1284–1292, 1979.
14. Weidmann S. The effect of the cardiac membrane potential on the rapid availability of the sodium carrying system. J Physiol *127*:213, 1955.
15. Hoffman BF, Cranefield PF. Physiologic basis of cardiac arrhythmias. Am J Med *37*:670, 1964.
16. Vassalle M. The relationship among cardiac pacemakers: overdrive suppression. Circ Res *41*:267–277, 1977.
17. Wit AL, Rosen MR, Hoffman BF. Relationship of normal and abnormal electrical activity of cardiac fibers to the genesis of arrhythmias. I. Automaticity. Am Heart J *88*:515, 1974.
18. Cranefield PF. Conduction of the Cardiac Impulse. Mt. Kisco, New York: Futura Publishing Co., Inc., 1975.
19. Wit AL, Cranefield PF. Reentrant excitation as a cause of cardiac arrhythmias. Am J Physiol *235*:H1–H17, 1978.
20. Cranefield PF, Hoffman BF. Reentry: slow conduction, summation and inhibition. Circulation *44*:309, 1971.
21. Cranefield PF, Wit AL, Hoffman BF. Genesis of cardiac arrhythmias. Circulation *47*:190, 1973.
22. Wit AL, Cranefield PF, Hoffman BF. Slow conduction and reentry in the ventricular conducting system. II. Single and sustained circus movement in networks of canine and bovine Purkinje fibers. Circ Res *30*:11, 1972.
23. Wit AL, Hoffman BF, Cranefield PF. Slow conduction and reentry in the ventricular conducting system. I. Return extrasystole in canine Purkinje fibers. Circ Res *30*:1, 1972.
24. Cranefield PF, Hoffman BF. Conduction of the cardiac impulse. II. Summation and inhibition. Circ Res *28*:220, 1971.
25. Cohen H, Langendorf R, Pick A. Intermittent parasystole—mechanism of protection. Circulation *48*:761, 1973.
26. Singer DH, Lazzara R, Hoffman BF. Interrelationship between automaticity and conduction in Purkinje fibers. Circ Res *21*:537–558, 1967.
27. Moe GK, Jalife J, Mueller WJ, Moe B. A mathematical model of parasystole and its application to clinical arrhythmias. Circulation *56*:968–979, 1977.
28. Michaelsson M, Engle MA. Congenital complete heart block: an international study of the natural history. *In*: Brest AN, Engle MA. eds. Cardiovascular Clinics, Philadelphia: F.A. Davis Company, 1972: 85.
29. McCue CM, Mantakas ME, Tingelstad JB, Ruddy S. Congenital heart block in newborns of mothers with connective tissue disease. Circulation *56*:82–90, 1977.
30. Driscoll DJ, Gillette PC, Hallman GL, et al. Management of surgical complete atrioventricular block in children. Am J Cardiol *43*:1175–1180, 1979.
31. Bigger JT Jr, Goldreyer BN. The mechanism of supraventricular tachycardia. Circulation *42*: 673–688, 1970.
32. Jacobsen JR, Garson A, Gillette PC, McNamara DG. Premature ventricular contractions in normal children. J Pediatr *92*:36–38, 1978.
33. Vincent GR, Abildskov JA, Burgess RJ. Q-T interval syndromes. Prog Cardiovasc Dis *16*:523, 1974.
34. Schwartz PJ, Periti M, Malliani A. The long Q-T syndrome. Am Heart J *89*:378, 1975.

35. James TN, Frogatt P, Atkinson WJ Jr, et al. De subtaneis mortibus. XXX. Observations on the pathophysiology of the long Q-T syndrome with special reference to the neuropathology of the heart. Circulation *57*:1221, 1978.
36. Sacks HS, Matisonn R, Kennelly BM. Familial paroxysmal ventricular tachycardia in two sisters. Am Heart J *87*:217, 1974.
37. McRae JR, Wagner GS, Rogers MC, Canent RV. Paroxysmal familial ventricular fibrillation. J Pediatr *84*:515, 1974.
38. Rozanski JJ, Dimich I, Steinfeld L, Kupersmith J. Maximal exercise stress testing in evaluation of arrhythmias in children: results and reproducibility. Am J Cardiol *43*:951–956, 1979.
39. Winkler RB, Freed MD, Nadas AS. Exercise induced ventricular ectopy in children and young adults with complete heart block. Am Heart J *99*:87, 1980.
40. Garson A, Gillette PC, Gutgesell HP, McNamara DG. Stress induced ventricular arrhythmia after repair of tetralogy of Fallot. Am J Cardiol *46*:1006–1012, 1980.
41. Goldreyer BN, Bigger JT. Site of reentry in paroxysmal supraventricular tachycardia in man. Circulation *43*:15–23, 1971.
42. Garson A, Gillette PC, McNamara DG. Supraventricular tachycardia in children: clinical features, response to treatment and long-term followup in 217 patients. J Pediatr *98*:875, 1981.
43. Harringan JT, Kangos JJ, Sikka A, et al. Successful treatment of fetal congestive heart failure secondary to tachycardia. N Engl J Med *304*:1527, 1981.
44. Gillette PC, Garson A. Electrophysiological and pharmacologic characteristics of automatic ectopic atrial tachycardia. Circulation *56*:571, 1977.
45. Garson A, Gillette PC. Junctional ectopic tachycardia in children: electrocardiography, electrophysiology and pharmacologic response. Am J Cardiol *44*:298, 1979.
46. Rosen MR, Fisch C, Hoffman BF, et al. Can accelerated atrioventricular junctional escape rhythms be explained by delayed afterdepolarizations? Am J Cardiol *45*:1272, 1980.
47. Radford DJ, Izukawa T. Atrial fibrillation in children. Pediatrics, *59*:250, 1977.
48. Tung KSK, James TN, Effler DB, McCormack LJ. Injury of the sinus node in open heart operations. J Thorac Cardiovasc Surg *53*:814, 1967.
49. El-Said G, Rosenberg JS, Mullins CE, et al. Dysrhythmias after Mustard's operations for transposition of the great arteries. Am J Cardiol *30*:526, 1972.
50. Greenwood RD, Rosenthal A, Sloss LJ, et al. Sick sinus syndrome after surgery for congenital heart disease. Circulation *52*:208, 1975.
51. Hayes CJ, Boxer RA, Krongrad E, Gersony WM. Cardiac rhythm after the Mustard operation for transposition of the great arteries. (Abstract) Am J Cardiol *45*:430, 1980.
52. Gillette PC, Kugler JO, Garson et al. Mechanism of cardiac arrhythmias after the Mustard operation for transposition of the great arteries. Am J Cardiol *45*:1225, 1980.
53. Ferrer, MI. The Sick Sinus Syndrome. Mt. Kisco, New York: Futura Publishing Co., Inc., 1974.
54. Lubbers WJ, Losekoot TG, Anderson RH, Wellens HJ. Paroxysmal supraventricular tachycardia in infancy and childhood. Eur J Cardiol *2*:91, 1974.
55. Gillette PC. The mechanisms of supraventricular tachycardia in children. Circulation *54*:133, 1976.
56. Gillette PC, Garson A, Kugler JD. Wolff-Parkinson–White syndrome in children: electrophysiologic and pharmacologic characteristics. Circulation *60*:1487, 1979.
57. Schiebler GL, Adams P, Anderson RC. The Wolff-Parkinson–White syndrome in infants and children. A review and a report of 28 cases. Pediatrics *24*:585, 1959.
58. Swiderski J, Lees MH, Nadas AS. The Wolff-Parkinson–White syndrome in infancy and childhood. Br Heart J *24*:567, 1962.
59. Giardina ACV, Ehlers KH, Engle MA. Wolff-Parkinson–White syndrome in infants and children. Br Heart J *34*:839, 1972.
60. Gallagher JJ, Pritchett ELC, Sealy WC, et al. The pre-excitation syndromes. Prog Cardiovasc Dis *20*:285, 1978.
61. Anderson RH, Becker AE, Brechenmacher C, et al. Ventricular preexcitation: a proposed nomenclature for its substrates. Eur J Cardiol *3*:27–35, 1975.
62. Tonkin AM, Wagner GS, Gallagher JJ, Wallace AG. Initial forces of ventricular depolarization in the Wolff-Parkinson-White syndrome. Circulation *52*:1020, 1975.
63. Sung RJ, Gelband H, Castellanos A, et al. Clinical and electrophysiologic observations in patients with concealed atrioventricular bypass tracts. Am J Cardiol *40*:839, 1977.
64. Gillette PC. Concealed anomalous cardiac conduction pathways: a frequent cause of supraventricular tachycardia. Am J Cardiol *40*:848–852, 1977.
65. Farshid A, Josephson MF, Horowitz LN. Electrophysiologic characteristics of concealed bypass tracts: clinical and electrocardiographic correlates. Am J Cardiol *41*:105, 1978.
66. Palaganas MC, Fay JE, Delahaye DJ. Paroxysmal ventricular tachycardia in childhood. J Pediatr *67*:784, 1965.
67. Videbaek J, Andersen E, Jacobsen J, et al. Paroxysmal tachycardia in infancy and childhood. II. Paroxysmal ventricular tachycardia and fibrillation. Acta Paediatr Scand. *62*:349, 1973.
68. Hernandez, A, Strauss A, Kleiger RE, Goldring D. Idiopathic paroxysmal ventricular tachycardia in infants and children. J Pediatr *86*:182, 1975.
69. James FW, Kaplan S, TeChuan C. Unexpected cardiac arrest in patients after surgical correction of tetralogy of Fallot. Circulation *52*:691, 1975.
70. Quattlebaum TG, Varghese PJ, Neill CA, Donahoo JS. Sudden death among postoperative patients with tetralogy of Fallot. Circulation *54*:289, 1976.
71. Gillette PC, Yeoman MA, Mullins CE, McNamara DG. Sudden death after repair of tetralogy of Fallot. Circulation *56*:566, 1977.
72. Horowitz LN, Vetter VL, Harleen AH, Josephson ME. Electrophysiologic characteristics of sustained ventricular tachycardia occurring after repair of tetralogy of Fallot. Am J Cardiol *46*:446, 1980.
73. Deanfield JE, McKenna WJ, Hallidie-Smith KA. Detection of late arrhythmia and conduction disturbance after correction of tetralogy of Fallot. Br Heart J *44*:248, 1980.
74. Kavey RE, Blackman MS, Sondheimer HM. Incidence and severity of chronic ventricular dysrhythmias after repair of tetralogy of Fallot. Am Heart J *103*:342, 1982.
75. Schamroth L, ed. Ventricular Tachycardia and Ven-

tricular Flutter. *In*: The Disorders of Cardiac Rhythm. Oxford: Blackwell Scientific Publishing, 1970:104–109.

76. Benson DW Jr, Smith WM, Dunnigan A, et al. Mechanisms of regular, wide QRS tachycardia in infants and children. Am J Cardiol *49*:1778, 1982.
77. Benditt DG, Pritchett ELC, Gallagher JJ. Spectrum of regular tachycardias with wide QRS complexes in patients with accessory atrioventricular pathways. Am J Cardiol *42*:828–838, 1978.
78. Gallagher JJ, Smith WM, Kasell JH, et al. Role of Mahaim fibers in cardiac arrhythmias in man. Circulation *64*:176–189, 1981.
79. Whitman V, Friedman Z, Berman W, Maisels MJ, Supraventricular tachycardia in newborn infants: an approach to therapy. J Pediatr *91*:304, 1977.
80. Bisset GS, Guam WE, Kaplan S. The ice bag: a new technique for interruption of supraventricular tachycardia. J Pediatr *97*:593–595, 1980.
81. Levy AM, Camm AJ, Keane JF. Multiple arrhythmias detected during nocturnal monitoring in patients with congenital complete heart block. Circulation *55*:247, 1977.
82. Kavey RE, Sondheimer HM, Blackman MS. Detection of dysrhythmia in pediatric patients with mitral valve prolapse. Circulation *62*:582, 1980.
83. Porter CJ, Gillette PC, McNamara DG. Twenty-four hour ambulatory ECG's in the detection and management of cardiac dysrhythmias in infants and children. Pediatr Cardiol *1*:203, 1980.
84. Valimaki I. Tape recordings of the electrocardiogram in newborn infants: section II. Long-term ECG tape recordings of the newborn infants. Acta Paediatr Scand (Suppl) *199*:1–75, 1969.
85. Southall, AP, Richards J, Mitchell P, et al. Study of cardiac rhythm in healthy newborn infants. Br Heart J *43*:14–20, 1980.
86. Scott O, Williams GJ, Fiddler GI. Results of 24-hour ambulatory monitoring of electrocardiogram in 131 healthy boys aged 10 to 13 years. Br Heart J *44*:304–308, 1980.
87. Southall DP, Johnston F, Shinebourne EA, Johnston PGB. 24-hour electrocardiographic study of heart rate and rhythm patterns in population of healthy children. Br Heart J *45*:281–291, 1981.
88. Garson A, Nihill MR, McNamara DG, Cooley DA. Status of the adult and adolescent after repair of tetralogy of Fallot. Circulation *59*:1232, 1979.
89. Lown B, Graboys TB. Management of patients with malignant ventricular arrhythmias. Am J Cardiol *39*:910–918, 1977.
90. Harrison DC, Fitzgerald JW, Winkle RA. Contribution of ambulatory electrocardiographic monitoring to antiarrhythmic management. Am J Cardiol *41*:996–1004, 1978.
91. James FW, Kaplan S, Schwartz DC, et al. Response to exercise in patients after total surgical correction of tetralogy of Fallot. Circulation *54*:671, 1976.
92. Rocchini AP, Chun PO, Dick M. Ventricular tachycardia in children. Am J Cardiol *47*:1091, 1981.
93. Goldberg SJ, Weiss R, Adams FH. A comparison of the maximal endurance of normal children and patients with congenital cardiac disease. J Pediatr *69*:46, 1966.
94. Goldberg SJ, Mendes F, Hurwitz R. Maximal exercise capability of children as a function of specific cardiac defects. Am J Cardiol *23*:349, 1969.
95. Thapar MK, Strong WB, Miller MD, et al. Exercise electrocardiography of healthy black children. Am J Dis Child *132*:592, 1978.
96. Rosing DR, Borer JS, Kent KM, et al. Long-term hemodynamic and electrocardiographic assessment following operative repair of tetralogy of Fallot. Circulation *58*: (Suppl)1–209, 1979.
97. Gillette PC, Garson A, Kugler JD, et al. Surgical treatment of supraventricular tachycardia in infants and children. Am J Cardiol *46*:281, 1980.
98. Gillette PC, Garson A, Hesslein PS, et al. Successful surgical treatment of atrial, junctional, and ventricular tachycardia unassociated with accessory connections in infants and children. Am Heart J *102*:984, 1981.
99. Hoffman BF, Singer DH. Effects of digitalis on electrical activity of cardiac fibers. Prog Cardiovasc Dis *7*:226–260, 1964.
100. Marks BH, Weissler AM, eds. Basic and Clinical Pharmacology of Digitalis. Springfield, Ill: Charles C Thomas Publisher, 1972.
101. Rosen MR, Wit AL, Hoffman BF. Electrophysiology and pharmacology of cardiac arrhythmias. IV. Cardiac antiarrhythmic and toxic effects of digitalis. Am Heart J *89*:391–399, 1975.
102. Seller TD, Bashore TM, Gallagher JJ. Digitalis in the preexcitation syndrome. Analysis during atrial fibrillation. Circulation *56*:260, 1977.
103. Ten Eick RE, Wyte RS, Ross MS, Hoffman BF. Post countershock arrhythmias in untreated and digitalized dogs. Circ Res *21*:375, 1967.
104. Kleiger R, Lown B. Cardioversion and digitalis. II. Clinical studies. Circulation *33*:878, 1966.
105. Porter CJ, Gillette PC, Garson A, et al. Effects of verapamil on supraventricular tachycardia. Am J Cardiol *48*:487, 1981.
106. Sapire DW, O'Riordan AC, Black IFS. Safety and efficacy of short and long term verapamil therapy in children with tachycardia. Am J Cardiol *48*:1091, 1981.
107. Gulamhusein S, Ko P, Carruthers SG, Klein GJ. Acceleration of the ventricular response during atrial fibrillation in the Wolff-Parkinson–White syndrome after verapamil. Circulation *65*:348–354, 1982.
108. Greco R, Musto B, Arienzo V, et al. Treatment of paroxysmal supraventricular tachycardia in infancy with digitalis, adenosine-5′-triphosphate, and verapamil: A comparative study. Circulation *66*:504–508, 1982.
109. Gutgessell HP, Tacker WA, Geldes LA, et al. Energy dose for ventricular defibrillation of children. Pediatrics *58*:989, 1976.
110. Chameides L, Brown GE, Raye JR, et al. Guidelines for defibrillation in infants and children: Report of the American Heart Association target activity group: cardiopulmonary resuscitation in the young. Circulation *56*:502A, 1977.
111. Waldo AL, Maclean WAH, Cooper TB, et al. Use of temporarily placed epicardial atrial wire electrodes for the diagnosis and treatment of cardiac arrhythmias following open heart surgery. J Thorac Cardiovasc Surg *76*:500, 1978.
112. Yabek SM, Akl BF, Berman W, et al. Use of atrial epicardial electrodes to diagnose and treat post-operative arrhythmias in children. Am J Cardiol *46*:285, 1980.
113. Waldo AL, Maclean WAH, Karp RB, et al. Entrainment and interruption of atrial flutter with atrial pacing: studies in man following open heart surgery. Circulation *56*:737–745, 1977.
114. Zipes DP, Troup PJ. New antiarrhythmic agents: amiodarone, aprinidine, disopyramide, ethmozin,

mexiletine, tocainide, verapamil. Am J Cardiol *41*:1005–1024, 1978.
115. Coumel P, Fidelle J. Amiodarone in the treatment of cardiac arrhythmias in children: one hundred thirty-five cases. Am Heart J *100*:1063, 1980.
116. Leahey EB Jr, Reiffel JA, Drusin RE, et al. Interaction between quinidine and digoxin. JAMA *240*:533–534, 1978.
117. Leahey EB Jr, Reiffel JA, Heissenbuttel RH, et al. Enhanced cardiac effect of digoxin during quinidine treatment. Arch Intern Med *139*:519–521, 1979.
118. Hager WD, Fenster P, Mayersohn M, et al. Digoxin-quinidine interaction: pharmacokinetic evaluation. N Engl J Med *300*:1238–1241, 1979.
119. Shakibi JG, Aryanpur I. Electrophysiologic effects of lidocaine in children. Jpn Heart J *20*:271, 1979.
120. Rosen MR, Hoffman BF, Wit AL. Electrophysiology and pharmacology of cardiac arrhythmias. V. Cardiac antiarrhythmic effects of lidocaine. Am Heart J *89*:526–536, 1975.
121. Hoffman BF, Rosen MR, Wit AL. Electrophysiology and pharmacology of cardiac arrhythmias. VII. Cardiac effects of quinidine and procaine amide. A. Am Heart J *89*:804–808, 1975.
122. Hoffman BF, Rosen MR, Wit AL. Electrophysiology and pharmacology of cardiac arrhythmias VII. Cardiac effects of quinidine and procaine amide. B. Am Heart J *90*:117–122, 1975.
123. Giardina EGV, Heissenbuttel RH, Bigger JT Jr. Intermittent intravenous procaine amide to treat ventricular arrhythmias. Ann Intern Med *78*:183, 1973.
124. Woosley RL, Shand DG. Pharmacokinetics of antiarrhythmic drugs. Am J Cardiol *41*:986–995, 1978.
125. Heissenbuttel RH, Bigger JT Jr. Bretylium tosylate: a newly available antiarrhythmic drug for ventricular arrhythmias. Ann Intern Med *91*:229–238, 1979.
126. Garson A, Kugler JD, Gillette PC, et al. Control of late postoperative ventricular arrhythmias with phenytoin in young patients. Am J Cardiol *46*:290, 1980.
127. Mortimer EA, Rakita L. Ventricular tachycardia in childhood controlled with large doses of procaine amide. N Engl J Med *262*:615, 1960.
128. Gelband H, Steeg CN, Bigger JT. Use of massive doses of procaine amide in the treatment of ventricular tachycardia in infancy. Pediatrics *48*:110, 1971.
129. Drayer DE, Hughes M, Lorenzo B, Reidenberg NM. Prevalence of high (35)-3-hydroxyquinidine/quinidine ratios in serum, and clearance of quinidine in cardiac patients with age. Clin Pharmacol Ther *27*:72, 1979.
130. Pickoff AS, Zies L, Ferrer PL, et al. High-dose propranolol therapy in the management of supraventricular tachycardia. J Pediatr *94*:144, 1979.
131. Reidenberg MM, Camacho M, Kluger J, et al. Aging and renal clearance of procainamide and acetylprocainamide. Clin Pharmacol Ther *28*:732, 1980.
132. Szefler SJ, Shen D, Gingell RL, et al. Quinidine elimination in pediatric patients. Pediatr Res *14*:473, 1980.
133. Keshani IA, Shakibi JG, Siassi B. Electrophysiologic effects of disopyramide in children. Jpn Heart J *21*:491, 1980.
134. Hordof A, Moak J, Steeg C, et al. Treatment of cardiac arrhythmias with disopyramide (Norpace). Pediatr Res *15*:465, 1981.
135. Singh S, Gelband HL, Mehta A, et al. Procainamide elimination kinetics in pediatric patients. Pediatr Res *15*:472, 1981.
136. Pickoff AS, Kessler KM, Singh S, et al. Age-related differences in the protein binding of quinidine. Dev Pharmacol Ther *3*:108, 1981.
137. Garson A. Evaluation and treatment of chronic ventricular dysrhythmias in the young. Cardiovasc Rev Rep *2*:1164, 1981.
138. Kavey REW, Blackman MS, Sondheimer HM. Phenytoin therapy for ventricular arrhythmias occurring late after surgery for congenital heart disease. Am Heart J *104*:794–798, 1982.
139. Dungan WT, Garson A, Gillette PC. Arrhythmogenic right ventricular dysplasia: a cause of ventricular tachycardia in children with apparently normal hearts. Am Heart J *102*:745, 1981.
140. Simcha A, Wells BG, Tynan MJ, Waterston AJ. Primary cardiac tumors in childhood. Arch Dis Child *46*:508, 1971.
141. Engle MA, Ebert PA, Jedo SF. Recurrent ventricular tachycardia due to resectable cardiac tumor. Circulation *50*:1052, 1974.
142. Caldwell PD, Ricketts HJ, Dillard DH, Guntheroth WG. Ventricular tachycardia in a child: an indication for angiocardiography? Am Heart J *88*:771, 1974.
143. Griffin JC, Mason JW, Calfee RV. Clinical use of an implantable automatic tachycardia-terminating pacemaker. Am Heart J *100*:1093, 1980.
144. Mirowski M, Reid PR, Mower MM, et al. Termination of malignant ventricular arrhythmias with an implanted automatic defibrillator in human beings. N Engl J Med *303*:322, 1980.
145. Dunnigan A, Benditt DG, Fetter J, et al. A patient activated radio frequency pacemaker system: therapy for recurrent ventricular tachycardia. J Pediatr *101*:403, 1982.

CHAPTER 14

Acute Renal Failure

Stephen G. Osofsky, M.D.
John E. Lewy, M.D.

Acute renal failure (ARF) is defined as a sudden deterioration in renal function usually associated with decreased or absent urinary output and concomitant fluid and electrolyte disturbances. The terms *acute tubular necrosis* and *acute renal failure* have incorrectly been used interchangeably. The former term connotes the histopathologic finding of tubular necrosis that is a frequent but not a consistent finding in ARF. ARF has multiple causes and pathogeneses, each of which will have a different prognosis. This chapter discusses ARF in the child, including pathophysiology, diagnosis, and management.[1–5]

CAUSES OF RENAL FAILURE

It is useful to discuss the etiology of ARF in terms of prerenal, intrinsic renal, and postrenal causes (Table 14–1).

Prerenal Failure

The term prerenal refers to underperfusion of functioning nephrons as is seen in hypovolemia and volume contraction. Patients with prerenal contractions respond to intravenous fluid challenges by increased urine output and corrected electrolyte disturbances. The causes of prerenal contraction include dehydration secondary to vomiting and diarrhea, inadequate oral intake during a febrile illness, sepsis, congestive heart failure, hemorrhagic volume contraction, and trauma. Prerenal failure can also occur in individuals who have obligatory salt and water or fluid losses with inadequate oral intake. Examples are children with cystic fibrosis,[6] sickle cell disease,[7] and nephrogenic diabetes insipidus during an illness in which there is inadequate fluid intake. The patient with obligatory salt wasting who takes adequate fluids but inadequate sodium chloride will develop hyponatremia and hypokalemia. If severe, this condition may also result in movement of fluid into cells to restore osmotic equilibrium. Hypovolemia from any of the previously mentioned causes results in renal underperfusion. If the circulation to the kidneys is not restored, continued renal ischemia often leads to intrinsic renal damage that will no longer respond to fluid challenge.

Intrinsic Renal Failure

In considering the causes of intrinsic ARF, we must separate those that have resulted in ARF because of prolonged hypoperfusion of the kidneys from those which have a glomerular, vascular, or other direct intrinsic basis. Those conditions in which there is prolonged hypoperfusion (severe asphyxia, volume contraction secondary to dehydration, hypotension, septicemia, volume contraction secondary to reduction in colloid oncotic pressure) result in ARF with the predominant disorder being in the tubules and interstitium. It is to these conditions that the term *acute tubular necrosis* has been applied. In acute tubular necrosis, the glomeruli are normal and there is a broad range of tubular injury seen by light and electron microscopy. In some renal biopsy specimens examined by light microscopy, tubulointerstitial architecture is well preserved and the tubules appear normal. In others there is significant tubular necrosis with shedding of the tubular epithelium and darkened nuclei. Electron microscopy usually reveals swollen tubular intracellular organelles and degeneration of nuclei even if appearance of light microscopy was normal.[8,9] Prolonged renal ischemia may result in cortical and medullary

Table 14–1. MAJOR CAUSES OF RENAL FAILURE IN CHILDREN

Prerenal Failure

- Hypovolemia and hypotension caused by:
  - Dehydration
    - Vomiting
    - Diarrhea
    - Febrile illness
    - Massive reduction in colloid oncotic pressure (protein losing enteropathy, nephrotic syndrome)
  - Septic shock
  - Congestive heart failure
  - Hemorrhage
  - Hyponatremia

Intrinsic Renal Failure

- Acute tubular necrosis
  - Prolonged secondary hypotension
    - Vomiting
    - Diarrhea
    - Shock
    - Nephrotoxins
    - Organ perfusion
- Glomerulonephritis
  - Primary
  - Secondary

Intrinsic Renal Failure *(Continued)*

- Interstitial nephritis
  - Primary
  - Secondary
    - Drugs
    - Toxins
- Vascular
  - Venous thrombosis
  - Cortical necrosis
  - Disseminated intravascular coagulation
- Pigmenturia (myoglobinuria, hemoglobinuria)

Postrenal Obstruction

- Urethral obstruction
  - Stricture
  - Posterior urethral valves
  - Diverticulum
- Ureterocele
- Solitary renal unit with ureterovesical or ureteropelvic juncture obstruction
- Extrinsic tumors compressing bladder outlet
- Intrinsic urinary tract tumors
- Neurogenic bladder

necrosis. Clinically, it may be seen in the young infant as a complication of severe dehydration, sepsis, and hemolytic-uremic syndrome. The kindeys are usually large; oliguria and gross hematuria are common. The pathology is highly variable. There may be diffuse or patchy involvement of one or both kidneys. In cortical necrosis there is frequently concurrent patchy infarction associated with hemorrhagic necrosis. There may be calcification of necrotic cortical tissue. Medullary necrosis results in the blunting of pyramids and in calyceal widening. It may be difficult to distinguish acute cortical and medullary necrosis from renal vein thrombosis.

ARF may also result from glomerulonephritis that may be a primary condition or secondary to a systemic disease. Post-infectious glomerulonephritis following a streptococcal infection,[10] hepatitis,[11] ventriculoatrial shunt infection,[12] infective endocarditis,[13] or osteomyelitis[14] may result in a mild to severe degree of acute renal insufficiency. Post-infectious glomerulonephritis is usually accompanied by the deposition of antigen-antibody in the glomerulus with an ensuing inflammatory process that in itself may reduce glomerular filtration rate substantially. Glomerulonephritis associated with connective tissue disease, such as systemic lupus erythematosus,[15] infrequently results in ARF and is more typically associated with a chronic course of renal failure. Similarly, neoplasia is infrequently associated with acute renal failure *per se.* ARF may be seen in association with secondary sepsis, dehydration, or hyperuricemia.[16, 17] Occasionally, ARF secondary to marked hyperuricemia will be the presenting finding in patients with leukemia or lymphoma.

The hemolytic-uremic syndrome is a more frequent cause of ARF in infancy and childhood.[18, 19] Its etiology is unknown and it is associated characteristically with a microangiopathic hemolytic anemia in which there are broken and fragmented erythrocytes in the peripheral smear and thrombocytopenia along with uremia. The condition affects small vessels in multiple organ systems, resulting in fibrin clots with platelet deposition and reduction in blood flow to the particular organ system. The hemolytic uremic syndrome is outlined in Table 14–2.

Henoch-Schoenlein purpura is associated with vasculitis in the skin, intestines, and kidneys (see Table 14–2). A patient with the most severe form of Henoch-Schoenlein purpura can present with ARF.[20, 21]

Nephrotoxins may produce interstitial nephritis and, on occasion, ARF. The term *interstitial nephritis* refers to an inflammatory process that often progresses to fibrosis of the interstitium and tubules of the kidneys. The glomeruli are involved secondarily because of interruption of vascular supply and nephron integrity. Heavy metals, hyperallergic responses to drugs (sulfonamides, furosemide,

Table 14–2. A COMPARISON OF THE CLINICAL FEATURES AND LABORATORY FINDINGS OF HEMOLYTIC UREMIC SYNDROME AND HENOCH-SCHOENLEIN PURPURA

Condition	Average Age of Patient	Antecedent Illness	Clinical Features	Laboratory Findings
Hemolytic-uremic syndrome[17, 18]	Infants and young children	Gastroenteritis (mild to severe); may mimic regional ileitis	Severe pallor Decreased urine output Obtundation, lethargy, irritability	Severe anemia Thrombocytopenia Broken RBCs (Burr cells, schistocytes) ↑ Reticulocyte count Proteinuria Hematuria ↓ Urine output ↑ Cr, ↑ BUN ↑ Uric acid, ↑ LDH
Henoch-Schoenlein purpura[19, 20]	Children more than 5 years old	Upper respiratory infection	Abdominal pain, diarrhea Purpuric rash of legs and buttocks Joint manifestations (arthritis, arthralgia)	Normal platelet count Proteinuria Hematuria RBC casts Normal serum C3 (complement)

phenytoin, penicillin, and its analogs), hyperparathyroidism, severe hyperuricemia, and oxalate deposition in association with methoxyflurane usage have occasionally been associated with interstitial nephritis.[22] Aminoglycoside antibiotics (gentamicin, tobramycin, amikacin, etc.) probably cause ARF by damaging proximal tubules (leading to enhanced reabsorption) and by decreasing glomerular permeability.[23] ARF following the injection of contrast media in diagnostic radiologic procedures rarely occurs.[24] The pathophysiologic mechanisms of ARF are not known, but it is clearly more prevalent in patients who already have renal insufficiency or dehydration.

Postrenal Failure

Postrenal renal failure is usually due to obstructive uropathy. It may result from severe urethral stricture, posterior urethral valves, ureterocele, tumors of the urinary tract, and ureteropelvic or ureterovesical junction obstruction in an individual with a solitary kidney or occlusive calculi. The risk is increased in a child who is immobile or in a cast, or who has metabolic abnormalities.[25]

Renal vein thrombosis is rarely seen in the child but when it is bilateral, it is usually associated with renal failure. Renal vein thrombosis may follow severe dehydration, hemorrhage, or sepsis and is usually a consequence of severe hypovolemia.[26] Clinically, in renal vein thrombosis there is usually a firm flank mass with scant and grossly bloody urine, hypertension, leukocytosis, thrombocytosis, and reduced renal function. Venography usually demonstrates the presence of a large thrombus in the renal vein.

PATHOPHYSIOLOGY OF ARF

Many theories have been advanced to explain the pathogenesis of ARF.[27–29] Several studies have evaluated prolonged hypoperfusion of the kidneys resulting in ARF. The *back-leak theory* suggests that relatively normal glomerular filtration persists, but because of damage to tubules and tubular epithelium, the glomerular filtrate is totally reabsorbed. The histopathologic findings of moderate to severe tubular necrosis in biopsy specimens of patients with clinical acute tubular necrosis and acute renal failure and in certain experimental nephrotoxic models support this theory. Experimental studies with substances such as inulin and Lissamine Green V dye (both are filtered but not secreted or absorbed) have demonstrated that the concentration of these markers increases along the length of the nephron as the glomerular filtrate is re-absorbed. The exception to this finding was in the mercuric chloride model in which an increase in the concentrations of Lissamine Green V dye and inulin was not seen. Further, tubular necrosis is not a consistently prominent feature in all forms of ischemia-induced renal failure. Infusions of saline, mannitol, or furosemide prevented ARF in certain models even though the histopathologic finding of tubular necrosis was evident.

In the *tubular obstruction theory,* tubular casts and debris lodge in the tubular lumen and increase intratubular back pressure, making the net glomerular filtration pressure zero. Although casts and debris are frequently associated with clinical and experimental renal failure, these pathologic findings are not found uniformly. In some cases of ARF, proximal tubule lumina are collapsed and there is normal or decreased intratubular pressure.

A popular theory holds that in ARF, afferent arteriolar constriction leads to a decrease in blood flow to the glomerulus with an attendant fall in glomerular filtration.[29] Other vascular theories propose that there is an efferent arteriolar dilatation that causes a marked decrease in glomerular filtration pressure.[29] Another theory holds that decreased glomerular permeability in ARF diminishes glomerular filtration.[29] Lending support to vascular theories of the pathogenesis of ARF is the finding of normal glomeruli and collapsed tubules in many cases of clinical and experimental ARF. Increased circulating vasoconstrictor substances, such as angiotensin, also often occur in ARF. Evidence against such theories is the observation that some nephrons are dilated and have increased intratubular pressures in experimental ARF.[29] Further, renal blood flow can be increased to normal levels with pharmacologic manipulation, and yet the ARF is not reversed.

It is likely that multiple factors contribute to ARF and no single hypothesis will explain the pathogenesis in all cases. It is likely that for different causes of ARF, different combinations of pathologic mechanisms are operative.

DIFFERENTIAL DIAGNOSIS OF PRERENAL, INTRINSIC RENAL, AND POSTRENAL FAILURE

The differential diagnosis and management of ARF should proceed simultaneously in order to lessen the morbidity and mortality associated with the condition. The mortality in ARF is dependent upon the underlying illness. Death has been reported in 25 to 65 per cent of post-operative and post-trauma patients with ARF.[30, 31] The mortality in other patients with ARF ranges from 10 to 35 per cent.[32] The prognosis for complete recovery is excellent in the child with ARF secondary to acute tubular necrosis when there is meticulous clinical management of the associated fluid, electrolyte, and metabolic abnormalities. The specific laboratory investigations that are performed are dependent upon the specific categories of diagnoses that are suspected. The history and physical examination are important in helping to identify factors that predispose to prerenal contraction (e.g., hypovolemia or hypotension). The history and physical examination also may give important clues for identifying drug ingestion, nephrotoxin exposure, or systemic disease.

The urinalysis may provide valuable clues as to the cause of ARF.[33] Hematuria and proteinuria with red blood cell casts suggest glomerulonephritis. Interstitial nephritis is seen more commonly with minimal to moderate proteinuria, few cells and casts, sodium wasting and increased urine volume, and a rather severe degree of anemia for the degree of renal insufficiency.[34] The presence of a flank mass in association with grossly bloody urine is most compatible with medullary necrosis, cortical necrosis, or renal vascular occlusion.[26] The complete blood count is important in suggesting the presence of the hemolytic-uremic syndrome (HUS), as there will usually be evidence of a microangiopathic hemolytic anemia and thrombocytopenia. The blood smear will show broken red blood cell forms, different shapes, and evidence of mechanical injury to RBCs within the circulation. Clotting studies in patients with HUS may reveal prolongation of PT and PTT, increased fibrin split products, but normal levels of factor V and VIII.[18, 19] In Henoch-Schoenlein purpura, although there may be purpura on the lower extremities, the platelet count will be normal.[20, 21] Electrolyte, BUN, and creatinine measurements are vital in defining the fluid and electrolyte abnormalities, acidemia, and degree of renal insufficiency. When post-infectious glomerulonephritis is suspected, serologic tests (antistreptolysin O tests, streptozyme, etc.) may reveal evidence of an antecedent streptococcal infection. Serum complement (CH50, C3) may be reduced when there has been deposition of immune complexes and complement on the glomerular basement membrane. It is important to remember that many organisms, other than streptococcus, are associated with post-infectious glomerulonephritis. If the child is suspected of having an infection, blood and urine cultures are indicated. A chest radiograph is helpful in the assessment of heart size, pleural effusion, and pulmonary edema. Renal ultrasonography is quite useful in the assessment of gross renal anatomy (size, presence or absence of hydronephrosis, etc.).[35, 36]

Table 14–3 summarizes pertinent features that should be elicited in the history and physical examination. Characteristic laboratory findings as they relate to the urinalysis, urine osmolality, and sodium concentration are presented. Urinary sodium concentration and urine osmolality are frequently (but not uniformly) useful when differentiating prerenal from intrinsic renal failure. In the child who has an illness with marked fluid and electrolyte losses and presumed prerenal failure, a fluid challenge can be used diagnostically to distinguish reversible prerenal failure from intrinsic renal failure. The fluid challenge is performed by the intravenous infusion of physiologic saline at a volume of 20 ml/kg of body weight over 60 to 120 minutes. It may be repeated once if the patient continues to appear dehydrated on physical examination. If oliguria persists at the end of the fluid challenge, 1–2 mg/kg of furosemide may be given intravenously. If there is no diuresis (urine output is < 2.0 ml/kg/hr) within 60 to 120 minutes of administration of furosemide, intrinsic renal damage should be suspected and fluids should be restricted to replacement of insensible water loss (see Table 14–4) plus urinary output.[37] If the patient responds to fluid challenge, prerenal oliguria is the most likely diagnosis. If this is the case, appropriate hydration should be continued, and careful observation of urine output, weight, and renal function maintained. If the patient is hypertensive or demonstrates evidence of volume overload (edema, congestive heart failure, and pulmonary edema), the administration of fluid and electrolytes must proceed with great care.

The pathophysiologic mechanisms of urinary tract obstruction have been well characterized and elucidated.[38] A list of causes of urinary tract obstruction that may lead to renal failure in children is given in Table 14–1. The history and physical examination gives valuable clues that may suggest the presence of a urinary tract obstruction. A distended bladder is readily detected on physical examination by palpation and percussion. The measurement of the large volume of residual urine that persists after the patient has voided confirms an obstruction or a neurogenic bladder. Nephrosonography is often a valuable diagnostic procedure in children with ARF.[35, 36] It is noninvasive and does not depend upon the presence of renal function for imaging the kidneys. It can accurately reveal the size of the kidneys and the collecting system, the presence of large cysts, hydronephrosis, or markedly dilated ureters. It can demonstrate whether two kidneys are present. Intravenous pyelography (IVP) is of limited value in the evaluation of kidney size and anatomy in established ARF. Visualization is often extremely poor or not possible because of the diminution of renal function. There is also a potential for nephrotoxicity from contrast agents used in such studies.[38] Thus, ultrasonography is a safer procedure that is better able to show the gross renal anatomy and help rule out severe obstructive uropathy.

MANAGEMENT OF ACUTE RENAL FAILURE

Diagnosis is essential in determining appropriate therapy. Reversible causes of ARF should be treated specifically. For example, in the child in whom obstructive uropathy has been identified, relief of the obstruction is essential. Hypovolemia should be corrected as described earlier. In the child with intrinsic renal failure, meticulous management of fluid, electrolytes, and blood pressure must take place.

Fluid Requirements

Once intrinsic ARF is confirmed, fluid intake should be restricted to replacement of insensible water loss plus renal and other losses that may occur from the gastrointestinal tract.[1] If the patient is not overloaded with fluid, urine losses should be measured and replaced with an equal volume for each interval. Catheterization should be avoided. Indwelling catheters are rarely needed. They markedly increase the risk of infection.[39] In patients who are volume-overloaded, the desired amount of weight loss should be subtracted from the total replacement fluids. Marked fluid overload associated with severe oliguria and evidenced by cardiac enlargement, pulmonary edema, and visceral organ enlargement is an indication for dialysis.

Maintenance fluid requirements for the infant, child, and adolescent are listed in Table 14–4. Maintenance electrolyte loss is from the skin and characteristically amounts to 0.5 mEq of sodium chloride and 0.5 mEq of potassium chloride per kilogram body weight per day.

Table 14–3. A COMPARISON OF CLINICAL FEATURES AND LABORATORY FINDINGS OF PRERENAL AND INTRINSIC RENAL FAILURE

Condition	History	Physical Examination	Urine Output	Laboratory Findings		
Prerenal failure	Febrile illness Vomiting Diarrhea Inadequate oral intake	Signs of dehydration Decreased weight, skin turgor, and BP Dry mucous membranes CNS signs Irritability Lethargy	Decreased	Urine osmolality significantly greater than serum osmolality	Urinary sodium low (<20 mEq/L)	Cells and casts: none or occasional
Intrinsic renal failure	Antecedent illness Pharyngitis Impetigo Gastroenteritis Known, severe, and prolonged hypoxemia Cardiac surgery Known drug or toxin exposure Changes in urine color, frequency of urination Development of edema Involvement of other organ systems Skin rashes Pulmonary abnormalities Pallor Joint manifestations	Signs of adequate or increased fluid status Increased weight, edema, BP Cardiac enlargement Gallop S3, S4 Passive congestion Liver Spleen Lungs (pulmonary edema) Signs of other systemic involvement Purpura Joint manifestations Heavy metal lines Severe anemia	Usually decreased	Urine osmolality variable	Urinary sodium high (>50 mEq/L)	Proteinuria Hematuria Leukocyturia RBCs, granular casts

Table 14–4. COMPONENTS OF MAINTENANCE FLUID LOSSES: AVERAGE DAILY FLUID NEEDS

Component	6 months–5 years (ml/kg/24 hr)	5–10 years (ml/kg/24 hr)	10 years to adolescence (ml/kg/24 hr)
Insensible	30	20	10
Urinary	60	50	40
Fecal	10	–	–
	—	—	—
Total	100	70	50

Urinary electrolyte losses are variable but average 3 mEq sodium and 2 mEq potassium per kilogram per day. The anion depends on the patient's acid-base status. Stool losses of electrolytes are high in the diarrheal state and must be considered,[40] but their values can be omitted when calculating maintenance needs in the non-diarrheal state. Thus, total maintenance electrolytes can usually be replaced by maintenance fluids given as 0.2 per cent saline in 5 to 10 per cent dextrose and water. Maintenance fluids must be reduced to replacement of insensible water loss plus measured urinary and non-renal output as described for intrinsic renal failure. It is most important that the child be weighed at least every 12 hours because weight most accurately reflects fluid status. An increase in weight reflects net water gain, and a decrease net water loss (intake minus output equals change in body weight). A daily loss of one per cent of body weight is expected owing to catabolism when the child in acute renal failure is not receiving an adequate intake of calories.[41] Once urine output begins to rise, fluid intake should be increased proportionately to allow for replacement of voided volume and electrolytes. Increased anabolic activity allows for the intracellular transfer of potassium, and hypokalemia may occur.

Hyperkalemia

Hyperkalemia is a life-threatening disturbance that may be seen in ARF. Close electrolyte monitoring and recognizing the presence of catabolism will lead to detection of impending or actual hyperkalemia. In the presence of ARF serum sodium, potassium, and CO_2 levels should be monitored every four to six hours until they are stabilized. Severe extracellular hyperkalemia results in depression of sinoatrial node activity, favoring ventricular arrhythmias or cardiac standstill. The electrocardiographic changes associated with hyperkalemia are initially tall peaked T waves followed by widening of the QRS complex and eventually by sine waves and cardiac arrest.

Serum potassium levels of 5.5–7.0 mEq/L without electrocardiographic changes may be treated with an ion-exchange resin (Kayexalate) by retention enema. Kayexalate is a cation-exchange resin that exchanges 1 mEq/L of potassium for 2–3 mEq/L of sodium. The usual dose is 1 gm/kg mixed with 10 per cent sorbitol (1 gm Kayexalate per 1–2 ml 10% sorbitol) and is given by enema. It should be retained for three hours to have maximal effect. This dose will usually reduce the serum potassium level by approximately 1 mEq/L in a 3 to 4 hour-period. In the volume-overloaded child with ARF, the continued use of Kayexalate enemas may result in hypernatremia and significant worsening of volume overload (severe vascular congestion, severe hypertension, or marked edema). If hypernatremia or severe edema is not present, Kayexalate enemas may be repeated every four to six hours. Hyperkalemia with associated evidence of peaked T waves on ECG (usually seen with potassium level at 7 mEq/L or greater) may be treated with 2 mEq per kilogram body weight of sodium bicarbonate given intravenously and Kayexalate enemas. The sodium bicarbonate begins to correct acidemia and leads to potassium movement into cells. This effect occurs rapidly (5–10 minutes). The Kayexalate enema removes potassium from the body slowly (2–4 hours). Severe hyperkalemia (>7.5–8.0 mEq/L) with major electrocardiographic changes (absent P waves, widened QRS complexes, ventricular arrhythmias) should first be treated with 0.5 ml/kg of ten per cent calcium gluconate given intravenously and cautiously under constant ECG monitoring. Calcium gluconate stabilizes membranes[32] and reduces the cardiotoxic effect of hyperkalemia. The calcium gluconate is followed by the intravenous administration of sodium bicarbonate (1–2 mEq/kg) to drive potassium intracellularly. Similarly, an intravenous solution of 25 to 50 per cent glucose accompanied by one unit regular insulin per five grams glucose transfers potassium to the intracellular compartment. It is preferable to omit the insulin to avoid the risk of hypoglycemia in infants.[37] The duration of the effect of sodium bicarbonate, calcium, glucose, and insulin is short, and dialysis should be instituted promptly to remove potassium from the body rather than redistribute it intracellularly.

If the measures discussed are successful,

serum potassium level should be evaluated every two to four hours until it is stabilized. There also should be constant monitoring of the ECG until the potassium level remains in the normal range and the catabolic process ceases. Once hyperkalemia is reversed, continuing but less frequent monitoring of the serum potassium level is indicated (q12–24h) until renal function is restored or long-term dialysis is instituted.

Hyponatremia

Hyponatremia in ARF is characteristically due to dilution of the sodium content of the extracellular space. It can usually be prevented or be slowly corrected by restricting fluid intake until the extracellular water content is normal. In severe hyponatremia (serum sodium level <120 mEq/L) or in symptomatic hyponatremia (which may include lethargy, coma, delirium, seizures, and muscle weakness), prompt (partial) correction is needed. Sodium can be infused (as saline) to bring the sodium concentration to 125–130 mEq/L. The amount of sodium needed is calculated by multiplying the concentration deficit (125 mEq/L minus measured serum sodium level) by 0.7 (distribution space for total body water) by body weight (kg). The amount of saline needed to accomplish this is calculated and the fluid infused over 60 to 120 minutes. If there is severe fluid overload or circulatory congestion, additional sodium may further impair cardiac output, and dialysis may be required. An example of the calculation follows: *A 1-year-old child who weighs 10 kilograms has ARF and a serum sodium level of 119 mEq/L. She requires 125 − 119 = 6 mEq/L Na × 0.7 × 10 kg = 42 mEq of sodium given as sodium chloride.* This concentration will be provided by infusing 270 ml of normal (0.9%) saline. Note that the sodium deficit is multiplied by the total body water. This calculation is necessary because infusion of sodium into the extracellular space is associated with water movement to maintain intra- and extracellular osmotic equilibrium. If fluid overload is present the sodium could be provided by infusing 84 ml of 3 per cent saline, but when fluid overload is severe dialysis is usually needed.

Hypernatremia

Hypernatremia in ARF occurs when water intake fails to keep pace with its excretion or when excess sodium is given intravenously or by Kayexalate enemas. At risk are the patients with enhanced urinary water losses and restricted intake (e.g., neurosurgical patients with diabetes insipidus), patients with large losses of water from the skin, and patients who cannot drink. Sodium is frequently given intravenously as sodium bicarbonate to correct acidosis or combat hyperkalemia. Hypernatremia is also a risk in these patients. Acidosis or hyperkalemia associated with hypernatremia is an indication for dialysis.

Hypertension

Hypertension in ARF may result from salt and water overload or because of increased release of renin by the underperfused kidney.[1–5] The management of fluid and electrolyte disturbances and overload was discussed earlier. Moderate hypertension (BP >2SDs but <3SDs above the mean) that is caused by such fluid overload usually normalizes when plasma volume returns to normal. Table 14–5 indicates the recommended antihypertensive drug therapy for the patient who has more severe hypertension or who is symptomatic (headache, vomiting, seizure). Other antihypertensive agents are available, but the ones listed are those for which dosages for children have been established and considerable experience has been accumulated.

Congestive Heart Failure

Circulatory congestion caused by salt and water overload or excessive fluid administration with resultant edema and pulmonary congestion is the predominant cardiovascular complication of ARF. Therapy, as described earlier, consists of meticulous management of fluid and electrolyte administration, control of hypertension, and dialysis therapy.

Nutrition

The basal caloric requirements for the child with ARF should be maintained predominantly by carbohydrate administration so as to minimize the rate of endogenous catabolism. At first, dietary protein should be restricted to no more than 1 g/kg/24 hours to slow the development of acidemia and azotemia. In patients who are severely catabolic with ARF, early use of intravenous hypertonic glucose

Table 14–5. A GUIDE TO ANTIHYPERTENSIVE AGENTS FOR THE MEDICAL MANAGEMENT OF HYPERTENSION IN CHILDREN WITH ACUTE RENAL FAILURE

	Agent	Dosage Range	Route and Frequency of Administration
Severe life threatening hypertension (severe headache, seizures, coma)	Diazoxide	3–5 mg/kg	IV by rapid injection May repeat at 4–24-hour intervals until oral regimen enables BP control
	Nitroprusside	0.5–10 μg/kg/min	IV pump infusion Requires constant BP monitoring Begin concomitant oral antihypertensive therapy and discontinue nitroprusside when it is effective Beware of any signs of cyanide toxicity and discontinue when present
Moderate hypertension Oral agents	Diuretics	mg/kg/day	
	Hydrochlorothiazide	1–4	PO daily or bid
	Chlorothiazide	10–40	
	Furosemide	1–5	
	Vasodilator		
	Hydralazine	0.7–7.5 (maximum 100–200 mg/day)	PO bid or tid
		0.15 mg/kg	IM; q4–6 h
	Anti-adrenergics		
	Methyldopa	10–60 (maximum 2 gm/day)	PO bid or tid
	Propranolol	1–10	PO bid or tid

and essential amino acid solutions may improve survival.[42]

Metabolic Acidosis

In ARF with increased catabolism, a profound acidemia may develop early in the clinical course. Usually, partial respiratory compensation with deep Kussmaul breathing occurs, along with resorption of calcium salts from bone, which partially buffers the circulating acids. Sodium bicarbonate or other alkali may be given to raise the blood pH level to between 7.25 and 7.30. The amount of sodium bicarbonate to be given is determined from the product of the base deficit concentration (calculated from readily available nomograms) times 0.3 (approximate distribution space of sodium bicarbonate), times body weight (kg), and infused over 12 hours. For example, in order to raise the total CO_2 level in a 10 kg 1-year-old child to the lower limit of normal (20 mEq/L), the following calculation is performed. The serum bicarbonate concentration is approximated from the total CO_2 level or preferably is calculated from the measurement of the serum pH and P_{CO_2} levels. If the total CO_2 level is 15 mEq/L, for example, correction is achieved by multiplying the deficit (20 mEq/L − 15 mEq/L) = 5 mEq/L × 0.3 × 10kg = 15 mEq, i.e., the deficit to be given. Excessive use of sodium bicarbonate results in hypernatremia and worsening of volume overload. The presence of severe acidemia that does not respond to sodium bicarbonate therapy or is associated with hypernatremia, is an indication for dialysis.

Hypocalcemia and Hyperphosphatemia

In acute renal failure, because of the characteristic breakdown of body tissues (hypercatabolism), there is an endogenous release of phosphate at a time when renal phosphate clearance is reduced or negligible.[43] Elevation of the serum phosphorus level will lead to proportionate depression of the serum calcium level. The serum phosphorus level can be reduced with dietary phosphate restriction and

ALGORITHM FOR THE MANAGEMENT OF ACUTE RENAL FAILURE

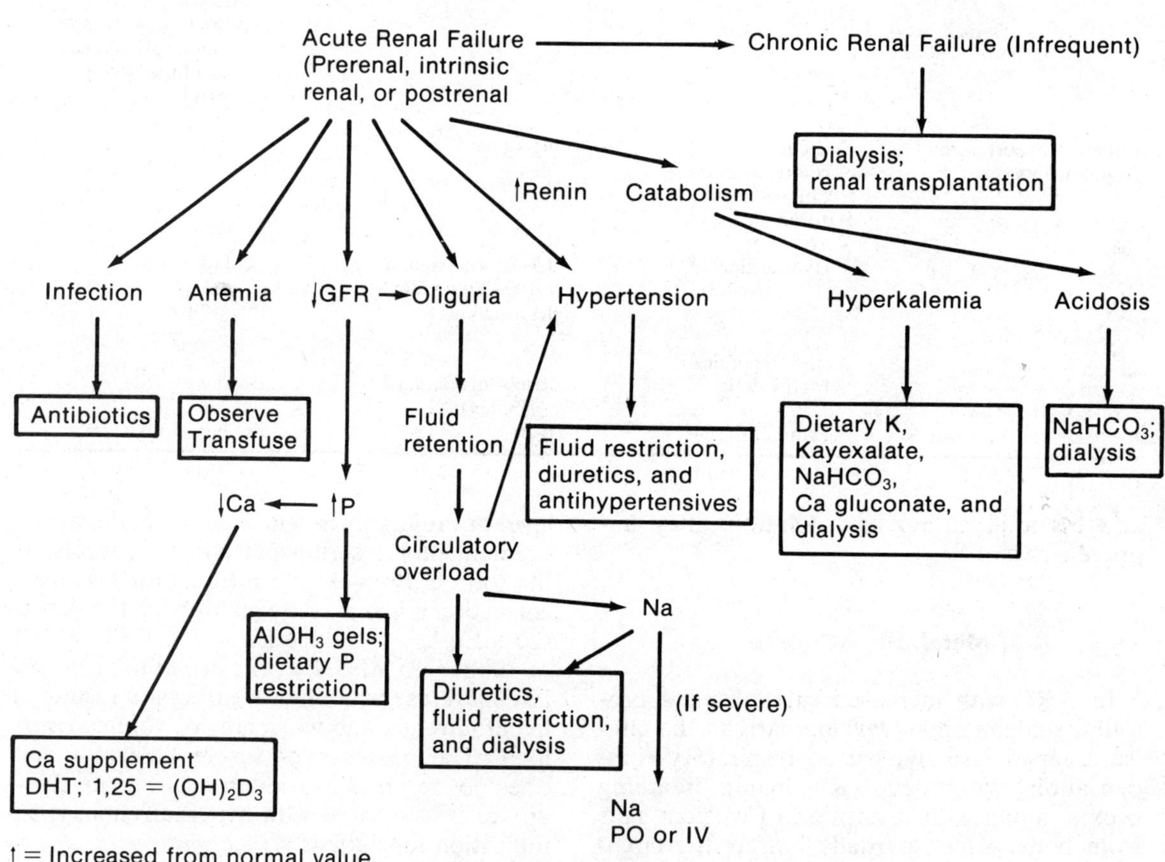

with oral administration of aluminum hydroxide. A starting dose of aluminum hydroxide is 60 mg/kg/day in 3 doses, given orally and adjusted to maintain the serum phosphorus level in the 5 to 6 mg/100 ml range. It is important to use only aluminum hydroxide gels because gels containing magnesium may cause hypermagnesemia. At present, the toxicity of aluminum is poorly understood and under study. If the patient is hypocalcemic and symptomatic (numbness, muscle cramps, tetany, laryngeal stridor, and seizures), 4 mg/kg/hr of elemental calcium (0.5 ml of 10% calcium gluconate per hour) is infused for 4 hours. Repeated doses are often needed to control recurrent hypocalcemia.

Anemia

Caution must prevail in the administration of blood or blood products to the patient with ARF. There is an increased risk, in the absence of renal function, of hyperkalemia and circulatory overload. If blood or blood products are necessary (symptomatic anemia, hematocrit <20%, cardiovascular instability) the minimal volume (usually 5–10 ml of packed cells/kg) of the freshest product should be utilized and administered slowly while one closely monitors clinical signs (blood pressure, pulse rate, breath sounds, liver size, etc.) and other parameters (serum potassium levels, ECGs).

Infection

Infection is a serious risk for all patients with ARF. All intravenous catheters should be removed as soon as possible, and indwelling bladder catheterization should be avoided. If infection is suspected, suitable cultures should be obtained and appropriate antibiotics should be given. The use of potentially nephrotoxic antibiotics should be avoided. If aminoglycosides are required, their peak and trough blood levels must be monitored closely. The dosages of antibiotics as well as other agents need to be examined because they are usually altered in frequency because of the presence of renal failure.

Dialysis

There are no absolute indications for dialysis, but relative indications include severe fluid overload (pulmonary edema), severe hyperkalemia (serum potassium levels > 7 mEq/L with ECG abnormalities that do not respond promptly to medical management) or hyperkalemia in the markedly catabolic patient (rapid tissue breakdown), acidosis or other electrolyte derangements not corrected by conservative methods, symptoms and signs of uremia (particularly evidence of CNS depression), and irreversible renal failure. Peritoneal dialysis is relatively safe and can be instituted rapidly. It can effect ultrafiltration with removal of excess fluid and improvement of metabolic parameters. Hemodialysis may be preferred in the patient who has marked tissue breakdown and is severely catabolic and hyperkalemic. Peritoneal dialysis is the preferred method in the patient who has severe fluid overload.

REFERENCES

1. Ellis D, Gartner JC, Galvis AG. Acute renal failure in infants and children: diagnosis, complications, and treatment. Crit Care Med 1981; *9*:607–617.
2. Hodson EM, Kjellstrand CM, Mauer SM. Acute renal failure in infants and children: outcome of 53 patients requiring hemodialysis treatment. J Pediatr 1978; *93*:756–761.
3. Gordillo PG, Valasquez JL. Acute renal failure. Pediatr Clin North Am 1976; *23*:817–828.
4. Chan JC. Acute renal failure in children: diagnosis and treatment. Va Med 1980; *7*:501–505.
5. Yahav J, Barzilay Z, Aladjem M, et al. Acute peritoneal dialysis in children. Int J Pediatr Nephrol 1981; *1*:33–35.
6. Rendle CF, Short J. Fibrocystic disease of the pancreas presenting with acute salt depletion. Arch Dis Child 1956; *31*:28–30.
7. Alleyne GAO, Statius Van Eps LW, et al. The kidney in sickle cell anemia. Kidney Int 1975; *7*:371–379.
8. Dunnill MS. A review of the pathology and pathogenesis of acute renal failure due to acute tubular necrosis. J Clin Pathol 1974; *27*:2–13.
9. Olsen S. Renal histopathology in various forms of acute anuria in man. Kidney Int 1976; *10* (4 Supp 6):S2–8.
10. McIntosh RM, Garcia R, Rubio L, et al. Evidence for an autologous immune complex pathogenic mechanism in acute poststreptococcal glomerulonephritis. Kidney Int 1978; *14*:501–510.
11. Kohler PF, Cronin FE, Hammond WS, et al. Chronic membranous glomerulonephritis caused by hepatitis B antigen-antibody immune complexes. Ann Intern Med 1974; *81*:448–451.
12. Beaufils M, Gibert C, Morel-Maroger L, et al. Glomerulonephritis in severe bacterial infection with and without endocarditis. Adv Nephrol 1977; *7*:217–234.
13. Bayer AS, Theofilopoulos AN, Eisenberg R, et al. Circulating immune complexes in infectious endocarditis. N Engl J Med 1976; *295*:1500–1505.

14. Boonshaft B, Maher JF, Schreiner GE. Nephrotic syndrome associated with osteomyelitis without secondary amyloidosis. Arch Intern Med 1970; *125*:322–323.
15. Fish AJ, Blau EB, Westberg NG, et al. Systemic lupus erythematosus within the first two decades of life. Am J Med 1977; *62*:99–114.
16. Kaplan BS, Klassen J, Gautt MH. Glomerular injury in patients with neoplasia. Annu Rev Med 1976; *27*:117–125.
17. Suki WN, Eknoyan G, eds. Renal involvement in Leukemia and Lymphoma. *In*: The Kidney in Systemic Diseases. New York: John Wiley & Sons, Inc., 1976.
18. Gianantonio CA, Vitacco M, Mendilaharzu F, et al. The hemolytic-uremic syndrome. Nephron 1973; *11*:174–192.
19. Kaplan BS, Thompson PD, de Chadarévian JP. The hemolytic uremic syndrome. Pediatr Clin North Am 1976; *23*:761–777.
20. Meadow SR, Glasgow EF, White RHR, et al. Schoenlein-Henoch nephritis. Q J Med 1972; *41*:241–258.
21. Meadow SR. The prognosis of Henoch Schoenlein nephritis. Clin Nephrol 1978; *9*:87–90.
22. Appel GB, Neu HC. The nephrotoxicity of antimicrobial agents (three parts). N Engl J Med 1977; *296*:663–670, 722–728, 784–787.
23. Hepatinstall RH. Interstitial nephritis. Am J Pathol 1976; *83*:213–236.
24. Ansari Z, Baldwin DS. Acute renal failure due to radio contrast agents. Nephron 1976; *17*:28–40.
25. Williams DI. Urology in Childhood. New York: Springer-Verlag, 1974.
26. Arneil GC, MacDonald A, Murphy A, Sweet EM. Renal venous thrombosis. Clin Nephrol 1973; *1*:119–131.
27. Flamenbaum W. Pathophysiology of acute renal failure. Arch Intern Med 1973; *131*:911–928.
28. Hanley MJ. Studies on acute disease models. Kidney Int 1982; *22*:536–545.
29. Schrier RW, Conger JC. Acute renal failure: Pathogenesis, diagnosis, and management. *In*: Schrier RW. ed. Renal and Electrolyte Disorders. Boston: Little, Brown & Company, 1980:375–408.
30. Abel RM, Buckley MJ, Austen WG, et al. Etiology, incidence and prognosis of renal failure following cardiac operations: results of a prospective analysis of 500 consecutive patients. J Thorac Cardiovasc Surg 1976; *71*:323–333.
31. Stott RB, Ogg CS, Cameron JS, Bewick M. Why the persistently high mortality in acute renal failure? Lancet 1972; *2*:75–79.
32. Minuth AN, Terrell JB, Suki WN. Acute renal failure: a study of the course and prognosis of 104 patients and of the role of furosemide. Am J Med Sci 1976; *271*:317–324.
33. Levinsky NG, Alexander EA. Acute renal failure. *In*: Brenner BM, Rector FC Jr. eds. The Kidney. Philadelphia: WB Saunders, 1976.
34. McMurray SD, Luft FC, Maxwell DR, et al. Prevailing patterns and predictor variables in patients with acute tubular necrosis. Arch Intern Med 1978; *138*:950–955.
35. Ellenbogen PH, Scheible FW, Talner LB, Leopold GR. Sensitivity of grey scale ultrasound in detecting urinary tract obstruction. AJR, 1978; *130*:731–733.
36. Sanders RC, Conrad MR. The ultrasonic characteristics of the renal pelvicalyceal echo complex. J Clin Ultrasound 1977; *5*:372–377.
37. Rahman N, Boineau FG, Lewy JE. Renal failure in the perinatal period. Clin Perinatol, 1981; *8*:241–250.
38. Teruel JL, Marcen R, Onaindia JM, et al. Renal function impairment caused by intravenous urography, a prospective study. Arch Intern Med 1981; *141*:1271–1274.
39. Garibaldi RA, Burke JP, Dickman ML, Smith CB. Factors predisposing to bacteriuria during indwelling urethral catherization. N Engl J Med 1974; *291*:215–219.
40. Dell RB. Pathophysiology of Dehydration in the Body Fluids. *In*: Pediatrics. Boston: Little, Brown, & Company, 1973:134–154.
41. Jones RWA, Rigden SP, Barratt TM, Chantler C. The effects of chronic renal failure in infancy on growth, nutritional status and body of composition. Pediatr Res 1982; *16*:784–791.
42. Feinstein EI, Blumenkrantz MJ, Healy M, et al. Clinical and metabolic responses to parenteral nutrition in acute renal failure: a controlled double-blind study. Medicine 1981; *60*:124–137.
43. Massry SG, Arieff AI, Coburn JW, et al. Divalent ion metabolism in patients with acute renal failure: studies on the mechanism of hypocalcemia. Kidney Int 1974; *5*:437–445.

CHAPTER

15

Status Asthmaticus

C. Warren Bierman, M.D.
Gail G. Shapiro, M.D.
Clifton T. Furukawa, M.D.
William E. Pierson, M.D.

Status asthmaticus is generally defined as asthma unresponsive or poorly responsive to oral, inhaled, and injected bronchodilator drugs. The severity and rapidity of worsening differs for various age groups. In a toddler, asthma can progress from mild wheezing to acute respiratory failure in hours despite optimal therapy. In adolescents, however, the same downhill course may take place but over a period of days. Whatever the time course and cause, status asthmaticus is a life-threatening medical emergency for which prompt, systematic, and aggressive management not only is lifesaving, but reduces the duration of hospitalization and the frequency of complications.[1]

PATHOLOGY AND PATHOPHYSIOLOGY

Pathology

Knowledge of the pathology of severe asthma has been obtained largely from postmortem examinations of adults who died of asthma.[2] Pulmonary biopsy specimens obtained by bronchoscopy from asthmatic patients are similar to those obtained from asthmatic patients who died. Pulmonary changes in children with asthma also are similar, though they are less likely to have evidence of chronic bronchitis that occurs frequently in adults.[4]

When the thoracic cage of a patient who died of asthma is opened at autopsy, the lungs are bulky and tense. They meet in the midline and fail to deflate to a third of the volume as do normal lungs. They cannot be deflated manually because air is trapped in the lungs by tenacious secretions in the airways. The lung surface appears normal, but patchy foci of airlessness and consolidation may be seen. On microscopic examination, layers of secretions can be distinguished that include sheets of eosinophils and shed surface epithelium.[5] Mucus is present in most layers. Charcot-Leyden crystals derived from eosinophilic basic protein and Curschmann's spirals of glycoprotein can be seen.[6] The mucus within the lumen is continuous with that in the ducts of the submucosal glands and that in the goblet cells of the surface epithelium.

In fatal cases of asthma, epithelium is shed over most of the airway lining. The shedding of these respiratory mucosal cells may be caused by the transudation of protein-laden exudate and is the source of Creola bodies found in the mucus. This disruption of epithelial cells causes a loss of "tight epithelial junctions,"[7] which permits antigen or irritant penetration to stimulate irritant nerve receptors directly and to come into direct contact with submucosal pulmonary mast cells. The result is more severe bronchospasm, secretion of additional inflammatory mediators, and further loss of tight junction protection. The basement membrane is very obviously thickened, a characteristic feature of asthma.[8] It may be present in mild as well as severe asthma and is due to deposition of collagen in this layer.

The eosinophil is the most numerous and characteristic cell in the inflammatory exudate. It is found throughout the airway wall and may be present in the alveolar region and in the lymph nodes. Plasma cells, polymorphonuclear leukocytes, and lymphocytes also infiltrate the exudate, though their relative numbers are quite variable.[9]

In a patient with asthma, the muscle of the bronchial wall is hypertrophied and hyperplastic. There is hypertrophy of the submucosal glands and an increase in the number of goblet cells in both central and peripheral airways.

During recovery from status asthmaticus, there is resolution and healing of many of these features. Phagocytosis of high-protein fluid and impacted mucus takes longer than clearance of edema—probably a week or more. After clinical "recovery," mucociliary clearance is still severely impaired because of loss of mucosal cells with their cilia. Remaining basal cells migrate to the basement membrane, multiply, form a stratified layer of cells, and differentiate to normal pseudo-stratified ciliated epithelium over two to four weeks. Coughing and the mechanical effects of lengthening and shortening of airways with respiration clears secretions during the period of mucociliary repair.

The basic pathology of asthma, i.e., thickening of the basement membranes, infiltration of eosinophils, hypertrophy of mucous glands, and submucosal smooth muscle with normal alveoli, is present in biopsy specimens obtained at bronchoscopy and even in children with asthma in remission who die of other causes.[10]

ETIOLOGY

In children, status asthmaticus may be induced by one or more of a number of factors. These include viral infections, inhalation of allergens, pollutants and irritants, and ill-defined factors such as a sudden change in barometric pressure and alterations in climatic conditions.[11, 12]

Viral Infections

Acute respiratory infections frequently induce severe asthma. In infancy, infectious bronchitis caused by a respiratory syncytial virus and possibly adenoviral infections and pertussis may induce airway hyper-reactivity that may persist long after recovery from the initial episode of small airway obstruction.[13] In some children such infections may result in lifelong bronchial hyper-reactivity. Other viral infections, such as parainfluenza virus and rhinovirus, can cause severe asthma in children who already have hyper-reactive airways.[14] Though the mechanism by which infectious agents induce obstruction of airways is still not clear, chemical mediators of inflammation produced by both non-immune and immune mechanisms are undoubtedly involved.[15]

While respiratory syncytial and parainfluenzal viral infections most frequently induce severe asthma in infants and young children, severe asthma in adults is associated more commonly with rhinovirus and influenza A infections. The severity of the viral illness appears to correlate with the severity of the associated asthma.[16]

Allergic Reactions

Allergic factors appear to play a role in asthma in a high proportion of asthmatic children.[17–19] In infancy and early childhood, allergic sensitivity tends to develop in response to the contents of house dust (especially house dust mites and cockroach feces), animal products (saliva, dander, urinary proteins), and common mold spores. With increasing age, the child becomes sensitive to seasonal pollen allergens. Severe asthmatic reactions to foods are most likely to occur in infancy and early childhood, principally to such foods as cow's milk, eggs, peanuts, and fish. In allergen-induced asthma, acute bronchospasm can occur within minutes and clear relatively rapidly, spontaneously, or with bronchodilator therapy, only to recur more severely a few hours later.[20] This "late" asthmatic attack responds poorly to bronchodilator drugs and may be especially important in the pathogenesis of status asthmaticus.[21] The probable mechanism involved in the late response is discussed in the section on inflammatory mediators of allergic inflammation.

Irritants, Weather, and Climatic Factors

Numerous irritating factors have also been implicated as precipitants of severe asthma, such as cigarette smoke and odors from paints and chemicals.[22] Weather and climatic changes, such as increased barometric pressure, temperature inversions, winds, moisture, ozone, and positive ions all have been associated with severe asthma.[23] An increase in emergency room visits[24] occurs during periods of thermal inversion and increased air pollution. Since these factors may co-exist at any given time, it is difficult to determine the relative importance of any one precipitating factor. Exercise during thermal inversions may lead to more severe exercise-induced asthma,[25] but there is little evidence to suggest that exercise *per se* can cause status asthmaticus.

Hypersensitivity to Drugs and Chemicals

Aspirin ingestion may cause a fall in pulmonary function in up to a third of adolescents with severe asthma.[26] In adults, aspirin and other non-steroidal anti-inflammatory agents such as indomethacin and ibuprofen can induce severe bronchial obstruction or even systemic anaphylaxis. A small proportion of aspirin-sensitive asthmatics also react to FD & C yellow No. 5 (tartrazine), which is commonly found in foods and drugs.[27] Other chemicals commonly used in the food industry, such as sodium metabisulfite and monosodium glutamate, have been incriminated recently as precipitants of acute asthma.

Emotional Factors

Psychological factors may play a role in many patients with asthma. The personality traits of patients, the coping styles of their families, and the behavior of their physicians have been shown to influence the severity of asthma.[28] Personality traits such as fearfulness, hostility, and dependency may also affect compliance. Lack of compliance, especially among adolescents, is often a major reason for hospital admission for asthma.[29]

Age-dependent Factors

Young children are particularly susceptible to status asthmaticus. Over a three-year period, 512 children were hospitalized for status asthmaticus in a major children's hospital.[30] Half of them were 3 years of age or less and two-thirds were less than 6 years of age.

The reasons for this predilection are primarily anatomic[31] and appear to be related to respiratory surface area, airway diameter, quantity of bronchial smooth muscle, and concentration of mucous glands in the airway.

At birth the lungs are relatively immature and the respiratory surface area is only a third that of a 3-year-old child. Hence, the younger the child, the smaller the reserve for gas exchange. Conducting airways are immature and increase in size from infancy to adulthood. Since airflow resistance is related to the fourth power of the radius of the bronchiole, a doubling of the radius decreases resistance to airflow to a sixteenth of that of the smaller airway. Thus, in children less than 5 years of age resistance to airflow in peripheral airways constitutes a much greater proportion of total respiratory resistance than that in children more than 5 years of age. For this reason the younger child with a predominance of small airways is at an extreme disadvantage in acute asthma. Not only does the child have little respiratory reserve, but airway resistance increases rapidly with even a slight decrease in airway caliber. The cause of airway obstruction is also age-dependent.[32] Since bronchial smooth muscle is relatively poorly developed in infants and children under 3 years of age, edema rather than bronchospasm is the predominant feature of asthma. The density of mucous glands is increased in the infant and the ratio of mucous gland to bronchial wall (the *Reid Index*) also is higher.[33] Asthma is thus related to increased quantities of secretions with consequent plugging of respiratory bronchioles and atelectasis to a much greater degree in the child less than 6 years old than in the child more than 6 years old. These factors account for the increased severity of asthma, the more frequent need for hospitalization, and the relatively poorer response to bronchodilator drugs in the child less than age 6 years and particularly in the child less than age 3 years.

Inflammatory Changes in Asthma

Asthmatic Inflammation—Mast Cell and Basophil

In status asthmaticus the interaction of cells and chemical inflammatory mediators, some of which are potent in nanogram or picogram quantities, produces acute inflammation of the airways. For three decades, the circulating basophil and the tissue mast cell have been known to contain histamine. With the discovery of IgE antibody, the mechanism by which IgE bound to the cell membrane interacts with specific antigen to induce histamine release has been elucidated. Specific antigen attaches to IgE antibody located on the surface of mast cells or basophils, activating the cellular receptors. This activation, in turn, leads to the activation of a chymotrypsin-like esterase and of methyl transferase in the cell membranes that leads to methylation of membrane phospholipids.[34] Calcium influx follows that permits secretion of histamine and activation of arachidonic acid metabolites. This secretory process is energy-dependent and does not destroy the cell. Cyclic nucleotides modify the process.[35] Increased intracellular cyclic AMP concentration inhibits mediator activation and secretion, whereas increased cyclic GMP concentration promotes it. Pharmacologic agents appear to modify this reaction by altering both intracellular concentration of cyclic nucleotides and metabolism of arachidonic acid. The list of recognized pharmacologically active agents, liberated or activated, grows yearly as new techniques are developed for their identification.

Inflammatory Mediators

Although histamine was the first of the mediators identified in the mast cell, more recently identified pre-formed and newly formed mediators are infinitely more important than histamine in allergic inflammation.

Arachidonic acid derived from cell membrane phospholipids is metabolized via the lipoxygenase pathway to form leukotrienes.[36] Leukotriene LTB_4 is a chemotatic factor, whereas leukotrienes LTC_4, LTD_4, and LTE_4 are the slow reactive substances of anaphylaxis (SRS-A).[37] Together, these mediators induce smooth muscle constriction, cause vasoconstriction, alter mucociliary clearance, stimulate vasopermeability, and depress the myocardium.

Alternatively, arachidonic acid may be metabolized via the cyclooxygenase pathway to form a cascade of thromboxanes and prostaglandins. These substances may cause vascular dilation, produce airway constriction, induce random migration of polymorphonuclear leukocytes (PMNs) and eosinophils, and stimulate mucus production. Prostaglandin-generating factor of anaphylaxis is particularly mucogenic.[38] Other mast cell components include β-hexosaminidase, β-glucoronidase, tryptase, and heparin.[39] These inflammatory mediators lead to proteoglycan degradation, collagenolysis, binding of antithrombin III, and inhibition of complement consumption, promoting further inflammation. Platelet-activating factor of anaphylaxis (PAFA)[40] and anaphylatoxins derived from other sources augment further the inflammatory response.[41]

Mediator Cellular Interaction

One of the most important features of mast cell stimulation is the recruitment and activation of immunoreactive cells.[42] Large numbers of eosinophils, PMNs, and monocytes are attracted by a variety of chemotactic factors secreted by or derived from chemicals released from the mast cell. Mast cells secrete such preformed substances as eosinophilic chemotactic factor of anaphylaxis (ECF-A), neutrophil chemotactic factor of anaphylaxis (NCF-A), neutrophil oligopeptides, and the strongly chemotactic LTB_4. Both histamine and prostaglandin D_2 stimulate random migration of cells.[43]

In severe asthma, the last phase of intense airway inflammation is associated with the infiltration of large numbers of cells. Eosinophilic basic protein, which is intensely toxic to cells, probably plays an important role in destruction of mucosal cells,[44] whereas a variety of proteolytic lysozymal enzymes derived from PMNs induce further inflammation. These enzymes may also activate kinins and arachidonic acid and generate additional leukotriene compounds. Numerous lymphokines are elaborated by lymphocytes that add to the inflammatory response. These lymphokines include mitogenic factors, interferon (which enhances antigen-induced mediator release), chemotactic factors, and substances that induce vasodilation and increase capillary permeability.[45]

Paradoxically, these cells are important inactivators of inflammatory mediators. Leukotrienes LTC_4, LTD_4, and LTE_4 are inactivated by polymorphonuclear leukocytes through the myeloperoxidase system outside the cell, and the chemotactic LTB_4 is inactivated within the cell. Eosinophils inactivate arylsulfatase and histamine.[46] Platelet-activating factor and anaphylatoxins are inactivated similarly by cells participating in the inflammatory response.

Pathophysiology

Pulmonary and metabolic changes that occur in acute asthma can cause homeostatic alterations in many organ systems.

Pulmonary

As airway obstruction progresses, forced vital capacity (FVC), forced expiratory volume at one second (FEV_1), and peak expiratory flow rate (PEFR) decrease while residual volume increases (RV).[47] These changes lead to hypoxemia and hyperventilation, which increase the work of breathing. With pneumonia, atelectasis, or extrapleural air, restrictive changes also occur. Mucus plugs and bronchospasms are distributed irregularly so that ventilation and perfusion abnormalities occur, causing arterial oxygen tensions to fall. Hypoxemia is accentuated when air is shunted to "dead spaces," i.e., poorly ventilated areas that are normally perfused.[48] Ultimately, this shunting of arterial blood to underventilated alveolae causes the blood that leaves the lungs to be so low in oxygen that it resembles mixed venous blood, in spite of oxygen administration.[49] This condition can progress to pulmonary hypertension, right ventricular hypertrophy, or cor pulmonale and cardiac failure.[50]

METABOLIC CHANGES

Acute asthma increases the work of breathing and increases tissue oxygen and energy consumption. In children, caloric expenditure may be increased further by fever from accompanying infections while caloric intake is reduced by vomiting or hypoxemia. Ketosis, resulting from depleted glycogen stores, leads to metabolic acidosis partially compensated by pulmonary hyperventilation and respiratory alkalosis. The combination of fatigue and progressive obstruction of pulmonary airways ultimately may lead to alveolar hypoventilation. Alveolar hypoventilation results in a rising arterial carbon dioxide tension (Pa_{CO2}) and respiratory acidosis.[51] Hence, an elevated or even "normal" Pa_{CO2} in severe asthma is an ominous sign. As Pa_{CO2} tensions rise, there is a further fall in Pa_{O2} values. Arterial pH values fall dramatically as respiratory acidosis is superimposed on metabolic acidosis.[52, 53] This process may progress to respiratory failure, cardiac arrhythmia, and cardiorespiratory arrest, which can lead to hypoxic brain damage or death.

DIAGNOSIS OF STATUS ASTHMATICUS

History

Patients with status asthmaticus can present in a number of ways, depending on both age and inciting events. The infant or toddler often presents with the fulminating symptoms of a viral respiratory infection associated with extreme respiratory distress, suprasternal, and infrasternal retractions, and paroxysmal coughing. Often these symptoms may develop abruptly over several hours. Sometimes the symptoms are those of acute croup that progresses to both inspiratory and expiratory obstruction. Occasionally, a pertussis-like syndrome associated with paroxysmal coughing and vomiting may herald asthma.

Older children usually have a more protracted course, though they may present to the emergency room with dyspnea, rapid respiration with use of all accessory respiratory muscles, and marked anxiety.[54] Vomiting and exhaustion often are overriding reasons for admission when an apparent response to bronchodilators would have otherwise justified a trial of home treatment.

On admission one should obtain detailed information concerning the acute illness, initiating factors, duration, progression, and specific respiratory signs and symptoms noted by the patient or by the parents. The patient's fluid balance over the preceding 24 hours should be ascertained, including intake, vomiting and urination. All medications administered should be recorded, including the specific drug or drugs, the exact quantity, and the exact time that they were given. This information is especially important if theophylline-containing drugs have been taken because some viruses such as influenza B, which may trigger severe asthma, may alter theophylline clearance as well.[73] The parents should be asked to bring in all medications that the patient has taken so that the exact doses administered can be verified.

The history of the child's asthma should be detailed. It should include the overall duration, descriptions of previous acute episodes, and information concerning the use of topical or oral corticosteroids. This last factor is of great importance because prolonged steroid administration may suppress adrenal function sufficiently that the patient is likely to develop adrenal failure unless supported by exogenous corticosteroids. One should also be certain to ask about any adverse effects from the medications.

Physical Examination

While the history is being elicited the physical examination may be carried out. The physician should note findings that relate to both the acute disease and the underlying chronic problem. One should note the patient's general appearance, degree of respiratory distress, respiratory rate, color of lips and nail beds, and use of accessory muscles in breathing. The skin turgor provides some information about fluid balance. Chest percussion gives evidence of the degree of hyperinflation. Particular note should be taken of the degree of pre-cardiac dullness, since its sudden disappearance may signal a complication such as pneumomediastinum. On auscultation, air exchange should be noted, as well as the relative ratio between inspiration and expiration. The degree of obstruction may be related to the degree of inspiratory and expiratory wheezing, though wheezing may decrease as air exchange is reduced. After the assessment of pulmonary status, an examination of growth and development, overall nutrition, and a search for evidence of other atopic disease or acute infections, such as otitis, is appropriate.

Differential Diagnosis

Although many disorders are associated with wheezing,[55] only a few can cause the kind of acute, severe respiratory distress seen in status asthmaticus. Wheezing itself if not necessary for establishing the diagnosis of status asthmaticus, since in severe stages so little air exchange occurs that wheezing actually may disappear. Thus, the differential diagnosis must include disorders in which the patient presents with acute respiratory distress.

Patients with airway infections such as croup, epiglottitis, bronchiolitis, and bronchopneumonia can present with acute respiratory distress.[56] Lateral neck x-rays and chest x-rays are helpful in differentiating asthma from diseases such as epiglottitis and aspiration of a foreign body.

Occasionally, cases of "asthma" will turn out to be, in fact, cases of aspiration of a foreign body and vice-versa. In older children, a history of acute gagging while eating peanuts or popcorn is almost diagnostic. The problem patient to diagnose is the child less than 4 years old, because only suspicion can lead to proper diagnosis. Inspiratory and expiratory chest x-rays or fluoroscopy can be helpful before bronchoscopy is considered.

Children with congenital disorders associated with obstructive airway disease (e.g., laryngotracheomalacia, anomalous subclavian artery syndrome) may worsen substantially during an acute viral illness and thus may appear to have severe asthma. Diagnosis is dependent upon careful history, physical and follow-up evaluations, and, sometimes, upon specialized procedures such as cinebronchography.

Clinical Studies

Pulmonary Function Testing and Response to Adrenergic Drugs

The diagnosis of status asthmaticus is often a clinical diagnosis based on failure of bronchodilator drugs to relieve severe respiratory obstruction.[57] While this may have to be ascertained by auscultation in the very young child, the index of improvement on auscultation can be very misleading. After a treatment with an aerosolized bronchodilator or an injection of epinephrine, the patient's air exchange may appear to improve. However, simultaneous pulmonary function tests may indicate only minimal improvement. Therefore, the clinical assessment of adrenergic responsiveness should be confirmed whenever possible by obtaining pulmonary function measurements before and after treatment with adrenergic drugs. In some children as young as 2 or 3 years, a peak expiratory flow measurement can be obtained as a means of documenting response. Most children who are 6 years of age or older are able to perform a forced vital capacity maneuver. Pulmonary function testing from which FEV_1 and $FEF_{25-75\%}$ can be observed before and after therapy is of great value in evaluating the degree of reversibility of airway obstruction.[58] The FEV_1/FVC percentage should not be used unless the FVC value is the *predicted normal,* not actual, value.

Table 15–1 shows an example of a child with acute asthma who is treated with a broncho-

Table 15–1. PULMONARY FUNCTION TEST RESULTS FOR A CHILD WITH ACUTE ASTHMA

Function	Predicted	Pre-bronchodilator	Post-bronchodilator
FVC (liters)	2.51	1.21 (48% predicted)	1.81 (72% predicted)
FEV_1 (liters)	2.01	0.61 (30% predicted)	0.81 (40% predicted)
FEV_1/FVC (%)	—	50%	44%
FEV_1/predicted normal FVC (%)	—	24%	32%

FVC—forced vital capacity.
FEV_1—forced expiratory volume in 1.0 second.
FEV_1/FVC—ratio of forced expiratory volume to forced vital capacity (%).

dilator. In this example, the pulmonary function has improved when compared with predicted normal values both in FVC and FEV_1. However, the FVC has improved to a greater degree than the FEV_1. Therefore, if one were to calculate the FEV_1/FVC percentage, the patient would have appeared to have worsened (from 50% to 44%); when the calculation was based on predicted FVC (from 24% to 32%) it indicated that he actually improved. Whenever possible, it is important to relate the post-therapy values to the patient's own optimal pulmonary function or at least to a table of normal values (Table 15–2). Often, the children whose bronchial obstructions appear to improve when evaluated by stethoscope will have post-treatment values so much lower than values obtained when they were well that hospitalization may be advisable.

SERUM THEOPHYLLINE LEVEL

A serum theophylline level should be obtained for any patient with poor response to bronchodilator, both as a guide to therapy if hospital admission is necessary, and to determine the need for additional theophylline. If the patient's theophylline level is low, a loading dose of 5 mg/kg theophylline may be administered to bring the serum concentration

Table 15–2. AVERAGE (50%) PULMONARY FUNCTION VALUES IN CHILDREN

Height		FVC (liters)		FEV_1	$FEF_{25-75\%}$		PEFR	
cm.	*in.*	*Boys*	*Girls*	*(liters)*	*L/min.*	*L/sec.*	*L/min.*	*L/sec.*
100	39.4	1.00	1.00	.70	55	.91	100	1.67
102	40.2	1.03	1.00	.75	60	1.00	110	1.83
104	40.9	1.08	1.07	.82	64	1.06	120	2.00
106	41.7	1.14	1.10	.89	70	1.17	130	2.17
108	42.5	1.19	1.19	.97	75	1.25	140	2.33
110	43.3	1.27	1.24	1.01	80	1.33	150	2.50
112	44.1	1.32	1.30	1.10	86	1.43	160	2.67
114	44.9	1.40	1.36	1.17	90	1.50	174	2.90
116	45.7	1.47	1.41	1.23	96	1.60	185	3.08
118	46.5	1.52	1.49	1.30	100	1.67	195	3.25
120	47.2	1.60	1.55	1.39	105	1.75	204	3.40
122	48.0	1.69	1.62	1.45	110	1.83	215	3.58
124	48.8	1.75	1.70	1.53	118	1.97	226	3.77
126	49.6	1.82	1.77	1.59	121	2.01	236	3.93
128	50.4	1.90	1.84	1.67	127	2.12	247	4.11
130	51.2	1.99	1.90	1.72	132	2.20	256	4.27
132	52.0	2.07	2.00	1.80	139	2.32	267	4.45
134	52.8	2.15	2.06	1.89	142	2.37	278	4.63
136	53.5	2.24	2.15	1.98	149	2.48	289	4.82
138	54.3	2.35	2.24	2.06	153	2.55	299	4.98
140	55.1	2.40	2.32	2.11	159	2.65	310	5.17
142	55.9	2.50	2.40	2.20	163	2.72	320	5.33
144	56.7	2.60	2.50	2.30	170	2.83	330	5.50
146	57.5	2.70	2.59	2.39	173	2.88	340	5.67
148	58.3	2.79	2.68	2.48	180	3.00	351	5.85
150	59.1	2.88	2.78	2.57	183	3.05	362	6.03
152	59.8	2.97	2.88	2.66	190	3.17	373	6.22
154	60.6	3.09	2.98	2.75	195	3.25	384	6.40
156	61.4	3.20	3.09	2.88	200	3.33	394	6.57
158	62.2	3.30	3.18	2.98	205	3.42	404	6.73
160	63.0	3.40	3.27	3.06	210	3.50	415	6.92
162	63.8	3.52	3.40	3.18	215	3.58	425	7.08
164	64.6	3.64	3.50	3.29	220	3.67	436	7.28
166	65.4	3.78	3.60	3.40	225	3.75	446	7.43
168	66.1	3.90	3.72	3.50	230	3.83	457	7.62
170	66.9	4.00	3.83	3.65	236	3.93	467	7.78
172	67.7	4.20	3.83	3.80	241	4.01	477	7.95
174	68.5	4.20	3.83	3.80	246	4.10	488	8.13
176	69.3	4.20	3.83	3.80	251	4.18	498	8.30

(Reproduced with permission from Polgar, G. and Promadhat, V.: Pulmonary Function Testing in Children: Techniques and Standards. Philadelphia: WB Saunders Company, 1971.)

FVC—forced vital capacity.

FEV_1—forced expiratory volume in 1.0 second.

$FEF_{25-75\%}$—forced expiratory flow at 25–75% vital capacity.

PEFR—peak expiratory flow rate (L/min).

into therapeutic range (10–20 μg/ml). The patient should be observed for an additional period. However, if the level is already therapeutic, more theophylline will not be helpful in promoting more bronchodilation, and the child should be admitted to the hospital.

ARTERIAL OR ARTERIALIZED BLOOD GAS LEVELS

The importance of obtaining arterial blood gas levels cannot be overemphasized as a guide to determining the adequacy of pulmonary gas exchange. However, it is a procedure frequently underutilized in children with asthma. Blood gas values provide information on the need for additional oxygen in the inspired air and are used to monitor carbon dioxide tension in arterial blood. Normally, the patient with airway-obstructive disease hyperventilates and Pa_{CO2} values will be in the high 20s or low 30s.[59] As airway obstruction increases, alveolar hypoventilation results in a rising Pa_{CO2} value. Hence, the patient with acute asthma who has a "normal" or elevated Pa_{CO2} tension ($\geq$ 40 mmHg) is in incipient respiratory failure, and should be admitted to the hospital at once for treatment.

Cyanosis is an alarming sign of severe respiratory distress. A cyanotic patient should be admitted to the intensive care unit immediately for treatment of acute respiratory failure with intubation and mechanical ventilation (see section on treatment of acute respiratory failure).

CHEST X-RAY

Children with asthma severe enough to require hospital admission should have a chest x-ray. Twenty-five per cent of children with acute asthma will have pulmonary infiltrates (atelectasis or viral pneumonia) and six per cent will have findings of pneumomediastinum or pneumothorax.[30] A "baseline" chest x-ray is useful also as a basis of comparison for children who develop pulmonary complications during hospitalization.

COMPLETE BLOOD COUNT

A red blood cell count and hematocrit determination will help assure adequate hemoglobin for maximal oxygen uptake. However, the white blood cell count may be a misleading indication of infection because both the stress of asthma and the treatment with epinephrine will induce leukocytosis with an increased number of PMNs.

Cytopathologic examinations of sputum or nasal mucus may provide a clue to the cause of the acute attack.[6] For example, a predominance of eosinophils suggests an allergic or "intrinsic" cause, while the predominance of PMNs or lymphocytes suggests an infectious cause.

Sputum samples are difficult to obtain from young children and therefore are rarely examined. However, sputum examination can be very useful. When sputum samples cannot be obtained, nasal secretions may be useful to help detect acute viral respiratory infections or acute infectious sinusitis. Layers of PMNs with ingested bacteria suggest a need to obtain sinus x-rays.

SERUM ELECTROLYTE LEVELS

Serum electrolyte levels should be obtained on admission as a guide to further therapy because many children with acute asthma may be dehydrated. An abnormally low or decreasing serum sodium level may indicate inappropriate ADH secretion (see section on extrapulmonary complications).

MANAGEMENT OF STATUS ASTHMATICUS

Pharmacology

OXYGEN

Though not ordinarily considered as a pharmacologic agent, humidified oxygen delivered at a final concentration (Fi_{O2}) to maintain Pa_{O2} $\geq$ 65 mmHg is an important adjunct in managing status asthmaticus. All patients who require hospitalization because of refractory asthma will have some degree of hypoxemia. Certain drugs that are employed frequently in treatment (e.g., epinephrine) may increase the myocardial oxygen need when arterial oxygen is already low. Leukotriene mediators,[60] which appear to be so important in severe asthma, may also reduce coronary artery blood flow and induce myocardial depression. The appropriate use of oxygen supports the myocardium and helps prevent arrhythmias.

INTRAVENOUS FLUIDS

Administration of intravenous fluids is essential for treatment of status asthmaticus, since the child is often dehydrated on admission because of vomiting, inadequate fluid intake, and greater insensible water loss from the increased work of breathing. Fluid therapy should be designed to replace fluid deficits as well as to provide for normal maintenance requirements. However, excessive fluid administration should be avoided, since pulmonary edema and hypovolemia with water intoxication may result.[62]

Overhydration may increase microvascular hydrostatic pressure and reduce plasma colloid osmotic pressure. These changes can lead to formation of pulmonary edema in the child who has asthma with substantial negative pleural pressure.[61] The problem of vasopressin excess and its relationship to hyponatremia and water intoxication is discussed on page 314.

If arterial pH is below 7.3 and the base deficit is greater than 5 mEq/L, intravenous sodium bicarbonate administration may be necessary to correct the metabolic acidosis of acute asthma.

Aminophylline (Theophylline Ethylene Diamine)

Aminophylline is an effective bronchodilator for children in status asthmaticus[63] and has become the keystone of intravenous drug therapy. It had been believed that aminophylline acted by increasing intracellular 3′,5′-cyclic adenosine monophosphate (cAMP) by inhibiting its phosphodiesterase degradation. This was thought, in turn, to promote bronchodilation by relaxing bronchial smooth muscle and inhibiting mediator secretion from mast cells. However, later studies have suggested that another mechanism or mechanisms may be involved. *In vitro* studies indicate that therapeutically effective theophylline levels do not inhibit cAMP degradation. Furthermore, papaverine, a far more active phosphodiesterase inhibiter, is not a bronchodilator.[64] Theophylline may act through inhibition of prostaglandin synthesis,[65] antagonism of adenosine receptors,[66] enhancement of cellular calcium uptake by smooth muscles,[67] stimulation of catecholamine secretion,[65] or increase of diaphragmatic contractibility.[69]

In status asthmaticus, aminophylline is usually administered as a loading dose in a volume of saline sufficient to dilute the drug 1:3, over 15 to 20 minutes. Its administration as a relatively rapid infusion will improve ventilation as measured by an increased FEV_1 while avoiding such adverse effects as cardiac arrhythmias.[70] Optimal bronchodilation occurs when the serum theophylline concentration is approximately 15 μg/ml.[71] With rapid infusion, this optimal range is quickly achieved. Once this concentration is reached, a maintenance infusion is administered at a rate suitable to match the disposition rate (zero-order kinetics).[72]

Aminophylline administration is complicated by a wide variety of factors that alter theophylline half-life. Individuals will clear the drug at their own rates. Viral infections,[73] fever,[74] concurrent medication usage,[75] and liver or heart disease[76] will alter an individual's clearance and, in turn, the theophylline dosage requirement. The theophylline half-life (T ½ is the time required to eliminate half of the dosage administered) is usually shorter in children than in adults.[77] Certain dosing guidelines have been established that help initiate aminophylline therapy. In general, each milligram per kilogram of aminophylline administered will increase its serum level by 2 μg/ml (until saturation kinetics are reached).[78] The loading dose in a patient not taking oral theophylline ranges from 5 to 7 mg/kg diluted in 25–50 ml of saline and given over 20 minutes. The maintenance infusion should be initiated at a rate of 0.85 mg/kg/hr for children 1–6 years old, 0.65 mg/kg/hr for children 7 to 16 years old, and 0.45 mg/kg/hr for patients older than 16 years. For infants less than 1 year of age, the maintenance dose can be derived from a regression formula, i.e., mg per day $= 0.3 \times$ age in weeks $+ 8$.[79] Intravenous aminophylline treatment consisting of a fourth of the calculated dosage of aminophylline administered intravenously every 6 hours may be preferred when constant infusion therapy is not practical.

During intravenous aminophylline therapy, the serum theophylline concentrations should be monitored for safety and effectiveness. An initial loading dose should not be administered to a patient who is receiving an oral theophylline preparation if the initial serum theophylline concentration is unknown. If this value cannot be obtained, the initial dosage must be adjusted on the basis of ingested theophylline administered over the 24 hours preceding admission. Serum theophylline concentrations should be obtained after the loading dose has equilibrated (approximately 1 hour after administration) and again after 6, 12, and 24 hours of intravenous therapy. Additional serum levels should be obtained if the patient has persistent heartburn, nausea, vomiting, or seizures, to rule out theophylline intoxication.[80, 81] Other adverse effects of theophylline include nervousness, anxiety and insomnia, headache, diarrhea, irritability, and cardiac arrhythmia at very high serum levels. If the serum concentration falls below 10 μg/ml, a booster dose of aminophylline should be administered and the serum concentration determined 1 hour later.

Whereas serum theophylline concentrations of 10–20 μg/ml provide maximal bronchodilation, levels close to 20 μg/ml may induce drug toxicity in some children but may be necessary for effectiveness in others.[82] If one wishes to maintain a level of 20 μg/ml with little fluctuation, a constant-infusion pump allows less variation than an ordinary controlled intravenous drip. Cardiac monitoring is advised when aminophylline is administered intravenously by continuous infusion. The chances of central nervous system irritability, headache, and gastrointestinal complaints increase when aminophylline level is more than 20 μg/ml. When levels are more than 40 μg/ml, life-threatening arrhythmias and seizures can occur. The consequences of inadvertent overdose are prolonged hospitalization or even seizures and irreversible brain damage.

After 24 to 48 hours of treatment, the patient's intravenous aminophylline therapy usually can be discontinued, and oral theophylline therapy can be initiated. The theophylline requirement for intravenous therapy can be used as a guideline for initiating oral therapy. In general, sustained-released theophylline preparations administered two or three times a day are most convenient.[83] The serum theophylline concentration should be determined during oral therapy once a steady-state level has been achieved.

β-Adrenergic Agents

β-adrenergic agents may be employed concurrently with aminophylline. Since they appear to act synergistically with theophylline, they add to the effectiveness of therapy. On admission, the child may respond poorly to β-adrenergic agents. However, aerosolized β-adrenergic agents become progressively more effective as the patient receives intravenous therapy. β-adrenergic agents bind to the β-adrenergic cellular receptor, which is thought to be adenylate cyclase the enzyme that converts ATP to 3′,5′-cyclic AMP. As intracellular cAMP increases, it promotes bronchodilation. Whereas subcutaneously injected epinephrine is commonly employed in treating acute asthma, its short duration of action and side effects (stimulation of α and β_1 as well as β_2 receptors) make it less desirable than drugs that can be administered by the aerosol route.[84]

Isoproterenol, which binds to both β_2 (lung) and β_1 (heart) receptors, has been used successfully for status asthmaticus. A 0.5% solution can be diluted ten-fold in saline and nebulized as a 0.05% solution with humidified oxygen at 6 L/min flow for 10 minutes for use in children. Effective bronchodilation can be achieved by administering it every 30 minutes for the first 2 hours and then as frequently as needed for bronchospasm. Because of its β_1 stimulation, cardiac monitoring should be employed, and administration of isoproterenol discontinued when the pulse rate exceeds 190 beats/min.[85] Pulmonary function tests performed immediately before and after aerosol therapy define the effectiveness of therapy and degree of reversibility of airway obstruction. The use of isoproterenol by intravenous administration is discussed in the section on the treatment of respiratory failure.

Isoetharine is an alternative catechol derivative with greater β_2 than β_1 selectivity. While it is one-tenth as active as isoproterenol on smooth muscle, it is one-fivehundredth as active on cardiac muscle.[86] Though isoetharine is a catechol compound and is degraded in the lung by catechol-O-methyltransferase (COMT), it has a slightly longer duration of action than isoproterenol. Unfortunately, pediatric dose-response studies for isoetharine have not been published. The adult dose of 2.5–5.0 mg diluted in saline and nebulized with oxygen at 6 L/min flow is modified arbitrarily for a child.

Metaproterenol, a resorcinol derivative, is not degraded by monamine oxidase (MAO) and COMT, making it both longer acting and more effective than isoetharine and isoproterenol.[85] In childhood status asthmaticus it has a slower onset of action than isoproterenol but has a substantially longer duration of action. Though pediatric dose-response studies have not been performed, metaproterenol can be used safely in a dosage of 0.1–0.2 ml (5–10 mg) of the five per cent solution diluted in 2 or 3 ml saline and nebulized with oxygen at 6 L/min flow. It can be repeated every 30 to 60 minutes during the first two hours and then as needed, provided that both cardiac rate and rhythm are monitored.

Terbutaline is another long-acting resorcinol derivative that appears to have greater β_2 selectivity than metaproterenol. Aerosolized terbutaline has been compared with metaproterenol and isoproterenol and appears to provide higher peak activity, longer duration of action, and less cardiac stimulation.[87, 88] Though terbutaline aerosol solution is not yet available, the parenteral solution can be employed by the aerosol route. This solution is available in a dose of 1 mg/ml, which is a lower dose than that recommended for pediatric use in Europe.

Metaproterenol is generally preferable for use in children because of its more appropriate concentration and substantially lower cost. Terbutaline should be reserved for special cases in which cardiac irritability is extreme or metaproterenol is ineffective. When terbutaline is used as an aerosol solution, it may be administered initially every 30 to 60 minutes and less frequently as the patient improves.

When the patient is well enough that intravenous therapy can be replaced by oral therapy, β-adrenergic agents can be administered orally or by aerosol nebulizer. The metaproterenol preparations commonly used are 10–20 mg orally every 4–6 hours or 5–10 mg (0.1–0.2 ml) diluted in normal saline as an aerosol every 2–4 hours.

Glucocorticosteroids

The use of intravenous glucocorticosteroids should be initiated promptly in status asthmaticus. Though the mechanism of action of steroids is not completely understood, several pharmacologic effects seem to be relevant. Corticosteroids increase the efficiency of the β-adrenergic system, restore responsiveness to β-adrenergic agents, and decrease pulmonary inflammation by diminishing migration and accumulation of neutrophil leukocytes. Corticosteroids also inhibit the synthesis of arachidonic acid–derived inflammatory mediators (lipoxygenase and cycloxygenase derivatives).[89] There is a delay of hours between the initiation of therapy and the beneficial effects to the asthmatic patient. Steroid molecules must diffuse into cells, bind to specific receptors, and be transferred to the nucleus where they interact with DNA to change its expression. New messenger RNA is then produced, and finally new protein is synthesized.[90] Both physiologic and metabolic changes can be detected approximately two hours after steroid administration.[91] While *in vitro* studies suggest that corticosteroid-induced changes occur within minutes, clinical studies show a delay of hours from time of administration to detection of physiologic effects.

Corticosteroids accelerate the recovery from status asthmaticus with a maximal effect occurring two to three days after beginning treatment. Pierson and coworkers[92] documented better arterial oxygen tensions in children who were treated with glucocorticosteroids compared with children who received placebo. In hospitalized infants with asthma, steroids have been shown to potentiate the effectiveness of β-adrenergic drugs.[93] In a recent study of children with acute asthma, steroid therapy improved small airway obstruction 24 hours after it was instituted but had minimal effectiveness on large airways as compared with the placebo-treated groups.[94] This finding may explain why several published studies have failed to show any beneficial effects of steroid therapy on lung function, since these studies employed measurements of only large airways.[95, 96]

Intravenous corticosteroid should be given as hydrocortisone hemisuccinate, dexamethasone phosphate, or betamethasone phosphate equivalent to 1–2 mg/kg of prednisone as a loading dose. It should be followed by an equivalent dosage over the next 24 hours by continuous infusion or by single dose every 4 to 6 hours. The use of higher dosages has not been beneficial.[97] When the patient is well enough to resume oral therapy, prednisone (1–2 mg/kg) in initiated as a single morning dose for at least 5 days or tapered gradually over 7 to 10 days.

Antibiotics

When respiratory infections cause status asthmaticus, they are almost always infections that will not respond to antibiotics. Antibiotics should be prescribed only when co-existing bacterial disease such as acute otitis media, acute or chronic sinusitis, or acute bacterial pneumonia is present. Randomized double-blind evaluations of broad spectrum antibiotic therapy compared to placebo have been carried out in children[98] and adults[99] with status asthmaticus. Not a single study has shown that antibiotics have benefited the patient who does not have a bacterial infection. When antibiotic therapy is necessary, the drug of choice and dosage will depend on the nature of the infection and the bacteria that are most likely involved.

Clinical Management[78]

General Treatment

The child with status asthmaticus should be managed in an intensive care unit or other facility where vital signs and overall condition can be monitored closely in a setting in which the physician, nurse, respiratory therapist, and consulting anesthesiologist can function as a team. Although the management of the child with status asthmaticus must be individualized, certain general principles apply to all patients.

Intravenous Fluids. Intravenous fluids should be administered to every patient with status asthmaticus. They are administered as 5 per cent glucose in normal saline for hydration with subsequent fluids for maintenance and depletion repair.

1. Initial hydration—12 ml/kg or 360 ml/m^2 for first hour (5% glucose in normal saline).
2. Maintenance—50 ml/kg/24 hours depending on age or 1500 ml/m^2/24 hours (5% glucose in water).
3. Depletion repair—normal saline, 10–15 ml/kg/24 hours or 300–500 ml/m^2 and water (5% glucose in water), 10–15 ml/kg/24 hours or 300–500 ml/m^2/24 hours.

Electrolytes

1. Potassium—2 mEq/100 ml of maintenance intravenous fluids
2. Sodium—3 mEq/100 ml of maintenance intravenous fluids

Buffers. If pH is below 7.30 and base deficit is greater than 5 mEq/L, correct to normal range with intravenous sodium bicarbonate as follows: mEq bicarbonate = (mEq) base excess × 0.3 × kg (body weight). Administer half the calculated dose initially and the other half after repeating blood gas determinations.

Intravenous Aminophylline (Theophylline Ethylenediamine).[63] Aminophylline is an effective agent for relieving bronchospasm when it is administered in sufficient concentration to achieve and maintain a serum level of 10–20 μg/ml. In the child who has not previously received theophylline, a loading dose should be administered followed by maintenance dosage with intravenous fluids. *Loading dosage* is 5–7 mg/kg diluted in 25–50 ml saline and given over 20 minutes by Vol-trol or infusion pump and modified on the basis of medication history or initial serum theophylline level. *Maintenance dosage* is 0.65 mg/kg/hr for children under 1 year of age, 0.85 mg/kg/hr for children 1 to 6 years of age, 0.65 mg/kg/hr for children 7 to 16 years of age, and 0.45 mg/kg/hr for patients more than 16 years of age. Aminophylline is administered by continuous-drip infusion (which is preferred) or given every 4 to 6 hours over 15 to 20 minutes.

Serum theophylline levels should be monitored, if possible, during therapy. An immediate theophylline serum level should be measured to determine the loading dose for patients who have received theophylline two hours before admission. If serum levels are not available, the loading dosage should be reduced appropriately, assuming an average theophylline half-life of three hours.

Corticosteroids. Intravenous corticosteroid therapy should be initiated immediately.[92] Short-term administration of steroids in high doses rarely, if ever, causes adverse effects. Dexamethasone phosphate (0.3 mg/kg stat and 0.3 mg/kg/24 hr), betamethasone (0.3 mg/kg stat and 0.3 mg/kg/24 hr by constant infusion or divided into four 6-hour doses), and hydrocortisone hemisuccinate (7 mg/kg stat and 7 mg/kg/24 hr) are all effective, although the first two appear to be more active.

Adrenergic Agents. After fluid, drug (aminophylline and corticosteroid), and oxygen therapy have been initiated, another trial of adrenergic agents by aerosol is appropriate, especially if acidosis has diminished and tachycardia has decreased. Aerosolized metaproterenol solution, 0.1 ml (5 mg)–0.2 (10 mg) in 2 ml saline or terbutaline (parenteral solution 1.0 mg in 2 ml saline), administered by a low-pressure ultrasonic or wall-mounted nebulizer may be given every half hour for the first two hours and at longer intervals as the patient improves. Adrenergic drugs (0.05% isoproterenol, 0.05% metaproterenol, 0.3% isoetharine, 0.5% salbutamol*, and 0.05% terbutaline†) are administered as adjuncts to theophylline therapy.[85] These drugs are administered by low-pressure ultrasonic or wall-mounted nebulizer for 5–10 minutes every half hour × 4, then as indicated by the patient's condition. The pulse should be monitored during each treatment. The treatment should be stopped when the pulse is ≥ 190 beats/minute.

Positive pressure ventilation should be avoided in children because of the danger of inducing greater bronchoconstriction, pneumomediastium, and pneumothorax.[100]

Cromolyn. The patient's use of cromolyn by turboinhaler is stopped at the time of admission because inhalation of the powder causes coughing.

Oxygen. Therapy is initiated with humidified oxygen delivered by Venturi mask, nasal prongs if tolerated, or appropriate oxygen tent (O_2 levels are monitored) and continued until Pa_{O_2} levels are stable in room air. The Fi_{O_2} should be adjusted to the patient's Pa_{O_2}.

---

*Not available in the United States.

†Available as a parenteral solution.

Antibiotics. Antibiotics are indicated only in children in whom bacterial disease is suspected.[97] There are no special indications for the use of antibiotics in asthma or other allergic disorders.

It is well to remember that:

Asthma is frequently accompanied by patchy atelectasis that is often misinterpreted on x-ray as bronchopneumonia.[30]

Leukocytosis of 15,000 WBC/mm^3 or more may occur in severe asthma in the absence of a demonstrable infection, particularly after administration of epinephine.

Sedatives. Patients with severe asthma have good reason to be extremely anxious, and their anxiety is the expression of their respiratory distress rather than the cause of it. *Sedatives are contraindicated in patients with status asthmaticus.*

Patient Monitoring

Clinical. Regular and systematic clinical, physiologic, and laboratory monitoring during therapy helps to ascertain the effectiveness of treatment and aids in early recognition of complications.[101]

Assessment of the patient's clinical course often is overlooked, but it is an important aspect of medical management of the patient with severe asthma. In order to make observations more objective and to aid in quantifying observations, a system similar to that devised by Silverman to score the progress of ideopathic respiratory distress syndrome of premature infants has been adapted for the clinical scoring of children being treated for status asthmaticus.[63] While this system is used in the United States to supplement other observations, it is a very useful tool in Third World countries when arterial blood gas studies and pulmonary function tests are difficult to obtain. The pulmonary index scoring system assigns numerial values to four physical signs: (1) respiratory rate, (2) ratio of inspirations to expirations, (3) presence or absence of accessory muscle utilization, and (4) presence of wheezing (Table 15–3).

Radiography. A chest x-ray should be performed on the patient at admission to identify the pulmonary factors that are complicating status asthmaticus and to serve as a baseline. Atelectasis and pulmonary infiltrates occur commonly (1 in 3 patients) and sometimes may involve an entire lobe. Pneumomediastinum, the next most common complication, may occur in 1 out of 20 children with status asthmaticus.[30] Pneumothorax occurs in approximately 1 out of 1000 patients admitted with acute asthma. Any patient who is doing poorly, or who suddenly begins to have increased respiratory distress, should have another chest x-ray to be compared with that obtained on admission.

Pulmonary Function Tests. Pulmonary function tests provide valuable data that cannot be obtained by physical examination. Children as young as 3 years of age can perform a peak expiratory flow rate maneuver (PEFR), which will provide a baseline measurement. As pulmonary obstruction is relieved by therapy, the PEFR should improve. A sudden worsening may be the first evidence of a pulmonary complication such as pneumomediastinum or atelectasis. Older children can usually perform a forced vital capacity (FVC) maneuver on a spirometer, which provides information concerning the forced vital capacity, forced expiratory volume in the first second of expiration (FEV_1), and forced expiratory flow during mid-expiration ($FEF_{25-75\%}$). The FEV_1 and $FEF_{25-75\%}$ measure the degree of airways ob-

Table 15–3. CLINICAL SCORING INDEX FOR FOLLOWING THE COURSE OF THERAPY OF STATUS ASTHMATICUS

Score	Respiratory Rate	Inspirations to Expirations Ratio	Accessory Respiratory Muscle Utilization	Wheezing*
0	<30	5:2	0	None
1	31–45	5:3–5:4	±	Terminal expirations or heard with stethoscope only
2	46–60	1:1	+ +	Entirely expirational or heard with stethoscope
3	>60	<1:1	+ + + +	Inspirational and expirational heard without stethoscope

*If no wheezing is audible owing to minimal air exchange, score 3.

struction in both small and large airways and are valuable objective measures of alterations in the degree of airway obstruction.

Pulmonary function should be assessed in the emergency room. Absence of a therapeutic response in the patient as measured by pulmonary function is the primary reason for hospital admission. After admission, spirometry should be used as another important measure of patient improvement. Ideally, it should be repeated every four to six hours during the first day of hospitalization and twice daily thereafter, until the patient's asthma is controlled. If FEV_1 and $FEF_{25-75\%}$ values begin to fall, spirometry should be performed more frequently to monitor the possible development of a pulmonary complication. Spirometric measurements before and after bronchodilation help to document the lack of reversibility of the airways, which is another parameter useful in determining the progress of the hospitalized patient.

Cardiovascular Monitoring. The physiologic consequence of acute asthma is hypoxemia.[48] While this condition by itself can produce adverse cardiovascular effects, the use of β-adrenergic drugs and aminophylline in the treatment of asthma stimulates the heart and increases its need for oxygen when the patient is relatively hypoxemic. Certain inflammatory mediators including the leukotrienes may induce coronary artery constriction that further decreases the blood flow to the cardiac muscle.[37] Arrhythmias may occur unexpectedly owing to these factors during the course of status asthmaticus, even in children. Continuous monitoring of heart rate and rhythm should be carried out during therapy of status asthmaticus until the patient's asthma has improved sufficiently to restore oral therapy.

Monitoring of Blood Gas and Serum Electrolyte Levels. Blood gas determinations are extremely important in the child with severe asthma in that they provide objective measurements of the adequacy of alveolar ventilation and blood oxygenation. Arterial blood gas analysis is most accurate, but for baseline or follow-up values "arterialized" blood (warming the hand for 10 minutes prior to drawing the capillary blood) can be a useful substitute in small children.[102] In the very sick patient, the insertion of an intra-arterial line facilitates repeated sampling without further discomfort to the child. If the initial Pa_{CO_2} is 40 mmHg or higher, the patient must be considered to be in impending respiratory failure. A Pa_{CO_2} value greater than 50 mmHg indicates respiratory failure and requires immediate provisions for assisted ventilation (see section on respiratory failure).

Serum electrolyte values should be obtained on admission as a guide to intravenous fluid therapy. They are especially important in a child who is vomiting or febrile. While unusual, "inappropriate" antidiuretic hormone response can occur in patients with severe asthma.[62] It is manifested by low urine output and reduced serum sodium concentration in association with excessive urinary sodium output (see section on complications of asthma).

Theophylline Monitoring. Therapeutic monitoring of serum theophylline levels is essential for patients with severe asthma, both to assure adequate therapy and to avoid theophylline toxicity. Since the majority of patients admitted with asthma have been receiving theophylline, an arbitrary "loading dose" should not be given without knowledge of the theophylline serum concentrations *on admission.* A number of factors may influence theophylline serum levels, even in patients whose pre-admission theophylline levels have been in steady state for weeks to months. Theophylline metabolism can be decreased by high fever,[74] liver disease,[76] and macrolide antibiotics, including erythromycin.[75] Influenza B infections may reduce metabolism for weeks to months, and even influenza immunizations may alter theophylline serum half-life.[73]

During intravenous therapy with aminophylline, periodic monitoring of theophylline levels is important, particularly in the child who is vomiting, who has cardiac arrhythmias, or who is not improving.

COMPLICATIONS OF ASTHMA

Complications of asthma may be pulmonary or extrapulmonary. Pulmonary complications include (1) acute respiratory failure, (2) atelectasis, (3) pneumomediastinum and pneumothorax, and (4) superimposed infections (pneumonia, empyema). Extra-pulmonary complications include (1) vasopressin excess, (2) flaccid paralysis of an arm or leg, (3) sudden alteration in theophylline metabolism, and (4) cardiac arrhythmia. Pulmonary and extrapulmonary factors may combine to cause acute respiratory failure accompanied by resulting cardiorespiratory arrest with brain damage or death.

Pulmonary Complications

Respiratory Failure

Respiratory failure occurs in a small but significant number of children admitted to the hospital with status asthmaticus.[103] It often occurs because the physician has failed to recognize the severity of the child's asthma. *The best treatment of respiratory failure is prevention by means of effective early treatment of asthma.* Signs of overt respiratory failure include decrease or absence of pulmonary breath sounds, severe intercostal retraction, pulsus paradoxus, use of accessory muscles of respiration, cyanosis in the presence of 40 per cent oxygen, reduced response to pain, poor skeletal muscle tone, and profuse diaphoresis.

These signs indicate an extreme emergency and mandate immediate treatment for acute respiratory failure with intravenous isoproterenol or mechanical ventilation.

The presence of a rising $Pa_{CO_2} > 45$ mmHg and a $Pa_{O_2} < 55$ mmHg in 40 per cent oxygen confirms the diagnosis of respiratory failure and the need for prompt emergency treatment.

Arterial blood gas tensions and pH must be monitored frequently in a distressed child. Impending respiratory failure cannot be diagnosed from clinical signs alone. For example, a rise of Pa_{CO_2} from 39 to 44 mmHg in one hour in an exhausted child who is receiving maximal therapy should be considered respiratory failure and treated as discussed later

Although several groups have reported extensive experience in management of respiratory failure with intravenous isoproterenol,[106, 107] they have had many treatment failures that have necessitated mechanical ventilation. In general, the use of intravenous isoproterenol remains controversial as a method of treating respiratory failure due to asthma in children. It is thought to be contraindicated in adults because of potentially serious cardiovascular side effects from intravenously administered isoproterenol. For completeness, we have included a proposed regimen for isoproterenol.

Intravenous isoproterenol therapy should never be initiated without all facilities and personnel for intubation and mechanical ventilation on hand.

Intravenous Isoproterenol. Therapy with intravenous isoproterenol must be carried out in a properly equipped intensive care unit with continuous cardiac monitoring and a calibrated constant-infusion pump. An intra-arterial catheter must be in place for monitoring blood gas tension. If the physician elects to treat the patient with intravenous isoproterenol, the anesthesiologist should be consulted first so that all facilities for mechanical ventilation are immediately available. This arrangement is especially important for the child who has received excessive quantities of β-adrenergic agents before admission, because isoproterenol may precipitate worsening of respiratory failure.[106] After an initial starting dose of 0.1 μg/kg/min delivered with a constant-infusion pump, the isoproterenol dosage is increased at the rate of 0.1 μg/kg/min every 15–20 minutes until there is clinical improvement, tachycardia of 200 beats/minute, or development of arrhythmia. Hazards include cardiac arrhythmia, myocarditis, and subendocardial necrosis. An essential part of therapy is a staff thoroughly familiar with this treatment. A proposed alternative to isoproterenol is constant nebulization with terbutaline, 1 mg/ml diluted in saline and aerosolized with oxygen. Again, cardiac monitoring should be continuous and arterial blood gas tensions should be monitored frequently.

Mechanical Ventilation. Mechanical ventilation requires endotracheal intubation, neuromuscular blockade, and sedation.[107] A volume-controlled ventilator with constant monitoring of ECG and an intra-arterial line for frequent blood gas determinations must be employed to ensure adequate alveolar ventilation. Once stabilized, the patient can be given intermittent mandatory ventilation and generally can be weaned in 24 to 48 hours. Pneumomediastinum, pneumothorax, cardiac arrhythmia, and unintentional extubation makes mechanical ventilation a complicated procedure that should be performed only in adequately equipped and staffed tertiary care centers.

Atelectasis

Approximately a third to a fourth of all hospitalized asthmatic children have pulmonary complications such as pneumonia and atelectasis.[30] In a study of 465 children admitted for asthma, 20 per cent had pulmonary infiltrates involving multiple lobes. Perihilar interstitial infiltrates varied in severity from increased bronchovascular markings to shaggy, diffuse peribronchial viral pneumonia. Atelectasis of all or part of a lobe was the next most common complication, occurring in 10 per cent of admissions and involving the right middle lobe most frequently. The right middle lobe is particularly susceptible to atelectasis because of anatomic factors, e.g., the right main-stem bronchus tends to twist with hyperinflation, resulting in its partial occlusion.[31] Why right-middle lobe atelectasis develops in girls more frequently than in boys is not clear.[108]

The treatment of atelectasis should be conservative. In most cases it will resolve when the asthma is controlled. Respiratory therapy consisting of postural drainage and clapping is helpful. Intermittent positive pressure breathing (IPPB) therapy should be avoided, since it is likely to induce pneumomediastinum or pneumothorax.[99] If atelectasis persists, the presence of a foreign body, an anatomic defect, or an obstructing peribronchial lymph node should be considered. Fiberoptic bronchoscopy may be useful if a foreign body is suspected.

Pneumomediastinum and Pneumothorax

In status asthmaticus, five per cent of patients may develop the complication of extrapulmonary air.[31] Shearing forces from coughing and bronchospasm superimposed on hyperinflation related to atelectasis or pneumonia and possible structural weakness cause air to rupture alveolar bases and to dissect along blood vessel sheaths.[109] This condition results in pulmonary interstitial emphysema. It manifests as a worsening clinical course associated with reduced venous return, decreased cardiac output, and lowered blood pressure. Air dissects along great vessel sheaths to the mediastinum, pericardium, and along the aorta to the intestinal wall or along fascial planes into the neck. While this air remains under high pressure, asthma symptoms worsen and pre-cardiac dullness disappears. The air may escape into the relatively low pressure subcutaneous tissue of the neck and axilla, resulting in crepitant subcutaneous emphysema.

Rarely, pneumothorax complicates childhood asthma. It may be self-limited if small or it may severely compromise breathing. Bilateral pneumothorax may be the cause of sudden death in asthma.[110] Tension pneumothorax that results from the rupture of a pleural bleb needs decompression with a chest tube and underwater suction. On the other hand, a pneumothorax secondary to air rupturing through parietal pleura into the pleural space from a pneumomediastinum is less serious and may be treated conservatively; often it will clear with treatment of the asthma.

Extrapulmonary Complications

Vasopressin Excess (Inappropriate ADH Secretion)

The release of ADH is regulated through such mechanisms as: (1) pain, fear, and drugs acting on higher CNS centers, (2) a drop in arterial pressure, (3) an increase in the plasma concentration of non-diffusible solute perfusing the hypothalamus ≥280 mOsm/L, and (4) a decreased stimulation of stretch receptors in the left atrium. When filling of the left atrium is reduced, the vagal nerve stimulates the hypothalamus to secrete vasopressin. In severe asthma, vasopressin levels are elevated regardless of the serum sodium concentrations, apparently because of the effect of severe asthma on the pulmonary circulation. Vasopressin levels fall as the patient improves.[62, 111]

The criteria for the diagnosis of vasopressin excess are:

1. Hyponatremia that is associated with plasma hypo-osmolality.
2. Continuing renal excretion of sodium in presence of hyponatremia.
3. Absence of any evidence of dehydration.
4. Urinary osmolality value that is greater than plasma osmolality value.
5. Normal kidney and adrenal function.

The treatment of vasopressin excess involves three general principles: First, severe asthma must be corrected with appropriate therapy. Second, water intake and body weight, plasma electrolyte concentration and osmolarity, and urine volume and osmolality must be monitored closely, and fluid intake should be restricted to the minimal amount compatible with control of asthma. Third, complications such as water intoxication with seizures should be treated with hypertonic saline (20 ml/100 kcal of 1.5% NaCl) plus furosemide. One rarely needs to use hypertonic saline and furosemide, if one corrects the underlying asthma.

Sudden Alteration in Theophylline Metabolism. Theophylline clearance may be decreased by fever or specific viral diseases such as influenza B[73] or infectious mononucleosis. Aminophylline should be used cautiously in febrile patients, and dosage should be regulated by serial therapeutic serum monitoring in order to avoid serious theophylline toxicity. The theophylline requirement may increase because of third compartment filling secondary to edema and inappropriate ADH secretion. This condition could lead to theophylline toxicity when the patient's pulmonary status improves.

ALGORITHM FOR THE TREATMENT OF ACUTE ASTHMA

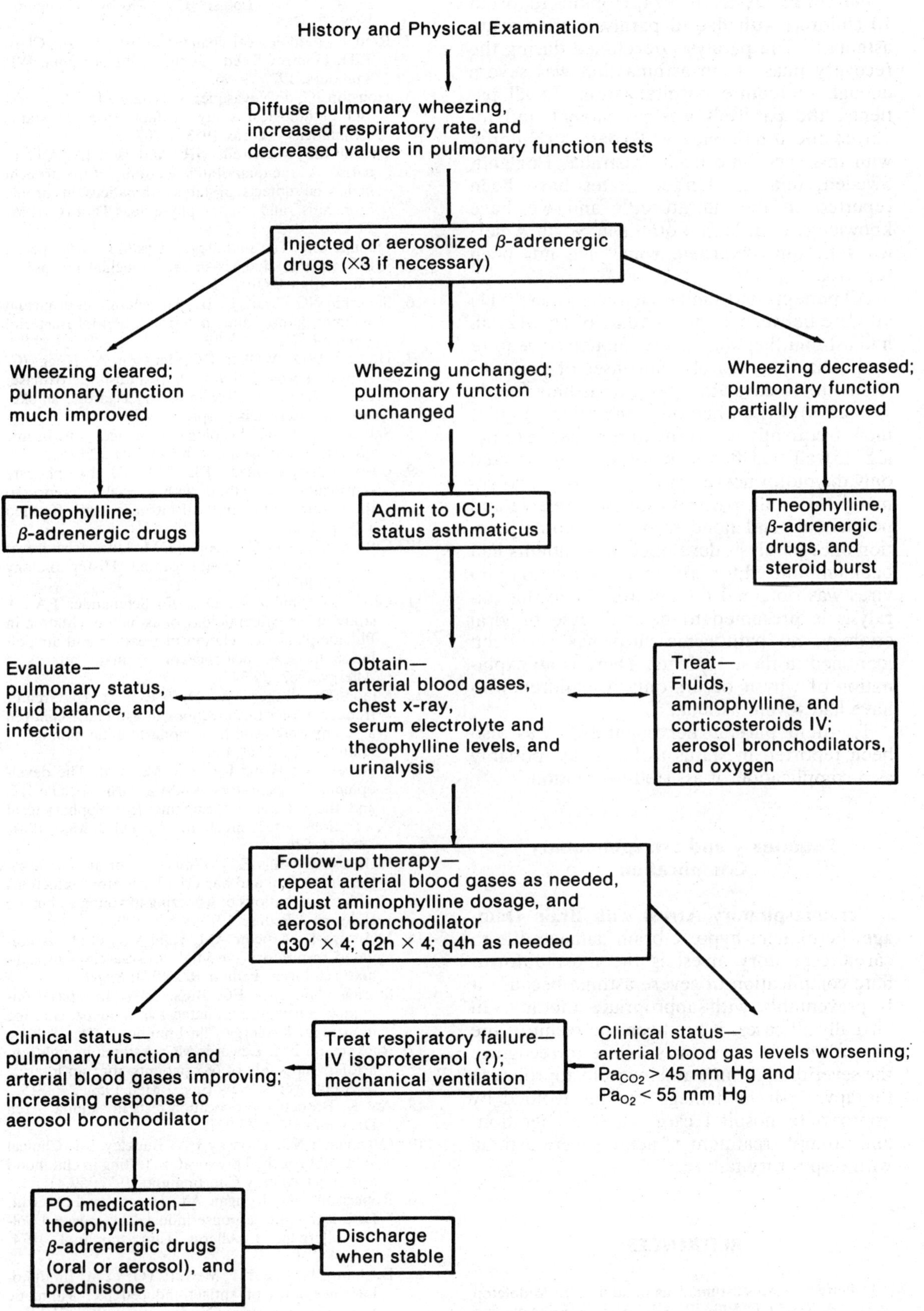

Flaccid Paralysis. In 1974, Hopkins reported 10 children with flaccid paralysis after acute asthma.[112] The paralysis developed during the recovery phase from asthma that was severe enough to require hospitalization. In all patients, the paralysis was permanent and involved one arm or one leg. To date, 19 children with this syndrome from Australia, England, Sweden, and the United States have been reported in the literature,[113] and we have knowledge of at least 4 others in North America with this syndrome who have not been reported.

All patients had similar characteristics:[114] (1) all were between 1 and 11 years of age, (2) all had asthma that was severe enough to require hospitalization, (3) all had onset of paralysis from 4 to 11 days after onset of asthma (mode = 5 days), (4) all had only one affected limb, more frequently it was the arm rather than the leg, (5) all had flaccid paralysis that affected only the motor nerves with no sensory involvement, (6) in all, paralysis was progressive and permanent; and none recovered motor function once paralysis developed. All patients had been immunized for poliomyelitis and no polio virus was obtained on culture. While this paralysis is presumed to be a disease of viral etiology, no pathogenic virus has yet been identified in these patients. There is no explanation of why it occurs only in children who have had severe asthma.

Transient phrenic nerve paralysis has also been reported in status asthmaticus, possibly as a complication of assisted ventilation.[115]

Pulmonary and Extrapulmonary Complication

Cardiorespiratory Arrest with Brain Damage. Permanent hypoxic brain damage due to cardiorespiratory arrest is the most unfortunate complication of severe asthma because it is preventable with appropriate therapy. In virtually all cases, it has been the result of the parent's or the physician's failure to recognize the severity of asthma and institute appropriate therapy.[116] Brain damage can be avoided by appropriate hospital care, early recognition, and prompt treatment of acute severe asthma with respiratory failure.

REFERENCES

1. Petty T. Status asthmaticus in adults. *In:* Middleton E, Reed CE, Ellis EF, eds. Allergy: Principle and Practice. St. Louis: CV Mosby Company, 1978:771–784.
2. Reid L. Pathological changes in asthma. *In:* Clark TJH, Godfrey S, eds. Asthma. Philadelphia: WB Saunders, 1977:79–96.
3. Houston JC, de Nevasquez S, Trounce JR. A clinical and pathological study of fatal cases of status asthmaticus. Thorax 1953; *8*:207.
4. Dunnill MS, Massarella GR, Anderson JA. A comparison of the quantitative anatomy of the bronchi in normal subjects, in status asthmaticus, in chronic bronchitis and in emphysema. Thorax 1969; *24*:176.
5. Dunnill MS. The pathology of asthma with special reference to changes in the bronchial mucosa. J Clin Pathol 1960; *13*:27.
6. Sanerkin NG, Evans DMD. The sputum in bronchial asthma: pathognomic patterns. J Pathol Bacteriol 1965; *89*:535.
7. Hulbert WD, Walker DC, Jackson A, Hogg JC. Airway permeability to horseradish peroxidase: the repair phase after injury by cigarette smoke. Am Rev Resp Dis (in press).
8. Salvato G. Some histological changes in chronic bronchitis and asthma. Thorax 1968; *23*:168.
9. Caspary EA, Feimann EL, Field EJ. Lymphocyte sensitization in asthma with special reference to the nature and identity of intrinsic form. Br Med J 1973; *1*:15.
10. Cutz E, Levison H, Cooper DM. Ultrastructure of airways in children with asthma. Histopathology 1978; *2*:407–421.
11. Girsh LS, Shubin E, Dick C, Schulander FA. A study of the epidemiology of asthma in children in Philadelphia: the relation of weather and air pollution to peak incidence of asthmatic attacks. J Allergy 1967; *39*:347.
12. Minor TE, Baker JW, Dick EC, et al. Greater frequency of viral infections in asthmatic children as compared with their nonasthmatic siblings. J Pediatr 1974; *85*:474.
13. Welliver RC, Wong DT, Sun M, et al. The development of respiratory syncytial virus specific IgE and the release of histamine in nasopharyngeal secretions after infection. N Engl J Med 1981; *305*:841–846.
14. McIntosh K, Ellis E, Hoffman LS, et al. The association of viral and bacterial respiratory infections with exacerbations of wheezing in young asthmatic children. J Pediatr 1973; *4*:578–590.
15. McIntosh K, Arbeter AM, Stahl MK, et al.: Attenuated respiratory syncytial virus vaccines in asthmatic children. Pediatr Res 1974; *8*:689.
16. Storms WW, Dick EC, Busse WW. Intranasal immunization with attenuated live influenza vaccine in asthma. J Allergy Clin Immunol 1976; *58*:284.
17. Rackemann FM, Edwards MC. Asthma in children: a follow-up study of 688 patients after an interval of twenty years. New Engl J Med 1952; *246*:815.
18. Aas K. Bronchial provocation tests in asthma. Arch Dis Child 1970; 45:221.
19. Cavanaugh MJ, Bronsky EA, Buckley JM. Clinical value of bronchial provocation testing in childhood asthma. J Allergy Clin Immunol 1977; 59:41.
20. Robertson DG, Kerigan AT, Hargreave FE, et al. Late asthmatic response induced by ragweed pollen allergen. J Allergy Clin Immunol 1974; *54*:244–254.
21. Durham SR, Lee TH, Merrett TG, et al. Immunological studies of antigen-induced late asthmatic responses. J Allergy Clin Immunol 1983; *71*:146.

22. Boushey HA, Holtzman MJ, Shelles JR, Nadel JA. State of the art: bronchial hyperreactivity. Am Rev Resp Dis 1980; *121*:384–413.
23. Lopez M, Salvaggio JE. Nonimmune Environmental Factors in Allergic Disease. *In:* Bierman CW, Pearlman DW, eds. Allergic Diseases of Infancy, Childhood and Adolescence. Philadelphia: WB Saunders, 1980:260–269.
24. Nadel JA. Autonomic control of airway smooth muscle and airway secretions. Am Rev Resp Dis 1977; *115*(Suppl 6, II):117.
25. Koenig JQ, Pierson WE, Horike M, Frank R. Bronchoconstrictor responses to sulfur dioxide or sulfur dioxide plus sodium chloride droplets in allergic nonasthmatic adolescents. J Allergy Clin Immunol 1982: *69*:339–344.
26. Rachelefsky GS, Coulsan A, Siegle SC, Stiehn ER. Aspirin intolerance in chronic childhood asthma: detected by oral challenge. Pediatrics 1975; *56*:443.
27. Szczeklik A, Gryglewski RJ, Czerniawska-Mysik G, et al. Aspirin-induced asthma. J Allergy Clin Immunol 1976; *58*:10.
28. Kinsman RA, Dahlem NW, Spector S, Standenmeyer H. Observations on subjective symptomology, coping behavior, and medical decision in asthma. Psychosom Med 1977; *39*:102.
29. Klieger JH, Dirks JF. Medication compliance in chronic asthmatic patients. J Asthma Res 1979; *16*:93.
30. Eggleston PA. Exercise-induced Asthma. *In:* Bierman CW, Pearlman DS, eds. Allergic Diseases of Infancy, Childhood and Adolescence. Philadelphia: WB Saunders Company, 1980:605–611.
31. Simons FER, Chernick V. Principles of Diagnosis and Treatment of Lower Respiratory Tract Disease. *In:* Bierman CW, Pearlman DS, eds. Allergic Diseases of Infancy, Childhood and Adolescence. Philadelphia: WB Saunders Company, 1980:535–549.
32. Hogg JC, Williams J, Richardson JB, et al. Age as a factor in the distribution of lower-airway conductance and in the pathologic anatomy of obstructive lung disease. N Engl J Med 1970: *282*:1283.
33. Field WE. Mucous gland hypertrophy in babies and children aged 15 years or less. Br J Dis Chest 1968; *62*:11.
34. Lauson D, Fewtrell C, Gamperts B, Roff MC. Anti-immunoglobulin induced histamine secretion of rat peritoneal mast cells studied by immunoferritin electron microscopy. J Exp Med 1975; *142*:391.
35. Bourne HR, Lichtenstein LM, Herney CS, et al. Modulation of inflammation and immunity by cyclic AMP. Science 1974; *184*:19.
36. MacGlashan DW Jr, Schleimer RP, Peters SP, et al. Generation of leukotrienes by purified human lung mast cells. J Clin Invest 1982; *70*:747–751.
37. Marom Z, Shelhamer JH, Bach MK, et al. Slow-reacting substances, leukotrienes C_4 and D_4, increase the release of mucus from human airways in vitro. Am Rev Respir Dis 1982; *126*:449–451.
38. Marom Z, Steel L. Shelhamer J, et al. Prostaglandin-generation factor of anaphylaxis increases mucous glycoprotein secretion and HETE formation from human airways. Clin Res 1982; *30*:479A.
39. Matthews KP. Respiratory Atopic Disease. *In:* Primer on allergic and immunologic diseases. JAMA 1982; *248*:2595–2598.
40. Schellenberg RR, Walker B, Snyder F. Platelet-dependent contraction of human bronchus by platelet activating factor. J Allergy Clin Immunol 1983; *71*:145.
41. Hugli TE. Human anaphylatoxin (C3a) from the third component of complement: primary structure. J Biol Chem 1975; *250*:8293–8305.
42. Snyderman R, Goetzel EJ. Molecular and cellular mechanisms of leukocyte chemotaxis. Science 1981; *213*:830–836.
43. Weissmann G. Eicosanoids of asthma. N Engl J Med 1983; *308*:454–455.
44. Ayers GH, Altman GL, Gleich GL, et al. Eosinophilic major basic protein causes pneumocyte cytolysis. J Allergy Clin Immunol 1983; *71*:139.
45. Cohen S, Pick E, Oppenheim JJ, eds. Biology of the Lymphokines. New York: Academic Press, 1979.
46. Weller PF, Goetzel EZ. The regulatory and effector roles of eosinophils. Adv Immunol 1979; *27*:339–371.
47. Ruth WE, Andrews CE. Airway resistance studies in bronchial asthma. J Lab Clin Med 1959; *54*:889.
48. McFadden ER Jr, Lyons HA. Airway resistance and uneven ventilation in bronchial asthma. J Appl Physiol 1968; *25*:365.
49. Mishkin FS, Wagner HN Jr, Tow DE. Regional distribution of pulmonary arterial blood flow in acute asthma. JAMA 1968; *203*:1019.
50. Griffin JT, Kass I, Hoffman MS. Cor pulmonale associated with symptoms and signs of asthma in children. Pediatrics 1959; *24*:54.
51. Weng TR, Langer HM, Featherby EA, Leison H. Arterial blood gas tensions and acid-base balance in symptomatic and asymptomatic asthma in childhood. Am Rev Resp Dis 1970; 101:274.
52. Rebuck AS, Read J. Assessment and management of severe asthma. Am J Med 1971; *51*:788.
53. Rees HA, Millar JS, Donald KW. A study of the clinical course and arterial blood gas tensions of patients in status asthmaticus. J Med 1968; *37*:541.
54. Banner AS, Ranchhodlal SS, Whitney WA. Rapid prediction of need for hospitalization in acute asthma. JAMA 1976; *235*:1335–1337.
55. Siegel SC, Katz RM, Rachelefsky GS. Asthma in Infancy and Childhood. *In:* Middleton E, Reed CE, Ellis EF, eds. Allergy: Principle and Practice. St. Louis: CV Mosby Company, 1978.
56. Paisley JW. Infection and Allergy. *In:* Bierman CW, Pearlman PS, eds. Allergic Diseases of Infancy, Childhood and Adolescence. Philadelphia: WB Saunders Company, 1980:270–281.
57. McFadden ER Jr, Kisir R, DeGroot WS. Acute bronchial asthma. N Engl J Med 1973; *288*:221–225.
58. Leffert F. The management of acute severe asthma. J Pediatr 1980: *96*:1–12.
59. McFadden ER Jr, Lyons HA. Arterial blood gas tensions in asthma. N Engl J Med 1968; *278*:1027.
60. Lewis RA, Austen KF. Mediation of local homeostasis and inflammation by leukotrienes and other mast cell-dependent compounds. Nature 1981; *293*:103–108.
61. Stalcup SA, Mellins RB. Mechanical forces producing pulmonary edema in acute asthma. New Engl J Med 1977; *297*:592–596.
62. Segar WE, Chesney RW. Disorders of electrolyte metabolism. Pediatr Ann 1981; *10*:288.
63. Pierson WE, Bierman CW, et al.: Double-blind trial of aminophylline in status asthmaticus. Pediatrics 1971; *46*:642.
64. Leoffler LJ, Lovenberg W, Sjordsma A. Effects of

dibutyryl 3'5' cyclic adenosine monophosphate, phosphodiesterase inhibitors and prostaglandin E, on compound 48/80-induced histamine release from rat peritoneal mast cells in vitro. Biochem Pharmacol 1971; *20*:2287–2297.

65. Horrobin OF, Marku JS, Franks DJ, Hamet P. Methyl xanthine phosphodiesterase inhibitors behave as prostaglandin antagonists in a perfused rat mesenteric artery preparations. Prostaglandins 1977; *13*:33.
66. Fredholm BB. Theophylline actions on adenosine receptors. Eur J Resp Dis 1980; *61*(Suppl 109):29.
67. Kolbeck RC, Speir WA, Carrier GO, Bransome ED Jr. Apparent irrelevance of cyclic nucleotides to the relaxation of tracheal smooth muscle induced by theophylline. Lung 1977; *156*:178.
68. Higbee MD, Kumar M, Galant SP. Stimulation of endogenous catecholamine release by theophylline: a proposed additional mechanism of action for theophylline effects. J Allergy Clin Immunol 1982; *70*:377–382.
69. Aubier M, DeTroyer A, Simpson M, et al. Aminophylline improves diaphragmatic contractility. N Engl J Med 1981; *305*:349–352.
70. Mitenko PA, Ogilvie RI. Rational intravenous doses of theophylline. N Engl J Med 1973; *289*:600–603.
71. Weinberger M. Theophylline for treatment of asthma. J Pediatr 1978; *92*:1–7.
72. Vozek S, Kewitz G, Perruchoud A, et al. Theophylline serum concentration and therapeutic effect in severe acute bronchial obstruction: the optimal use of intravenously administered aminophylline. Am Rev Resp Dis 1982; *125*:181–184.
73. Kraemer MJ, Furukawa CT, Kaup JR, et al. Altered theophylline clearance during an influenza B outbreak. Pediatrics 1982; *69*:476–480.
74. Chang KC, Bell T, Laver BA, et al. Altered theophylline pharmacokinetics during acute respiratory viral illness. Lancet 1978; *1*:1132–1134.
75. Weinberger M, Hudgel D, Spector S, et al. Inhibition of theophylline clearance by troleandomycin. J Allergy Clin Immunol 1977; *59*:228–231.
76. Mangione A, Imhoff TE, Lee RV, et al. Pharmacokinetics of theophylline in hepatic disease. Chest 1978; *73*:616–622.
77. Ellis EF, Kaysooko R, Levy G. Pharmacokinetics of theophylline in children with asthma. Pediatrics 1976; *58*:542–547.
78. Easton J, Hillman B, Shapiro GG, Weinberger M. American Academy of Allergy, Section on Allergy and Immunology: Management of Asthma. Pediatrics 1981; *68*(6):874–879.
79. Maselli R, Casal GL, Ellis EF. Pharmacologic effects of intravenously administered aminophylline in asthmatic children. J Pediatr 1970; *76*:777–782.
80. Weinberger MW, Matthay RA, Ginihansky EJ, et al. Intravenous aminophylline dosage: use of serum theophylline measurement for guidance. JAMA 1976; *235*:2110–2113.
81. Fox J, Hicks P, Feldman BR, et al.: Theophylline blood levels as a guide to intravenous therapy in children. Am J Dis Child 1982; *136*:928–930.
82. Ahrens RC, Hendeles L, Weinberger M. The clinical pharmacology of drugs used in the treatment of asthma. *In* Yaffe SJ, ed. Pediatric Pharmacology. New York: Grune & Stratton, Inc. 1980:243–259.
83. Weinberger M, Hendeles L, Bighley L. Relationship of product formulation to absorption of oral theophylline. N Engl J Med 1978; *299*:852–857.
84. Becker AB, Nelson NA, Simons FER. Inhaled salbutamol (albuterol) vs. injected epinephrine in the treatment of acute asthma in children. J Pediatr 1983; *102*:465–469.
85. Garra B, Shapiro GG, Dorsett CS, et al. A double-blind evaluation of the use of nebulized metaproterenol and isoproterenol in hospitalized asthmatic children and adolescents. J Allergy Clin Immunol 1977; *60*:63–68.
86. Herschtus J, Bresnick E, Levinson L, et al. A new sympathomimetic amine in the treatment of bronchial asthma. Ann Allergy 1951; *9*:769–773.
87. Roth MJ, Wilson AF, Novey HS. A comparative study of the aerosolized bronchodilators isoproterenol, metaproterenol and terbutaline in asthma. Ann Allergy 1977; *38*:16–21.
88. Chester EH, Doggett WE, Montenegro HD, et al. Bronchodilating effect of terbutaline aerosol. Clin Pharmacol Ther 1978; *23*:630–634.
89. Shapiro GG. Corticosteroids in the treatment of allergic disease: principles and practice. Pediatr Clin North Am 1983; *30*:995–971.
90. Morris HG. Factors that influence clinical responses to administered corticosteroids. J Allergy Clin Immunol 1980; *66*:343–346.
91. Subcommittee on Clinical Trials, British Medical Research Council: Controlled trial of effects of cortisone acetate in status asthmaticus. Lancet 1956; *2*:803–806.
92. Pierson WE, Bierman CW, Kelly VC. A double-blind trial of corticosteroid therapy in status asthmaticus. Pediatrics 1974; *54*:282–288.
93. Tal A, Barilski C, Yohai D, et al. Dexamethasone and salbutamol in the treatment of acute wheezing in infants. Pediatrics 1983; *71*:13–18.
94. Shapiro GG, Furukawa CT, Pierson WE, et al. Double-blind evaluation of methylprednisolone versus placebo for acute asthma episodes. Pediatrics 1983; *71*:510–514.
95. Luksza ARP. Acute severe asthma treated without steroids. Br J Dis Chest 1982; 76:15–19.
96. Kattan M, Gurwitz D, Levison H. Corticosteroids in status asthmaticus. J Pediatr 1980; *96*:596–599.
97. Harfi H, Hanissian AS, Crawford LV. Treatment of status asthmaticus in children with high doses and conventional doses of methylprednisolone. Pediatrics 1978; *61*:829–831.
98. Graham VAL, Knowles GK, Milton AR, Davies RJ. Routine antibiotics in hospital management of acute asthma. Lancet 1982; *1*:418–421.
99. Shapiro GG, Eggleston PA, Pierson WE, et al. Double-blind study of the effectiveness of a broad spectrum antibiotic in status asthmaticus. Pediatrics 1974; *53*:867–873.
100. Alveolar rupture (commentary). Lancet 1978; *2*:137.
101. Bierman CW, Pierson WE. The pharmacologic management of status asthmaticus in children. Pediatrics 1974; *54*:245–247.
102. Stamm SJ. Reliability of capillary blood for measurement of paO_2 Pa_{O_2} and O_2 saturation. Dis Chest 1967; *52*:191–194.
103. Simons FER, Pierson WE, Bierman CW. Respiratory failure in childhood status asthmaticus. Am J Dis Child 1977; *131*:1097.
104. Pearlman DS, Bierman CW. Asthma. *In:* Bierman CW, Pearlman DS, eds. Allergic Diseases of Infancy, Childhood and Adolescence. Philadelphia: WB Saunders Company, 1980:602–604.
105. Wood DW, Downes JJ, Schemkoph H, et al. Intra-

venous isoproterenol in the management of respiratory failure in childhood status asthmaticus. J Allergy Clin Immunol 1972; *50*:75.
106. Parry WH, Martorano F, Cotton EIC. Management of life threatening asthma with intravenous isoproterenol infusions. Am J Dis Child 1976; *130*:39–46.
107. Simons FER, Pierson WE, Bierman, CW. Respiratory failure in childhood status asthmaticus. Am J Dis Child 1977; *131*:1097–1101.
108. Dees SC, Spock A. Right middle lobe syndrome in children. JAMA 1966; *197*:8.
109. Bierman CW. Pneumomediastinum and pneumothorax complicating asthma in children. Am J Dis Child 1967; *114*:42.
110. Jorgensen JR, Fallure CJ, Bukantz SC. Pneumothorax and mediastinal and subcutaneous emphysema in children with bronchial asthma. Pediatrics 1963; *31*:824.
111. Benfield QF, Odoherty K, Davies BH. Status asthmaticus and the syndrome of inappropriate secretion of antidiuretic hormone. Thorax 1982; *37*(2):147–148.
112. Hopkins IJ. A new syndrome: poliomyelitis-like illness associated with acute asthma in childhood. Aust Paediatr J 1974; *10*:273–276.
113. Shapiro GG, Chapman JT, Pierson WE, Bierman CW. Poliomyelitis-like illness after acute asthma. J Pediatr 1979; *94*:767–768.
114. Post-asthmatic pseudopolio in children (commentary). Lancet 1980; *1*:860.
115. Rohatigi N, Fields A, Sly RM. Status asthmaticus complicated by phrenic nerve paralysis. Ann Allergy 1980; *45*:177–178.
116. Bierman CW, Pierson WE, Shapiro GG, Simons FER. Brain damage from asthma in children. J Allergy Clin Immunol 1975; *55*:126.

CHAPTER

16

Congestive Heart Failure

Welton M. Gersony, M.D.
Carl N. Steeg, M.D.

Heart failure is a condition in which the heart cannot produce the cardiac output required to sustain the metabolic needs of the body without evoking certain compensatory processes. When these responses are no longer effective, increasingly severe clinical manifestations result.

Cardiac output is defined as the product of heart rate and stroke volume (HR × SV). There are several types of pathophysiologic derangements that, when sufficiently severe, can compromise stroke volume and thus lead to cardiac decompensation. First is the failure of the heart to respond adequately to an increase in pressure work, i.e., *afterload.* An example of a lesion in which an increase in pressure work is required in order to eject sufficient blood during systole is aortic stenosis. A second mechanism leading to heart failure is excessive volume work, i.e., *preload.* Lesions that require greater volume work by the heart include left to right shunts and valvular insufficiency. Third, severe *abnormalities in myocardial contractility* can result in reduced cardiac output even in the absence of defects causing increased preload or afterload. In pediatric cases, metabolic or inflammatory cardiomyopathies are the most common examples of intrinsic myocardial failure. Cardiac failure may also ensue, with disturbances in heart rate. *Cardiac tachyarrhythmias* shorten diastolic filling of the ventricles and compromise stroke volume. On the other hand, if the cardiac rate is sufficiently slow, an adequate cardiac output may not be maintained even with an increase in stroke volume. Clinically, heart failure is caused principally by abnormalities in one of these areas, and combined mechanisms are common.

The physician caring for a critically ill child must understand basic physiologic processes in order to recognize and evaluate clinical manifestations of heart failure as reflections of pathophysiologic events. Sound principles of management can then be defined, and therapeutic regimens instituted on a rational basis for individual patients.

PATHOPHYSIOLOGY

The heart can be viewed as a pump whose output is directly proportional to its filling volume. This is a basic concept best expressed by the Frank-Starling principle. As end-diastolic volume rises, the healthy heart will increase cardiac output in a linear fashion until a maximum is reached, and cardiac output can no longer be augmented. The increased stroke volume obtained in this manner is explained on the basis of greater myocardial contractility associated with stretching of muscle fibers, but also requires increased wall tension and higher myocardial oxygen requirements. A normal heart will generate the classic Frank-Starling curve, but hearts functioning under various types of stress will produce different types of abnormal curves (Fig. 16–1). Cardiac muscle whose contractility is compromised will require greater dilatation to produce increased stroke volume but will not achieve the cardiac output of the normal myocardium. If a cardiac chamber is already dilated because of a lesion causing an increased preload (e.g., left to right shunt, valve insufficiency, anemia), there is little room for further dilatation and augmentation of cardiac output. The presence of severe afterload-inducing lesions will also markedly compromise the usual Frank-Starling relationship between filling volume and cardiac output.

Ventricular function can be defined in terms of the velocity of shortening of the sarcomere as it is stretched and is affected by three

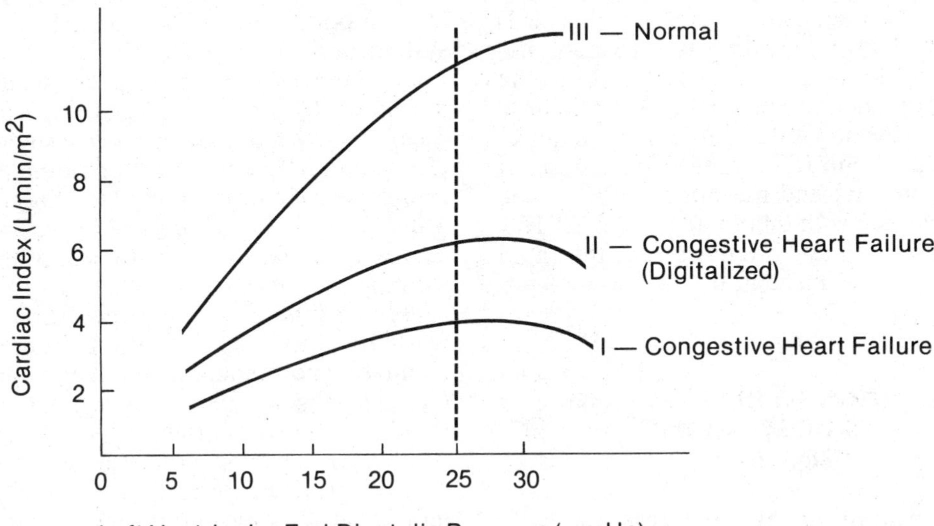

Figure 16–1. As the left ventricular end-diastolic pressure (LVED) increases, cardiac index increases, even in the presence of congestive heart failure until a critical level of LVED is reached. Adding an inotropic agent (digoxin) shifts the curve from I to II.

factors: preload, afterload, and myocardial contractility.[1] *Preload* in the intact heart refers to the diastolic volume that results from filling of the ventricle with blood. An increase in preload causes the sarcomeres to lengthen, and under normal circumstances, this results in an increase in cardiac output (Frank-Starling curve).

Afterload is the force against which the heart muscle must pump. The instantaneous shortening velocity of the sarcomere decreases as afterload is increased.[1] Afterload, as applied to the intact left ventricle, is primarily defined by aortic pressure and peripheral vascular resistance. Obstruction to left ventricular emptying will significantly increase afterload. The sum total of the afterload effects on the heart is best expressed by left ventricular wall stress during ventricular contraction.

Myocardial contractility, or the inotropic state of the myocardium, is the third determinant of ventricular function. It can be defined as the maximal force of contraction (shortening velocity of sarcomeres) that can be developed independent of either volume or afterload. The contractile or inotropic state of the myocardium, although not altered by preload or afterload, is affected by various circulating or intrinsic humoral substances (e.g., norepinephrine, angiotensin II, epinephrine).

BIOCHEMICAL MECHANISMS

The major biochemical abnormality in ventricular failure is the depression of excitation-contraction coupling. *Excitation-contraction coupling* is the process that begins with impulse generation via the specialized conduction system and progresses to depolarization of the myocardial muscle cells. The ultimate cellular mechanism for this reaction is considered to be related to ionic calcium flux, resulting in contraction of the myocardium.[2] The sarcolemma, or cardiac cellular membrane, binds calcium in great quantity. With depolarization, calcium ions cross the cell membrane and are also released from the sarcoplasmic reticulum. The latter response is mediated by a calcium-ATPase system. These ions are necessary for the activation of the contractile protein actomyosin. It is postulated that when the heart fails, ineffective pumping by the sarcoplasmic reticulum causes a decrease in the amount of intracellular calcium available to enhance excitation-contraction coupling. Although calcium is also stored in mitochondria, transport of these calcium stores into the sarcomere has not been definitely proven.[3–6] It has been shown, however, that calcium uptake by mitochondria in heart failure is below that found in normal hearts, perhaps causing less calcium to be available to the sarcomere.

In the adult heart, energy requirements are primarily met by the conversion of fatty acids to glucose. However, owing to enzymatic deficiencies in the utilization of fatty acids, fetal and newborn hearts appear to rely primarily on stored carbohydrates for energy requirements. Mitochondrial oxygen consumption is enhanced in fetal and newborn lambs' hearts when compared with that of adult hearts.[7] This higher capacity may be required for the rapid growth that takes place in the newborn.

ADAPTATION TO HEART FAILURE: COMPENSATORY MECHANISMS (Fig. 16–2)

Adrenergic Mechanisms

The heart is directly affected by stellate ganglia adrenergic nerve endings. Stimulation of these nerve endings via the central nervous system serves to augment cardiac performance, increasing conduction velocity, heart rate, and ventricular contractility. The direct cardiac effects are augmented by peripheral adrenergic effects on the systemic vascular bed, and these, together, contribute to regulation of cardiac output.

The transmission of adrenergic neural stimulation occurs via the neurotransmitter norepinephrine, which is activated when it is bound to specific receptor sites in the innervated tissues. These receptor sites are of two types, alpha (α) and beta (β). *α-Adrenergic receptors* are principally located in the arteriolar smooth muscle of the peripheral vascular system and are responsible for vasoconstriction. The *β-adrenergic receptors* are classified as either β_1 or β_2 subtypes. β_1-Adrenergic receptors predominate in cardiac smooth muscle; β_2-adrenergic receptors predominate in the smooth muscle of the peripheral vascular bed. Stimulation of the β_1-adrenergic receptors causes an increase in ventricular contractility; stimulation of the β_2-adrenergic receptors causes peripheral vascular relaxation. Sympathetic nerve endings may also be stimulated by circulating norepinephrine and epinephrine released by the adrenal medulla. Stimulation via the direct neural transmitter is more rapid but of shorter duration, whereas stimulation by way of the circulating adrenal medullary hormones causes a more protracted effect.

Plasma and urinary concentrations of norepinephrine in patients with congestive heart failure are significantly higher than in controls and show an even greater increase during exercise.[8–9] Furthermore, myocardial biopsy specimens from patients with congestive heart failure have shown a significant depletion of myocardial norepinephrine stores.[10] The exact mechanism for depletion is unknown. It has been postulated that it may be related to exhaustion through markedly increased activity at the nerve endings in patients with heart failure or, perhaps, related to a deficiency in the re-uptake of norepinephrine by the nerve terminals.[11] Some investigators have postu-

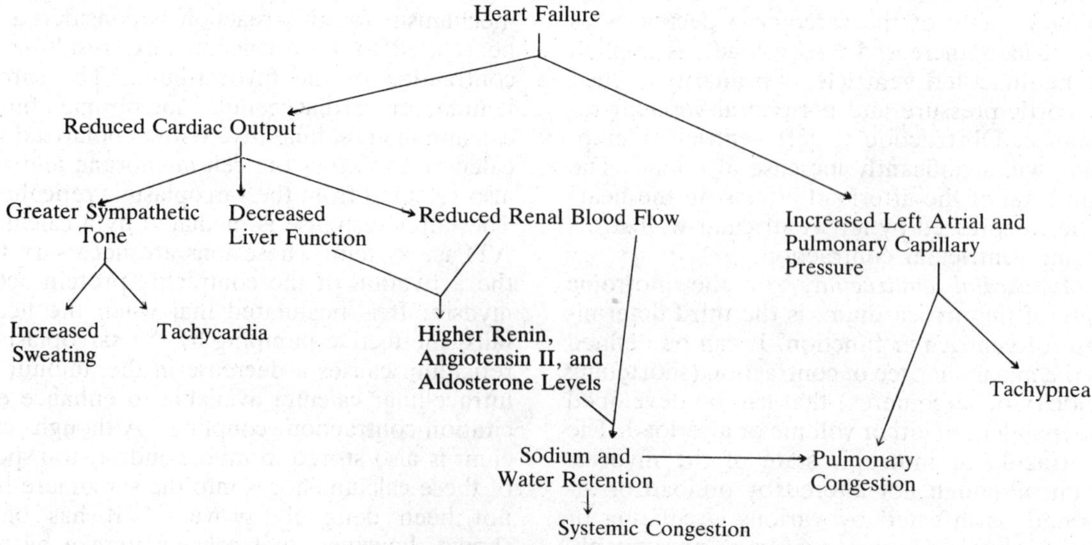

Figure 16–2. Pathophysiologic effects of congestive heart failure.

lated a deficiency in norepinephrine stores due to a reduction in the precursor tyrosine hydroxylase.[12, 13] The depletion of norepinephrine stores appears to be balanced by a striking increase in the contribution by the adrenal medullary hormones to the general level of adrenergic tone. It appears from these data that patients in congestive heart failure rely primarily on adrenergic stimulation to maintain cardiac output.

In profound heart failure, despite very high levels of circulating catecholamines, cardiac stimulation via myocardial receptors seems to be deficient.[14] This deficiency may be related to β_2-adrenergic receptor "burn out" as a result of prolonged high levels of norepinephrine over long periods.[15] The administration of beta agonists, such as isoproterenol, to patients with heart failure does not promote the secretion of cyclic AMP, a hormone that is released by the normally functioning β_2-adrenergic receptors. This fact may be related to a smaller number of binding sites. The development of radioligand binding studies has allowed investigators to evaluate the number of myocardial receptors available for stimulation by adrenergic agents. Several of these studies have demonstrated drug tachyphylaxis and a decreased number of receptor sites in cardiac tissue exposed to chronically high levels of circulating adrenergic agonists.[16, 17] There is some evidence that this lack of available β_2-adrenergic receptors results in a chronically failing heart that is no longer receptive to adrenergic stimulation.[15] Thus, in congestive heart failure, lack of myocardial stimulation by norepinephrine may be explained by (1) norepinephrine stores' depletion, (2) inadequate receptor function, and (3) fewer receptor sites. These new concepts have raised interesting clinical implications and may explain the predictable decrease in drug effect with adrenergic agonists during long-term treatment of congestive heart failure.

Renin-Angiotensin System

Renin is a proteolytic enzyme secreted by the juxtaglomerular apparatus of the kidney and is responsible for the conversion of angiotensinogen to angiotensin I. Angiotensin-converting enzyme (ACE) then converts angiotensin I to angiotensin II by the removal of two amino acids. Angiotensin II is a powerful vasoconstrictor that also stimulates the production of aldosterone. Initially, the vasoconstrictive effects of angiotensin II in patients with congestive heart failure serve to maintain adequate blood pressure, but in patients with chronic cardiac failure, the increased afterload is deleterious. The greater production of aldosterone leads to sodium and water retention and a subsequent increase in ventricular filling. However, in the chronically failing heart, the ensuing elevated diastolic pressures and hypervolemia cause peripheral and pulmonary edema.

Renin levels are significantly elevated in most patients with congestive heart failure.[18–20] The secretion of renin is stimulated by a number of factors, including (1) an increase in plasma catecholamine levels, (2) a decrease in renal blood pressure and perfusion, and (3) an increase in sodium intake. In addition, there is reduced hepatic clearance of renin in patients with advanced congestive heart failure. Agents such as teprotide and captopril inhibit the production of angiotensin-converting enzyme, significantly lowering the levels of circulating angiotensin II despite the excess availability of the renin substrate. The consequent vasodilatory effect and lowered aldosterone production are the mechanisms by which such agents assist in the management of chronic congestive heart failure.

Salt and Water Retention

Salt and water retention in patients with congestive heart failure is due to a number of interrelated factors, including decreased renal perfusion, increased levels of circulating antidiuretic hormones, active retention of sodium and water by muscles, hypoproteinemia, and higher aldosterone levels.

When renal plasma flow is diminished in the presence of low cardiac output, salt and water are retained as a compensatory mechanism to increase intravascular volume and therefore renal perfusion. In addition, venous return is greater and subsequent elevation of end-diastolic volume can potentially increase cardiac output on the basis of the Frank-Starling concept. The renal mechanism appears to be that of higher proximal tubular reabsorption of sodium as well as greater sodium reabsorption in the distal tubular and collecting duct. The latter appears to be due to the effects of hyperaldosteronism as stimulated via the renin-angiotensin mechanism.[21]

A high concentration of sodium in the body has been found to increase the level of circulating antidiuretic hormone and this increase appears to augment water retention in patients with congestive heart failure. Recent experimental studies have also implied that muscle cell edema is important in the origin of fluid retention. It has been shown that prior to a demonstrable decrease in renal blood flow, muscle cells undergo an increase in osmolality. Active retention of sodium and water by muscle cells in congestive heart failure occurs during times of anaerobic metabolism (e.g., exercise). Edema persisting during aerobic metabolism (e.g., rest) is an indication that congestive heart failure has been complicated by reduced renal perfusion.

Pulmonary and Peripheral Edema

When water moves into the pulmonary interstitial spaces of the alveoli to the extent that it cannot be eliminated by lymphatic flow, pulmonary congestion or edema or both will ensue. In the presence of left ventricular failure, pulmonary venous hypertension leads to increased capillary pressure and fluid retention in the extravascular space of the lung. In the presence of hypervolemia and hypoproteinemia, the accumulation of lung fluid is augmented. A high rate of formation of interstitial edema may eventually exceed the capacity of the lymphatic system to remove fluid, and alveolar and bronchial edema will result if the process is not reversed. Interstitial edema alone will result in diminished pulmonary compliance and the clinical manifestations of dyspnea and tachypnea. In the presence of alveolar edema, more acute symptoms will occur, gas exchange will eventually become impaired, and the $Pa{O_2}$ will fail.

When capillary pressure rises in the systemic venous system, fluid will flow into the tissues and edema may become clinically apparent. If liver function is compromised, hypoproteinemia will contribute to the accumulation of fluid. Edema may occur in dependent areas in older children, but the fluid is well distributed throughout the tissues of the body in most infants, so that the typical features of peripheral edema may not be obvious. In infants, the flexible capsule of the liver allows accumulation of fluid, resulting in hepatomegaly. Under exceptional circumstances, anasarca can occur in the presence of severe right-sided heart failure.

High Output Failure

High output failure is defined as the development of signs and symptoms of congestive heart failure in which there is no basic abnormality in myocardial function, and the cardiac output is greater than normal. Heart failure in the presence of increased cardiac output can be caused by conditions such as profound anemia, severe hyperthyroidism, and large systemic arteriovenous fistulae. The fundamental cardiovascular physiologic consequences of these disease states are a decrease in peripheral vascular resistance, a reduction in cardiac afterload, and an enhancement of myocardial contractility. Heart "failure" results from the greater demands for cardiac output that strip the ability of the system to respond. Chronic, severe "high output failure" may eventually result in a lessening of myocardial performance as the metabolic requirements of the myocardium itself are not met, which in turn can result in further physiologic deterioration.

CAUSES OF HEART FAILURE

Cardiac failure occurs most often in children who are less than 1 year of age, the great majority of cases within the first three months. The differential diagnosis varies with age, and heart failure can be recognized even in a fetus. However, most congenital heart lesions, even those with severe hemodynamic derangements, are well compensated *in utero* as a result of the fetal circulation. For example, transposition of the great arteries has no detrimental effect on the cardiopulmonary system of the fetus. It is, however, a devastating lesion after birth, when the neonate's oxygen requirements depend on blood flow through the lungs rather than the placenta, and the transposed aorta no longer receives blood supplied with oxygen from the maternal circulation. Prior to birth, in the presence of left or right ventricular outflow stenosis, the ductus arteriosus allows blood to bypass even the most severe obstructive lesions. In addition, abnormal intracardiac communications between the left and right sides of the heart do not interfere with systemic delivery of oxygenated blood to the fetus. The major causes of *intrauterine* heart failure include arrhythmias, profound anemia, and infection.

Congestive heart failure *at birth* is uncommon. The diagnostic possibilities include (1) systemic arteriovenous fistulae, (2) severe tricuspid or pulmonary valvular regurgitation or both, (3) severe anemia of any cause, (4) cardiac arrhythmias, (5) birth asphyxia with left or right ventricular ischemia or both, (6) severe cardiomyopathy, and, rarely, (7) hypoplastic left heart syndrome.

Within the infant's *first week of life,* variations of hypoplastic left heart syndrome and coarctation complexes with ventricular septal defects are the most likely lesions causing heart failure. Truncus arteriosus, total anomalous pulmonary venous drainage, complete atrioventricular canal, transposition of the great arteries with ventricular septal defect, and various forms of single ventricle, often in the presence of the asplenia or polysplenia syndromes, also may cause heart failure during this period.

Severe isolated aortic or pulmonary stenosis can cause signs of decompensation during the infant's first week but may not be clinically evident until the *second or third week.* Large left to right shunts without significant valvular abnormalities do not become clinically evident until the infant is *two to six weeks of age.* Patent ductus arteriosus associated with respiratory distress syndrome in the premature infant, however, may be recognized as early as the first few days after birth.

Heart failure secondary to the cardiomyopathies of infancy usually does not occur until later in the *first year.* In general, *it is extremely rare for an infant, who demonstrates normal growth and development and absence of symptoms of cardiac dysfunction during the first five or six months, to develop congestive heart failure.* In most cases, when heart failure is initially diagnosed later in the child's first year, early symptoms were present but unrecognized. Failure of compensatory mechanisms to operate under the stress of even a minor infection may result in what appears to be sudden cardiac failure but in reality is often the culmination of a chronic process.

DIAGNOSIS

The clinical manifestations of congestive heart failure depend on the degree of cardiac reserve under various conditions. Critically ill infants or children who have exhausted their compensatory mechanisms to the point where they no longer achieve sufficient cardiac output to meet the basal metabolic needs of the body will be symptomatic even at rest. Other patients may be comfortable when quiet but are incapable of increasing cardiac output in response to even mild activity without developig significant symptoms. On the other hand, it may take rather vigorous exercise to elucidate abnormal cardiac function in children who have less severe heart disease.

A thorough history is extremely important both in making the diagnosis of heart failure and in evaluating the possible causes. A number of special areas must be singled out for specific questioning, and the physician must be aware, at the onset, that parents who observe their infant on a daily basis may not recognize subtle changes that have occurred over the course of days or weeks. They may consider cyanosis merely "a deep coloring" and not recognize it as abnormal. Eliciting a history of fatigue in an older child requires specific questions about activity, including stair climbing, walking various distances, bicycle riding, and so forth. Information should also be obtained regarding more severe manifestations, such as orthopnea and nocturnal dyspnea. The history obtained from the parents for a young infant should focus on the feeding process. The baby with congestive heart failure will often take less volume per feeding, become dyspneic while sucking, and perhaps perspire profusely. After falling into an exhausted sleep, the inadequately fed baby will soon awake for the next feeding. This cycle continues around the clock and must be carefully differentiated from feeding disorders and colic.

Physical examination must include an assessment of growth and development. Severe cardiac disease may lead to failure to thrive as manifested by poor weight gain. Baby length remains relatively unaffected. An infant with severe chronic heart failure usually appears to be undernourished. In contrast, an infant with cyanotic heart disease unaccompanied by cardiac decompensation may display a more normal growth pattern. Failure to thrive, tachycardia, tachypnea, and liver enlargement are the major signs of heart failure on physical examination. Pulmonary rales and peripheral edema are less often noted. Cyanosis may be absent or only minimally present.

Careful evaluation of the character of the pulses is an important component of the physical examination of the cardiovascular system. A wide pulse pressure with bounding pulses in the presence of other signs of congestive heart failure may suggest an aortic runoff lesion such as a patent ductus arteriosus, aortic insufficiency, or an arteriovenous communication. In most instances, however, severe congestive heart failure is associated with normal or diminished pulses.

Blood pressures in both upper and lower extremities should be measured, and the presence or absence of neck vein distension should be determined. Cardiac examination should not be focused only on findings consistent with heart failure (e.g., gallop rhythm, tachycardia, and signs of cardiac enlargement) but should also be regarded as an important step in delineating the nature of the underlying lesion. This process is accomplished by the careful evaluation of the heart sounds and precordial murmurs.

SIGNS AND SYMPTOMS OF CONGESTIVE HEART FAILURE

The signs and symptoms of congestive heart failure not only are the result of insufficient cardiac output per se, but also are manifestations of the adverse physiologic effects of extreme conpensatory mechanisms.

Tachycardia

A basic compensatory mechanism in the presence of cardiac failure is an increase in cardiac rate. This increase is mediated by the autonomic nervous system in response to a fall in cardiac output. Stroke volume falls with a rise in heart rate, but minute output will increase to the physiologic limit. After infancy, when the rate increases to more than 140 per minute, the accompanying decrease in diastolic filling time results in lower stroke volume and cardiac output. Prolonged tachyarrhythmia (>240/min) of itself, even in a patient with a normal heart, will eventually result in cardiac failure.

Cardiomegaly

Classic heart failure is invariably associated with higher diastolic volume and consequent cardiac dilatation. On physical examination, enlargement of the heart is determined by eliciting a point of maximum impulse beyond the mid-clavicular line in the fifth or sixth intercostal space. In addition, a diffuse overactive left, right, or mixed cardiac impulse can be palpated, depending on the basic cause of the cardiac failure. Correlation of such findings with the chest x-ray is important. Some patients with large left to right shunts display a hyperdynamic cardiac impulse without cardiac decompensation. In infants and children with primary myocardial or pericardial diseases, the precordium may be quiet even when other signs of heart failure are evident.

Gallop Rhythm

A prominent third heart sound in the presence of tachycardia and in association with other signs of myocardial failure defines a gallop rhythm. This clinical sign is associated with poor ventricular function and indicates greater diastolic filling pressure. A prominent third heart sound may be part of the normal examination findings in a healthy child, so it is important to further differentiate a gallop rhythm by the heart rate and the presence of other manifestations of heart failure. A short mid-diastolic rumble at the apex may suggest a gallop rhythm but does not necessarily indicate heart failure. This murmur is associated with increased diastolic blood flow across an atrioventricular valve and is heard in the presence of a large left to right shunt at the ventricular or ductal level and with mitral insufficiency.

Peripheral Pulses

An infant with severe congestive heart failure and low cardiac output at rest may show signs of cardiovascular collapse, including weakness or absence of peripheral pulses, cold extremities, and hypotension. In most instances, however, pulses are normal. When peripheral pulses remain bounding in the presence of other signs of advanced heart failure, the presence of an aortic run off lesion, such as patent ductus arteriosus, aortic insufficiency, truncus arteriosus, or arteriovenous fistula, should be suspected. Certain non-cardiac abnormalities, such as severe anemia, hyperthyroidism, and arteriovenous malformations, require a high cardiac output to provide adequate oxygen to meet the needs of the body, and brisk peripheral pulses are noted in their presence. Absence or weakness of pulses in the lower extremities suggests the diagnosis of coarctation of the aorta. Pulsus alternans, a phenomenon in which systolic pressure varies from beat to beat, is a finding associated with poor myocardial performance.

Cyanosis

Congestive heart failure causes mild cyanosis with a pulmonary basis. Ventilation and perfusion inequalities resulting from severe pulmonary congestion lead to oxygen desaturation of the left atrial blood supply and lowered peripheral arterial and capillary PaO_2. This cyanosis must be differentiated from the cyanosis based on true right to left shunts due to cyanotic congenital heart lesions. Cyanosis secondary to true right to left shunts will not resolve with the administration of 100 per cent oxygen, whereas cyanosis secondary to pulmonary congestion will resolve, and the PaO_2 will rise significantly. Some patients with cyanotic heart disease (e.g., total anomalous pulmonary venous return, truncus arteriosus, single ventricle, and transposition of the great vessels with ventricular septal defect) may have concomitant heart failure, which may further lower arterial PaO_2 on the basis of pulmonary congestion.

Fatigue and Sweating

When cardiac output cannot be increased to match the greater demand, the patient will manifest symptoms of fatigue with activity and may sleep excessively. Infants will become markedly tachypneic with feeding and will take small amounts of food despite obvious signs of hunger. Sweating during feeding is most likely a sign of higher autonomic nervous system activity provoked by myocardial dysfunction.

Growth Retardation

An infant or a child with chronic congestive heart failure is almost invariably undernourished. Infants with tachypnea and increased autonomic nervous system activity require a greater than normal caloric intake to sustain higher demands and also allow for growth. However, intake is actually reduced because of fatigue and dyspnea during feedings. Height is maintained, whereas weight gain is inadequate; this growth pattern is similar to that displayed by children with chronic malnutrition.

Systemic Venous Congestion

Left- or right-sided heart failure results in hepatomegaly, especially in infants, in whom fluid retention is reflected by rapid changes in liver size. The liver is usually tender and relatively soft. Systolic pulsations of the liver may suggest tricuspid valve insufficiency. With severe hepatic congestion, jaundice may be noted, but normal liver function will almost invariably return as congestive heart failure is controlled. Hepatic enlargement also occurs in the presence of severe pericardial disease. Frank peripheral edema or anasarca is noted more often in older children and adults than in infants. Neck vein distension may be observed in older children, but this sign is difficult to recognize in infants.

Pulmonary Congestion

Tachypnea is a universal sign of left heart failure. An increase in the rate of respiration is usually related to a decrease in pulmonary compliance resulting from interstitial congestion or pulmonary edema. Chronic wheezing in this context occurs as a result of bronchial constriction caused by bronchial edema (cardiac asthma) and should not be confused with bronchospasm caused by reactive airway disease or bronchiolitis. In both of these latter conditions, the liver may appear to be enlarged secondary to flattening of the diaphragms, but the chest x-ray reveals a normal-sized heart. Pulmonary rales indicate the presence of significant fluid in the alveolar spaces, but this finding is often not detectable in infants. Bronchial compression from a large heart and pulmonary arteries, resulting in atelectasis or emphysema or both, may also cause tachypnea, coughing, and respiratory distress. A higher incidence of pulmonary infection may occur in the presence of cardiac failure with pulmonary congestion.

NON-INVASIVE DIAGNOSTIC TECHNIQUES

A number of non-invasive techniques are helpful in elucidating the presence of congestive heart failure and providing qualitative and quantitative diagnostic data regarding severity.

Chest X-ray

X-ray films of the chest are very helpful in the diagnosis of congestive heart failure. Cardiac enlargement is evident. The appearance of the pulmonary vascularity is variable, depending on the cause of the heart failure. Infants and children with congestive heart failure associated with large left to right shunts have exaggeration of the pulmonary arterial vessels to the periphery of the lung fields, whereas those with cardiomyopathy may have a relatively normal pulmonary vascular bed early in the course of the disease. The fluffy pulmonary markings suggestive of venous congestion and acute pulmonary edema are often not seen in children, except in the most extreme circumstances. Specific chamber enlargement may be diagnosed relatively easily in adults but is less well defined in children even when the clinical findings suggest predominant left or right ventricular decompensation.

Electrocardiogram (ECG)

The finding of specific chamber enlargement may be helpful in assessing the etiology of congestive heart failure but does not establish the diagnosis. Left or right ventricular ischemic changes may correlate well with clinical and other non-invasive parameters of ventricular function. Low-voltage QRS morphology with ST-T wave abnormalities may suggest myocardial inflammatory disease and may also suggest pericarditis. The ECG is the best tool for evaluation of rhythm disorders that cause cardiac failure.

Echocardiography

Echocardiographic techniques to evaluate myocardial function have been intensely studied in recent years.[22–24] The relationship between end-systolic and end-diastolic diameters (shortening fraction) is useful in the assessment of ventricular function.[25] The normal shortening fraction should be 28 to 36 per cent as compared with the normal ejection fraction of 55 to 65 per cent, as measured by angiography. A second method useful in the echocardiographic evaluation of myocardial function is the pre-ejection/ejection-period ratio (PEP/EP). The PEP/EP ratio should be less than 40 per cent. A long pre-ejection period with a very short ejection period usually denotes myocardial failure.[25]

Radionuclide Techniques

Radionuclide techniques have had significant use in the evaluation of myocardial function.[26] Ejection fraction is determined by injecting a radioisotope (e.g., ^{99m}Tc) into a vein and measuring end-diastolic volume, end-systolic volume, and stroke volume by counts per unit time over the ventricles. The ejection fraction is calculated utilizing the standard formula, i.e., ejection fraction = stroke volume/end-diastolic volume. This method is advantageous in that cardiac catheterization is not required and radiation exposure is minimal. Radionuclide techniques can be carried out to evaluate the performance of the myocardium while a patient is exercising or resting.

Arterial Blood Gas and Electrolyte Levels

Arterial blood oxygen levels may be reduced when ventilation/perfusion inequalities occur secondary to pulmonary edema. When heart failure is severe, mild respiratory acidemia may be present. Infants with severe heart failure and decreased cardiac output demonstrate metabolic acidemia. In contrast, infants with marked tachypnea associated with lowered pulmonary compliance secondary to interstitial congestion without alveolar edema may have mild respiratory alkalosis.

Infants with congestive heart failure often display hyponatremia as a result of water retention. Although serum sodium concentration is low, total body sodium level actually is increased because of sodium retention. An abnormal steady state is reached in which relatively more water is retained. Greater secretion of antidiuretic hormone or exaggerated proximal renal tubular reabsorption of glomerular filtrate may explain this finding. Later in extreme heart failure, hyperkalemia occurs as a result of intracellular release of potassium secondary to impaired tissue perfusion with oxygen and usually is associated with decreased renal blood flow.

EVALUATION OF VENTRICULAR FUNCTION

Pressure Volume Measurements

Standards for evaluation of ventricular function are based on cardiac catheterization and angiographic data. Increased end-diastolic volume, as calculated from angiocardiographic images, is a reflection of poor ventricular function. High diastolic volume results in a rise in end-diastolic pressure, but the relationship is not linear. Analysis of pressure-volume curves offers a sensitive assessment of ventricular performance in the failing heart.[27] However, with only minimal left ventricular dysfunction, pressure volume curves may be normal at rest. In such situations, it may be necessary to further evaluate myocardial function by means of exercise or pharmacologic stress studies.

Ejection Fraction

Ejection fraction represents the percentage of end-diastolic volume that is ejected per stroke. This measurement is one of the most practical and commonly utilized indicators of myocardial function and can be evaluated while patients rest or exercise.

Ventricular volumes are calculated from angiographic data, and the ejection fraction is determined by the ratio of total stroke volume to end-diastolic volume (normal 55–65%).[28, 29] Ejection fraction is an indicator solely of myocardial function and not of forward stroke output. When atrioventricular valve insufficiency exists, a proportion of ejectate is regurgitant. In such cases, cardiac failure is present even when the ejection fraction is normal.

Isovolumetric Phase Indices

The maximum rate of rise of the left ventricular pressure, i.e., rate of pressure increase/time (dp/dt), has also been utilized as an indicator of myocardial function and is measured by catheter tip transducers.[1] Dp/dt is influenced not only by contractility but is also affected by preload and afterload. The absolute indicator of myocardial contractility (V_{max}) can be determined by measuring dp/dt at different intraventricular pressures throughout the period of isovolumic systole and extrapolating these measurements to zero pressure.[1] This calculation theoretically eliminates afterload as a factor and is an attempt to assess the true inotropic state of the myocardium.

TREATMENT OF CONGESTIVE HEART FAILURE (Table 16–1)

Digitalis

Digitalis glycosides have been the mainstay of management for cardiac failure over the years, and a great deal of investigation has been carried out to determine the mechanism of action of these substances. Digitalis has been shown to inhibit sodium and potassium transport across the plasma membrane of the cardiac muscle cell by interfering with sodium-potassium ATPase. This interaction appears to increase the availability of calcium to the contracting sarcomere at the cellular level and is thought to be the mechanism by which digitalis exerts a positive inotropic effect on the myocardium.[30] The velocity and force of myocardial contraction are enhanced by digitalis in both the normal and failing heart. However, a significant increase in cardiac output is demonstrated only when digitalis is administered in the presence of myocardial failure. Cardiac output is not affected by digitalis in the normal heart, since the homeostatic adjustments of the peripheral circulation regulate total cardiac output within the normal range.

Digoxin is the digitalis glycoside most often used in the pediatric patient.The one half-life of 36 hours is long enough to allow once daily or twice daily administration and short enough to limit toxic effects from overdoses. Digoxin is absorbed by the gastrointestinal tract. When digoxin is taken with or after meals, the rate of absorption may be somewhat retarded, but the amount of digoxin absorbed is almost always unchanged. Following oral administration, approximately 60 to 85 per cent of digoxin is absorbed. Absorption is greater for the elixir than for the tablet. The peak effect for oral digoxin is approximately 2 to 6 hours; an initial effect can be seen as early as 30 minutes. When the drug is administered intravenously, the initial effect is seen in 15 to 30 minutes, and the peak effect is from 1 to 4 hours. The drug crosses the placenta, and therefore, a fetus can be treated via administration to the mother. Digoxin is eliminated by the kidney, and the rate of excretion is proportional to the glomerular filtration rate. After intravenous administration, 50 to 70 per cent is excreted unchanged in the urine. In subjects with normal renal function, the one half-life of digoxin

Table 16–1. TREATMENT OF CONGESTIVE HEART FAILURE*

Severity of CHF	Physical Activities	Digoxin	Sodium Restriction	Diuretics	Vasodilators	Non-glycoside Inotropic Agents	Surgical Correction of Underlying Lesions
Mild	Restrict from sports and heavy work	Maintenance digoxin dosage ↓	No added salt ↓				
Moderate	Frequent test periods			Moderate dosage of chlorothiazide or furosemide (qod) ↓			
Severe	Bed rest	Maximum digoxin dosage	Low sodium diet	Maximum dosage with spironolactone and/or KCl	Prazosin with diuretic or hydralazine	Dopamine, dobutamine, etc.	

*Not all modes of therapy are always utilized. Treatment depends on cause of CHF.

is 1 to 2 days, but may be six days in patients with renal shutdown.

Rapid digitalization of infants and children with congestive heart failure may be carried out intravenously. The dose is dependent on the patient's weight, and various regimens are utilized (Table 16–2). The recommened schedule of administration is to give a third of the total digitalizing dose immediately and the succeeding 2 doses 8 and 16 hours later. In cases of profound congestive heart failure, more rapid digitalization, using shorter intervals and a larger initial loading dose, may be required. The ECG must be closely monitored and rhythm strips obtained prior to each of the 3 digitalizing doses. Digoxin should be discontinued if a new rhythm disturbance is noted. A prolongation of the PR interval is not in itself an indication to withhold digitalis, but a delay in administration of the next dose or reduction in dosage should be considered, depending on the patient's clinical status. Serum digoxin level determination is helpful when digitalis toxicity is suspected. ST segment or T-wave changes are commonly noted with digitalis administration and should not affect the digitalization regimen. Serum electrolyte levels should be measured before and after digitalization.

Table 16–2. DOSAGE OF DRUGS COMMONLY USED FOR THE TREATMENT OF CONGESTIVE HEART FAILURE

Drug	Dosage
Digoxin	
Digitalization (IV)	0.03–0.04 mg/kg, 3 doses, 8 hr apart
Digitalization (po)	0.04–0.05 mg/kg, 3 doses, 8 hr apart
Maintenance (po)	0.01–0.02 mg/kg/day, q12h
Furosemide	
IV	1–2 mg/dose, prn
po	1–4 mg/kg/day, qd, bid, or qod
Chlorothiazide (po)	20–50 mg/kg/day, bid, or qod
Spironolactone (po)	2–3 mg/kg/day, bid
β-Agonists (IV)	
Isoproterenol	0.01–0.5 μg/kg/min
Dopamine	2–20 μg/kg/min
Dobutamine	2–20 μg/kg/min
Afterload reducing agents	
Nitroprusside (IV)	0.5–8 μg/kg/min
Hydralazine	
(IV)	0.5 mg/kg
(po)	0.5–7.5 mg/kg/day, tid
Prazosin (po)	
Starting dose	0.2–0.4 mg/kg/day or 1–3 mg/day, qid
Chronic dose	6–15 mg/day, qid
Captopril (po)	0.5–6 mg/kg/day, qid

μ = micro

Maintenance digitalis therapy is started approximately 12 hours after full digitalization. The daily dosage is divided in two and given at 12 hour intervals for more consistent blood levels and more flexibility in case of toxicity. The dosage is a fourth to a third of the full digitalizing dose. For patients who are initially digitalized intravenously, maintenance digoxin can be given orally, once oral feedings are tolerated. Since absorption from the gastrointestinal tract is less certain, the oral maintenance dose is approximately 25 per cent higher than the parenteral dose (see Table 16–2). The normal daily dosage of digoxin for older children (>5 years of age) should not exceed the normal daily dosage for adults, 0.2–0.5 mg/day.

Patients who are not critically ill may be digitalized initially using an oral regimen (see Table 16–2), and in most instances, digitalization is completed within 24 hours, as with the parenteral regimen. When slow digitalization is appropriate, initiation of a maintenance digoxin schedule, without a loading dose, will achieve full digitalization in seven to ten days. This regimen often can be carried out on an outpatient basis.

If an infant improves significantly on a digitalis regimen over a period of a few months, and the need for the drug appears to be lessening (e.g., a ventricular septal defect becomes smaller) he or she may be permitted to "outgrow" the dose. Dosage is not increased as the child gains weight, and if the clinical status warrants, the drug is eventually discontinued.

If the effectiveness or toxicity of digitalis is in question, plasma digoxin levels should be measured. Blood must be drawn at least 4 hours after the last dose so that tissue-to-plasma equilibration has occurred. A normal blood level in an infant is approximately 2–4 ng/ml and in older children, 1–2 ng/ml. Exceeding this level will not generally improve the control of congestive failure.[31]

Serum digoxin levels are useful under three circumstances: (1) when a standard dose of digoxin is not resulting in signs of beneficial therapeutic effects; (2) when an unknown amount of digoxin is administered or ingested accidentally and (3) when a toxic response is suspected. It must be emphasized that in the last situation, *elevated serum digoxin levels are not of themselves diagnostic of toxicity but must be interpreted as an adjunct to other clinical and electrocardiographic findings.*[32] Effects of toxicity are primarily related to rhythm and conduction disturbances. The clinical symptoms of nausea and vomiting do not occur frequently in the pediatric patient. Serum electrolyte abnormalities such as hypokalemia and hypercalcemia, cardiac inflammation, and prematurity potentiate the possibility of digoxin toxicity.

A cardiac arrhythmia that develops in a child with congestive heart failure who is taking digitalis may be related to cardiac disease rather than to the drug. However, *any form of arrhythmia noted to occur following the institution of digitalis therapy must be considered to be drug related until proven otherwise.* Succeeding doses should be withheld until the problem is resolved.

Diet

Infants with congestive heart failure are calorically deprived because of both increased metabolic requirements and decreased caloric intake.[33, 34] Raising daily caloric intake is an important aspect of the management of such patients. Often, as other therapeutic measures take effect, the child's appetite will improve in parallel with the regression of other signs of heart failure. However, increasing calories per ounce of feeding may still occasionally be beneficial. Formulas containing 24 calories per ounce can be substituted for standard formulas containing 20 calories per ounce. Some infants cannot tolerate excessive concentrations of calories in this manner because of gastrointestinal disturbances, particularly diarrhea. Furthermore, these formulas may also provide too large a solute load, creating further difficulty for the already compromised kidneys, which may then fail to maintain adequate sodium and water balance.

Severely ill infants in congestive heart failure may lack sufficient strength for effective sucking because of extreme fatigue, rapid respirations, and generalized weakness. It may be helpful to initiate nasogastric feedings to provide adequate nutrition. When congestive heart failure continues unabated, however, an increased caloric diet will frequently be of no avail. Indeed, unresolved malnutrition may be an important factor in deciding for early surgical intervention in patients who have an operable congenital heart lesion associated with heart failure and who are being managed medically.

The use of formulas very low in sodium in the routine management of infants with congestive heart failure is no longer emphasized. These preparations are often poorly tolerated, and thus, although sodium intake is decreased, caloric needs are less well met than with standard formulas. The advent of more potent diuretic agents allows more palatable standard formulas to be utilized for nutrition while controlling salt and water balance with long-term diuretic administration. Some infants and children can be managed with "no added salt" diets and abstinence from high-sodium containing foods. A "strict," extremely low sodium diet is rarely required.

Diuretic

Diuretic agents contribute to the management of congestive heart failure by interfering with reabsorption of water and sodium by the kidneys. Effective diuresis results in the reduction of circulating blood volume and thereby reduces ventricular filling pressures. These agents are most often utilized in conjunction with digitalis therapy in patients with severe congestive heart failure.

Furosemide is now the most commonly used diuretic for patients with cardiac failure. This potent agent inhibits the reabsorption of sodium and chloride not only in the distal tubules but also in the loop of Henle. Patients requiring acute diuresis are managed with intravenous or intramuscular furosemide at an initial dose of 1–2 mg/kg (see Table 16–2). This treatment often results in rapid diuresis and prompt improvement in clinical status, particularly if symptoms of pulmonary congestion are present. Long-term furosemide therapy is then prescribed at a dosage of 1–4 mg/kg/day or every other day, usually as a single oral dose in the morning. Careful monitoring of serum electrolyte levels is necessary with long-term diuretic therapy, since there may be significant potassium loss. Potassium chloride supplementation or spironolactone or both may be administered in conjunction with long-term diuretic therapy to preserve potassium. Spironolactone is given orally in divided doses of 2–3 mg/kg/day. The effect of this agent is twofold, enhancement of potassium retention and competitive inhibition of aldosterone. When furosemide is administered every other day, dietary potassium supplementation may be adequate to maintain normal serum potassium levels. Long-term administration of furosemide may cause contraction of the extracellular fluid compartment, resulting in a "contraction alkalosis." When this occurs, the medication should be discontinued and acetazolamide, a carbonic anhydrase inhibitor, substituted until the metabolic disturbance has been corrected.

Chlorothiazide is occasionally used for diuresis in children with less severe chronic congestive heart failure. This medication, which is less immediate in action and less potent than furosemide, affects the reabsorption of electrolytes in the renal tubules only. The usual dosage is 20–50 mg/kg every day or every other day in divided doses. Potassium supplementation may also be utilized concurrently with this diuretic.

Afterload Reducing Agents

Over the past several years, pharmacologic manipulation of the peripheral vascular system in order to affect cardiac preload and afterload has been used for the treatment of selected patients with congestive heart failure. A group of drugs are available that reduce ventricular afterload by reducing peripheral vascular resistance, thereby improving myocardial contractility. Some agents also decrease systemic venous tone, significantly reducing preload. Afterload reducing agents have been of most benefit in children with congestive heart failure secondary to a cardiomyopathy but also are effective in patients with severe mitral regurgitation or aortic insufficiency. Congestive heart failure secondary to left to right shunts or stenotic lesions is treated less often with afterload reducing agents. Questions regarding effects on pulmonary vascular resistance have made this type of therapy controversial in the management of large left to right shunts.[35, 36] If heart failure is the result of a fixed obstructive cardiac lesion, peripheral vasodilation beyond the site of stenosis will not significantly affect total ventricular afterload. Afterload reducing agents are most often used in conjunction with other anticongestive drugs, such as digoxin and diuretics. In pediatrics, these drugs are rarely used first, but are added to treatment regimens in specific situations when decreasing peripheral vascular resistance will add significantly to optimal management. A number of afterload reducing agents are available, but only a few have been utilized extensively in children.

Nitroprusside

Nitroprusside directly dilates arterial and venous vessels and is a potent intravenous medication that should be administered only in an intensive care setting.[36, 37] Peripheral arterial vasodilation and afterload reduction are the major effects of nitroprusside, but venodilation, causing a decrease in venous return, is also beneficial because it reduces preload.

The initial infusion rate of nitroprusside is 0.5 μg/kg/min and can be increased to a maximum of 8 μg/kg/min if necessary. Blood pressure must be continuously monitored by means of an intra-arterial line, since sudden hypotension can occur with overdose. Nitroprusside is contraindicated in cases of pre-existing hypotension.

Toxicity occurs as a result of accumulation of cyanide. As the drug is metabolized, small amounts of circulating cyanide can be detoxified in the liver, and the metabolite, thiocyanate, is excreted in the urine. However, when high doses of nitroprusside are administered for several days, toxic symptoms related to thiocyanate poisoning may occur. These symptoms include fatigue, nausea, disorientation, and muscular spasm. If the use of nitroprusside is to be prolonged, levels of blood thiocyanate should be monitored. Values of 5 to 10 μg/100 ml are consistent with clinical symptoms of toxicity. Nitroprusside is a potent intravenous vasodilator that should be utilized only in the most critically ill patients for as short a period as possible.

Hydralazine

Hydralazine is a direct arteriolar smooth muscle relaxant and has virtually no effect on preload.[38, 39] Therefore, it is occasionally administered together with a venodilating agent, such as a nitrate derivative. The usual oral dosage of hydralazine is 0.5–5 mg/kg/day in 3 divided doses. In some cases, it may be advantageous to study the immediate effects of intravenous hydralazine in the cardiovascular laboratory. If positive responses including increased cardiac output, decreased peripheral vascular resistance, and reduced left ventricular filling pressure are observed, then long-term oral therapy is instituted. One of the major disadvantages of hydralazine is tachyphylaxis. Thus, increasing dosage over time will be required in order to maintain the peripheral dilating effects in many patients.

Adverse reactions with hydralazine include

headache, palpitations, nausea, and vomiting. In addition, systemic lupus erythematosus occasionally occurs after administration of large doses of hydralazine over prolonged periods. The manifestations of lupus are reversible when the drug is discontinued.

Prazosin

Prazosin is a postsynaptic α-adrenergic blocking agent that affects the arterial and venous systems and thereby reduces both preload and afterload.[40] Cardiac output increases and systemic venous return decreases. Treatment with this agent is especially beneficial when cardiomyopathy or left heart valve insufficiency is associated with pulmonary edema. The usual starting dosage for children is 0.2–0.4 mg/kg/day in 4 divided doses. Total daily dosage of 6–15 mg may be given to the adolescent patient. However, a dosage of more than 20 mg/day does not significantly increase efficacy.

Adverse reactions to prazosin include dizziness, drowsiness, and palpitations. There also may be excessive postural hypotension with syncope, so that monitoring of blood pressure during the administration of prazosin is mandatory. In most instances, side effects completely disappear when dosage is reduced.

Captopril

Captopril is an orally active angiotensin-converting–enzyme inhibitor that produces marked arterial dilatation by blocking the production of angiotensin II, resulting in significant afterload reduction.[41] Venodilation and consequent preload reduction have also been reported.[42] This agent has the additional advantage of interfering with aldosterone production, and thereby also helps control salt and water retention. The oral dose of captopril is 0.5–6 mg/kg/day given in 2 to 4 divided doses. Some patients who initially do not show significant improvement with captopril therapy nevertheless display clinical benefits when the drug is administered on a long-term basis. In some patients, however, the converse has been found to be true.

Adverse reactions to captopril are hypotension and its sequelae (e.g., syncope, weakness, and dizziness). A maculopapular pruritic rash occurs in 5 to 8 per cent of patients, but the drug may be continued, since the rash often disappears spontaneously with time. Neutropenia and proteinuria have also been reported as complications of captopril therapy.

β-Adrenergic Agonists

Isoproterenol

Isoproterenol is an intravenous preparation used for treating low cardiac output. This agent has central and peripheral β-adrenergic effects and therefore both enhances myocardial contractility and reduces cardiac afterload. The drug is administered intravenously in an intensive care setting and the dosage is adjusted to between 0.01 and 0.5 μ/kg/min, depending on heart rate response. Continuous determinations of arterial blood pressure and heart rate are mandatory, and measurement of cardiac output at the bedside also may be helpful in assessing the efficacy of this drug. Since isoproterenol has a marked chronotropic effect, it should not be used in patients who have significant tachycardia. Children receiving isoproterenol must be carefully monitored for the development of atrial or ventricular premature depolarizations, because they may lead to supraventricular or ventricular tachycardia. As the patient's clinical condition improves, the dosage is gradually tapered, usually over one or two days. As isoproterenol treatment is withdrawn, digoxin therapy is often added for continued inotropic effect.

Dopamine

Dopamine is an effective β-adrenergic agent that has the advantage of being less chronotropic and arrhythmogenic than isoproterenol. In addition, it is a selective renal vasodilator and has particular use in patients with the compromised kidney function that is often associated with low cardiac output. At a dosage of 2–10 μg/kg/min, dopamine results in both inotropism and peripheral vasodilatation. However, if the dosage must be increased to more than 10 μg/kg/min, peripheral α-adrenergic effects may result in vasoconstriction rather than in vasodilation.

Dobutamine

Dobutamine, a derivative of dopamine, is another agent that is utilized for the treatment of low cardiac output. It has the advantage of causing direct inotropic effects without dose-related variations in peripheral vascular resistance. It can be an effective substitute for high-dose dopamine therapy in order to avoid vasoconstrictive effects. Furthermore, dobutamine is unlikely to cause cardiac rhythm disturbances even at maximal dosage. The usual dose is similar to that of dopamine (2–20 μg/kg/min).

REFERENCES

1. Braunwald E, Ross J Jr, Sonnenblick EH. Mechanisms of contraction of the normal and failing heart. N Engl J Med 1967; *277*:853.
2. Schwartz A, Sordahl LA, Entman ML, et al. Abnormal biochemistry in myocardial failure. Am J Cardiol 1973, *32*:407.
3. Plaut GWE, Gertler MM. Oxidative phosphorylation studies in normal and experimentally produced congestive heart failure in the guinea pig: a comparison. Ann NY Acad Sci 1959; *72*:515.
4. Szekeres L, Schein M. Cell metabolism of the overloaded mammalian heart in situ. Cardiologia (Basel) 1959; *34*:18.
5. Schwartz A, Lee KS. Study of heart mitochondria and glycolytic metabolism in experimentally induced cardiac failure. Circ Res 1962; *10*:321.
6. Sobel BE, Spann JF Jr, Pool PE, et al. Normal oxidative phosphorylation in mitochondria from failing hearts. Circ Res 1967; *21*:355.
7. Su JY, Friedman WF. Comparison of the responses of fetal and adult cardiac muscle to hypoxia. Am J Physiol 1973; *224*:1249.
8. Chidsey CA, Braunwald E, Morrow AG. Catecholamine excretion and cardiac stores of norepinephrine in congestive heart failure. Am J Med 1965; *39*:442.
9. Lees MH. Catecholamine metabolite excretion of infants with heart failure. J Pediatr 1966; *69*:259.
10. Bristow MR, Ginsburg R, Minobe W, et al. Decreased catecholamine sensitivity and beta adrenergic receptor density in failing human hearts. N Engl J Med 1982; *307*:205.
11. Rutenberg HL, Spann JF Jr. Alterations of cardiac sympathetic neurotransmitter activity in congestive heart failure. Am J Cardiol 1973; *32*:472.
12. Pool PE, Covell JW, Levitt M, et al. Reduction of cardiac tyrosine hydroxylase activity in experimental congestive heart failure: its role in depletion of cardiac norepinephrine stores. Circ Res 1967; *20*:249.
13. Krakoff LR, Buccino RA, Spann JF Jr, DeChamplain J. Cardiac catechol O-methyltranasferase and monamine oxidase activity in congestive heart failure. Am J Physiol 1968; *215*:549.
14. Spann JF Jr, Buccino RA, Sonnenblick ER, Braunwald E. Contractile state of cardiac muscle obtained from cats with experimentally produced ventricular hypertrophy and heart failure. Circ Res 1967; *21*:341.
15. Heinsimer JA, Lefkowitz RJ. The beta-adrenergic receptor in heart failure. Hosp Pract 1983; *18*:103.
16. Colucci WS, Alexander RW, Williams GH, et al. Decreased lymphocyte beta-adrenergic-receptor density in patients with heart failure and tolerance to the beta-adrenergic agonist pirbuterol. N Engl J Med 1981; *305*:185.
17. Fraser J, Nadeau J, Robertson D, Wood AJJ. Regulation of human leukocyte beta receptors by endogenous catecholamines: relationship of leukocyte beta receptor density to the cardiac sensitivity of isoproterenol. J Clin Invest 1981; *67*:1777.
18. Merrill AJ, Morrison JL, Brannon ES. Concentration of renin in venous blood in patients with chronic heart failure. Am J Med 1946; *1*:468.
19. Brown JJ, Davies DL, Johnson VW, et al. Renin relationship in congestive cardiac failure, treated and untreated. Am Heart J 1970; *80*:329.
20. Vandongen R, Gordon RD. Plasma renin in congestive heart failure in man. Med J Aust 1970; *1*:215.
21. Baylen BG, Johnson G, Tsang R, et al. The occurrence of hyperaldosteronism in infants with congestive heart failure. Am J Cardiol 1980; *45*:305.
22. Meyer RA, Stockert J, Kaplan S. Echocardiographic determination of left ventricular volumes in pediatric patients. Circulation 1975; *51*:297.
23. Kaye HH, Tynan M, Hunter S. Validity of echocardiographic estimates of left ventricular size and performance in infants and children. Br Heart J 1975; *37*:371.
24. Blatt DR, Isabel-Jones JB, Villoria GJ, et al. Accuracy of echocardiography in assessing left ventricular dimensions and volume. Circulation 1978; *57*:699.
25. Gutgesell HP, Paquet M, Duff DF, McNamara DG. Evaluation of left ventricular size and function by echocardiography. Results in normal children. Circulation 1977; *56*:457.
26. Treves S, Fogle R, Lang P. Radionuclide angiography in congenital heart disease. Am J Cardiol 1980; *46*:1247.
27. Ross J Jr. The failing heart and the circulation. Hosp Pract 1983; *18*:151.
28. Dodge HT. Angiographic evaluation of ventricular function. N Engl J Med 1977; *296*:551.
29. Graham TP Jr, Jarmakani MM, Canent RV Jr, et al. Characterization of left heart volumes and mass in normal children and in infants with intrinsic myocardial disease. Circulation 1968; *38*:826.
30. Lee KS, Klaus W. The subcellular basis for the mechanism of inotropic action of cardiac glycosides. Pharmacol 1971; *23*:193.
31. Sandor GGS, Bloom KR, Izukawa T, et al. Noninvasive assessment of left ventricular function related to serum digoxin levels in neonates. Pediatrics 1980; *65*:541.
32. Hayes CJ, Butler VP, Gersony WM. Serum digoxin studies in infants and children. Pediatrics 1973; *52*:561.
33. Lees MH, Bristow JD, Griswold HE, Olmstead RW. Relative hypermetabolism in infants with congenital heart disease and undernutrition. Pediatrics 1965; *36*:183.
34. Fomon SJ, Ziegler EE. Nutritional management of infants with congenital heart disease. Am Heart J 1972; *83*:581.
35. Synhorst OP, Lauer RM, Doty DD, Brody MJ. Hemodynamic effects of vasodilator agents in dogs with experimental ventricular septal defect. Circulation 1976; *54*:472.

36. Beekman RH, Rocchini AP, Rosenthal A. Hemodynamic effects of nitroprusside in infants with a large ventricular septal defect. Circulation 1981; *64*:553.
37. Guiha NH, Cohn JN, Mikulic E, et al. Treatment of refractory heart failure with infusion of nitroprusside. N Engl J Med 1974; *291*:587.
38. Chatterjee K, Parmley WW, Massie B, et al. Oral hydralazine therapy for chronic refractory heart failure. Circulation 1976; *54*:879.
39. Fried R, Steinherz LF, Levin AR, et al. Use of hydralazine for intractable cardiac failure in childhood. J Pediatr 1980; *97*:1009.
40. Miller RR, Awan NA, Maxwell K, Mason DT. Sustained reduction of cardiac impedance and preload in congestive heart failure with the antihypertensive vasodilator prazosin. N Engl J Med 1977; *297*:103.
41. Vidt DG, Bravo EL, Fouad FM. Captopril. N Engl J Med 1982; *306*:214.
42. Tarazi RC, Bravo EL, Fouad FM, et al. Hemodynamic and volume changes associated with captopril. Hypertension 1980; *2*:576.

Index

Note: Page numbers in italics refer to figures; page numbers followed by (t) refer to tables.